Uveitis

George N. Papaliodis
Editor

Uveitis

A Practical Guide to the Diagnosis and Treatment of Intraocular Inflammation

Springer

Editor
George N. Papaliodis, MD
Director of the Ocular Immunology
and Uveitis Science
Massachusetts Eye and Ear Infirmary,
Harvard Medical School
Boston, MA
USA

ISBN 978-3-319-09125-9 ISBN 978-3-319-09126-6 (eBook)
DOI 10.1007/978-3-319-09126-6

Library of Congress Control Number: 2016952816

Printed on acid-free paper

This Springer imprint is published by Springer Nature
The registered company is Springer International Publishing AG
The registered company address is: Gewerbestrasse 11, 6330 Cham, Switzerland

I dedicate this book to my daughter Alexandra Papaliodis.
I never knew how much I could love anything until I held you in my arms. You are the reason for my existence...

Acknowledgements

When Springer Publishing approached me about writing a textbook on uveitis, I envisioned this to be a collaborative endeavor involving many of my colleagues and those with an interest in this field. I am deeply indebted to each of my contributing authors who devoted so much time and effort to make this book a success. I am similarly appreciative of Jessica Gonzalez, Kevin Wright, and Rebekah Amos from Springer who assisted in every phase of production of this book. Thank you for your support and patience.

On a personal note, I am rarely granted such a public forum to thank the people who have supported me in my career and personal life. I thank Dr. C. Stephen Foster, my former mentor at the Massachusetts Eye and Ear Infirmary (MEEI), for introducing me to this incredible realm and allowing me to recognize that I could practice both ophthalmology and internal medicine. I also thank my department chair Dr. Joan W. Miller who entrusted me as the director of the Harvard Medical School/MEEI Ocular Immunology and Uveitis Service in 2005. Dr. Miller embodies every professional and personal characteristic I associate with success and I am honored to call her my friend.

I am blessed that my parents, Nick and Georgia Papaliodis, encouraged their three sons to never settle for anything less than the best (a common mantra around the Papaliodis household). The ingredients for producing successful children (per my parents) are: unwavering support, infinite love, and great Greek food. My brothers, Louis Papaliodis and Dean Papaliodis, are my best friends, business associates, and constant confidants. No task or challenge is too formidable to overcome with those two by my side. My wife, Sofia Lingos-Papaliodis, has supported and loved me while tolerating my insanely busy schedule between two academic institutions (and writing this textbook) all while juggling the management her own law firm, teaching, and raising our rambunctious little toddler. There are no words to adequately describe how fortunate I am to have Sofia as my partner in everything.

Contents

Contributors

Jessica Ackert MD Department of Ophthalmology, Drexel College of Medicine, Philadelphia, PA, USA

Scott M. Barb MD Department of Ophthalmology, Massachusetts Eye and Ear Infirmary, Boston, MA, USA

Miriam B. Barshak MD Department of Medicine, Massachusetts General Hospital, Harvard Medical School, Massachusetts Eye and Ear Infirmary, Boston, MA, USA

Soumyava Basu MS Retina-Vitreous and Uvea Service, L V Prasad Eye Institute, Bhubaneswar, Odisha, India

Durga S. Borkar MD Department of Ophthalmology, Veterans Affairs Boston Healthcare System, Jamaica Plain, MA, USA

Katarzyna Brodowska MD Department of Ophthalmology, Harvard Medical School, Massachusetts Eye and Ear Infirmary, Boston, MA, USA

Nicholas J. Butler MD Department of Ophthalmology, Veterans Affairs Boston Healthcare System, Jamaica Plain, MA, USA

Dean M. Cestari MD Department of Neuro-Opthalmology, Massachusetts Eye and Ear Infirmary, Boston, MA, USA

Victoria Chang MD Department of Ophthalmology, Harvard Medical School, Massachusetts Eye and Ear Infirmary, Boston, MA, USA

Emmett T. Cunningham Jr MD, PhD, MPH California Pacific Medical Center, San Francisco, CA, USA; Stanford University School of Medicine, Stanford, CA, USA; UCSF School of Medicine, San Francisco, CA, USA; West Coast Retina Medical Group, San Francisco, CA, USA

Mark Dacey MD Colorado Retina Associates, P.C, Denver, CO, USA

Jose Daniel Diaz MD Department of Ophthalmology, Massachusetts Eye and Ear Infirmary, Boston, MA, USA

Sonam Dilwali PhD Medical School, UT Southwestern Medical Center, Dallas, TX, USA

Marlene L. Durand MD Department of Medicine, Massachusetts General Hospital, Harvard Medical School, Massachusetts Eye and Ear Infirmary, Boston, MA, USA

Khayyam Durrani MD Division of Ophthalmology, Cornea & External Disease, and Ocular Immunology & Uveitis Services, University of Connecticut Health Center, Farmington, CT, USA

Dean Eliott MD Department of Ophthalmology, Massachusetts Eye and Ear Infirmary, Boston, MA, USA

Thomas Flynn MD Ellsworth, ME, USA

Russell N. Van Gelder MD, PhD Department of Ophthalmology, University of Washington, Seattle, WA, USA

Lindsay Grotting MD Department of Ophthalmology, Massachusetts Eye and Ear Infirmary, Boston, MA, USA

Bradley A. Hansen MD Department of Ophthalmology, New England Eye Center, Tufts University School of Medicine, Boston, MA, USA

Rebecca Hunter MD Department of Ophthalmology, Harvard Vanguard Medical Associates, Boston, MA, USA

Eleni Konstantinou MD Department of Ophthalmology, Massachusetts Eye and Ear Infirmary, Boston, MA, USA

Erik Letko MD Deparment of Ophthalmology, Colorado Permanente Medical Group, Denver, CO, USA

Stephanie M. Llop MD Department of Uveitis, Massachusetts Eye and Ear Infirmary, Boston, MA, USA

Ann-Marie Lobo MD Department of Ophthalmology, Harvard Medical School, Massachusetts Eye and Ear Infirmary, Boston, MA, USA

Alice Lorch MD Department of Opthalmology, Harvard Medical School, Massachusetts Eye and Ear Infirmary, Boston, MA, USA

Anna Marmalidou MD Department of Ophthalmology, Massachusetts Eye and Ear Infirmary, Harvard Medical School, Boston, MA, USA

John B. Miller MD Retina Service, Massachusetts Eye and Ear Infirmary, Boston, MA, USA

Humzah Nasir Department of Ophthalmology, Harvard Medical School, Massachusetts Eye and Ear Infirmary, Boston, MA, USA

Milka C. Nova MD Immunology Uveitis Service, MEEI, Boston, MA, USA

Chukwuemeka Nwanze MD Department of Ophthalmology, Boston Medical Center, Boston, MA, USA

George N. Papaliodis MD Department of Ophthalmology, Harvard Medical School, Massachusetts Eye and Ear Infirmary, Boston, MA, USA

Evangelia Papavasileiou MD Department of Ophthalmology, Harvard Medical School, Massachusetts Eye and Ear Infirmary, Boston, MA, USA

Louis R. Pasquale MD, FARVO Massachusetts Eye and Ear Infirmary, Harvard Medical School, Boston, MA, USA

Avni Patel MD Department of Ophthalmology, Massachusetts Eye and Ear Infirmary, Boston, MA, USA

Kathryn L. Pepple MD, PhD Department of Ophthalmology, University of Washington, Seattle, WA, USA

Parvathy Pillai MD Sinai Hospital of Baltimore, The Krieger Eye Institute, Baltimore, MD, USA

Cynthia X. Qian MD Department of Ophthalmology, Retina Service, Massachusetts Eye and Ear Infirmary, Boston, MA, USA

Safa Rahmani MD Department of Ophthalmology, Massachusetts Eye and Ear Infirmary, Boston, MA, USA

Narsing A. Rao MD Department of Ophthalmology, The Keck School of Medicine, USC Eye Institute, University of Southern California, Los Angeles, CA, USA

Olga Rosenvald MD Department of Neurology, Massachusetts General Hospital and Brigham and Women's Hospital, Boston, MA, USA

Sergio Schwartzman MD Rheumatology, Hospital for Special Surgery, New York Presbyterian Hospital, Weill Medical College of Cornell University, New York, NY, USA

Nathan Scott MD Massachuetts General Hospital, Boston, MA, USA

Carol L. Shields MD Ocular Oncology Service, Thomas Jefferson University, Philadelphia, PA, USA; Ocular Oncology Service, Wills Eye Hospital, Philadelphia, PA, USA

Jerry A. Shields MD Ocular Oncology Service, Thomas Jefferson University, Philadelphia, PA, USA; Ocular Oncology Service, Wills Eye Hospital, Philadelphia, PA, USA

Lucia Sobrin MD, MPH Department of Opthalmology, Harvard Medical School, Massachusetts Eye and Ear Infirmary, Boston, MA, USA

Sarkis H. Soukiasian MD Department of Ophthalmology, Lahey Health Systems, Tufts University of Medicine, Burlington, MA, USA

Eduardo Uchiyama MD Retina Group of Florida, Fort Lauderdale, FL, USA

Sonia Utley Ocular Immunology and Uveitis Service, Massachusetts Eye and Ear Infirmary, Boston, MA, USA

Demetrios G. Vavvas MD, PhD Department of Ophthalmology, Massachusetts Eye and Ear Infirmary, Massachusetts General Hospital, Boston, MA, USA

Jay Wang MD Department of Ophthalmology, Massachusetts Eye and Ear Infirmary, Boston, MA, USA

Robert Wang MD Department of Ophthalmology, Texas Retina Associates, UT Southwestern, Dallas, TX, USA

Lucy Young MD Department of Ophthalmology, Massachusetts Eye and Ear Infirmary, Boston, MA, USA

Jing Zhang MD Department of Ophthalmology, Massachusetts Eye and Ear Infirmary, Boston, MA, USA

Part I
General Principles

Introduction

1

George N. Papaliodis

The term uveitis is broadly defined as inflammation of the uveal tract comprised by the iris, ciliary body, and choroid. In practice, this term has been more broadly applied to any inflammatory state involving the interior of the eye including iritis, intermediate uveitis, pars planitis, vitritis, retinal vasculitis (phlebitis and arteritis), choroiditis, and papillitis. This area of ophthalmology encompasses multiple pathologic processes that can induce aberrant or exuberant inflammation within the eye such as infections of the eye, autoimmune disorders, trauma to the eye, certain medications which can incite ocular inflammation, and rarely malignancies.

The practitioner in this realm must

- perform a careful history with review of systems as this can often lead to a differential diagnosis and direct subsequent investigations. The adage that "if you listen to the patient, they will very likely give you their diagnosis" is more pertinent in this realm than practically any other in ophthalmology.
- examine the patients' eyes CAREFULLY documenting: visual acuity, pupillary responses, extraocular muscle movements, confrontational or automated visual field testing, the areas of the eye with inflammation (anterior, intermediate, posterior), presence of cells and/or flare (quantified and characterized as granulomatous or non-granulomatous), iris pathology (transillumination defects, nodules, peripheral anterior synechiae, posterior synechiae), lens changes, intraocular pressure, clarity of the vitreous, appearance of the optic nerve and retinal vasculature, and choroidal pathology.
- examine other areas of the patient's body for pertinent findings (joint swelling, rashes, heart murmur, etc.).
- evaluate the information obtained by history, review of systems, and physical exam to parsimoniously order supportive laboratory and radiographic studies. Every patient with uveitis does NOT require complete serologic testing and MRI of the brain/orbit.
- prescribe the most effective and least toxic medication to treat the ocular pathology. This may merely require the use of topical steroids for an episode of iritis or could necessitate intravenous Infliximab or cyclophosphamide for Adamantiades-Behçet's associated retinal vasculitis. The decision of which medication to use should be evidenced based. Are there double-blinded, placebo controlled trials demonstrating safety and efficacy for this indication? If not, are there large cohort series or published reports in this realm? Additionally, the physician must be cognizant of the overall health of the patient and especially comorbidities when prescribing systemic medications (e.g., avoiding methotrexate in

G.N. Papaliodis (✉)
Department of Ophthalmology, Harvard Medical School, Massachusetts Eye and Ear Infirmary, 243 Charles Street, Boston, MA 02114, USA
e-mail: George_Papaliodis@meei.harvard.edu

G.N. Papaliodis (ed.), *Uveitis*,
DOI 10.1007/978-3-319-09126-6_1

the alcoholic cirrhotic or cyclosporine in the patient with renal dysfunction).

- refer the patient to the appropriate practitioner if the patient's condition requires care outside of one's area of expertise or seek a second opinion. It entails a generous level of humility to admit to the patient that despite years in medical education and training their ocular problem requires a different specialist with greater experience or unique expertise. A second opinion may merely provide a fresh perspective on a problem and direct therapy or diagnosis in an alternative direction.
- remain current. Since approval of etanercept in 1998, the TNF alpha inhibitors have altered the course of inflammatory disease management and proven to be invaluable therapies in those with recalcitrant ocular inflammatory disease. In 2009, the global market for TNF alpha inhibitors was $22 billion [1]. This is but one example of the explosion in targeted immunomodulatory therapy directed toward specific cytokines, interleukins, cell surface markers, etc. This trend will invariably progress as our knowledge of the immune system and disease mechanisms are further elucidated. It will require that the physician dedicate time to continuing medical education to remain on the cutting edge of therapeutic options.

This is a daunting list to say the least, and I am reminded of the sixteenth century ophthalmologist, Dr. George Bartish, who wrote about the qualities of a "good" ophthalmologist. In Dr. Bartish's era, a "good" ophthalmologist was defined as having descended from religious parents; studied Latin; training by a well-respected ophthalmologist; not being motivated by financial rewards; never promising more than one can deliver. After reviewing his own criteria, Dr. Bartish realized that there were indeed very few well trained ophthalmologists meeting those standards [2]. Similarly, those who treat uveitis patients have considerable expectations, and the risk in performing below standard can have sight threatening and at times life threatening ramifications. The reward of this field is the constant intellectual stimulation, diversity of diseases, and the appreciation of patients and colleagues alike for the skills and knowledge necessary to deter the effects of these infirmities.

Epidemiology

Uveitis can affect patients of any age and is one of the leading causes of preventable blindness in the world accounting for approximately 10 % of blindness worldwide [3]. The worldwide prevalence of uveitis is estimated to be 115–204/100,000 people, and the incidence is estimated at 17–52/100,000 people per year [4]. The mean age of patients with uveitis is 40 years old, thus this disease has a significant impact on patients' productivity in the work force and their long-term health care costs [5].

The prevalence of uveitis in the United States is 38 per 100,000 with an incidence of approximately 15 cases per 100,000 population per year [6]. Uveitis is estimated to be responsible for approximately 10–20 % of the blindness in the United States [7].

The male to female ratio is approximately equal when grouping all uveitic diagnoses in aggregate. There is considerable variability depending upon specific diagnosis (e.g., ankylosing spondylitis is 2.5 fold more common in men than women).

Signs and Symptoms

The signs and symptoms produced by active uveitis are dependent upon the anatomic location of the inflammation in the eye, rapidity of onset of the inflammation, and duration and course of disease.

The signs of ocular inflammation involving the anterior segment of the eye include the following:

- Cells
- Flare
- Fibrin
- Hypopyon
- Synechiae (both anterior and posterior)
- Iris nodules
- Iris atrophy
- Keratic precipitates
- Band keratopathy

The signs of ocular inflammation involving the intermediate segment of the eye include the following:

- vitreal cells
- "snowball" opacities in the vitreous
- exudates over the pars plana (snowbanking)
- neovascularization of the pars plana

The signs of ocular inflammation involving the posterior segment of the eye include the following:

- Vascular sheathing (arteries, veins, or both)
- Retinal pigment epithelial hypertrophy or atrophy
- Cystoid macular edema
- Atrophy or swelling of the retina, choroid, or optic nerve head
- Exudative, tractional, or rhegmatogenous retinal detachment
- Retinal or choroidal neovascularization

The symptoms of uveitis are similarly dependent upon the location of involvement in the eye and include the following:

- Anterior segment (ocular injection, light sensitivity, pain, blurry vision, epiphora)
- Intermediate and posterior segment (floaters, flashing lights, blurry vision)

When counseling patients regarding the symptoms of ocular inflammation, the abbreviation "RSVP" commonly used by primary care physicians in deciding when to refer a patient to an ophthalmologist is simple to remember (**R**edness, Light **S**ensitivity, Change in **V**ision, and **P**ain). Although nonspecific, any of these symptoms should prompt the patient to seek medical attention.

Classification of Uveitis

The classification of uveitis is important for multiple reasons that are as follows:

- The location of ocular inflammation may assist in diagnosis or at least narrow the potential etiologies (e.g., Fuch's heterochromic iridocyclitis involves the anterior chamber; ocular toxoplasmosis primarily effects the retina with significant inflammatory spillover into the choroid and vitreous)
- Uveitis may be a manifestation of an underlying serious or potentially lethal systemic disease. The correct diagnosis can be sight- and on occasion life-preserving.
- Uveitis may be caused by a vast number of conditions including infections, autoimmune disorders, medication induced, traumatic, and neoplastic. The correct characterization of the ocular manifestations may assist in identifying an underlying etiology.

There are several classification models in existence (International Uveitis Study Group, Standardization of Uveitis Nomenclature Working Group). Historically, the variability between the various classification schemes lead to some degree of confusion, and there was a need for an accepted system to improve the comprehension of the disease course, prognosis, and scientifically scrutinize the efficacy of various treatments. The Standardization of Uveitis Nomenclature (SUN) Working Group in 2005 developed an anatomical classification system, standard grading systems, and accepted terminology to use for evaluating patients with uveitis (Tables 1.1, 1.2 and 1.3).

The grading of anterior chamber inflammation is determined via a 1 mm × 1 mm slit beam and the rheostat adjusted to the brightest setting (Table 1.4).

Table 1.1 SUN working group anatomical classification of uveitis

Type of uveitis	Primary site of inflammation	Includes
Anterior uveitis	Anterior chamber	Iritis Iridocyclitis
Intermediate uveitis	Vitreous	Pars planitis Posterior cyclitis Hyalitis
Posterior uveitis	Retina or choroid	Focal, multifocal, or diffuse choroiditis Chorioretinitis Retinochoroiditis Retinitis Neuroretinitis
Panuveitis	Anterior chamber, vitreous, and retina or choroid	

Jabs DA, et al. [10: Table 1]

Table 1.2 The SUN working group descriptors in uveitis

Category	Descriptor	Comment
Onset	Sudden Insidious	
Duration	Limited Persistent	≤3 months duration >3 months duration
Course	Acute Recurrent Chronic	Episode characterized by sudden onset and limited duration Repeated episodes separated by periods of inactivity without treatment ≥3 months duration Persistent uveitis with relapse in <3 months after discontinuing treatment

Jabs DA, et al. [10: Table 2]

Table 1.3 The SUN working group activity of uveitis terminology

Term	Definition
Inactive	Grade 0 cells (anterior chamber)
Worsening activity	2 Step increase in level of inflammation (e.g., anterior chamber cells, vitreal haze) or increase from grade 3+ to 4+
Improved activity	2 Step decrease in level of inflammation (e.g., Anterior chamber cells, vitreous haze) or decrease to grade 0
Remission	Inactive disease for ≥3 months after discontinuing all treatment for eye disease

Jabs DA, et al. [10, Table 5]

Anterior chamber flare is more difficult to objectively quantify at the slit lamp without the use of a laser flare photometer. This instrument can measure the back-scattered light from small molecules such as proteins in the anterior chamber. There is a highly significant linear relationship between laser flare intensity and protein concentration which has been shown both in vitro and in vivo [8, 9]. Without the use of a laser flare photometer, the SUN Working group chose the grading system shown in Table 1.5 which employs a more qualitative metric.

The chapters that follow will provide a basis for evaluating, diagnosing, and treating patients with uveitis. This is not an "all inclusive" reference guide but a reasonable synopsis by experts

Table 1.4 Grading of anterior chamber cell

Grade	Number of cells
0	<1 cell
0.5+	1–5 cells
1+	6–15 cells
2+	16–25 cells
3+	26–50 cells
4+	>50 cells

Jabs DA, et al. [10]

Table 1.5 Grading of anterior chamber flare

Grade	Description
0	None
1+	Faint
2+	Moderate (iris and lens details clear)
3+	Marked (iris and lens details hazy)
4+	Intense (fibrin or plasmoid aqueous)

Jabs DA, et al. [10, Table 4]

in the field to provide adequate depth of information to the practitioner faced with these challenging patients. As with all textbooks, the information contained herein constantly evolves and may not completely represent the latest advances in this realm.

References

1. http://knol.google.com/k/top-ten-twenty-best-selling-drugs-2009#Best_selling_therapeutic_categoriesBest_selling_therapeutic_categoriesef.
2. Tower Paul. Notes on the life and work of George Bartisch. AMA Arch Ophthalmol. 1956;56(1):57–70. doi:10.1001/archopht.1956.00930040063009.
3. Nussenblatt RB. The natural history of uveitis. Int Ophthalmol. 1990;14(5–6):303–8.
4. Jabs DA. Epidemiology of uveitis. Ophthalmic Epidemiol. 2008;15(5):283–4.
5. Hunter RS, Lobo AM. Dexamethasone intravitreal implant for the treatment of noninfectious uveitis. Clin Ophthalmol. 2011;5:1613–21.
6. Silverstein A. Changing trends in the etiological diagnosis diagnosis of uveitis. Doc Ophthalmol. 1997;94:25–37.
7. Gritz, D. Incidence and prevalence of uveitis in Northern California—The Northern California Epidemiology of Uveitis Study. Ophthalmology. 2004;111(3):491–500.
8. Shah SM, Spalton DJ, Taylor JC. Correlations between laser flare measurements and anterior chamber protein concentrations. Invest Ophthalmol Vis Sci. 1992;33(10):2878–84.
9. el-Maghraby A, Marzouki A, Matheen TM, Souchek J, Van der Karr M. Reproducibility and validity of laser flare/cell meter measurements as an objective method of assessing intraocular inflammation. Arch Ophthalmol. 1992;110(7):960–962.
10. Jabs DA, Nussenblatt RB, Rosenbaum JT. The Standardization of Uveitis Nomenclature (SUN) Working Group. Standardization of nomenclature for reporting clinical data: results of the First International Workshop. Am J Ophthalmol. 2005;140:509–16.

Approach to the Laboratory, Imaging, and Molecular Work-up for Uveitis

2

Bradley A. Hansen and Sarkis H. Soukiasian

Introduction

The work-up and diagnosis of uveitic diseases can be a challenge. Evolving nomenclature and classifications as well as a limited understanding of the utility and limitations of diagnostic tests may lead to confusion, unnecessary testing, and inaccurate or delayed diagnosis. In this chapter, we hope to clarify the goals of diagnosis and present a systematic approach for the diagnostic work-up in patients with uveitis. In order to appropriately discuss this work-up, we will briefly review current nomenclature, emphasize the importance of history, present a few important discriminating exam findings, and highlight the utilization of an anatomic classification system. In addition, we will highlight the utility, indications, and complementary role of laboratory, radiographic, and molecular testing. With this review, we hope to remove some of the uncertainty that comes when approaching these often complicated patients.

Goal of Testing

There is little consensus among providers about which testing should be ordered for a uveitic evaluation. This fact highlights the importance of defining specific goals for initiating a work-up. It may be helpful to ask the questions: Will the results of this test affect my clinical decision making and change my management? Will the results affect the patient's visual or systemic prognosis? Traditionally, when defining uveitic disease, there has been an emphasis on the search for the "etiologic diagnosis" of the inflammation [1, 2]. One problem with this approach, is that even after exhaustive testing, many uveitic disorders do not have a known systemic association and are ultimately termed "idiopathic" or "undifferentiated" [1, 3]. Thus, this search may lead to "shot-gun" testing that may not affect treatment or prognosis. Jabs et al. suggest that except for infectious diseases, Mendelian genetic disorders, and toxic or allergic reactions, most uveitic disorders are not amenable to a simple unifying "etiology" [4]. With this in mind, our diagnostic philosophy places a strong emphasis on history and physical examination findings. This is to be followed by focused, complementary testing with the primary goal of ruling out diseases not treated

B.A. Hansen
Department of Ophthalmology, New England Eye Center, Tufts University School of Medicine, 260 Tremont St., Boston, MA 02116, USA
e-mail: bhansen@tuftsmedicalcenter.org

S.H. Soukiasian (✉)
Department of Ophthalmology, Lahey Health Systems, Tufts University of Medicine, 41 Mall Rd, Burlington, MA 01803, USA
e-mail: s.soukiasian@lahey.org

G.N. Papaliodis (ed.), *Uveitis*,
DOI 10.1007/978-3-319-09126-6_2

with immunomodulators (i.e., infections—particularly those that cannot be identified by unique exam features, and masquerade syndromes) and systemic diseases that may have an impact on the patient's systemic health, prognosis, or treatment plan. This approach helps to limit unnecessary testing and facilitates critical treatment decisions early in the disease course. As a secondary concern, each clinician should further consider the cost of each test and try to improve the financial burden on the patient and the health care system. Finally, it is best for the examining ophthalmologist to order and interpret the appropriate testing. The primary care provider or rheumatologist will not be familiar with the ocular differential diagnosis, so a referral for testing may lead to inappropriate testing. An unnecessary or incomplete work-up can cloud the clinical picture further and ultimately lead to testing results that are misleading.

Nomenclature and Classification

In 1996, Rosenbaum et al. highlighted the gross inconsistencies in the use of vocabulary among uveitis specialists. In this editorial, members of the American Uveitis Society were given clinical vignettes and informally surveyed about terms that were deemed appropriate in describing the vignette. Only one-third of specialists agreed on descriptive terminology [5]. Some of this confusion invariably contributes to the uncertainty that many clinicians have when approaching patients with uveitis. The International Uveitis Study Group (IUSG) and the Standardization of Uveitis Nomenclature (SUN) Working Group have worked to unify inflammatory grading, outcome measurements, and disease classification. The classification established by the IUSG in 1987 [6] is based on the anatomic location of inflammation (see Table 2.1). This includes anterior uveitis (iritis, iridocyclitis, and anterior cyclitis), intermediate uveitis (pars planitis, posterior cyclitis, hyalitis/vitritis), posterior uveitis (focal, multifocal, or diffuse choroiditis, chorioretinitis, retinitis, and neuroretinitis), and panuveitis (anterior, vitreous, retina, and choroid). In 2005, the SUN Working Group came to the consensus that this IUSG anatomic classification should be used as a global standard [7]. In 2008, the IUSG designed an additional clinical classification system for uveitis based on disease etiology [8]. This was defined in 3 main categories: Infectious (bacterial, viral, fungal, parasitic, and others), non-infectious (with known systemic association, or no known systemic association), and masquerade syndromes (neoplastic, non-neoplastic). Between 2009 and 2013, the SUN Working group continued to further unify classification criteria by "mapping" terms into the description of 28 major uveitic diseases [9, 10]. Other proposed dimensions in characterizing uveitis include course (acute, monophasic vs. recurrent acute vs. chronic), laterality (unilateral vs. unilateral alternating vs. bilateral asynchronous vs. bilateral simultaneous), morphology (retinitis vs. choroiditis, paucifocal vs. multifocal), host (child vs. adult)

Table 2.1 Uveitic diseases by anatomic classification

Classification	Related conditions
Anatomic	• Anterior—iritis, iridocyclitis, anterior cyclitis • Intermediate—pars planitis, posterior cyclitis, vitritis/hyalitis • Posterior—focal, multifocal, or diffuse choroiditis, chorioretinitis, retinitis, neuroretinitis • Panuveitis—anterior, vitreous, retina, and choroid
Etiology	• Infectious—bacterial, viral, fungal, parasitic, and others • Non-infectious—known versus unknown systemic association • *Masquerade syndromes*—neoplastic, non-neoplastic
Additional dimensions	• *Course*—acute monophasic versus recurrent acute versus chronic • *Laterality*—unilateral versus unilateral alternating versus bilateral asynchronous versus bilateral simultaneous • *Morphology*—retinitis versus choroiditis paucifocal versus multifocal • *Host*—child versus adult immunocompromised versus immunocompetent

and immune status (immunocompromised vs. immunocompetent) [10].

In summary, based on the uveitis working groups described above each patient with uveitis should have a descriptive diagnosis based on anatomic location. Then using standardized examination reporting, additional disease dimensions (course, laterality, morphology, host, and immune status) should be assigned to create a differential of major uveitic diseases. Narrowing the possible diagnosis in this way will lead to a focused laboratory evaluation and greatly increase the utility of each test ordered.

The Importance of History and Examination

One cannot emphasize enough that ancillary testing should only be a supplement to the most important initial components of the uveitis work-up, the history and physical examination. In a busy ophthalmology practice it may be tempting to marginalize these steps and even have a reflex "uveitis panel" of testing regardless of the history and exam. This approach is costly, exposes patients to unnecessary testing, and may also produce testing results that confuse the diagnostic picture with false positives or negatives.

History: As with all aspects of clinical medicine, an essential first step when establishing a differential diagnosis is a thorough history [11, 12]. This becomes increasingly essential in our modern world of wide spread travel and globalization. We suggest utilizing a questionnaire for new patients with uveitis. This provides a thorough and time affective way to elicit important historical details that may otherwise be missed. An example of one such questionnaire is seen in Fig. 2.1a–d. To date, there has not been a standardized questionnaire established. Details such as age, gender, race, social history (residence, occupation, diet, travel, sexual history, drug abuse), past medical history, family history, and review of systems will help to narrow the differential diagnosis [13–20] (see Table 2.2).

Exam Findings: There is a tremendous amount of cross-over in exam findings between uveitic diseases. However, some diseases are clinically identifiable, and specific exam findings provide important clues into the possible diagnosis limiting the need for additional work-up. Particularly, a combination of specific findings may be syndromic for a specific diagnosis. For example, a patient with anterior uveitis, elevated intraocular pressure, and sectoral iris atrophy makes a diagnosis of herpetic uveitis very likely. Below, we highlight a few key exam findings that may help to further focus the work-up.

Intraocular Pressure: Both ocular hypertension and hypotony can result from intraocular inflammation. Elevated intraocular pressure in uveitis has been estimated to occur in nearly 42 % of patients [21]. Diseases thought to have a higher rate of ocular hypertension include Fuch's heterochromic iridocyclitis (FHIC), glaucomatocyclitic crisis or Posner-Schlossman syndrome, sarcoidosis, juvenile rheumatoid arthritis, VKH, toxoplasmosis, and herpetic keratouveitis.

Keratic precipitates—The presence of keratic precipitates may be helpful in defining between acute versus chronic inflammation, and based on the appearance, may also give clues into the pathogenesis [1]. Fine precipitates are thought to be more common in spondyloarthropathies and juvenile arthropathies. Stellate precipitates that may be seen involving the superior cornea (as opposed to the typical inferior corneal base down triangular appearance of most precipitates) are often seen with Fuch's heterochromic iridocyclitis. "Mutton fat" prescipitates are larger and are formed from macrophages and epithelioid cells. These may be indicative of a granulomatous disease (see Table 2.3).

Hypopyon—This layering of leukocytes is indicative of not only the number of cells in the anterior chamber, but also the presence of enough fibrin to cause the cells to clump. A limited number of etiologies may present with a hypopyon. The most common etiologies include infectious (both bacterial and viral), HLA-B27 associated uveitis, and Behcet's disease. With infectious endophthalmitis the patient will typically have a history of recent surgery, trauma, or

Fig. 2.1 a–d Example questionnaire. Modified from questionnaire created by Dr. Stephen Foster at the Massachusetts eye and ear infirmary. Available at http://www.uveitis.org/uveitis-questionnaire

(a)
Example Questionnaire

Modified from Questionnaire created by Dr. Stephen Foster at the Massachusetts Eye and Ear Infirmary. Available at http://www.uveitis.org/uveitis-questionnaire

FAMILY HISTORY

These questions refer to your grandparents, parents, aunts, uncles, brothers, and sisters, children, or grandchildren

Has anyone in your family had any of the following? PLEASE CIRCLE YES or NO

Cancer	Y/N	Diabetes	Y/N
Allergies	Y/N	Arthritis or rheumatism	Y/N
Syphilis	Y/N	Tuberculosis	Y/N
Sickle Cell disease or trait	Y/N	Lyme disease	Y/N

Has anyone in your family had medical problems listed below? PLEASE ANSWER YES or NO
Eyes
Skin
Kidneys
Lungs
Stomach or bowel
Nervous system or brain

SOCIAL HISTORY
Age:______________ Current
Job:____________________________________

Where were you born?__________________________
Have you lived outside of the USA?
If yes, where?________________________
Have you ever owned a dog?_______ a cat?_______
Have you ever eaten raw meat or uncooked sausage?
Have you ever had unpasteurized mild or cheese?
Have you ever been exposed to sick animals?
Do you drink untreated stream, well or lake water?
Do you smoke cigarettes?
Have you ever used intravenous drugs?
Have you ever had a bisexual or homosexual relationship?
Have you ever taken birth control pills?

have risk factors for endogenous infection (e.g., intravenous drug use). Ocular involvement in these patients will typically be diffuse. Very fibrinous aqueous exudate and dense hypopyon are more commonly seen with infections and HLA-B27-associated disease. In contrast, the hypopyon seen with Behcet's typically has much less fibrin and may shift with the patient's head position. A hypopyon may also be seen in patients with rifabutin toxicity [22, 23]. Pseudohypopyon, composed of tumor cells and debris can occur in some of the masquerade syndromes. Triamcinolone layering may also present as a pseudohypopyon.

Iris Changes—Sectoral iris atrophy is more commonly seen with herpes simplex, varicella zoster, and cytomegalovirus infections. As mentioned above, if accompanied by elevated intraocular pressure one should be suspicious of a herpetic etiology. Nodule formation from the

Fig. 2.1 (continued)

(b) **PERSONAL MEDICAL HISTORY**

Are you allergic to any medications?
If yes, which medications?___________________________
Please list your current medications including non-prescription drugs such as aspirin, Advil, antihistamines etc.

____

____

____

____

____

____

____

PAST MEDICAL HISTORY

Please list all surgeries you have had (including laser surgery)

____
_Date______________

____
_ Date______________

____
_ Date______________

____
_Date______________

(c) **Have you ever had any of the following conditions? PLEASE CIRCLE YES or NO**

Anemia (low blood counts)	Y/N	Cancer	Y/N
Diabetes	Y/N	Hepatitis	Y/N
High Blood pressure	Y/N	Pleurisy	Y/N
Pneumonia	Y/N	Ulcers	Y/N
Herpes (cold sores)	Y/N	Chicken pox	Y/N
Shingles (Zoster)	Y/N	German measeles (Rubella)	Y/N
Mumps	Y/N	Chlamydia or Trachoma	Y/N
Syphilis	Y/N	Gonorrhea	Y/N
Any other sexually transmitted disease	Y/N	Tuberculosis	Y/N
Leprosy	Y/N	Leptospirosis	Y/N
Lyme disease	Y/N	Histoplasmosis	Y/N
Candida or Moniliasis	Y/N	Coccidiomycosis	Y/N
Sporotrichosis	Y/N	Toxoplasmosis	Y/N
Toxocariasis	Y/N	Cysticercosis	Y/N
Trichinosis	Y/N	Whipples disease	Y/N
AIDS	Y/N	Hay Fever	Y/N
Allergies	Y/N	Vasculitis	Y/N
Arthritis	Y/N	Rheumatoid arthritis	Y/N
Lupus (Systemic Lupus Erythematosus)	Y/N	Scleroderma	Y/N

Have you ever had any of the following illnesses? PLEASE ANSWER YES or NO

Reiter's Syndrome	Y/N	Colitis	Y/N
Crohn's disease	Y/N	Ulcerative Colitis	Y/N
Behcet's disease	Y/N	Sarcoidosis	Y/N
Ankylosing spondylitis	Y/N	Erythema Nodosa	Y/N
Temporal Arteritis	Y/N	Multiple Sclerosis	Y/N
Serpiginous Choroidopathy	Y/N	Fuchs' Heterochromic iridocyclitis	Y/N
Vogt/Koyanagi-Harada Syndrome	Y/N		

Fig. 2.1 (continued)

(d) **Have you had any of the following symptoms in the past year? PLEASE CIRCLE YES or NO**

GENERAL			
Chills	Y/N	Fevers (persistent or recurrent)	Y/N
Night Sweats	Y/N	Fatigue	Y/N
Poor appetite	Y/N	Unexplained weight loss	Y/N
HEAD			
Frequent headaches	Y/N	Fainting	Y/N
Numbness/tingling	Y/N	Paralysis in parts of your body	Y/N
Seizures or convulsions	Y/N		
EARS			
Hard of hearing or deafness	Y/N	Ringing or noises in your ears	Y/N
Frequent or severe ear infections	Y/N	Painful or swollen ear lobes	Y/N
NOSE AND THROAT			
Sores in your nose or mouth	Y/N	Severe or recurrent nosebleeds	Y/N
Frequent sneezing	Y/N	Sinus trouble	Y/N
Persistent hoarseness	Y/N	Tooth and gum infections	Y/N
SKIN			
Rashes	Y/N	Skin Sores	Y/N
Sunburn Easily	Y/N	White patches of skin or hair	Y/N
Loss of hair	Y/N	Tick or insect bites	Y/N
Painfully cold fingers	Y/N	Severe Itching	Y/N

RESPIRATORY			
Severe or frequent colds	Y/N	Constant coughing	Y/N
Coughing up blood	Y/N	Recent flu or viral infection	Y/N
Wheezing or asthma attacks	Y/N	Difficulty breathing	Y/N
BLOOD			
Frequent or easy bruising	Y/N	Frequent or easy bleeding	Y/N
Have you had a blood transfusion?	Y/N		
GASTROINTESTINAL			
Trouble swallowing	Y/N	Diarrhea	Y/N
Bloody stools	Y/N	Stomach ulcers	Y/N
Jaundice or yellow skin	Y/N		
BONES AND JOINTS			
Stiff joints	Y/N	Painful or swollen joints	Y/N
Stiff lower back	Y/N	Stiff lower back	Y/N
Other back pain	Y/N	Muscle aches	Y/N
GENITOURINARY			
Kidney problems	Y/N	Bladder trouble	Y/N
Blood in your urine	Y/N	Urinary discharge	Y/N
Genital sores or ulcers	Y/N	Prostatitis	Y/N
Testicular pain	Y/N		

Table 2.2 Uveitic diseases by demographics

History	Related conditions
Age	
• Age < 5	• Juvenile arthropathies, masquerade (retinoblastoma, juvenile xanthogranuloma)
• Age 5–25	• Juvenile arthropathies, post-viral neuroretinitis, parasitic (e.g., toxocariasis), TINU, masquerade (retinoblastoma, juvenile xanthogranuloma), sarcoidosis, acute retinal necrosis, HLA-B27, toxoplasmosis, Fuch's uveitis
• 25–45	• HLA-B27, CMV retinitis, acute retinal necrosis, ankylosing spondylitis, Behcet's, Vogt Koyanagi Harada's (VKH), sarcoidosis, toxoplasmosis, serpiginous choroidopathy, white dot syndromes, idiopathic
• 45–65	• HLA-B27, Behcet's, birdshot retinochoroiditis, serpiginous choroidopathy, idiopathic
• >65	• Serpiginous choroidopathy, masquerade syndromes (lymphoma), herpes zoster, idiopathic
Gender	
• Male	• Ankylosing spondylitis, reactive arthritis, Behcet's, sympathetic ophthalmia
• Female	• Juvenile arthropathies
Race/ancestry	
• Caucasian	• Ankylosing spondylitis, reactive arthritis
• African American	• Sarcoidosis
• Asian	• VKH, Bechet's
• Central/South America	• Toxoplasmosis, cysticercosis, onchocerciasis
Social history	
• Endemic location	• Histoplasmosis, tuberculosis, toxoplasmosis, Lyme
• Tick/insect or water borne	• Leptospirosis, treamtode granulomas, Lyme
• Animal exposure	• Toxoplasmosis, toxocariasis, leptospirosis, cysticercosis
• Immunosuppresion	• HIV, opportunistic infections

Table 2.3 Conditions causing granulomatous inflammation

Sarcoidosis
Sympathetic ophthalmia
Vogt-Koyanagi-Harada syndrome
Syphilis
Tuberculosis
Herpetic
Uveitis associated with multiple sclerosis
Intraocular foreign body

accumulation of inflammatory cells on or within the iris is more commonly seen with diseases causing granulomatous inflammation (see Table 2.3). Heterochromic iris changes are often, but not always, observed in Fuch's heterochromic uveitis.

Retinal/Choroidal findings—The diagnosis of posterior uveitis may be recognizable clinically based on vascular and chorioretinal lesion characteristics. Ocular imaging techniques such as fluorescein angiogram are essential in characterizing these changes. Pattern recognition is important and a few key findings may be seen more commonly with specific diagnosis. Serous retinal detachments are classically associated with VKH syndrome (particularly if bilateral). Dalen-Fuchs nodules (small, discrete, deep, yellow-white chorioretinal lesions) may be associated with VKH and sympathetic ophthalmia. Acute retinal necrosis (ARN) is a type of necrotizing retinitis most commonly caused by herpetic viruses (HSV, VZV). The classic posterior appearance includes vitritis, retinal vascular arteriolitis, and peripheral retinitis. Typically, the retinitis begins as peripheral areas of multifocal retinal yellowing, often flat with scalloped edges. This can eventually progress into confluent whitening extending into the posterior pole. Cytomegalovirus (CMV) retinitis may also be identified clinically and should be suspected in patients that are immunosuppressed. The classic exam findings in CMV retinitis are peripheral or posterior yellow-white lesions that follow the retinal vasculature centripetally, vasculitis with a "frosted branch" appearance, and retinal hemorrhages. This constellation of findings has been described as a "scrambled eggs or cottage cheese with ketchup" appearance. There may be little to no vitritis, given the immunocompromised state of these patients. Classic toxoplasmosis lesions present as focal and white with overlying vitritis with a "headlight in the fog" appearance, often with adjacent pigmented retinochoroidal scarring. Other diagnosis that may be clinically identifiable include white dot syndromes, ocular histoplasmosis syndrome, and serpiginous choroidopathy.

Optic Nerve—Disc hyperemia, papillitis or papilledema can occur in many uveitic disorders, However, classically prominent disc hyperemia is noted in VKH.

Principles of Diagnostic Testing

As emphasized above, all testing should be complementary to the history and exam, not an alternative. Patient work-up should focus on ruling out infectious diseases that may respond to antimicrobial therapy and systemic disorders that may affect the patients overall health.

It is important to understand several key concepts when discussing diagnostic testing. Knowing how pre- and post-test probabilities and predictive values change based on Bayesian principles can help direct when a test should be ordered. Additionally, the utility of each test can be clarified by acknowledging the difference between targeted versus screening tests as well as understanding when different tests are helpful for ruling in disease versus ruling out disease.

Pre-test probability is defined as the likelihood that a patient has the disease in question prior to testing. It can be estimated based on history, exam, the incidence of disease in the population, and the sensitivity and specificity of the test (see Fig. 2.2). To illustrate how this value changes from patient to patient we will use the example of a male patient with no risk factors, from a non-endemic area presenting with intermediate uveitis. The clinician is considering sending Lyme testing (specificity 50–95 %, sensitivity 99–100 % [24, 25]). For purposes of

$$\text{Post-test probability} = \frac{\text{Pretest probability x sensitivity}}{\text{(Pre-test probability x sensitivity) + (1-pretest probability)(1-specificity)}}$$

Fig. 2.2 Post-test probability formula

this illustration we will say the overall incidence for the patient's geographic location is 1:1000. The patient has no risk factors on history and no other findings on exam so we would estimate the pre-test probability to be approximately 1:1000 (0.1 %). Using a specificity and sensitivity of 90 %, we can calculate the post-test probability using the formula in Fig. 2.2. This calculation estimates the post-test probability as only 0.9 %. In other words, if this patient's serology testing came back positive, there would still only be a 0.9 % chance of having Lyme disease and ultimately a positive value may be misleading. Testing may likewise be unhelpful if the pre-test probability is very high (i.e., the patient recently went hiking in the northeast, was bitten by a tick, and has a new "bulls-eye" rash). In this case, the post-test probability would nearly equal the pre-test probability. This also makes the test minimally useful as the patient would likely receive treatment regardless of the results.

Positive predictive value defines the likelihood that a person with a positive test has the disease in question. It is a function of the test itself and is also dependent on disease prevalence in the population being tested. Thus, if a test is performed on a population with a very low prevalence of disease, the positive predictive value declines substantially. The alternative is true, the more prevalent the disease, the more likely a positive test accurately indicates that the patient has the disease in question (high positive predictive value). An example of this can be demonstrated with tuberculosis testing. In the general population of the United States, tuberculosis accounts for 0.1–0.5 % of uveitis cases [26–29]. The reported sensitivity and specificity of purified protein derivative (PPD) ranges from 75–89 % and 85–86 %, and for Quantiferon-gold 70–81 %, 97–99 % [27–30], respectively. If all patients are screened for tuberculosis, the positive predictive value is 1 % for the PPD test and 11 % for Quantiferon-gold [26, 27]. However, in a patient from an endemic area with exam findings concerning for possible tuberculosis (e.g., differential of serpiginous choroiditis vs. serpiginous-like choroiditis) the positive predictive value of the PPD and Quantiferon-gold increase to 82 and 96 %, respectively [1, 31]. Thus the utility of each test can vary remarkably based on which patients are tested. The same concept applies when defining disease by anatomical location of the inflammation (see below). For example, the utility of HLA-B27 testing in a patient with bilateral posterior uveitis is poor and a positive test would confuse the diagnostic picture and likely represent a false positive (can be positive in up to 8 % of Caucasians and 4 % of African Americans [32]) and should, in general, be performed only in patients with acute, recurrent anterior uveitis. Likewise, positive HLA-A29 or toxoplasmosis testing will likely represent false positivity in a patient with anterior uveitis and should generally be restricted to selective cases with posterior uveitis. Table 2.4 illustrates how positive predictive values are affected by disease prevalence.

Targeted versus Screening tests—After addressing the importance of a focused or targeted laboratory work-up, it is important to acknowledge that there are a few infectious uveitic diseases that cannot be defined by their clinical findings and may present in various anatomical locations. These are important to

Table 2.4 The affect of disease prevalence on positive predictive value

Disease prevalence (%)	Positive predictive value (%)
1	16
10	68
20	83
50	95

Modified from https://www.ncbi.nlm.nih.gov/pmc/articles/PMC2636062/

highlight as they are not treated with immunomodulators, and if left untreated can lead to a poor visual and in some cases systemic prognosis. Generally, these diseases include Lyme disease, syphilis, and tuberculosis. The appropriate timing for Lyme testing can be elicited by the patient's history and risk factors, and thus should not be ordered on every patient. We do, however, suggest that it may be warranted to send a screening syphilis test on all patients requiring laboratory work-up. Although this infection is rare, the incidence of primary and secondary disease has doubled in the US since 2000 [33]. Screening is warranted given that risk factors may be difficult to illicit, testing is inexpensive and very sensitive and specific, it is easily treatable, and there is significant morbidity associated if left untreated. There are differing opinions on whether or not tuberculosis testing should be sent as a screening test on all patients. Rosenbaum et al. [26] concluded that routine screening in the general US population with purified protein derivative (PPD) is not warranted based on the low positive predictive value. Hong et al. [34] more recently suggested that screening in certain geographic areas in the US that are known to have a large immigrant population (such as the Los Angeles County hospital cited in the study) may be useful. It is important to highlight that in the latter study the only risk factor found to significantly predict PPD positivity was a history of being born outside of the United States. Thus, a thorough history may help guide the decision about screening for tuberculosis. In practice, many uveitis specialists advocate for screening tuberculosis testing citing the importance of confirming negativity prior to starting systemic immune modulation therapy, especially if an anti-TNF (anti-Tissue Necrosis Factor) medication may be utilized [35].

Several non-specific tests may also be appropriate as screening tools. A complete blood count (CBC) with differential may be useful for identifying more urgent diagnosis such as patients with systemic infection (leukocytosis or eosinophilia), malignancy (leukemia), or who are immunocompromised. Likewise, a comprehensive metabolic panel (CMP) and urinalysis (UA) may reveal renal or hepatic dysfunction or hyperglycemia. This information may also be important when making decisions about starting oral immunomodulators.

Tests that rule in disease versus ruling out disease—In some cases, a test being negative may be just as important as positive testing. An example is seen with toxoplasmosis titers. A positive value does not mean a patient has toxoplasma retinochoroiditis, since nearly 30 % of the population may have been exposed to toxoplasma at some point in their life. Specifically, seropositivity in the US has been reported as >20 % (higher in males, nonhispanic blacks, those not born in the US, elderly) [36, 37]. In contrast, a negative test is sensitive for the exclusion of toxoplasmosis. HLA-A29 is another test that, if negative, may be helpful in ruling out Birdshot chorioretinopathy in patients with multiple white chorioretinal lesions.

Individual Tests

We will now briefly review the sensitivities and specificities of commonly ordered diagnostic testing. It is important to keep in mind the above concepts that despite sensitivity and specificity, the utility of each test may vary greatly dependent on the patient's risk factors, population prevalence, and exam findings. A summary of the discussed tests including their estimated costs, sensitivities, and specificities can be found in Table 2.5. Additionally, it is important to note that much of the research regarding sensitivity and specificities of the following tests are based on non-ophthalmologic literature.

Laboratory

Tuberculin Skin Test and Interferon Gamma Release Assays

Tuberculin is a glycerol extract derived from the precipitate of sterilized, concentrated cultures of the tubercle bacillus. The skin test, also known as the purified protein derivative (PPD), or Mantoux

Table 2.5 Summary of important testing modalities

Test	% Positivity (in uveitis patients)	[a]Estimated cost	Sensitivity/specificity disease prevalence dependent	Possible indications
Tuberculin skin test	0.2–1 %	$18	75–89 %/85–86 %	Tuberculosis, immunomodulatory therapy
Interferon gamma release assay—*Quantiferon-gold*		$243	70–81 %/97–99 %	Tuberculosis, immunomodulatory therapy
Lyme serology	Geographic dependent	$56-screening $193-confirmatory	59–99 %/81–100 %[b]	Lyme disease
Angiotensin converting enzyme	3-7 %	$56	60–90 %/83–95 %[d]	Sarcoidosis
Lysozyme		$75	60 %/76 %	Sarcoidosis
Antinuclear antibodies	0.1–1 %	$48	95 %/68–97 %[e]	JIA, vasculitis, connective tissue disease
VDRL	1.6–4.5 %	$27	Primary 78–86 %/85–99 % Secondary 100 %/85–99 % Tertiary 95–98 %/85–99 % Neurosyphilis/ocular 69 %/85–99 %	Syphilis
FTA-ABS		$60	Primary 84 %/96 % Other stages 100 %/96 %	Syphilis
HLA-B27	50–80 % of acute anterior uveitis	$105	99 %/99 %	Seronegative spondyloarthropathy
Complete blood count		$27		Overall health, immunomodulatory therapy, masquerade syndromes
Complete metabolic panel		$92		Overall health, immunomodulatory therapy, sarcoidosis, masquerade syndromes
Urinalysis		$40		Vasculitis, TINU
Chest X-ray—*Sarcoidosis*		$156[c]	79 %/99 %	Sarcoidosis, tuberculosis, Wegener's
Chest X-ray—*Tuberculosis*		$156[c]	86.8 %/89.4 %	
Chest computed tomography—*Sarcoidosis*		$975[c]	85–95 %/53 %	Sarcoidosis
Magnetic resonance imaging—head		$2,785[c]		Multiple sclerosis, CNS lymphoma, cysticercosis
Gallium scan		$695[c]		Sarcoidosis

[a]Estimated from the Lahey clinic laboratories 2009–2014. These are charges and do not reflect what may be collected. Radiologic datat from 2009
[b]Dependent on when in the disease course the tests were done
[c]Professional fee included
[d]Depdendent on active versus inactive disease
[e]Dependent on titer values used—note very low positive predictive value (<1 %)

Table 2.6 Positivity classification of the tuberculin skin test reaction

Diameter of induration	Persons for whom reaction is considered positive
Induration of ≥5 mm	HIV infected, recent contact of person with TB, fibrotic changes on X-ray consistent with prior TB, immunosuppressed (history of organ transplant, taking the equivalent of >15 mg/day of prednisone for ≥1 month; taking TNF-α antagonists)
Induration of ≥10 mm	Recent immigrants (<5 years) from high prevalence countries, Injection drug users, Nursing home/correctional facility residents and employees, healthcare workers, Mycobacteriology laboratory personnel, Age >70 or <18 years old, medical condition associated with increased TB risk (diabetes, corticosteroid use, gastrectomy, malabsorption, silicosis, malnutrition)
Induration of ≥15 mm	All others

Modified from Centers for disease control, tuberculosis, publications and products, fact sheets testing & diagnosis, tuberculin skin testing, classification of the tuberculin skin test reaction. Available at http://www.cdc.gov/tb/publications/factsheets/testing/skintesting.htm

skin test, is performed when tuberculin is injected intradermally and then skin induration is measured at 24–48 h based on a host type IV Hypersensitivity reaction. The extent of skin induration indicates test positivity (see Table 2.6). It is important to note that certain conditions can suppress this reaction leading to false negative results (see Table 2.7). The test was established in 1908 and remained the foremost means of screening for tuberculosis for nearly a century. In 2005, the CDC released guidelines for use of FDA approved interferon gamma release assays. These tests are ELISA assays that measure the interferon gamma produced when the patient's peripheral blood leukocytes are purified and mixed with three different tuberculosis antigens from a whole blood sample. There are currently two FDA approved tests, the Quantiferon TB-gold test, and the T-SPOT TB test. A recent head-to-head prospective study demonstrated the Quantiferon TB-gold test to be more specific but slightly less sensitive than the T-SPOT TB [38, 39]. However, the Quantiferon test was significantly more accurate in identifying true-positive tuberculous uveitis than T-SPOT TB in discordant cases (98 % vs. 76 %) [39]. The Quantiferon-gold is more readily available and used more extensively in the US. Latent versus active TB cannot be differentiated from a positive result for skin testing or for ELISA assays. It is not recommended that these be used as the sole method for diagnosis. Microbiologic sampling remains the gold standard for diagnosis. However, culture or tissue sampling is often difficult to obtain in an ocular specimen and analysis may be limited in its availability.

Table 2.7 Conditions that suppress PPD hypersensitivity reaction

Infectious mononucleosis
Live virus vaccine—if given within 3 weeks of testing
Sarcoidosis
Hodgkin's disease
Corticosteroids/immune suppression
Malnutrition
Upper respiratory tract infection

There are certain limitations to both the tuberculin skin test and ELISA assays. Skin testing is limited by poor inter-reader reliability (e.g., 9 mm negative vs. 10 mm positive), low specificity (e.g., prior BCG vaccination), poor predictive value in low prevalence populations (see example mentioned above), and it requires patient reliability to return to read the test. Thus, interferon gamma release assays may be more useful for poorly reliable patients or immigrants from endemic areas that may have a false positive PPD from previous BCG vaccination. There are conflicting reports about the sensitivities and specificities of purified protein derivative versus Quantiferon-gold. Reported sensitivities and specificities range from 75–89 % and 85–86 % for the PPD test and 70–81 %, 97–99 % for Quantiferon-gold, respectively [27–30]. Another recent study by McMullen et al. indicates that in the correct population, PPD screening is still highly specific with a specificity of 99.7 % versus 91.4 % for Quantiferon-gold ($p < 0.0001$) [40]. Cost continues to be an important disparity between these two screening methods. One study focusing on the cost-effectiveness of Quantiferon versus PPD measured the number of averted TB cases in two years. This study estimated the cost for the screening of latent TB and treatment of a hypothetical cohort to be $16,021 per averted case for PPD versus $227,977 per averted TB case for Quantiferon [41].

As mentioned above, the role of tuberculosis testing as a screening tool for all patients is debated among uveitis specialists. Given the varied population presenting at our clinic, it is generally our practice to selectively send this as a screening test for patients with intermediate or posterior/panuveitis, any patient with suggestive exposure history or risk, and those we are anticipating the initiation of systemic immune modulation therapy (especially with TNF alpha inhibitors).

Syphilis Testing (Non-specific and Specific)

Syphilis is rarely diagnosed by dark field microscopy or immunofluorescence from a tissue biopsy. Thus, the mainstays of testing are specific (direct) and non-specific (indirect) treponemal antibody tests. Indirect tests such as the Venereal Disease Research Laboratory (VDRL) and rapid plasma reagin (RPR) measure IgG and IgM antibodies directed to cardiolipin that is released during cellular damage that occurs during active infection. These antibodies are not specific for *Treponemal pallidum.* These tests typically become non-reactive with time and following adequate treatment. The sensitivities for the indirect tests for syphilis are reported to be 78–86 % for detecting primary syphilis, 100 % for detecting secondary syphilis, and 95–98 % for detecting tertiary syphilis [42]. Sensitivity, however, decreases significantly for detection of neurosyphilis to 69 % [43]. Specificity ranges from 85 to 99 %. False positives can be seen with systemic lupus erythematosus, biliary cirrhosis, rheumatoid arthritis, pregnancy, intravenous drug use, advanced malignancy, tuberculosis, malaria, Lyme, HIV, hepatitis, viral diseases. Confirmation for any positive or equivocal non-treponemal test result are traditionally followed with a specific or direct treponemal test, such as the fluorescent treponemal antibody absorption (FTA-ABS), quantitative VDRL/RPR, microhemagglutination assay *T. pallidum* (MHA-TP), *T. pallidum* hemagglutination (TPHA), or *T. pallidum* particle agglutination (TPPA) test. Direct treponemal tests detect antibodies specific to *T. pallidum* (and a few other treponemal subspecies that are rarely seen in the US). This test stays reactive for life and indicates that infection has occurred but does not distinguish active versus latent or treated infection. Thus, a positive direct test will indicate whether the patient has been exposed to syphilis in the past and a positive indirect test such as the RPR or VDRL will indicate active untreated infection. FTA-ABS is the most commonly used confirmatory test following positive VDRL or RPR test findings. FTA-ABS has a sensitivity of 84 % for detecting primary syphilis infection and almost 100 % sensitivity for detecting syphilis infection in other stages. Its specificity is 96 % [42]. Possible causes for a positive direct test and negative indirect are latent syphilis, previously treated infection, neurosyphilis, or false positive direct test.

Of note, it has been reported that nearly 30 % of ocular syphilis cases test negative to non-specific testing [44]. Thus, we strongly advocate using direct testing for initial screening. Many laboratory protocols have been trending toward this approach as well. Treponemal Enzyme Immunoassays (EIA) are a type of automated direct treponemal test, where reactive results are subsequently followed by indirect testing. Reports indicate that this approach is highly cost effective, slightly decreases the sensitivity, but improves specificity [45–47]. This protocol is now the standard at many academic laboratories, including ours. Ophthalmologists should become familiar with their local laboratory testing algorithm for syphilis, so if needed, it can be specified that you would like direct testing done first.

It is our practice to send for syphilis testing on all patients with uveitis (excluding HLA-B27 positive anterior uveitis—*see targeted versus screening* section above).

Lyme Testing

The most accepted laboratory analysis for Lyme disease is based on a two-step approach. The first screening test is a serology test looking at serum IgG and IgM antibodies. The host antibody response to *B. burgdorferi* infection develops slowly so both the IgG and IgM antibodies take weeks to appear (2–4 weeks and 4–6 weeks, respectively). Thus, if serology alone is performed early in the disease course the sensitivity and specificity are 59 and 93 %, respectively [24]. Considering this delayed response, if suspicion for infection is high, tests may need to be repeated later in the disease course for confirmation. If testing is performed after 2–4 weeks the sensitivity and specificity increases to 95 and 81 %, respectively [24]. The two-step approach recommended by the CDC describes that positive or indeterminate serologies should be followed by a Western blot test [25]. This approach increases specificity to 99–100 % [24, 25]. It is worth emphasizing again the importance of pre- and post-test probabilities with this disease in particular as there are rather well defined endemic areas within the US (see Fig. 2.3). Despite the two-step testing approach the guidelines for the diagnosis of Lyme disease as described by the American College of Physicians is based primarily on clinical findings [24]. More recent tests have been developed in an effort to obviate the need for western blot confirmatory testing. Two of these tests include the C6 and VlsE antibody tests. These detect both IgG and IgM antibodies specific to portions of the *B. burgdorferi* organism. There are several advantages to the use of these newer tests, including no interference in patients who have been vaccinated with the available Lyme antigen, detection of antibodies to the European strains of *B. burgdorferi*, and high specificity [48, 49]. These tests currently are not widely available and have limited clinical data.

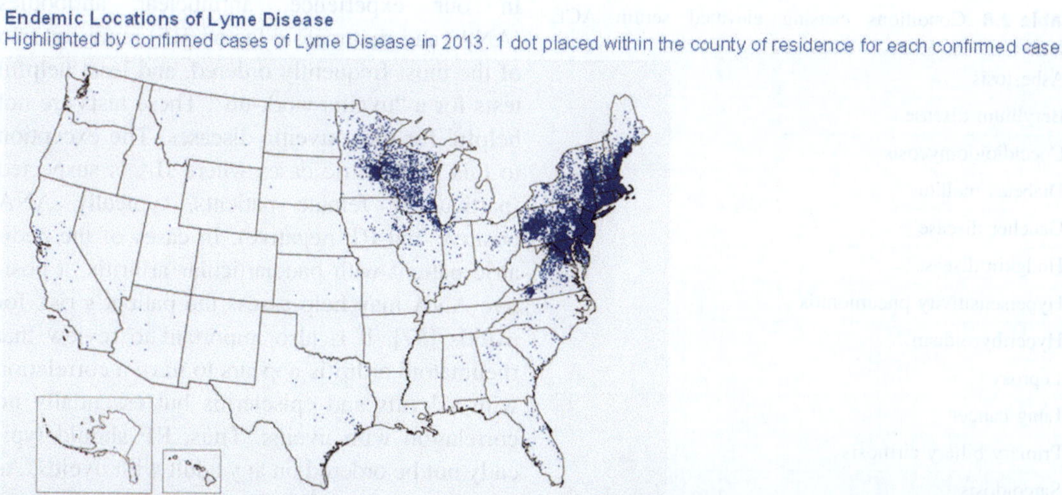

Fig. 2.3 Endemic locations of Lyme disease

Angiotensin Converting Enzyme and Lysozyme

Angiotensin converting enzyme is secreted in the lungs and kidneys by the pulmonary endothelium and activated macrophages (epithelioid cells). Measurements of serum ACE may be elevated in multiple systemic disorders (see Table 2.8). It is proposed that the elevation of ACE in sarcoidosis specifically, is related to the abundance of epithelioid cells and macrophages in sarcoid granulomas. In addition to ACE, sarcoid granulomas also secrete lysozyme, glucuronidase, collagenase and elastase. Despite certain limitations, elevated ACE levels have been found to be a useful *adjunct* to the diagnosis and assessment of disease activity and management of sarcoidosis. Reference values for serum ACE is age dependent and it is important to note that healthy children have ACE levels that are 40–50 % higher than adults [50]. The sensitivities have been reported with a rather broad range of 59 % for inactive disease and 60–90 % in active disease [51, 52]. Specificity ranges from 83 to 95 % [53, 54]. In one report, the sensitivity increases to 85.9 % when looking only at patients with a clinical suspicion of sarcoidosis and 92.1 % if only those with a known diagnosis of sarcoidosis are included [29]. Reports specifically focusing on patients with uveitis found sensitivities of 73–84 % and specificities of 83–95 % but with a predictive value of 47 % [54, 55].

Table 2.8 Conditions causing elevated serum ACE levels

Asbestosis
Beryllium disease
Coccidioidomycosis
Diabetes mellitus
Gaucher disease
Hodgkin disease
Hypersensitivity pneumonitis
Hyperthyroidism
Leprosy
Lung cancer
Primary biliary cirrhosis
Sarcoidosis
Silicosis
Tuberculosis

Lysozyme, like ACE is an enzyme produced by epithelioid cells, giant cells, and macrophages found in granulomas. It is often increased in the serum and tears of sarcoid patients. Serum levels are age dependent with levels increasing with age above 60 years. Levels may also be increased in patients with kidney dysfunction. Baarsma et al. found a sensitivity of 60 % and a specificity of 76 % and a mean predictive value of only 12 % in patients with uveitis [54]. This test should not be used in isolation, as it has poor sensitivity and specificity. However, this test may be a useful adjunctive test when combined with serum ACE, where the predictive value when both are positive will be over 70 %.

It is important to note that in patients suspected of having sarcoidosis, other than with tissue confirmation of sarcoidosis (see Tissue Sampling), there are no definitive diagnostic blood, skin, or radiologic imaging tests specific for this disorder and the diagnosis is made based on a constellation of findings [56].

Antinuclear Antibodies and Rheumatoid Factor

In our experience, antinuclear antibodies (ANA) and rheumatoid factor (RF) represent two of the most frequently ordered, and least helpful tests for a "uveitis work-up". These tests are not helpful for most uveitic diseases. The exception to this is pediatric cases where JIA is suspected (particularly female patients, typically ANA positive and RF negative). In cases of the pediatric patient with pauciarticular arthritis, a positive ANA may help assess the patient's risk for uveitis [57]. It is also important to review that rheumatoid arthritis appears to have a correlation with scleritis and episcleritis but essentially no correlation with uveitis. Thus, RF should typically not be ordered on any adult with uveitis. As with the other testing described above, the sensitivity and specificity of ANA varies greatly depending on the pre-test probability of the

Table 2.9 Conditions causing elevated serum ANA

Hashimotos thyroiditis
Graves disease
Autoimmune hepatitis
Primary biliary cirrhosis
Primary autoimmune cholangitis
Idiopathic pulmonary arterial hypertension
Infectious mononucleosis
Hepatitis C
Subacute bacterial endocarditis
Tuberculosis

population being evaluated. Levels of ANA may be elevated in a number of systemic disorders (see Table 2.9).

The specificity of ANA testing has been reported to range from 68 to 97 % (dependent on titer levels) [58]. Based on the high false positive rates among healthy individuals, ANA testing is not recommended as a *screening* test for autoimmune disorders. When applying the use of ANA testing to the disease prevalence seen in uveitis patients, Rosenbaum et al. found that patients with uveitis and a positive ANA have <1 % chance of having systemic lupus erythematosus (SLE). Thus, it is important to emphasize that even in patients with uveitis and *positive* ANA the chance of then having an underlying systemic diagnosis of SLE is <1 %. Thus, the utility of this test in the work-up of uveitis is very limited [26].

Less Frequently Used Laboratory Tests

Based on the clinical presentation, some less common laboratory tests should be considered. Urinary β2-microglobulin may be of value in detecting tubulointerstitial nephritis and uveitis syndrome (TINU) and should be considered in pediatric and young patients presenting with acute anterior uveitis [59]. Bartonella henselae should be considered in patients with a history of a cat scratch or significant cat exposure, especially when presenting with neuroretinitis [60].

Molecular

HLA-Typing

Several uveitic diseases have been found to be associated with specific human leukocyte antigen types (see Table 2.10). The most studied antigen type is HLA-B27. It has been shown that patients with recurrent, acute unilateral, alternating

Table 2.10 HLA associations in uveitic disease

Disease	HLA association
Acute anterior uveitis	HLA-B27
Reactive arthritis	HLA-B27
Juvenile idiopathic arthritis	HLA-DR, Dw2
Behcet syndrome	HLA-B51
Birdshot retinochoroiditis	HLA-A29
Intermediate uveitis	HLAB8, B51, DR2, DR15
Sympathetic ophthalmia	HLA-DR4
VKH syndrome	HLA-DR4
Sarcoidosis	HLA-BA, B13
Multiple sclerosis	HLA-B7, DR2
Ocular histoplasmosis syndrome	HLA-B7, DR2
Retinal vasculitis	HLA-B44

Modified from Intraocular inflammation and uveitis, basic and clinical science course, 2003–2004. American Academy of Ophthalmology, 2003. p. 92

anterior uveitis have nearly an 80 % chance of being HLA-B27 positive [61]. Of those patients that are positive for HLA-B27, 66–75 % will have an associated spondyloarthropathy [62–64]. It has been reported that up to 50 % of these arthropathies are either misdiagnosed or undiagnosed [65]. Thus, HLA-B27 testing may be helpful as an adjunct for the patient's systemic health. Based on the typical presentation of HLA-B27 associated anterior uveitis, this should *not* be ordered for patients with intermediate or posterior disease. As a *diagnostic* test, however, the utility of HLA-typing is limited. This is demonstrated by applying Bayes theorem when using HLA-A29 typing to diagnose Birdshot Chorioretinopathy (BSCR). HLA-A29 has one of the highest associations between HLA type and disease with nearly 85–95 % of BSCR patients being HLA-A29 positive (vs. 4–8 % of the general population) [32, 61]. However, when applied as a screening test in *all* patients with posterior uveitis the positive predictive value is only 47 % [61]. This predictive value would increase if applied to only patients with multiple white chorioretinal lesions. It does, however, and retain high sensitivity (99 %) when applied exclusively to patients with posterior uveitis [61, 66]. Thus, it may be a useful to aid in exclusion of disease. In HLA-types that are not as tightly associated to a specific uveitic disease, the utility for use as a diagnostic test is significantly decreased.

Imaging

Chest X-Ray

Chest radiography is often used as an adjunctive screening test for both sarcoidosis and tuberculosis. Important findings for sarcoidosis include hilar or mediastinal nodal enlargement, interstitial "air-space like" opacities and peripheral cavitation [67]. For tuberculosis, findings include patchy consolidation or poorly defined linear and nodular opacities often located in the posterior or superior segments of the lung [68]. Studies have estimated that 90–95 % of patients with sarcoidosis have pulmonary findings on chest X-ray [69–71]. In one representative study, 8 % of patients presented at radiologic stage zero (no visible changes on plain film chest X-ray), 40 % presented at stage 1 (bilateral hilar lymphadenopathy), and 37 % present at stage 2 (bilateral hilar lymphadenopathy and diffuse pulmonary infiltration) [69]. The utility of the chest X-ray for sarcoid has been well established and the reported sensitivity is 79 % [72, 73]. It is important to note, however, that these estimates may have a selection bias for patients that were ultimately diagnosed with pulmonary sarcoid. In our experience, it is not uncommon for patients to present with extrapulmonary sarcoidosis (uveitis) and have an unremarkable chest X-ray.

A review looking at chest X-ray as an additional screening tool for active tuberculosis (specifically reporting "abnormalities suggestive of TB"), estimated sensitivity and specificity as 86.8 and 89.4 %, respectively [74]. When comparing chest X-ray and symptoms (e.g., prolonged cough) in parallel, the sensitivity was improved by 0–9 % and specificity by 2–5 % [74]. It is important to recognize, however, that most cases of ocular TB from paucibacillary or miliary disease are not accompanied by pulmonary findings. Thus, positive testing in a patient with suspicious ocular findings but a negative chest X-ray does not rule out TB infection. In such cases appropriate tissue sampling through culture or PCR analysis (e.g., anterior chamber or vitreous sampling) should be considered.

Chest Computed Tomography

Computed tomography is a more sensitive but less specific modality for detecting mediastinal lymphadenopathy in sarcoid patients, particularly in the elderly [75]. Some studies suggest that chest computed tomography (CT) may not add significant additional clinical information for the initial diagnosis of sarcoidosis and is generally not a helpful adjunctive test [76]. However, one study looking specifically at elderly women with chronic uveitis found a chest CT useful in identifying mediastinal lymphadenopathy and helped to guide tissue confirmation [77]. According to the American Thoracic Society, European Respiratory Society, and the World Association of Sarcoidosis and Other Granulomatous Disorders, chest CT can be justified in the following circumstances: 1—Atypical clinical and/or chest radiograph findings, 2—normal chest radiograph but a strong clinical suspicion of the disease, 3—Detection of complications of the lung disease [78, 79]. Additional limitations of this modality include significant cost and radiation exposure. The typical chest CT will expose the patient to 2 millisieverts (mSv) of radiation versus the 0.05 mSv of a chest X-ray. Thus, a chest CT should be used as an adjunctive test only if it will impact a patient's systemic health or the treatment paradigm.

Magnetic Resonance Imaging

Magnetic resonance imaging (MRI) of the brain may be warranted in the work-up of uveitis in very select cases. Examples may include patients (particularly elderly) in whom CNS lymphoma is suspected. Additionally, for the evaluation of intermediate uveitis in a patient with other neurologic symptoms concerning for possible multiple sclerosis (e.g., numbness, tingling, weakness, muscle spasms), MRI of the brain and neurologic consultation should be considered. This is particularly important given recent data suggesting that early initiation of disease-modifying therapy may improve prognosis and reduce neurologic damage [80].

Tissue Sampling

Polymerase Chain Reaction

The polymerase chain reaction is an important biologic test that is used to amplify an infinitesimal amount of sampled DNA into analytic quantities. This test utilizes thermal cycling, where the nucleic acid sequence is repeatedly heated and cooled, allowing replicating enzymes and primers to exponentially amplify the sequence. This test provides a method for minimally invasive tissue sampling through aqueous and vitreous extraction. The sensitivity of PCR for the detection of DNA is astounding and estimated to be nearly 1×10^{-21} molar [81]. This sensitivity also leads to a potential pitfall of false positivity with amplification of contaminated samples. Indications for PCR testing include media opacity, irregular or unanticipated disease course, disease unresponsive to therapy, or diagnosis confirmation. This test should also be considered when viral or fungal retinitis is suspected where the typical yield of culture alone is poor or results may be delayed. Much of the utility of sampling depends on laboratory handling. Generally, approximately 0.05 cc of fluid is required for analysis, which should be placed immediately on ice, followed by freezing on dry ice, then sent to a PCR laboratory. Improper handling can lead to false negative or positive results. A list of organisms available for PCR analysis can be seen in Table 2.11. The broad utility of PCR testing is still under investigation. Rothova et al. examined the usefulness of aqueous humor analysis for the diagnosis of posterior uveitis. In their report, 29 % of patients had positive PCR results to at least one diagnostic assay and 24 % of patients required a change of treatment based on their assay findings [82]. Additional studies have shown that PCR diagnostic testing correlates with improved clinical outcomes [83, 84]. Given that PCR analysis may be costly and not widely available, alternative methods for DNA amplification are currently being explored [85].

Table 2.11 Organisms available for testing by PCR

Viral: CMV, HSV, VZV, EBV, HIV, HTLV-1, Rubella, HHV-6, HHV-8
Bacteria: All (using 16S ribosomal DNA sequencing)—including TB
Protozoans: *Toxoplasma gondii, Oncocerca*
Fungi: All (using 18S/28S ribosomal DNA sequencing)

Biopsy/Cytology

Tissue biopsy accompanied with cytologic examination plays an important role in the diagnosis of specific uveitic entities. Examples of important biopsy and sampling procedures that may be utilized include anterior chamber paracentesis, vitreous tap and diagnostic vitrectomy, iris and ciliary body biopsy, choroidal and retinochoroidal biopsy and fine needle aspiration biopsy. Given the invasive nature of this testing, indications are often limited to clinical presentations suspicious for vision or life threatening etiologies, diseases with an unanticipated course, or that are unresponsive to therapy. These may include masquerade syndromes such as leukemia, lymphoma, or metastatic disease. A ratio measurement in the aqueous humor of the cytokines IL-10 (elevated in non-Hodgkins lymphoma) and IL-6 (elevated with intraocular inflammation) show promise as an adjunctive measure for intraocular lymphoma but is currently not widely utilized. Additional indications for sampling and cytology include concern for infectious endophthalmitis, necrotizing retinitis, delayed endophthalmitis, or parasitic uveitis.

Biopsy also plays an important diagnostic role in sarcoidosis with the sample exhibiting noncaseating epithelioid granulomas. The most common biopsy site is to the intrathoracic lymph nodes (transbronchial). Yield of these biopsies have been found to be 60 % in patients with a normal chest X-ray and 90 % if parenchymal disease is present [86]. Conjunctival, lacrimal gland, cutaneous lesions or extrathoracic nodes have also been utilized for diagnosis. The yield of conjunctival and lacrimal biopsies without a discrete lesion is controversial and reports of positive yield range from 10 to 55 %. This has been shown to improve in the presence of follicles, when bilateral biopsies are taken, and when multiplane sectioning techniques are utilized [87–90]. Thus, the yield for biopsy is low if there is no discrete lesion or if there is no other imaging modality indicating infiltration of that tissue (e.g., Gallium-67 scanning may show lacrimal gland uptake and can guide where to biopsy [91]). Our recommendation when considering tissue biopsy for sarcoid is to perform a thorough physical exam and consider biopsy if there is an abnormal lesion.

Suggested Testing Algorithm by Anatomic Classification

As described earlier in the chapter, the SUN working group established an anatomic classification for uveitis in 1987 that was later proposed as being the global standard in 2005. Thus, our classification scheme generally follows this standard. Grouping each uveitic patient into an anatomic class is important when deciding about what and when testing should be ordered. For example, the first episode in a patient with isolated mild to moderate acute anterior uveitis and an unremarkable history generally does not require *any* work-up. Alternatively, patients with intermediate, posterior, or panuveitis should *always* have testing done. The anatomic location will also direct what tests to order. For example, you would not send HLA-B27 testing on a patient with posterior uveitis. Likewise, you would not send HLA-A29 or Toxoplasmosis testing on a patient with isolated anterior uveitis. Possible diagnosis and associated testing based on anatomic classification can be seen in Fig. 2.4a–d and are briefly discussed below.

Anterior uveitis—This includes terms such as iritis, irdocyclitis and anterior cyclitis. We further divide these patients into acute versus chronic and unilateral versus bilateral simultaneous versus bilateral alternating. Common etiologies for anterior uveitis can be seen in Fig. 2.4a. As mentioned above, testing is not necessary in patients with a single episode of mild to moderate anterior uveitis and an unremarkable history. However, in patients with anterior uveitis that is recurrent, bilateral, chronic, granulomatous, associated with a questionable history, or are unresponsive to treatment, additional testing should be considered. Suggested work-up for these patients includes HLA-B27 (if acute unilateral or alternating bilateral). If this test is negative, additional testing may include, syphilis, PPD/Quantiferon-gold, chest X-ray, Lyme titers,

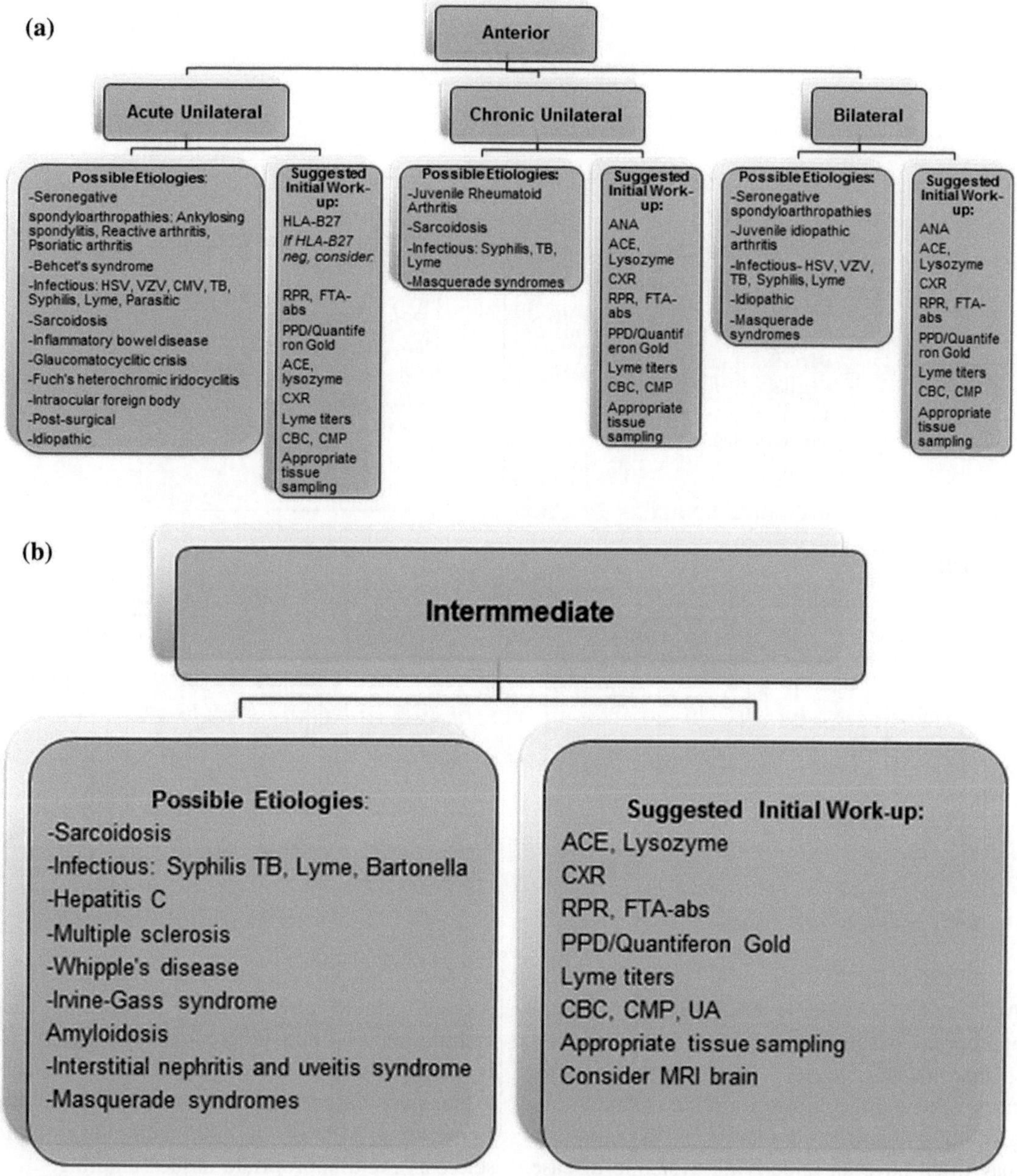

Fig. 2.4 a–d Note this is list by no means all-inclusive. *Abbreviations* HSV-herpes simplex virus, VZV-varicella zoster virus, CMV-cytomegalovirus, TB-tuberculosis, VKH-Vogt-Koyanagi-Harada syndrome, HLA-human leukocyte antigen, RPR-rapid plasma reagin, FTA-fluorescent treponemal antibody absorption, ACE-angiotensin converting enzyme, PPD-purified protein derivative, CXR-chest X-ray, CBC-complete blood count, CMP-complete metabolic panel

(c)

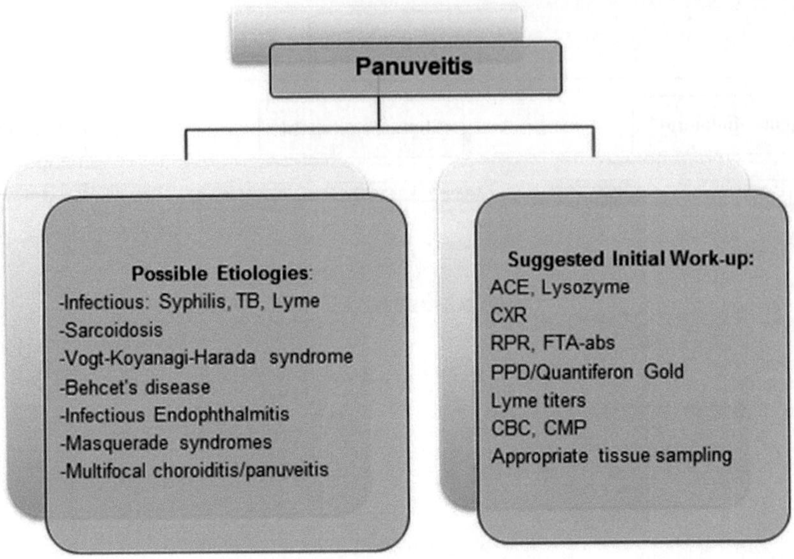

(d)

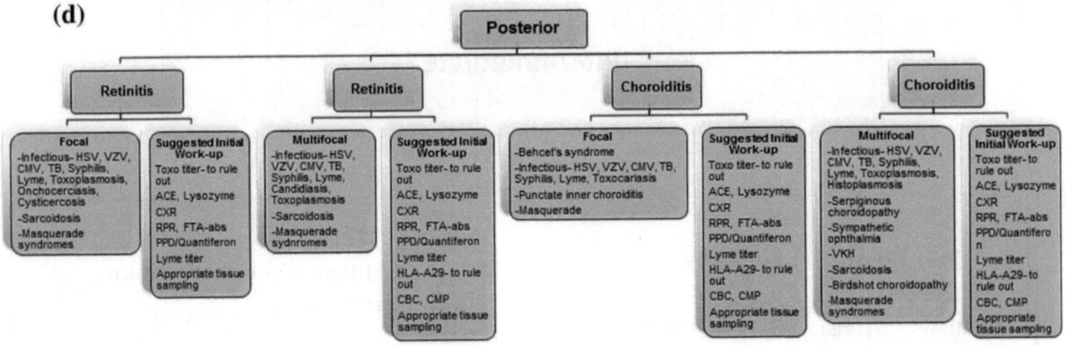

Fig. 2.4 (continued)

ACE and lysozyme levels, CBC, CMP, and appropriate tissue sampling.

Intermediate uveitis—This diagnosis often causes the most confusion among ophthalmologists but is important to identify as these patients may often have an underlying systemic disease. The inflammation in intermediate uveitis primarily affects the vitreous and at times the peripheral retina. Terminology used to describe this inflammation includes pars planitis, posterior cyclitis, vitritis, and hyalitis. Additional terms frequently used to describe aggregates of inflammatory cells in the inferior vitreous and along the pars plana/ora serrata are "snowballs" and "snowbanks", respectively. The most common etiologies are seen in Fig. 2.4b. These patients should always have a work-up that include syphilis and tuberculosis testing, ACE, lysozyme, chest X-ray, CBC, CMP. Other tests to consider based on history and exam include Lyme titers, MRI of the brain (rule out multiple sclerosis), and appropriate tissue sampling.

Posterior and Panuveitis

Many of the entities considered in posterior and panuveitis pose a unique diagnostic challenge in that most of them have no clear etiology and thus no specific applicable laboratory test. Thus, our goal of diagnosis is to rule out entities not treated with immunomodulators (infections and masquerade syndromes) or other diagnosis that affect systemic prognosis. Pattern recognition and additional modalities such as fluorescein angiography are essential in characterization of these entities. Examples not amenable to laboratory diagnosis include Behcet's, VKH, sympathetic ophthalmia, multifocal choroiditis with panuveitis, white dot syndromes, acute posterior multifocal placoid pigment epitheliopathy, serpiginous choroiditis, punctate inner choroidopathy, and relentless placoid chorioretinitis.

Posterior uveitis—This refers to inflammation limited primarily to the retina and choroid. The potential causes are rather vast, so this category is defined as retinitis, choroiditis; then further divided into focal or multifocal disease. A list of potential causes is seen in Fig. 2.4c. Suggested work-up includes syphilis and tuberculosis testing, toxoplasma titers (primarily to rule out in atypical cases), ACE, lysozyme, chest X-ray, CBC, CMP, UA (if evidence of vasculitis), HLA-A29, and appropriate tissue sampling. Testing for Lyme may be sent based on appropriate history.

Panuveitis—This classification refers to diseases that involve inflammation of all segments of the eye. The most common entities are listed in Fig. 2.4d. Suggested work-up includes syphilis and tuberculosis testing, ACE, lysozyme, chest X-ray, CBC, CMP, UA and appropriate tissue sampling.

Testing for Masquerade Syndromes

Although much less common than other etiologies, each clinician should be vigilant for the exclusion of masquerade syndromes. Non-malignant causes that can mimic uveitic disorders include intraocular foreign body, retinal detachments, myopic degeneration, pigment dispersion syndrome, retinal degeneration, ocular ischemia and drug reactions. Malignant masqueraders include intraocular/central nervous system lymphoma, leukemia, uveal melanoma, metastasis, paraneoplastic syndromes, cancer-associated retinopathy, and retinoblastoma. These syndromes should be considered in patients with concerning systemic symptoms and chronic uveitis that shows minimal response to aggressive medical therapy. Careful history and exam coupled with screening CBC, CMP, UA and appropriate tissue sampling are important steps in appropriately diagnosing these patients.

Particularly, in elderly patient with chronic posterior or panuveitis that shows minimal response to steroid treatment, lymphoma should be considered. Intraocular lymphoma typically occurs as an extension of central nervous system (CNS) lymphoma. Thus, additional appropriate testing would include an MRI of the head and possible lumbar puncture. The gold standard for confirmation, however, is vitreous biopsy for cytology and immunohistochemistry. It is important to confirm that the pathology lab receiving the specimen is familiar with the diagnosis of intraocular lymphoma so appropriate markers can be tested. As mentioned earlier in the chapter, aqueous measurements of IL-10 and IL-6 may be sent as an adjunctive means for diagnosis.

In a child with decreased red reflex and a hypopyon or vitritis clinicians should consider seeding from retinoblastoma. This diagnosis is made primarily by clinical findings, B-mode ultrasonography, and/or CT imaging. Biopsy is contraindicated for fear of seeding the tumor systemically.

Tests of Limited Utility and Additional Testing

There are certain tests that are commonly ordered both by ophthalmologists and non-ophthalmologists that have little to no role in the diagnosis of uveitis. The confusion may lie in separating the work-up for uveitis versus scleritis and peripheral ulcerative keratitis. The latter two entities yield a different differential diagnosis and

Table 2.12 Less common testing for specific clinical scenerios

Disease	Typical findings	Testing
Toxocariasis	Unilateral posterior uveitis in child with history of dog/cat exposure. Posterior pole or peripheral granuloma, often with a grey center and adjacent retinal folds	Serology
Onchocerciasis	Unilateral panuveitis in patient from endemic region, possible visualization of microfilaria in anterior chamber. Distinct skin findings of freely mobile subcutaneous nodules over bony prominences (hips, lower limbs), dermatitis, lymphadenitis, depigmentation	Skin biopsy, Filarial screening Serology
Cysticercosis	Panuveitis with subretinal or vitreal translucent potentially mobile cyst with dense white spot in one region	CBC, Serology, CT/MRI brain
Bartonella	History of exposure to cats, tender regional lymphadenopathy, unilateral exudative optic neuritis with transudation into the macula forming a macular star	Serology, PCR, culture
TINU	Bilateral sudden-onset anterior uveitis in young patient	CBC, CMP, Urinalysis, Non-specific: Beta-2 microglobulin, ANA, Lysozyme, CXR
Isolated retinal vasculitis		CBC, CMP, ANA, complement 3 and 4 levels, urinalysis, Antiphospholipid antibodies, ESR/CRP, Anti-dsDNA, Anti-RoSSA/La/SSB, ANCA

work-up that would include testing for rheumatoid arthritis, granulomatosis with polyangiitis (GPA previously known as Wegener's Granulomatosis), polyarteritis nodosa, and relapsing polychondritis. Generally, ANA, rheumatoid factor, anti-CCP, and antineutrophil cytoplasmic antibody (ANCA) should *not* be ordered on patients with uveitis. Exceptions to this would include children, where a positive ANA may supplement the work-up for suspected JIA [57]. Additionally, ANCA may be considered in patients with retinal signs of vasculitis accompanied with other findings concerning for GPA. HLA-B27 should not be ordered on patients with intermediate, posterior, or panuveitis. Pathergy testing has been used to aid in the diagnosis of Behcet's disease. This test has poor sensitivity (35.8 %) but high specificity (98.4 %) [92]. In our experience, the diagnosis of Behcet's is based on the clinical presentation, and this test is rarely performed.

Less common testing that should be reserved for very specific patient presentations are listed in Table 2.12.

Conclusion

Making decisions about the appropriate work-up in patients with uveitis can be a challenge. In this chapter we highlighted a few key points that may help guide this process:

1. Remember the goal of testing is not necessarily to find an "etiology" but should be to rule out diseases not treated with immunomodulators (i.e., infections—particularly those that cannot be identified by unique exam features, and masquerade syndromes) and systemic diseases that may have an impact on the patient's systemic health, prognosis, or treatment plan.

2. The history and physical exam is the first and most important step in deciding which testing may be appropriate.
3. Laboratory, imaging, and molecular testing should be a supplement to and not a replacement for a thorough history and physical exam.
4. To facilitate limitation of the differential and further guide testing, each patient should be defined into an anatomic classification.
5. When deciding when to order testing, consider the pre- and post-test probabilities and potential for false positives and negatives.
6. With only a few exceptions ANA, rheumatoid factor, anti-CCP, ANCA testing should not be included in the work-up for uveitis.

References

1. Jabs DA, Busingye J. Approach to the diagnosis of the uveitidies. Am J Ophthalmol. 2013;156:228–36.
2. Silverstein, et al. Changing trends in the etiologic diagnosis of uveitis. Doc Ophthalmol. 1997;94(1–2):25–37.
3. Smith NE, Nozik RA. Uveitis: a clinical approach to diagnosis and management. 3rd ed. Michigan: Lippincott Williams & Wilkins; 2003.
4. Jabs DA, Nussenblatt RB, Rosenbaum JT. Standardization of uveitis nomenclature (SUN) working group. Standardization of uveitis nomenclature for reporting clinical data. Results of the first international workshop. Am J Ophthalmol. 2005;140(3):509–16.
5. Rosenbaum JT, Holland GN. Uveitis and the tower of babel. Arch Ophthalmol. 1996;114(5):604–5.
6. Bloch-Michael E, Nussenblatt RB. International uveitis study group recommendations for the evaluation of intraocular inflammatory disease. Am J Ophthalmol. 1987;103:234–5.
7. Jabs DA, Nussenblatt RB, Rosenbaum JT. Standardization of uveitis nomenclature (SUN) working group. standardization of uveitis nomenclature for reporting clinical data. Results of the first international workshop. Am J Ophthalmol. 2005;140:509–16.
8. Deschenes J, Murray PI, Rao NA, Nussenblatt RB. International uveitis study group. International uveitis study group (IUSG): clinical classification of uveitis. Ocul Immunol Inflamm. 2008;16:1–2.
9. Okada AA, Jabs DA. The standardization of uveitis nomenclature project: the future is here. JAMA Ophthalmol. 2013;131(6):787–9.
10. Trusko B, Thorne J, Jabs D, et al. The standardization of uveitis nomenclature (SUN) project. Development of a clinical evidence base utilizing informatics tools and techniques. Methods Inf Med. 2013;52(3):259–65 Epub 8 Feb 2013.
11. Cunningham ET, Nozik RA. Duane's clinical ophthalmology. Vol. 37. Philadelphia: Lippincott-Raven; 1997. Uveitis: Diagnostic approach and ancillary analysis. p. 58–68.
12. Harper SL, Chorich LJ, Foster CS. Diagnosis of uveitis. In: Foster CS, Vitale AT, editors. Diagnosis and treatment of uveitis. Philadelphia: W.B. Saunders; 2002. p. 79–103.
13. Cunningham ET. Uveitis in children. Ocul Immunol Inflamm. 2000;8:251–61.
14. Rathinam SR, Namperumalsamy P. Global variation and pattern changes in epidemiology of uveitis. Indian J Ophthalmol. 2007;55:173–83.
15. Jones NP. The manchester uveitis clinic: the first 3000 patients-epidemiology and casemix. Ocul Immunol Inflamm. 2013;23:118–26.
16. Rathinam SR, Babu M. Algorithmic approach in the diagnosis of uveitis. Indian J Ophthalmol. 2013;61(6):255–62.
17. Chang JH, McCluskey PJ, Wakefield D. Acute anterior uveitis and HLA-B27. Surv Ophthalmol. 2005;50:364–88.
18. McCannel CA, Holland GN, Helm CJ, et al. Causes of uveitis in the general practice of ophthalmology. UCLA community-based uveitis study group. Am J Ophthalmol. 1996;121:35–46.
19. Reeves SW, Sloan FA, Lee PP, Jaffe GJ. Uveitis in the elderly. Epidemiological data from the national long-term care survey medicare cohort. Ophthalmology. 2006;113:302–7.
20. Yanoff M, Duker JS. Ophthalmology. 3rd ed. Elsevier; 2009. Uveitis and other intraocular inflammations; 7.3, p. 784.
21. Herbert HM, Viswanathan A, Jackson H, Lightman SL. Risk factors for elevated intraocular pressure in uveitis. J Glaucoma. 2004;13(2):96–9.
22. Bhagat N, Read RW, Rao NA, et al. Rifabutin-associated hypopyon uveitis in human immunodeficiency virus-negative immunocompetent individuals. Ophthalmol. 2001;108(4):750–2.
23. Petrowski JT 3rd. Uveitis associated with rifabutin therapy: a clinical alert. J Am Optom Assoc. 1996;67(11):693–6.
24. Tugwell P, Dennis DT, Weinstein A, Wells G, Shea B, Nichol G, et al. Laboratory evaluation in the diagnosis of Lyme disease. Ann Intern Med. 1997;127:1109–23.
25. Ledue TB, Collins MF, Craig WY. New laboratory guidelines for serologic diagnosis of Lyme disease: evaluation of the two-test protocol. J Clin Microbiol. 1996;34:2343–50.
26. Rosenbaum JT, Wernick R. The utility of routine screening of patients with uveitis for systemic lupus erythematosus or tuberculosis. A Bayesian analysis. Arch Ophthalmol. 1990;108(9):1291–3.

27. Albini TA, Karakousis PC, Rao NA. Interferon-gamma release assays in the diagnosis of tuberculosis uveitis. Am J Ophthalmol. 2008;146 (4):486–8.
28. Streeton, JA, Desem N, Jones SL. Sensitivity and specificity of a gamma interferon blood test for tuberculosis infection. Int J Tuberc Lung Dis Off J Int Union Tuberc Lung Dis. 1998;2(6):443–50.
29. Mazurek GH, Jereb J, et al. Updated guidelines for using interferon gamma release assays to detect mycobacterium tuberculosis infection—centers for disease control. United states, 2010. MMWR Recomm Rep. 2010;59(RR05):1–25.
30. McMullen SE, Pegues DA, et al. Performance of QuantiFERON-TB gold and tuberculin skin test relative to subjects' risk of exposure to tuberculosis. Clin Infect Dis. 2014;58(9):1260–6 Epub 27 Feb 2014.
31. Vasconcelos-Santos DV, Rao PK, et al. Clinical features of tuberculous serpiginous like choroiditis in contrast to classic serpiginous choroiditis. Arch Ophthalmol. 2010;128(7):853–8.
32. Kahn MA. Thoughts concerning the early diagnosis of ankylosing spondylitis and related diseases. Clin Exp Rheumatol. 2002;20(Suppl. 28):S6–10.
33. Patton ME, Su JR, Nelson R, et al. Primary and secondary syphilis—United states, 2005–2013. MMWR Morb Mortal Wkly Rep Cent Dis Control Prev. 2014;63(18):402–6.
34. Hong BK, Khanamiri HN, Bababeygy SR, Rao NA. The utility of routine tuberculosis screening in county hospital patients with uveitis. Br J Ophthalmol. 2014;98:1091–5.
35. Cush JJ, Winthrop K, Dao K, et al. Screening for mycobacterium tuberculosis infection: questions and answers for clinical practice. Drug Saf Quart. 2010; Spring 1(2):1–4.
36. National Health and Nutrition Examination Survey III (NHANES III), series 11 Data Files 1988–1994. Available online at http://www.cdc.gov/nchs/nhanes/nh3data.htm.
37. Jones JL, Kruszon-Moran D, Sanders-Lewis K, et al. Toxoplasma gondii infection in the United states, 1999 2004, decline from the prior decade. Am J Trop Med Hyg. 2007;77(3):405–10.
38. Ang M, Htoon HM, et al. Diagnosis of tuberculous uveitis: clinical application of an interferon-gamma release assay. Ophthalmology. 2009;116(7):1391–6.
39. Ang M, Wong WL, Kiew SY, et al. Prospective head-to-head study comparing 2 commercial interferon gamma release assays for the diagnosis of tuberculous uveitis. Am J Ophthalmol. 2014;157 (6):1306–14.
40. McMullen SE, Pegues DA. Performance of QuantiFERON-TB gold and tuberculin skin test relative to subjects' risk of exposure to tuberculosis. Clin Infect Dis. 2014;58(9):1260–6. doi:10.1093/cid/ciu119 Epub 27 Feb 2014.
41. Steffen RE, Caetano R, et al. Cost-effectiveness of quantiferon®-TB gold-in-tube versus tuberculin skin testing for contact screening and treatment of latent tuberculosis infection in Brazil. PLoS One. 2013;8 (4). Print 2013.
42. U.S. Preventive Services Task Force. Screening for syphilis infection. Recommendation statement. 2004.
43. Larsen SA, Hambie EA, Wobig GH, Kennedy EJ. Cerebrospinal fluid serologic tests for syphilis: treponemal and nontreponemal tests. In: Morisset R, Kurstak E, editors. Advances in sexually transmitted diseases. Utrecht, The Netherlands: VNW Science Press; 1986. p. 157–62.
44. Tamesis RR, Foster CS. Ocular syphilis. Ophthalmology. 1990;97(10):1281–7.
45. Schmid GP. Serologic screening for syphilis. Rationale, cost, and realpolitik. Sex Transm Dis. 1996;23 (1):45–50.
46. Reisner BS, Mann LM, Tholcken CA, et al. Use of the treponema pallidum-specific captia syphilis IgG assay in conjunction with the rapid plasma regain to test for syphilis. J Clin Microbiol. 1997;35(5):1141–3.
47. Wong EH, Klausner JD, Caguin-Grygiel G. Evaluation of an IgM/IgG sensitive enzyme immunoassay and the utility of index values for the screening of syphilis infection in a high-risk population. Sex Transm Dis. 2011;38(6):528–32.
48. Fawcett PT, Rose CD, Budd SM, Gibney KM. Effect of immunization with recombinant OspA on serologic tests for Lyme borreliosis. Clin Diagn Lab Immunol. 2001;8(79–84):50.
49. Mogilyansky E, Loa CC, et al. Comparison of western immunoblotting and the C6 Lyme antibody test for laboratory detection of Lyme disease. Clin Diagn Lab Immunol. 2004;11(5):924–9.
50. Beneteau-Burnat B, Baudin B, Morgant G, Baumann FC, Giboudeau J. Serum angiotensin-converting enzyme activity in normal children and in those with sarcoidosis. Clin Chem. 1990;36: 344–6.
51. Tomita H, et al. Serum lysozyme levels and clinical features of sarcoidosis. Lung. 1999;177:161–7.
52. Weinreb RN, Tessler H. Laboratory diagnosis of ophthalmic sarcoidosis. Surv Ophthalmol. 1984;28:653–64.
53. Ainslie GM, Benatar SR. Serum angiotensin converting enzyme in sarcoidosis: sensitivity and specificity in diagnosis: correlations with disease activity, duration, extra-thoracic involvement, radiographic type and therapy. Q J Med. 1985;55 (218):253–70.
54. Baarsma GS, La Hey E. The predictive value of serum angiotensin converting enzyme and lysozyme levels in the diagnosis of ocular sarcoidosis. Am J Ophthalmol. 1987;104(3):211–7.
55. Power WJ, Neves RA, et al. The value of combined serum angiotensin-converting enzyme and gallium scan in diagnosing sarcoidosis. Ophthalmology. 1995;102(12):2007–11.
56. Newman LS, Rose CS, Maier LA. Sarcoidosis. N Engl J Med. 1997;336:1224–34.

57. Cassidy JT, Levinson JE, Bass JC, et al. A study of classification criteria for a diagnosis of juvenile rheumatoid arthritis. Arthritis Rheum. 1986;29:274–81.
58. Tan EM, Feltkamp TE, et al. Range of antinuclear antibodies in "healthy" individuals. Arthritis Rheum. 1997;40(9):1601.
59. Hettinga YM, Scheerlinck LME, Lilein MR, et al. The value of measuring urinary β2-microglobulin and serum creatinine for detecting tubulointerstitial nephritis and uveitis syndrome in young patients with uveitis. JAMA Ophthalmol. Published online, 30 Oct 2014. doi;10.1001/jamaophthalmol.2014.4401.
60. Reed JB, Scaled DK, Wong MT, et al. Bartonella henselae neuroretinitis in cat scratch disease. Diagnosis management and sequelae. Ophthalmology. 1998;105(3):459–66.
61. Zamecki KJ, Jabs DA, et al. HLA typing in uveitis: use and misuse. Am J Ophthalmol. 2010;149:189–93.
62. Rosenbaum JT. Characterization of uveitis associated with spondyloarthritis. J Rheumatol. 1989;16:792–6.
63. Monnet D, Breban M, et al. Ophthalmic findings and frequency of extraocular manifestations in patients with HLA-B27 uveitis: a study of 175 cases. Ophthalmology. 2004;111:802–9.
64. Linssen A, Meenken C, et al. Outcomes of HLA-B27 positive and HLA-B27 negative acute anterior uveitis. Am J Ophthalmol. 1995;120:351–61.
65. Tay-Kearney ML, Schwam BL, et al. Clinical features and associated systemic diseases of HLA-B27 uveitis. Am J Ophthalmol. 1996;121:47–56.
66. Nussenblatt RB, Mittal KK. Birdshot retinochoroidopathy associated with HLA-A29 antigen and immune responsiveness to retinal s-antigen. Am J Ophthalmol. 1982;94(2):147–58.
67. Miller BH, Rosado-de-christenson ML, Mcadams HP, et al. Thoracic sarcoidosis: radiologic-pathologic correlation. Radiographics. 1995;15(2):421–37.
68. Müller NL, Franquet T, Lee KS, et al. Imaging of pulmonary infections. Lippincott Williams & Wilkins; 2007.
69. Yeager H, Rossman MD. Pulmonary and psychosocial findings at enrollment in the ACCESS study. Sarcoidosis Vasc Diffuse Lung Dis. 2005; 22 (2):147–53.
70. Disayabutr S, Pattanaprichakul P. A case series of sarcoidosis with pulmonary involvement: various clinical and radiographic manifestations. J Med Assoc Thai. 2013;96(8):888–97.
71. Criado E, Sanchez M. Pulmonary sarcoidosis: typical and atypical manifestations at high-resolution CT with pathologic correlation. Radiographics. 2010;30 (6):1567–86.
72. Klech H, Kohn H, Pohl W, et al. Diagnosis in sarcoidosis. Sensitivity and specificity of 67-gallium scintigraphy, serum angiotensin converting enzyme levels, thoracic radiography and blood lymphocyte subpopulations. Wien Med Wochenschr. 1983;133 (17):425–32 (article in German).
73. Silva M, Nunes H, Valeyre D, et al. Imaging of sarcoidosis. Clin Rev Allergy Immunol. 2015;49(1) 1:45–53.
74. Van't Hoog AH, Langendam MW, et al. A systematic review of the sensitivity and specificity of symptom- and chest-radiography screening for active pulmonary tuberculosis in HIV-negative persons and persons with unknown HIV status. Cochrane Database Syst Rev Infect Dis Group. Published online, 2 Jan 2014.
75. Takada K, Matsumoto S, et al. Diagnostic management of patients with suspected ocular sarcoidosis. J Thorac Dis. 2013;5(2):135–40.
76. Mana J, Teirstein AS, et al. Excessive thoracic computed tomographic scanning in sarcoidosis. Thorax. 1995;50(12):1264–6.
77. Kaiser PK, Lowder CY, Sullivan P, et al. Chest computerized tomography in the evaluation of uveitis in elderly women. Am J Ophthalmol. 2002;133 (4):499–505.
78. Statement on sarcoidosis. Joint statement of the american thoracic society (ATS), the European respiratory society (ERS), and the world association of sarcoidosis and other granulomatous disorders (WASOG) adopted by the ATS board of directors and by the ERS executive committee, February 1999. Am J Respir Crit Care Med. 1999;160:736–55.
79. Nunes H, Brillet PY, et al. Imaging in sarcoidosis. Semin Respir Crit Care Med. 2007;28(1):102–20.
80. Noyes K, Weinstock-Guttman B, et al. Impact of diagnosis and early treatment on the course of multiple sclerosis. Am J Manag Care. 2013;19 (Suppl. 17):s321–31.
81. Zhao Y, Xu L, Ma W, et al. Shell-engineered chiroplasmonic assemblies of nanoparticles for zeptomolar DNA detection. Nano Lett. 2014;14 (7):3908–13.
82. Rothova A, de Boer JH, Ten Dam-van Loon NH, et al. Usefulness of aqueous humor analysis for the diagnosis of posterior uveitis. Ophthalmology. 2008;115(2):306–11.
83. Knox CM, Chandler D, Short GA, et al. Polymerase chain reaction-based assays of vitreous samples for the diagnosis of viral retinitis. Use in diagnostic dilemmas. Ophthalmology. 1998;105:37–44.
84. Chan CC, Shen D, Tuo J, et al. Polymerase chain reaction in the diagnosis of uveitis. Int Ophthalmol Clin. 2005;45(2):41–55.
85. Balne PK, Barik MR, Sharma S, et al. Development of a loop-mediated isothermal amplification assay targeting the mpb64 gene for the diagnosis of intraocular tuberculosis. J Clin Microbiol. 2013;51 (11):3839–40.
86. Fanburg BL: Sarcoidosis. In: Wyngaarden JB, Smith LH, Jr., Bennett JC, editors. Cecil textbook of medicine. 19th ed. Philadelphia: W.B. Saunders; 1992:430–5.

87. Nichols CW, Eagle RC, Yanoff M, et al. Conjunctival biopsy as an aid in the evaluation of the patient with suspected sarcoidosis. Ophthalmology. 1980;87:287–91.
88. Bui KM, Garcia-Gonzales JM, Pael SS, et al. Directed conjunctival biopsy and impact of histologic sectioning methodology on the diagnosis of ocular sarcoidosis. J Ophthalmic Inflam Infect. 2014;4:8.
89. Karcioglu AZ, Brear R. Conjunctival biopsy in sarcoidosis. Am J Ophthal. 1985;99:68–73.
90. Spaide RF, Ward DL. Conjunctival biopsy in the diagnosis of sarcoidosis. Br J Ophthalmol. 1990;74:469–71.
91. Sulavik SB, Palestro CF, et al. Extrapulmonary sites of radiogallium accumulation in sarcoidosis. Clin Nucl Med. 1990;15:876–8.
92. Davatchi F, Chams-Davatchi C, et al. Diagnostic value of pathergy test in Behcet's disease according to the change of incidence over the time. Clin Rheumatol. 2011;30(9):1151–5.

Part II
Causes-Infectious Uveitis

Bartonella

3

Humzah Nasir and George N. Papaliodis

Introduction

The genus *Bartonella* is an alpha proteobacterium [1]. They are gram negative, facultative, intracellular organisms, and the genus encompasses around 20 species and subspecies [2, 3]. *Bartonella henselae* is the species that accounts for most human illnesses with manifestations including lymphadenopathy, neuroretinitis, bacteremia, endocarditis, bacillary angiomatosis, and other localized infections [4]. The origins of most *Bartonella henselae* infections can be traced back to exposure to cats (especially kittens), particularly when scratched, and also possibly dogs [1, 2, 5–7].

Bartonella henselae are especially prevalent in the feline population with the cat's fleas playing the role of transmitting the agent between cats [2]. Cat flea feces, which are usually the source of *Bartonella*, can accumulate onto the cat's claws which allow the pathogen to then be accidentally transmitted to humans when scratched [1, 2]. This condition called Cat Scratch Disease (CSD) often manifests as subacute, regional lymphadenopathy [4]. While Cat Scratch Disease is often regarded as benign and manifesting as a flu-like illness, it has the potential to induce ocular inflammation including neuroretinitis, choroidal nodules, and disciform keratitis [8, 9].

Unlike *Bartonella henselae*, which has a worldwide presence, *Bartonella quintana* has been predominantly observed in the head or body lice of infected homeless populations of the US and Europe [4]. In addition to Europe and the US, *Bartonella quintana* has also been isolated from lice collected from the heads of poor and homeless people from the Nepal, Senegal, Ethiopia, and the Democratic Republic of the Congo [10]. Although *Bartonella quintana* is strongly associated with the presence of head lice, it has yet to be detected in the head lice of school children [10].

Epidemiology

Infections involving *Bartonella henselae* are relatively common in the United States with approximately 3.7 cases per 100,000 [3]. Multiple published series have estimated 5–25 % of patients infected with *Bartonella henselae* develop ocular manifesations [9, 11, 12]. The incidence of *Bartonella quintana* is rather

H. Nasir (✉) · G.N. Papaliodis
Department of Ophthalmology, Harvard Medical School, Massachusetts Eye and Ear Infirmary, Boston, MA 02114, USA
e-mail: hnasir@email.wm.edu

G.N. Papaliodis
e-mail: George_Papaliodis@meei.harvard.edu

G.N. Papaliodis (ed.), *Uveitis*,
DOI 10.1007/978-3-319-09126-6_3

difficult to determine as only a small proportion of those affected exhibit noticeable symptoms indicative of disease [4]. Nonetheless, chronic and acute effects of *Bartonella quintana* infection have included chronic bacteremia and trench fever, respectively [4]. Of the 20 known species and subspecies of *Bartonella,* five have been discovered to be highly associated with the occurrence of human disease in North America [3].

Clinical Manifestations

Ocular manifestations that can occur due to *Bartonella henselae* include neuroretinitis with or without macular involvement, acute multifocal retinitis, intermediate uveitis with retinal vasculitis, choroiditis, iridocyclitis, and papillitis [9, 12–14]. The most common ocular manifestation of *Bartonella henselae* infection is Parinaud's oculoglandular syndrome (POGS) [2, 9, 12]. POGS is a syndrome that occurs in approximately 5 % of patients who contract cat scratch disease, the usual symptoms include unilateral ocular injection, foreign body sensation and epiphoria [2, 11].

Neuroretinitis occurs in around 1–2 % of patients with *Bartonella henselae* infection causing optic nerve head swelling with incomplete (Fig. 3.1) or complete macular star formation (Fig. 3.2) [2, 9]. In 2008, Donnio and colleagues reported a case whereby a patient who had neuroretinitis due to *Bartonella henselae* had developed a macular hole within twelve days of presentation of the infection [8].

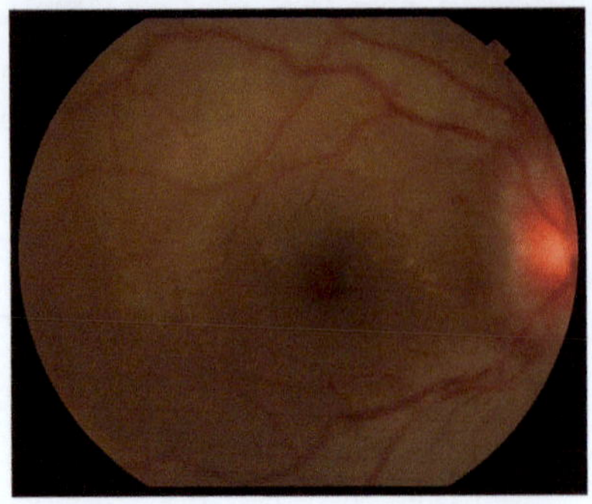

Fig. 3.1 Patient with neuroretinitis from CSD demonstrating incomplete macular star and marked optic nerve swelling

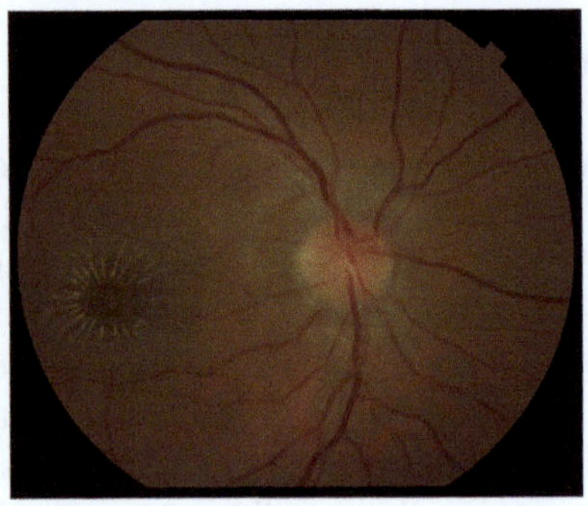

Fig. 3.2 Patient with neuroretinitis from CSD and complete macular star

Diagnosis

The diagnosis of CSD is based on supportive clinical findings and serologic testing. Indirect fluorescence assay (IFA) and enzyme-linked immunosorbent assay (ELISA) testing can detect serum antibodies to *Bartonella henselae.* An antibody titer that exceeds 1:64 suggests recent *Bartonella* infection. Polymerase chain reaction (PCR) testing can also detect the presence of *Bartonella* infection in serum.

Treatment

There are no specific guidelines for the treatment of CSD or the associated ocular manifestations as there are no randomized, controlled trials to assess the multiple therapeutic options. Many physicians will not offer therapy for mild to moderate systemic CSD. Various antimicrobial agents have demonstrated efficacy against infections caused by *Bartonella henselae* including erythromycin, chloramphenicol, rifampin, gentamicin, trimethoprim–sulfamethoxazole, doxycycline, and ciprofloxacin [7, 11].

In those who receive treatment, doxycycline is the antimicrobial agent most commonly used (there are case reports using doxycycline 100 mg orally BID and as high as 250 mg orally QID). An alternative therapy is Ciprofloxacin 500 mg orally BID. The duration of treatment is typically 10–14 days. In patients with *Bartonella henselae* infection with compromised visual acuity from neuroretinitis, there are case reports/series recommending doxycycline 100 mg every 12 h along with rifampin 300 mg every 12 h [10]. The benefit of systemic corticosteroids is unknown.

Conclusion

The genus Bartonella comprises approximately 20 species of gram negative, intracellular organisms that can cause human disease. *Bartonella henselae* is the most common cause of ocular associated manifestations with 5–25 % of those infected demonstrating some degree of ocular inflammation [15]. There are no clear guidelines for therapy but most patients who are treated receive Doxycycline 100 mg BID for 10–14 days. The role of systemic corticosteroids is unknown.

References

1. Gil H, Escuerdo R, Pons I, Vargas M, Esteban C, Moreno I, Amil C, Lobo B, Valcarcel F, Perez A, Jimenez S, Jado I, Juste R, Segura F, Anda P. Distribution of *Bartonella henselae* variants in patients, reservoir hosts and vectors in Spain. PLoS. 2013;8 (7):e68248.
2. Kalogeropoulos C, Koumpoulis I, Mentis A, Pappa C, Zafeiropoulos P, Aspiotis M. *Bartonella* and intraocular inflammation: a series of cases and review of literature. Clin Ophthalmol. 2011;5: 817–29.
3. Iralu J, Bai Y, Crook L, Tempest B, Simpson G, McKenzie T, Koster F. Rodent-associated *Bartonella* febrile illness Southwestern United States. Emerg Infect Dis. 2006;12(7):1081–6.
4. Prutsky G, Domecg J, Mori L, Bebko S, Matzumura M, Sabouni A, Shahrour A, Erwin P, Boyce T, Montori V, Malaga G, Murad M. Treatment outcomes of human bartonellosis: a systematic review and meta-analysis. J Infect Dis. 2012;17(10):811–9.
5. Im J, Baek J, Lee H, Lee J, Chung M, Kim M, Lee S, Kang J. First case of *Bartonella henselae* bacteremia in Korea. Infect Chemoteherapy. 2013;45(4):446–50.
6. Marcarelli P, Maggi R, Hopkins S, Mozayeni R, Trull C, Bradley J, Hegarty B, Breitscherdt E. Bartonella henselae infection in a family experiencing neurological and neurocognitive abnormalities after woodlouse hunter spider bites. Parasites Vectors. 2013;6:98.
7. Kordick D, Papich M, Breitschwerdt E. Efficacy of Enrofloxacin or Doxycycline for treatment of *Bartonella Henselae* or *Bartonella Clarridgeiae* infection in cats. Antimicrob Agents Chemother. 1997;41 (11):2448–55.
8. Donnio A, Charles A, Merle H. Macular hole following *Bartonella henselae* neuroretinitis. Eur J Ophthalmol. 2008;18(3):456–8.
9. Kawaski A, Wilson D. Mass lesions of the posterior segment associated with *Bartonella henselae*. Br J Ophthalmol. 2003;87(2):248–9.
10. Drali R, Sangare A, Boutellis A, Angelakis E, Veracx A, Socolovschi C, Brouqui P, Raoult D. *Bartonella* quintana in body lice from scalp hair of homeless persons France. Emerg Infect Dis. 2014;20 (5):907–8.
11. Ahmadi S, Azizi B, Tsang AC, Coupland S, Gottlieb C, Zackon D. Neuroretinitis with branch retinal artery occlusion in a 15-year-old female. Case Rep Ophthalmol. 2013;4(3):265–8.
12. Tager F, Jahnsen K, Marisol R, Burgos R. Ocular bartonellosis: report of three cases. Chilean J Infect. 2008;25(1):58–63.
13. Goldstein D, Mouritsen L, Friedlander S, Tessler H, Edward D. Acute endogenous endophthalmitis due to bartonella heselae. Clin Infect Dis. 2001;33(5):718–21.
14. Martínez-Osorio H, Calonge M, Torres J, González F. Cat-scratch disease (ocular bartonellosis) presenting as bilateral recurrent iridocyclitis. Clin Infect Dis. 2005;40(5):e43–5.
15. Jackson LA, Perkins BA, Wenger JD. Cat Scratch disease in the United States. An analysis of three national databases. Am J Public Health. 1993;83:1707–11.

Candida

4

Sonam Dilwali and George N. Papaliodis

Introduction

Candidiasis is a fungal infection caused by yeasts under the genus *Candida*. *Candida* yeasts normally live on the skin and mucous membranes; however, aberrant overgrowth or invasive spread of these organisms can cause symptomatic infection [1].

Invasive candidiasis is the most common fungal disease in hospitalized patients in the developed world [2], being especially prevalent in the immunocompromised and critically ill populations [1]. The majority of invasive *Candida* infections have been attributed to intensive care unit (ICU)-related exposures such as indwelling central venous catheters, total parental nutrition, recent surgery or broad-spectrum antibiotics [1, 3, 4]. Both candidaemia, the most common form of invasive candidiasis, and localized invasive candidiasis are associated with significantly increased morbidity and mortality [1, 5]. It is therefore crucial to rapidly identify and treat these infections as well as their associated complications [6].

Although the incidence and the distribution of candidaemia vary substantially by geographic location and by patient population [7], incidence rates have been cited between 2 and 29 cases per 100,000 persons in population-based studies [1, 7, 8]. There are currently 15 identified infectious species of *Candida*. Up to 95 % of all invasive *Candida* infections in the US are ascribed to five species of *Candida*: *C. albicans*, *C. glabrata*, *C. parapsilosis*, *C. tropicalis*, and *C. krusei* [9, 10]. *C. albicans* has historically been implicated as the most common species causing candidaemia, although non-*C. albicans* species now comprise up to two-thirds of invasive *Candida* infections in the US [9, 10]. Interestingly, a study has shown that patients with ocular candidiasis were more often infected with *C. albicans* and less often with *C. parapsilosis* than patients without retinal lesions [11].

Clinical Manifestations

Candida can seed various organ systems leading to infections such as urinary tract infections, peritonitis, endocarditis, meningitis, and chorioretinitis [1]. In the eye, *Candida* infections can arise following trauma, eye surgery, or through hematogenous seeding of the retina and choroid

S. Dilwali (✉)
Medical School, UT Southwestern Medical Center, 5323 Harry Hines Boulevard, Dallas, TX 75390, USA
e-mail: sonam.dilwali@utsouthwestern.edu

G.N. Papaliodis
Department of Ophthalmology, Harvard Medical School, Massachusetts Eye and Ear Infirmary, 243 Charles Street, Boston, MA 02114, USA
e-mail: George_Papaliodis@meei.harvard.edu

G.N. Papaliodis (ed.), *Uveitis*,
DOI 10.1007/978-3-319-09126-6_4

as a complication of candidaemia. Eight to 16 % of candidaemic patients present with ocular complications [11, 12]. Interestingly, the duration of candidaemia is significantly longer in patients who develop ocular involvement suggesting a more aggressive systemic infection [11, 13]. One study found that fungi, with *Candida* being the most common culprit, cause over 60 % of the cases of endogenous endophthalmitis due to hematogenous seeding [16].

The major ocular presentations of candidaemia are chorioretinitis and endophthalmitis (see Fig. 4.1). Patients with chorioretinitis typically have white chorioretinal infiltrates noted on funduscopic exam. Progression to vitritis and endophthalmitis occurs in approximately 10 % of *Candida* chorioretinitis patients [6, 11]. Clinically patients with endophthalmitis present with blurred vision and/or floaters [6, 14]. Two-thirds of patients with symptomatic ocular candidiasis have bilateral ocular disease, with over half demonstrating multiple lesions and vitreous involvement [15]. Long standing endophthalmitis can result in retinal necrosis and detachment with substantial permanent vision loss [6]. Therefore, early identification and adequate treatment is critical for long-term vision preservation [6, 16].

Diagnosis

The pursuit of a diagnosis of invasive candidiasis is largely driven by clinical suspicion and supportive exam findings. Blood cultures/fungal isolators are commonly utilized, although they have been shown to have a wide range of sensitivities ranging from 21 to 71 % [17]. Additionally, whole-blood, multiplex polymerase chain-reaction (PCR) assay (currently only validated in independent laboratories) can detect the five clinically most important *Candida* species as well as several other fungal and bacterial organisms; this modality of testing has demonstrated a high sensitivity ranging from 85 to 95 % in candidaemic patients [17, 18].

For ocular involvement, the guidelines of the Infectious Diseases Society of America (IDSA) recommend that all candidaemic patients undergo a dilated funduscopic exam to screen for endophthalmitis [19]. Special emphasis should be placed on routine, dilated fundoscopy for candidaemic patients with visual symptoms or inability to report these symptoms [13]. Cultures of vitreous samples confirm the diagnosis [12].

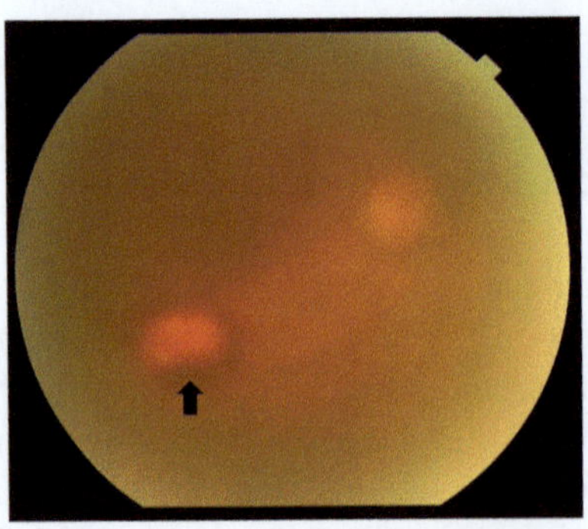

Fig. 4.1 Patient with *Candida* endophthalmitis demonstrating chorioretinal infiltrate (*arrow*) and dense vitritis

Treatment

Treatment for candidaemia requires systemic antifungal agents, with an echinocandin or liposomal amphotericin B being first choice medications. Treatment duration should be at least 4–6 weeks and continue for 2 weeks after negative blood cultures [19]. Daily blood cultures and fundoscopic exams should be used to track efficacy of treatment [19].

For ocular manifestations, *Candida* chorioretinitis is typically treated adequately with systemic antifungal therapy [11, 12, 19]. *Candida* endophthalmitis with vitreous involvement commonly warrants pars plana vitrectomy with or without intravitreal antifungal administration [15, 19].

Conclusion

Candida associated uveitis occurs due to localized candidiasis or candidaemia, usually in immunocompromised or hospitalized patients. Ocular manifestations include chorioretinitis and progression to vision-threatening endophthalmitis. Diagnosis of candidaemia can be made using blood cultures or PCR assay. Ocular manifestations are diagnosed and followed via fundoscopic exams. Therapeutic guidelines recommend 4–6 weeks of systemic antifungal treatment that should continue for 2 weeks after documented *Candida*-negative blood cultures. More aggressive intraocular antifungal treatment and pars plana vitrectomy are recommended for endophthalmitis.

References

1. Kullberg BJ, Arendrup MC. Invasive candidiasis. N Engl J Med. 2015;373(15):1445–56. doi:10.1056/NEJMra1315399.
2. Wisplinghoff H, Bischoff T, Tallent SM, Seifert H, Wenzel RP, Edmond MB. Nosocomial bloodstream infections in US hospitals: analysis of 24,179 cases from a prospective nationwide surveillance study. Clin Infect Dis. 2004;39(3):309–17. doi:10.1086/421946.
3. Arendrup MC. Epidemiology of invasive candidiasis. Curr Opin Crit Care. 2010;16(5):445–52. doi:10.1097/MCC.0b013e32833e84d2 PubMed PMID: WOS:000281621000008.
4. Chow JKGY, Ruthazer R, Karchmer AW, Carmeli Y, Lichtenberg DA, Chawla V, Young JA, Hadley S. Risk factors for albicans and non-albicans candidemia in the intensive care unit. Crit Care Med. 2008;36(7):1993–8. doi:10.1097/CCM.0b013e31816fc4cd.
5. Oude Lashof AML, Donnelly JP, Meis JFGM, Meer JWM, Kullberg BJ. Duration of antifungal treatment and development of delayed complications in patients with candidaemia. Eur J Clin Microbiol Infect Dis. 2003;22(1):43–8. doi:10.1007/s10096-002-0854-6.
6. Khalid A, Clough LA, Symons RCA, Mahnken JD, Dong L, Eid AJ. Incidence and clinical predictors of ocular candidiasis in patients with *Candida* fungemia. Interdisc Perspect Infect Dis. 2014;2014:6. doi:10.1155/2014/650235.
7. Pfaller MA, Diekema DJ. Epidemiology of invasive candidiasis: a persistent public health problem. Clin Microbiol Rev. 2007;20(1):133–63. doi:10.1128/cmr.00029-06.
8. Cleveland AA, Harrison LH, Farley MM, Hollick R, Stein B, Chiller TM, et al. Declining incidence of candidemia and the shifting epidemiology of *Candida* resistance in two US metropolitan areas, 2008–2013: results from population-based surveillance. PLoS One. 2015;10(3):e0120452. doi:10.1371/journal.pone.0120452.
9. Yapar N. Epidemiology and risk factors for invasive candidiasis. Ther Clin Risk Manag. 2014;10:95–105. doi:10.2147/TCRM.S40160 PubMed PMID: PMC3928396.
10. Lockhart SR, Iqbal N, Cleveland AA, Farley MM, Harrison LH, Bolden CB, et al. Species identification and antifungal susceptibility testing of *Candida* bloodstream isolates from population-based surveillance studies in two U.S. cities from 2008 to 2011. J Clin Microbiol. 2012;50(11):3435–42. doi:10.1128/jcm.01283-12.
11. Oude Lashof AML, Rothova A, Sobel JD, Ruhnke M, Pappas PG, Viscoli C, et al. Ocular manifestations of candidemia. Clin Infect Dis. 2011;53(3):262–8. doi:10.1093/cid/cir355.
12. Shah CP, McKey J, Spirn MJ, Maguire J. Ocular candidiasis: a review. Br J Ophthalmol. 2008;92(4):466–8. doi:10.1136/bjo.2007.133405.
13. Brooks RG. Prospective study of *Candida* endophthalmitis in hospitalized patients with candidemia. Arch Intern Med. 1989;149(10):2226–8. doi:10.1001/archinte.1989.00390100056014.
14. Vinikoor MJ, Zoghby J, Cohen KL, Tucker JD. Do all candidemic patients need an ophthalmic examination? Int J Infect Dis. 2013;17(3):e146–8. doi:10.1016/j.ijid.2012.12.014.
15. Khan FA, Slain D, Khakoo RA. *Candida* endophthalmitis: focus on current and future antifungal treatment options. Pharmacother J Hum Pharmacol Drug Ther. 2007;27(12):1711–21. doi:10.1592/phco.27.12.1711.
16. Schiedler V, Scott IU, Flynn HW, Jr., Davis JL, Benz MS, Miller D. Culture-proven endogenous endophthalmitis: clinical features and visual acuity outcomes. Am J Ophthalmol.137(4):725–31. doi:10.1016/j.ajo.2003.11.013.
17. Clancy CJ, Nguyen MH. Finding the "missing 50 %" of invasive candidiasis: how nonculture diagnostics will improve understanding of disease spectrum and transform patient care. Clin Infect Dis. 2013;. doi:10.1093/cid/cit006.
18. Lucignano B, Ranno S, Liesenfeld O, Pizzorno B, Putignani L, Bernaschi P, et al. Multiplex PCR allows rapid and accurate diagnosis of bloodstream infections in newborns and children with suspected sepsis. J Clin Microbiol. 2011;49(6):2252–8. doi:10.1128/jcm.02460-10.
19. Pappas PG, Kauffman CA, Andes DR, Clancy CJ, Marr KA, Ostrosky-Zeichner L, et al. Clinical practice guideline for the management of candidiasis: 2016 update by the infectious diseases society of America. Clin Infect Dis. 2015;62:e1–50. doi:10.1093/cid/civ933.

CMV Retinitis

5

Avni Patel and Lucy Young

Introduction

Cytomegalovirus (CMV), a double-stranded DNA virus in the herpesvirus family, is a major cause of morbidity and mortality in severely immunocompromised patients. This population includes those with acquired immune deficiency syndrome (AIDS) and those with iatrogenic immune suppression such as chemotherapy, solid organ transplant recipients, and bone marrow transplantation recipients.

CMV is a fairly ubiquitous infection with an estimated 60 % or more of the general adult population in the United States showing serologic evidence of prior CMV infection [1]. Following the primary infection, CMV then remains latent in the infected host throughout life and reactivates only to cause illness in immunocompromised hosts. CMV infection is more prevalent in populations at risk for HIV infection with more than 75 % of IV drug users and more than 90 % of homosexual men having detectable IgG antibodies to CMV [2].

Retinitis is the most common clinical manifestation of CMV infection. However, systemic CMV manifestations in immunocompromised hosts also include esophagitis, colitis, pneumonitis, and neurologic disease such as encephalitis and polyradiculopathy.

There is some data to suggest that recent progress in bone marrow transplantation including increased transplantation from HLA-matched unrelated or mismatched donors, new preconditioning regimens, more aggressive treatment of graft-versus-host disease, and prolonged survival rate after bone marrow transplantation may prolong hematopoietic stem cell recipient survival and result in a growing incidence of CMV retinitis [3]. One study suggests the cumulative incidence of CMV retinitis in transplant recipients reaches greater than 2 % [4].

While the advent of highly active antiretroviral therapy has significantly decreased the incidence of CMV retinitis in the AIDS population, it continues to be an important major sight-threatening conditions in the severely immuno suppressed.

Clinical Presentation

Patients with retinitis most often present with symptoms such as decreased visual acuity, floaters, photopsia, eye pain, and scotomas.

A. Patel · L. Young (✉)
Department of Ophthalmology, Massachusetts Eye and Ear Infirmary, 243 Charles Street, Boston, MA 02114, USA
e-mail: lhyoung@meei.harvard.edu

A. Patel
e-mail: Avni_patel@meei.harvard.edu

G.N. Papaliodis (ed.), *Uveitis*,
DOI 10.1007/978-3-319-09126-6_5

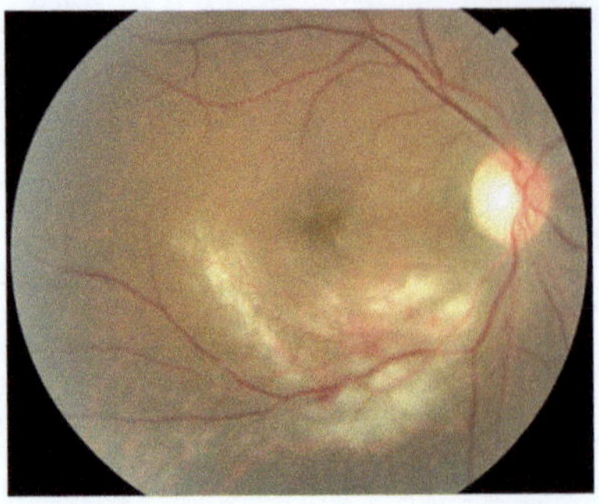

Fig. 5.1 Classic appearing CMV retinitis with white retinal lesions and hemorrhages along the arcades of the posterior pole

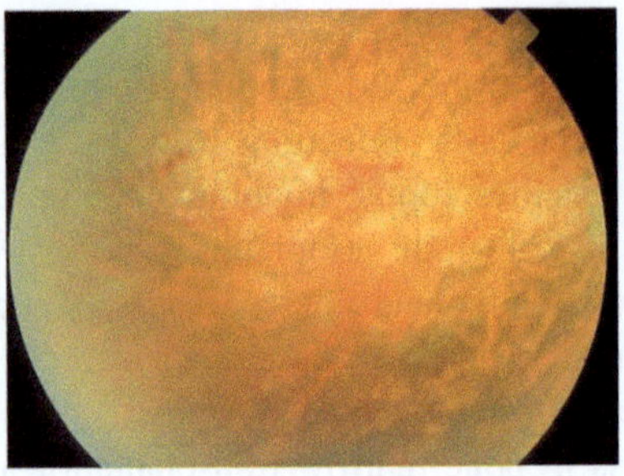

Fig. 5.2 Granular peripheral lesions that are typically seen in the peripheral retina

Photopsia and floaters are both independently significant predictors of CMV retinitis in patients with AIDS [5].

The external appearance of an eye with active CMV infection is usually white and quiet. Slit lamp exam may reveal mild inflammation including fine, stellate keratic precipitates, anterior chamber cells and a mild vitritis may be present on posterior examination.

CMV infection causes a full-thickness necrotizing retinitis that may affect the posterior pole, periphery, or both, and it can be either unilateral or bilateral. The appearance of the retinitis may be variable though the most characteristic ophthalmologic appearance consists of perivascular fluffy whitish yellow retinal lesions with intraretinal hemorrhages [6]. Early on, retinal lesions may be small, white infiltrates resembling large cotton wool spots (Fig. 5.1). These may evolve into larger creamy white geographic lesions. Retinal hemorrhages are often present along the leading edge of or within a necrotic area. Peripheral lesions may appear more granular and may not be associated with retinal hemorrhages (Fig. 5.2). Other features that may be present on retinal examination include vascular sheathing with a so-called "frosted branch angiitis" and papillitis, which may be present in 4 % of CMV patients and spread either by primary optic nerve involvement of spread from the peripapillary retina [7, 8].

Diagnosis

The differential diagnosis for CMV retinitis includes other viral retinitides, particularly those in the herpesvirus family such as acute retinal necrosis (ARN) and progressive outer retinal necrosis (PORN) as well as toxoplasmosis, candidiasis, syphilis, and Behcet's disease. These can often be distinguished from CMV retinitis by clinical history and ophthalmologic evaluation.

ARN and PORN are much more rapidly progressive and present with fulminant retinal necrosis. Unlike ARN and PORN, however, CMV retinitis is usually localized to one quadrant initially and progresses more slowly. The amount of intraocular inflammation associated with CMV retinitis is minimal to nonexistent, while there is often significant intraocular inflammation associated with ARN, toxoplasmic retinitis, Candida endophthalmitis, and Behcet's disease. In addition to being marked by intraocular inflammation, even in an immunocompromised host, toxoplasmosis is generally confined to a limited portion of the retina. Moreover, in cases of reactivation, a pigmented chorioretinal scar is often found adjacent to the area of active toxoplasmic retinitis.

However, should there be uncertainty regarding the diagnosis, a polymerase chain reaction (PCR) analysis of vitreous or aqueous samples can be performed. In making the diagnosis of CMV retinitis, PCR-based analysis of vitreous tap is highly sensitive and specific; however, it is usually reserved for patients with atypical lesions or those unresponsive to treatment. The specificity of PCR testing for the detection of CMV in vitreous and aqueous samples has a specificity of 93 % and a sensitivity of 67 % for vitreous samples and 37 % for aqueous samples according to one study [9].

The presence of CMV serum antibodies is not diagnostically useful as this only confirms prior exposure to the infection. Additionally, urine is CMV culture positive in the majority of AIDS patients, including many without CMV retinitis, rendering the test poorly specific for CMV infections.

Treatment

There are several effective pharmaceutical agents which may be administered systemically or locally for the treatment of cytomegalovirus retinitis. The choice of initial therapy for CMV retinitis should be individualized to each patient and based on several clinical factors including antiretroviral history, underlying degree and reason for immunosuppression, location of lesion, ability to adhere to treatment, and patient preference.

Ganciclovir was the first anti-CMV drug, approved for use in 1989, and it acts via competitive inhibition of CMV DNA polymerase following phosphorylation in CMV-infected cells. To achieve high tissue concentrations of the drug in the induction phase, ganciclovir must be infused intravenously at a dose of 5 mg/kg every 12 h for at least 14 days. After induction, a 5 mg/kg daily dose of intravenous ganciclovir is given indefinitely. On discontinuation of the drug, CMV retinitis can recur as early as 10–21 days at the borders of previously healed areas. Researchers have found recurrences even during maintenance therapy in about 30 % of patients [10] and a 100 % recurrence in patients with discontinuation or delay in ganciclovir therapy. [11, 12] Oral ganciclovir can be used as maintenance therapy though it is less effective than intravenous ganciclovir. Oral ganciclovir for prophylaxis or long-term maintenance treatment of CMV retinitis has been replaced with valganciclovir, which provides greater bioavailability.

Ganciclovir is excreted by the kidneys, and those with renal insufficiency need appropriate dosage adjustments. Notable medication-induced side effects include granulocytopenia, abnormal liver function tests, neurologic dysfunction, and thrombocytopenia [13–15].

Valganciclovir is an orally administered prodrug form of ganciclovir which provides greater bioavailability. It is used for both induction and maintenance therapy of CMV retinitis and is administered in a dose of 900 mg twice daily for three weeks as induction therapy followed by 900 mg daily as maintenance therapy. Orally administered valganciclovir has been shown to be as effective as intravenously administered ganciclovir for induction treatment and is an effective maintenance therapy for CMV retinitis [15, 16]. Its pharmacologic safety profile and side effects are similar to that of intravenously administered ganciclovir given it is concerted to ganciclovir in the bloodstream.

Foscarnet is a pyrophosphate analog approved for use in 1993 with broad antiviral activity against CMV and other herpes viruses as well as HIV. It is useful against strains of ganciclovir-resistant CMV due to its different mechanism of action [15, 17]. In a large, randomized trial comparing ganciclovir to foscarnet in the treatment of CMV retinitis, no difference in the rate of progression of retinitis was demonstrated in the two groups; however, foscarnet was found to offer a slight survival benefit [18]. Induction therapy with foscarnet is 90 mg/kg given intravenously over 1 h, every 12 h, for 2–3 weeks or until retinitis stabilizes. Maintenance therapy is 90–120 mg/kg given IV over 2 h, once per day. Renal function must be closely monitored and patients must be adequately hydrated while receiving the medication as the most frequently reported adverse effect with foscarnet administration is nephrotoxicity. Other adverse effects of foscarnet include abnormalities in phosphorous and calcium handling, including symptomatic hypocalcemia which can lead to arrhythmias and seizures. Other less common side effects are nausea, genital ulcers, anemia, hypokalemia, and hypomagnesemia [19].

Cidofivir is a nucleotide analog with a longer intracellular half-life which is used intravenously and is active against a broad spectrum of herpes viruses, including CMV. Standard dosing of cidofivir is induction with weekly 5 mg/kg intravenous infusion for 2 weeks followed by maintenance therapy with 5 mg/kg every two weeks. The main side effect of the drug is nephrotoxicity, thus it is administered in conjunction with oral probenecid to reduce renal uptake of cidofivir and IV saline hydration [20, 21]. Cidofivir can also cause anterior uveitis and hypotony, thought due to its toxic effects on the ciliary body [22]. This severe renal and ocular toxicity has limited the use of cidofivir in clinical practice.

Systemic therapy reduces the likelihood of involvement of the contralateral eye and improves survival [15, 23, 24]. However, intravitreal therapy is often used to have maximal drug affect in the retina without systemic side effects. Intravitreal injections of ganciclovir or foscarnet may be used in conjunction with oral valganciclovir. This may provide for higher immediate intraocular levels of the drug and faster control of retinitis that is macula-threatening.

The ganciclovir implant, which is no longer manufactured, was able to provide control of retinitis for 6–8 months [11, 24]. Intravitreal ganciclovir is used less frequently since the introduction of HAART as the majority of patients respond to systemic anti-CMV treatment alone.

Other options for intravitreal therapy include foscarnet and cidofivir. Foscarnet is given as a 2.4 mg injection one or two times weekly and has been shown to be a safe and effective alternative treatment in patients resistant to intravenous therapy [25]. Cidofivir is injected at a 20 Âµg dose every 5–6 weeks and has been shown to be as effective as induction therapy with only rare episodes of reactivation and progression, though the known ocular complications of hypotony and iritis limit its use [26–28].

Fomivirsen is an antisense oligonucleotide that prohibits the production of messenger RNA and thus inhibits CMV replication. This drug is solely approved for intravitreal injection for CMV retinitis that has not been controlled well with other medications [29]. The drug has several toxic side effects including anterior and posterior uveitis, transient elevation in intraocular pressure, retinal pigment epitheliopathy, and bull's eye maculopathy [30].

CMV Retinitis in the Era of HAART

Highly active antiretroviral therapy (HAART) has dramatically altered not only the incidence of CMV retinitis in patients with AIDS but it has also affected the presentation and course of CMV infection.

Highly active antiretroviral therapy consists of three or more antiretroviral drugs and is composed of one or more protease inhibitor (PIs), nucleoside or nucleotide reverse transcriptase inhibitors (NRTIs), non-nucleoside reverse transcriptase inhibitors (NNRTIs), and an integrase or entry inhibitor as the third agent.

HAART has led to a reduction of morbidity and mortality in HIV-infected patients through immune reconstitution in HIV patients with increased CD4 + T cell counts and decreased HIV replication [31]. CMV retinitis was the most common cause of visual impairment and vision loss in HIV-infected patients prior to the advent of HAART in 1995. Prior to this, about 25–42 % of HIV-infected patients with AIDS developed CMV retinitis and the incidence of cytomegalovirus retinitis in patients with CD4 + T cell counts less than 50 cells/mm^3 was approximately 20 % per year [32, 33]. Widespread use of HAART has led to a decrease in the annual number of new cases of CMV by more than 50 % [34].

HAART has not only reduced the risk of CMV retinitis in patients with HIV but has also altered the course. Prior to HAART, CMV retinitis, even with appropriate anti-CMV treatment, often progressed to blindness. Bilateral disease occurs less frequently in patients on HAART and anti-CMV treatment, 26 % per person-year compared with approximately 60 % per person-year in those patients not on HAART or CMV therapy [35]. Prior to the advent of HAART, time to progression of CMV retinitis was approximately 2 months in patients treated with intravenous ganciclovir or foscarnet [36], 2–

4 months with intravenous cidofivir [37], and up to 7 months with the ganciclovir intravitreal implant [24].

The advent of HAART and its resulting aid in the recovery of immune function in HIV patients has even allowed patients to discontinue their CMV treatment, whereas prior to the HAART era long-term maintenance treatment was necessary. Discontinuation of maintenance therapy has been shown to be safe in a subset of patients. Patients should have sustained CD4 count elevation of at least 100 cells/mm^3 for at least 3–6 months before discontinuing anti-CMV treatment and should be monitored carefully for reactivation [12, 38–40].

One study showed that if retinitis has adequately resolved with antiviral treatment and immune function has recovered (two consecutive CD4 + T cell counts of ≥100 cells/mm^3 at least 6 months apart) CMV therapy may be discontinued [36]. Another study showed that with discontinuation of anti-CMV therapy after persistent CD4 + T cell count over 50 cells/mm^3, 19 of 22 patients remained healed without CMV recurrence at the end of the study and the three patients who progressed had CD4 cell counts that dropped below 50 cells/mm^3 and viral loads in the hundreds of thousands, representing HAART failure [38]. This emphasizes the importance of periodic ophthalmologic monitoring in all patients, even those with successful immune recovery on HAART, as the HAART-induced elevation in CD4 count can fall allowing the recurrence of CMV infection.

Complications Related to CMV Retinitis

Retinal Detachment in CMV Retinitis

Retinal detachment is a common cause of vision loss in patients affected by cytomegalovirus retinitis. In the pre-HAART era the incidence of retinal detachment in CMV retinitis was approximately 33 % per eye per year [41]. Greater involvement of the peripheral retina and active retinitis are two significant risk factors for the development of retinal detachment in these patients [42]. Rhegmatogenous retinal detachment is associated with active retinitis due to breaks in necrotic retina. The use of HAART has resulted in a 60 % decrease in the rate of retinal detachment in AIDS patients with CMV retinitis [23]. The standard approach for the repair of these retinal detachments is a pars plana vitrectomy removal of posterior hyaloid and intraocular tamponade with silicone oil or a long-acting gas due to the propensity for multiple breaks which may not be apparent until the time of vitrectomy [41, 43]. Studies have shown no statistically significant difference in the rate of retinal reattachment or macular reattachment in patients where scleral buckle was used versus vitrectomy and silicone oil tamponade [44]. Visual acuity may continue to be compromised by silicone oil, resulting cataract formation from the oil or optic atrophy due to the disease.

Immune Recovery Uveitis

While HAART has significantly improved prognosis in HIV-infected patients, the immune reconstitution associated with antiretroviral therapy also presents additional ocular complications, most importantly immune recovery uveitis (IRU).

IRU is a syndrome that may develop in patients with cytomegalovirus retinitis who have responded to antiretroviral therapy with immune recovery and increase in CD4 + T cells. Immune recovery uveitis was first described in 1998 in patients with cytomegalovirus who experienced immune reconstitution due to highly active antiretroviral therapy [45, 46]. The incidence rate of IRU has varied among different reports from 15 to 37.5 % [12, 47].

The primary signs and symptoms of IRU include decreased vision and floaters. Clinically, this entity is characterized by signs of inflammation including iritis, vitritis, papillitis, and macular changes.

Pathogenesis of IRU is unknown, however it is hypothesized that this is an immunologic reaction to cytomegalovirus antigens in retinal tissues caused by HAART-mediated recovery in immune status. Another hypothesis is that the control of CMV retinitis is actually incomplete and the recovered immune system is mounting an inflammatory response to virus or viral proteins. Previous treatment with cidofivir may be a risk factor for the development of IRU [48]. Similar reactions have occurred in other organs, such as fever and lymphadenitis in patients with Mycobacterium avium complex or meningitis in patients with latent cryptococcal CNS infection after the initiation of HAART [49].

Vision loss in these patients occurs from long-term complications associated with IRU. These may include posterior subcapsular cataracts, cystoid macular edema, epiretinal membrane, proliferative vitreoretinopathy, neovascularization of the disc, vitreomacular traction, and severe postoperative inflammation [50–52].

Conclusion

Cytomegalovirus retinitis may lead to significant ocular morbidity in immunocompromised patients that are not readily diagnosed and treated. The advent of HAART has transformed one of the most common intraocular infections within the United States to an entity that may be rarely seen by an ophthalmology resident during a three-year training program. Despite these advances for AIDS patients, CMV retinitis remains a concern for HIV-infected individuals not on treatment or those who have failed anti-HIV treatment as well as those immunocompromised by other means such as chemotherapy, organ transplantation, and bone marrow transplantation. With the advancement in medical therapies prolonging survival and increasing the number of these immunocompromised hosts, physicians should continue to remain vigilant and screen these patients for CMV retinitis. Regular dilated exams are recommended for these immunocompromised hosts, particularly those with CD4 + T cell counts less than 50 cells/mm^3, as these patients may remain asymptomatic due to the lack of intraocular inflammation unless a lesion involves the macula or the optic nerve. Early detection not only reduces visual loss by reducing the risk of retinal detachment and other associated ocular complications, but also decreases overall morbidity and mortality in these patients.

References

1. Krech U. Complement-fixing antibodies against cytomegalovirus in different parts of the world. Bull World Health Organ. 1973;49(1):103–6.
2. Jackson JB, Erice A, Englund JA, Edson JR, Balfour HH. Prevalence of cytomegalovirus antibody in hemophiliacs and homosexuals infected with human immunodeficiency virus type 1. Transfusion. 1988;28(2):187–9.
3. Jeon S, Lee WK, Lee Y, Lee DG, Lee JW. Risk factors for cytomegalovirus retinitis in patients with cytomegalovirus viremia after hematopoietic stem cell transplantation. Ophthalmology. 2012;119(9):1892–8.
4. Xhaard A, Robin M, Scieux C, et al. Increased incidence of cytomegalovirus retinitis after allogeneic hematopoietic stem cell transplantation. Transplantation. 2007;83(1):80–3.
5. Hodge WG, Boivin J-F, Shapiro SH, et al. Clinical risk factors for cytomegalovirus retinitis in patients with AIDS. Ophthalmology. 2004;111(7):1326–33.
6. Wiegand TW, Young LHY. Cytomegalovirus retinitis. Int Ophthalmol Clin. 2006;46(2):91–110.
7. Walker S, Iguchi A, Jones NP. Frosted branch angiitis: a review. Eye (Lond). 2004;18(5):527–33.
8. Mansour AM. Cytomegalovirus optic neuritis. Curr Opin Ophthalmol. 1997;8(3):55–8.
9. Pathanapitoon K, Ausayakhun S, Kunavisarut P, Pungrasame A, Sirirungsi W. Detection of cytomegalovirus in vitreous, aqueous and conjunctiva by polymerase chain reaction (PCR). J Med Assoc Thai. 2005;88(2):228–32.
10. Henderly DE, Freeman WR, Causey DM, Rao NA. Cytomegalovirus retinitis and response to therapy with ganciclovir. Ophthalmology. 1987;94(4):425–34.
11. Anand R, Font RL, Fish RH, Nightingale SD. Pathology of cytomegalovirus retinitis treated with sustained release intravitreal ganciclovir. Ophthalmology. 1993;100(7):1032–9.
12. Jabs DA, Bolton SG, Dunn JP, Palestine AG. Discontinuing anticytomegalovirus therapy in patients with immune reconstitution after combination antiretroviral therapy. Am J Ophthalmol. 1998;126(6):817–22.
13. Noble S, Faulds D. Ganciclovir. An update of its use in the prevention of cytomegalovirus infection and disease in transplant recipients. Drugs. 1998;56(1):115–46.
14. McGavin JK, Goa KL. Ganciclovir: an update of its use in the prevention of cytomegalovirus infection

and disease in transplant recipients. Drugs. 2001;61 (8):1153–83.
15. Huynh N, Daniels AB, Kohanim S, Young LHY. Medical treatment for cytomegalovirus retinitis. Int Ophthalmol Clin. 2011;51(4):93–103.
16. Martin DF, Sierra-Madero J, Walmsley S, et al. A controlled trial of valganciclovir as induction therapy for cytomegalovirus retinitis. N Engl J Med. 2002;346(15):1119–26.
17. Ohta H, Matsuda Y, Tokimasa S, et al. Foscarnet therapy for ganciclovir-resistant cytomegalovirus retinitis after stem cell transplantation: effective monitoring of CMV infection by quantitative analysis of CMV mRNA. Bone Marrow Transplant. 2001;27(11):1141–5.
18. Studies of Ocular Complications of AIDS Research Group. Mortality in patients with the acquired immunodeficiency syndrome treated with either foscarnet or ganciclovir for cytomegalovirus retinitis. N Engl J Med. 1992;1992(326):213–20.
19. Jacobson MA, Wulfsohn M, Feinberg JE, et al. Phase II dose-ranging trial of foscarnet salvage therapy for cytomegalovirus retinitis in AIDS patients intolerant of or resistant to ganciclovir (ACTG protocol 093). AIDS Clinical Trials Group of the National Institute of Allergy and Infectious Diseases. AIDS. 1994;8(4):451–9.
20. Lalezari JP, Stagg RJ, Kuppermann BD, et al. Intravenous cidofovir for peripheral cytomegalovirus retinitis in patients with AIDS. A randomized, controlled trial. Ann Intern Med. 1997;126(4):257–63.
21. Polis MA, Spooner KM, Baird BF, et al. Anticytomegaloviral activity and safety of cidofovir in patients with human immunodeficiency virus infection and cytomegalovirus viruria. Antimicrob Agents Chemother. 1995;39(4):882–6.
22. Akler ME, Johnson DW, Burman WJ, Johnson SC. Anterior uveitis and hypotony after intravenous cidofovir for the treatment of cytomegalovirus retinitis. Ophthalmology. 1998;105(4):651–7.
23. Kempen JH, Jabs DA, Dunn JP, West SK, Tonascia J. Retinal detachment risk in cytomegalovirus retinitis related to the acquired immunodeficiency syndrome. Arch Ophthalmol. 2001;119 (1):33–40.
24. Martin DF, Parks DJ, Mellow SD, et al. Treatment of cytomegalovirus retinitis with an intraocular sustained-release ganciclovir implant. A randomized controlled clinical trial. Arch Ophthalmol. 1994;112 (12):1531–9.
25. Diaz-Llopis M, España E, Muñoz G, et al. High dose intravitreal foscarnet in the treatment of cytomegalovirus retinitis in AIDS. Br J Ophthalmol. 1994;78 (2):120–4.
26. Kirsch LS, Arevalo JF, de la Paz EC, Munguia D, de Clerq E, Freeman WR. Intravitreal cidofovir (HPMPC) treatment of cytomegalovirus retinitis in patients with acquired immune deficiency syndrome. Ophthalmology. 1995;102(4):533–43.
27. Banker AS, Arevalo JF, Munguia D, et al. Intraocular pressure and aqueous humor dynamics in patients with AIDS treated with intravitreal cidofovir (HPMPC) for cytomegalovirus retinitis. Am J Ophthalmol. 1997;124(2):168–80.
28. Chavez-de la Paz E, Arevalo JF, Kirsch LS, et al. Anterior nongranulomatous uveitis after intravitreal HPMPC (cidofovir) for the treatment of cytomegalovirus retinitis. Analysis and prevention. Ophthalmology. 1997;104(3):539–44.
29. De Smet MD, Meenken CJ, van den Horn GJ. Fomivirsen - a phosphorothioate oligonucleotide for the treatment of CMV retinitis. Ocul Immunol Inflamm. 1999;7(3–4):189–98.
30. Amin HI, Ai E, McDonald HR, Johnson RN. Retinal toxic effects associated with intravitreal fomivirsen. Arch Ophthalmol. 2000;118(3):426–7.
31. Palella FJ, Delaney KM, Moorman AC, et al. Declining morbidity and mortality among patients with advanced human immunodeficiency virus infection. HIV Outpatient Study Investigators. N Engl J Med. 1998;338(13):853–60.
32. Bloom JN, Palestine AG. The diagnosis of cytomegalovirus retinitis. Ann Intern Med. 1988;109(12):963–9.
33. Pertel P, Hirschtick R, Phair J, Chmiel J, Poggensee L, Murphy R. Risk of developing cytomegalovirus retinitis in persons infected with the human immunodeficiency virus. J Acquir Immune Defic Syndr. 1992;5(11):1069–74.
34. Jabs DA, Bartlett JG. AIDS and ophthalmology: a period of transition. Am J Ophthalmol. 1997;124 (2):227–33.
35. Jabs DA, Holbrook JT, Van Natta ML, et al. Risk factors for mortality in patients with AIDS in the era of highly active antiretroviral therapy. Ophthalmology. 2005;112(5):771–9.
36. Holbrook JT, Colvin R, van Natta ML, Thorne JE, Bardsley M, Jabs DA. Evaluation of the United States public health service guidelines for discontinuation of anticytomegalovirus therapy after immune recovery in patients with cytomegalovirus retinitis. Am J Ophthalmol. 2011;152(4):628–37.
37. Lalezari JP, Drew WL, Glutzer E, et al. (S)-1-[3-hydroxy-2-(phosphonylmethoxy)propyl]cytosine (cidofovir): results of a phase I/II study of a novel antiviral nucleotide analogue. J Infect Dis. 1995;171 (4):788–96.
38. Macdonald JC, Torriani FJ, Morse LS, Karavellas MP, Reed JB, Freeman WR. Lack of reactivation of cytomegalovirus (CMV) retinitis after stopping CMV maintenance therapy in AIDS patients with sustained elevations in CD4 T cells in response to highly active antiretroviral therapy. J Infect Dis. 1998;177(5):1182–7.
39. Curi AL, Muralha A, Muralha L, Pavesio C. Suspension of anticytomegalovirus maintenance therapy following immune recovery due to highly active antiretroviral therapy. Br J Ophthalmol. 2001;85 (4):471–3.

40. Whitcup SM, Fortin E, Lindblad AS, et al. Discontinuation of anticytomegalovirus therapy in patients with HIV infection and cytomegalovirus retinitis. JAMA. 1999;282(17):1633–7.
41. Freeman WR, Henderly DE, Wan WL, et al. Prevalence, pathophysiology, and treatment of rhegmatogenous retinal detachment in treated cytomegalovirus retinitis. Am J Ophthalmol. 1987;103(4):527–36.
42. Freeman WR, Friedberg DN, Berry C, et al. Risk factors for development of rhegmatogenous retinal detachment in patients with cytomegalovirus retinitis. Am J Ophthalmol. 1993;116(6):713–20.
43. Irvine AR, Lonn L, Schwartz D, Zarbin M, Ballesteros F, Kroll S. Retinal detachment in AIDS: long-term results after repair with silicone oil. Br J Ophthalmol. 1997;81(3):180–3.
44. Nasemann JE, Mutsch A, Wiltfang R, Klauss V. Early pars plana vitrectomy without buckling procedure in cytomegalovirus retinitis-induced retinal detachment. Retina. 1995;15(2):111–6.
45. Karavellas MP, Lowder CY, Macdonald C, Avila CP, Freeman WR. Immune recovery vitritis associated with inactive cytomegalovirus retinitis: a new syndrome. Arch Ophthalmol. 1998;116(2):169–75.
46. Zegans ME, Walton RC, Holland GN, O'Donnell JJ, Jacobson MA, Margolis TP. Transient vitreous inflammatory reactions associated with combination antiretroviral therapy in patients with AIDS and cytomegalovirus retinitis. Am J Ophthalmol. 1998;125(3):292–300.
47. Arevalo JF, Mendoza AJ, Ferretti Y. Immune recovery uveitis in AIDS patients with cytomegalovirus retinitis treated with highly active antiretroviral therapy in Venezuela. Retina. 2003;23(4):495–502.
48. Song M-K, Azen SP, Buley A, et al. Effect of anti-cytomegalovirus therapy on the incidence of immune recovery uveitis in AIDS patients with healed cytomegalovirus retinitis. Am J Ophthalmol. 2003;136(4):696–702.
49. Woods ML, MacGinley R, Eisen DP, Allworth AM. HIV combination therapy: partial immune restitution unmasking latent cryptococcal infection. AIDS. 1998;12(12):1491–4.
50. Karavellas MP, Song M, Macdonald JC, Freeman WR. Long-term posterior and anterior segment complications of immune recovery uveitis associated with cytomegalovirus retinitis. Am J Ophthalmol. 2000;130(1):57–64.
51. Sanislo SR, Lowder CY, Kaiser PK. Optic nerve head neovascularization in a patient with inactive cytomegalovirus retinitis and immune recovery. Am J Ophthalmol. 1998;126(2):318–20.
52. Canzano JC, Reed JB, Morse LS. Vitreomacular traction syndrome following highly active antiretroviral therapy in AIDS patients with cytomegalovirus retinitis. Retina. 1998;18(5):443–7.

Herpes Simplex and Herpes Zoster

6

Thomas Flynn and Jessica Ackert

Anterior Segment Disease

Anterior uveitis remains the most common form of uveitis, and herpes virus associated anterior segment inflammation is a common infectious etiology. The herpes virus family was first implicated in the 1950s as a cause of anterior uveitis [1]. The presenting symptoms may differ based on the specific virus involved and the immune status of the host. Treatment regimens for different viruses, sites of infection, and host factors also vary. In all cases, recurrent disease is not uncommon and this constitutes a significant potential for visual compromise in inadequately treated or monitored patients.

Herpes Simplex Virus

Herpes simplex virus, type 1 (HSV-1) is the most common infectious cause of anterior uveitis. Though the initial presentation is often that of a dendritic epithelial keratitis, there can be an associated stromal keratitis with accompanying anterior chamber inflammation. The finding of an associated uveitis is more common in recurrent episodes rather than primary disease and may occur in the absence of active corneal involvement [2]. Patients afflicted with HSV uveitis tend to be younger than those with VZV associated anterior uveitis.

Classically, patients present with a red, painful eye, photophobia, decreased vision, and often increased intraocular pressure. The disease is most often unilateral. A vesicular rash may be present in cases of primary infection but is generally absent in recurrent disease. There are often associated fine or granulomatous keratic precipitates (KP's) occurring either centrally on the corneal endothelium or localized to Arlt's triangle [3]. Patchy iris transillumination defects are considered to be a hallmark finding of the herpes simplex (see Fig. 6.1). Patients are at high risk of glaucoma-associated vision loss due to the possibility of severely increased intraocular pressures (IOP) due to concomitant trabeculitis. Previous reports have indicated 50–90 % of patients will have increased intraocular pressure during the course of active infection and inflammation [3, 4]. The pupil is often distorted with poor dilation even in the absence of posterior synechiae [5]. The disease is most commonly isolated to the anterior chamber and does not typically affect the posterior segment of the eye.

T. Flynn (✉)
35 Eastward Ln, Ellsworth, ME 04605, USA
e-mail: tomflynn@ix.netcom.com

J. Ackert
Department of Ophthalmology, Drexel College of Medicine, 219 N Broad Street, 3rd Floor, Philadelphia, PA 19106, USA

G.N. Papaliodis (ed.), *Uveitis*,
DOI 10.1007/978-3-319-09126-6_6

However, the presence of a co-existent viral retinitis must be considered in all patients. It is important to monitor the posterior segment regularly in affected patients. There is a small cohort of infants infected with Herpes simplex (type 2) during delivery who also manifest severe retinal and ocular involvement: the mortality rate for these infants is quite high and this presentation is unlikely to be seen in an ambulatory patient population.

Diagnosis of HSV is often based on the clinical presentation and examination of the patient. The presence of a dendritic epithelial keratitis, stromal disease, iris transillumination defects, and elevated IOP are highly suggestive of herpetic disease. A corneal swab with positive culture proven to be HSV is helpful to confirm the diagnosis in most patients. In cases with atypical findings or poor response to empiric treatment, PCR testing of aqueous humor can be performed via an anterior chamber tap to confirm the etiology and direct appropriate treatment.

The propensity for HSV to manifest as recurrent episodes is common and can lead to severe visual impairment due to a combination of corneal scarring, cataract, and secondary glaucoma. The development of cataract and glaucoma are also related to the chronic use of strong topical steroids to suppress the anterior uveitis.

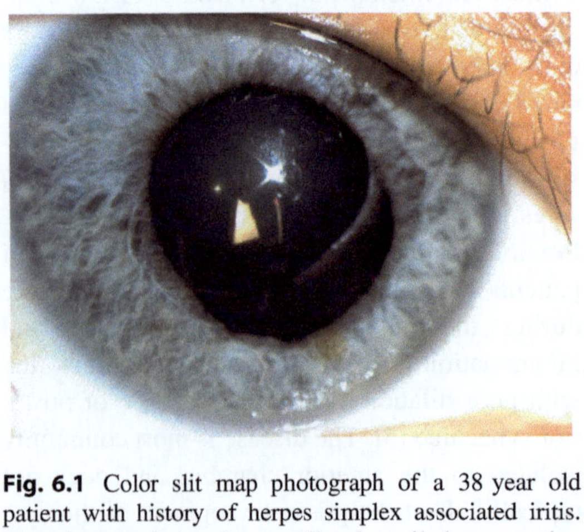

Fig. 6.1 Color slit map photograph of a 38 year old patient with history of herpes simplex associated iritis. The photograph is of an undilated pupil demonstrating inferior iris atrophy

Treatment

Treatment of the virus often includes a combination of systemic and topical antiviral medications. Much of the evidence-based guidelines for treatment emerged from the randomized, prospective Herpetic Eye Disease Study (HEDS). Presence of an active keratitis should be aggressively treated with topical antiviral therapy. Generally either topical trifluridine 1 % ophthalmic solution (Viroptic) 8–9 times daily or vidarabine ointment (Vira A) every 3 h is prescribed. More recently, a topical ganciclovir 0.15 % gel (Zirgan) has been used with good therapeutic success and less corneal toxicity. Though oral antiviral therapy did not improve outcome in patients with only an epithelial keratitis, it did lessen the risk of recurrent disease [6].

The associated uveitis is treated with a combination of cycloplegia and topical Prednisolone acetate 1 %. This drop is necessary initially to speed resolution of the anterior chamber reaction and stromal inflammation, but its use should be delayed until the epithelial surface is adequately healed [7]. Once started, Prednisolone acetate is typically prescribed every 1–2 h frequency based on the severity of the cellular reaction and tapered according to clinical response. Escalation of therapy to difluprednate (Durezol) may be necessary for those cases with difficult to control anterior segment inflammation. Close monitoring of the intraocular pressure is necessary given the propensity for the disease and the most commonly employed therapy to elevate intraocular pressure. Most authors suggest avoiding the use of prostaglandin analogs given the association with inflammation and possible risk of recurrent herpetic keratitis.

Oral antiviral therapy seems to improve the course of the disease in patients with concomitant uveitis though data from the HEDS study did not reach a level of statistical significance for that contention. However, oral acyclovir was found to be effective in preventing recurrent herpes simplex in patients undergoing penetrating keratoplasty with a history of prior herpetic eye disease [8]. For these reasons, most specialists often prescribe either oral Acyclovir 800 mg 3 times daily or Valtrex 1 gm twice daily for the treatment of active disease. Although the duration of treatment has classically been 7–10 days, there is increasing anecdotal evidence that a longer duration of therapy using lower doses of antivirals may prevent recurrences [9]. The treatment of chronic or recurrent herpes simplex uveitis may require long-term use of oral antivirals, topical steroids, and intraocular pressure lowering agents for an indefinite period of time.

Varicella Zoster Virus

Patients at risk for ophthalmic varicella zoster virus (VZV) classically present with a painful vesicular rash in the V1 or V 2 dermatome. While the initial rash typically clears in 2–4 weeks [10], associated ocular inflammation can take significantly longer to resolve fully. Patients typically are older than 50 years of age at presentation, although herpes zoster can present at any age. Patients who are immunocompromised are at greater risk for systemic involvement, and without timely diagnosis and treatment, infection with VZV can be fatal [11].

The initial dermatological manifestations may, and often do, precede ophthalmological findings. Unilateral involvement is the rule, with poor dilation of the pupil even in the absence of posterior synechiae. Traditionally there are zonal or sectoral transillumination defects in the iris, though patchy defects have been reported as well. Granulomatous KP's are often found either centrally or in Arlt's triangle [3]. Like patients with HSV, decreased corneal sensation is common as is elevated intraocular pressure. Posterior segment involvement is uncommon, but cases of acute retinal necrosis (ARN) can occur concomitantly even in immunocompetent individuals, and it is important to monitor for any evidence of vitritis or retinitis. The course of VZV associated keratouveitis tends to be chronic in contrast to the acute, recurrent course typical of HSV-associated uveitis [12].

While the clinical history and ocular findings generally confirm the diagnosis, sampling of aqueous fluid via an anterior chamber tap with subsequent PCR testing can be utilized in cases where the diagnosis is unclear or the uveitis does not respond adequately to appropriate treatment [13].

Treatment

There is minimal role for topical antivirals in the treatment of herpes zoster ophthalmicus. However, systemic antivirals play a critical role in the management of both the dermatological and ophthalmic manifestations of the infection. The treatment dose of Acyclovir is 800 mg dosed five times daily, Valacyclovir (Valtrex) 1gm dosed three times daily, or Famciclovir (Famvir) 500 mg dosed three times daily. While all three are affective in the treatment of varicella zoster virus, the ocular bioavailability of valacyclovir and famciclovir are superior to that of acyclovir. Traditionally treatment is continued for 10–14 days, which is the time frame for resolution of the dermatological manifestations [10]. However, in patients with chronic or recurrent ocular disease, there is a role for extended duration of systemic antiviral therapy.

Concomitant uveitis is treated with a tapering dose of topical corticosteroids. Prednisolone acetate 1 % is generally the first line agent. Patients who have persistent inflammation despite maximum doses of topical prednisolone acetate may benefit from difluprednate (Durezol) due to its efficacy as an emulsion. Strong steroids will require close follow up (every week to 2 weeks) to assess clinical effect and monitor intraocular pressure. Cycloplegia is often used both for patient comfort and prevention of development of posterior synechiae. Intraocular pressure is controlled with use of topical IOP lowering agents. Prostaglandins are preferentially avoided due to the potential risk of reactivation of herpes virus replication and reports of association with episodes of uveitis/development of macular edema.

Posterior Segment Disease

One of the most feared and devastating manifestations of herpetic eye disease is retinal necrosis. In the immunocompetent patient, this is often referred to as acute retinal necrosis (ARN) or bilateral ARN (BARN); while in the immunocompromised patient (patients with human immunodeficiency virus, s/p organ transplantation, etc.), the infection may manifest as ARN or progressive outer retinal necrosis (PORN).

Acute Retinal Necrosis

Acute retinal necrosis (ARN) is a devastating retinal infection most commonly caused by a member of the herpes virus family. The herpes simplex virus (HSV-1 and HSV-2) and varicella zoster virus (VZV) are the most common etiologies. Much less frequently, cytomegalovirus (CMV) and Epstein–Barr virus (EBV) have been reported to cause ARN.

ARN was initially described in 1971 by Urayama et al. [14] as an intraocular inflammatory event, and named as Krieye's disease, but it was not until 1982 that an infectious etiology was identified. Culbertson and colleagues performed histopathological analysis of enucleated eyes from this condition and demonstrated the herpes virus in all layers implicating an infectious etiology [15]. Case series published in the 1970s and 1980s described cases of both unilateral ARN and bilateral ARN (BARN) [16, 17]. These series found a high incidence of combined mechanism tractional and rhegmatogenous retinal detachments that proved difficult to repair with most patients requiring silicone oil tamponade and extensive laser demarcation. The patients' visual prognosis was uniformly poor due to a combination of retinal detachment, silicone oil tamponade, occlusive retinal vasculitis, and optic neuropathy. This condition occurs equally in men and women and occurs at any age.

Clinical Presentation

ARN can present with unilateral or bilateral disease and can occur with or without an antecedent Herpetic rash. Exposure to any member of the herpes virus family in the patient's lifetime is thought to be sufficient to confer risk of this disorder. Most commonly patients present with unilateral disease, though nearly 33 % will ultimately progress to bilateral involvement. Patients typically report an acute onset of a red, painful eye associated with blurry vision, and floaters. Clinical examination classically reveals an aggressive anterior chamber reaction, vitritis, vitreous haze, and areas of peripheral retinal necrosis which spread circumferentially and posteriorly (see Fig. 6.2). There may be associated arteritis, retinal vascular occlusions, retinal thinning, and extensive retinal pigment epithelial changes often appearing as a deep white or yellow choroiditis. Histopathological analysis of the vitritis shows a predominantly chronic granulomatous inflammation characterized by clusters of lymphocytes and plasma cells [15]. Fischer et al. [18] first described the classic triad of necrotizing retinitis, vitritis, and retinal vasculitis in immunocompetent patients considered pathognomonic for ARN.

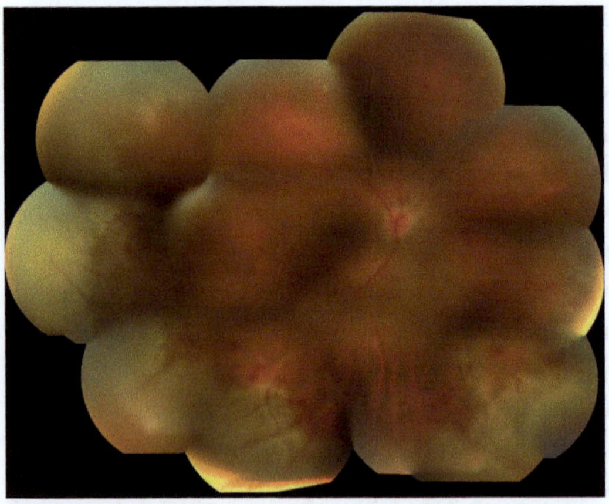

Fig. 6.2 Color fundus photograph montage of a 21 year old college student with acute retinal necrosis OD. The patient had diffuse, necrotizing retinal vasculitis on presentation and was admitted for IV Acyclovir therapy

ARN has traditionally been a clinical diagnosis though PCR testing via an aqueous or vitreous sample is increasingly utilized for diagnostic confirmation given its high sensitivity and rapid test results. Diagnostic criteria for ARN were first proposed in 1994 by the American Uveitis Society (AUS) which broadly included full thickness necrotizing retinitis, arteritis, and severe inflammation of the anterior chamber and vitreous cavity [19]. More specific criteria include the following:

(1) one or more discrete foci of retinal necrosis located in the peripheral retina,
(2) rapid progression in the absence of antiviral therapy
(3) circumferential spread
(4) evidence of occlusive vasculopathy with arterial involvement
(5) a prominent inflammatory reaction in the vitreous and anterior chambers.

Although the diagnostic criteria listed above are valuable for the clinician, the advent of PCR testing has confirmed the diagnosis of ARN both in patients who demonstrate the aforementioned inflammatory findings and in those who do not [20, 21]. There are multiple case series reporting patients with unusual or atypical presentations of PCR-confirmed ARN with minimal posterior necrotizing findings [22, 23]. Some authors suggest that the clinical presentation may vary depending upon the causative strain of virus and the underlying host characteristics; more investigation is required to confirm this hypothesis. A high degree of suspicion regarding the possibility of this diagnosis is critical for prompt diagnosis and rapid initiation of therapy given the relentless progression of the retinitis.

Treatment

Despite advanced therapeutic and surgical management for this disorder, the visual prognosis for ARN remains poor with a high percentage of patients failing to achieve acuities better than 20/200. In a study of 58 patients, Tibbets et al. [24] report 50 % failed to achieve vision of 20/200 or better at 3 months.

Systemic antivirals are the mainstay of therapy. In addition to arresting progression of retinal necrosis in the affected eye, these agents are considered critical to the prevention of contralateral eye involvement [25–30]. Patients are typically hospitalized for treatment with intravenous acyclovir dosed at 10 mg/kg every 8 h (or 1500 mg/m^2 per day) for 5–10 days. Recent data indicates that oral valacyclovir (dosed at 1–2 gm three times daily) and oral famciclovir (dosed at 500 mg three times daily) are also able to rapidly achieve the same ocular bioavailability in the vitreous cavity as intravenous acyclovir. Oral acyclovir's vitreous bioavailability is inferior to both oral valacyclovir and famiclovir; thus, this drug is less frequently used for treatment of acute ARN [31]. Patients initially treated with intravenous acyclovir therapy are often converted after 5–10 days to oral valacyclovir or famciclovir due to their superior bioavailability for more extended therapy. Antiviral medication is generally continued for 3 months. Some physicians, including the authors of this chapter, advocate for a longer duration of therapy in order to minimize the risk of recurrence. For patients with HIV/AIDS, the duration of therapy is life-long.

In addition to systemic therapy, many physicians will also initially treat with intravitreal injection of either ganciclovir (200–2000 μg per 0.1 ml) or foscarnet (1.2–2.4 mg per 0.1 ml) [32]. Recent work by Flaxel et al. [33] suggests a slightly improved visual outcome and decreased risk of RD in patients receiving both systemic and intravitreal therapies compared with systemic therapy alone. However, other data suggests the adjunctive use of intravitreal agents does not appear to alter the clinical outcome [24]. Despite this, many specialists tend to treat extensive retinal necrosis with a combination of systemic and intravitreal antivirals, though the choice of drug, injection frequency, and duration of the course of injections is subjective. No published definitive therapeutic protocol exists. Given that foscarnet attacks the herpes virus at a different target point than ganciclovir, valacyclovir or famciclovir, there is a hypothesis that injection of foscarnet may be superior to ganciclovir as a therapeutic adjuvant [34]. This remains to be proven as there is no definitive head to head comparison trial.

Systemic corticosteroids are frequently used to treat the inflammatory sequelae of ARN and minimize the associated tissue damage, though these are reserved for use only after an adequate vitreous concentration of antivirals have been reached. Most authors defer use of corticosteroids for a minimum of 24 h after initiation of antiviral therapy. Use, duration, and dosage of systemic corticosteroids also remain highly variable among practitioners.

Combined rhegmatogenous and tractional retinal detachment unfortunately occurs in a high percentage, 50 % or greater, of patients with ARN [24]. Some studies suggest that risk of retinal detachment may be lowered in patients receiving intravitreal therapy in addition to systemic antivirals; a definitive comparative study has not yet been done. Many practitioners advocate for the placement of prophylactic laser barricade surrounding the involved peripheral retina in an attempt to decrease the risk of detachment. Although many physicians still offer this intervention due to the relatively low-risk profile of the laser treatment, there is data to suggest that laser has minimal effectiveness in preventing retinal detachments [35]. Retinal detachments can occur months or years after the initial presentation, however, the majority of patients who detach commonly do so in the first 6 months following diagnosis. Retinal detachments secondary to ARN are difficult to effectively repair given the combined tractional and rhegmatogenous components and require vitrectomy, endolaser, and tamponade with silicone oil to effectively flatten the retina and relieve the traction.

Additional adjuvant therapies that have been considered include aspirin and warfarin to counteract the occlusive retinal vasculitis. No therapeutic benefit has been demonstrated, and thus there remains no evidence-based rationale for using either therapy.

Progressive Outer Retinal Necrosis

Progressive outer retinal necrosis (PORN) is the most aggressive entity in the subset of viral retinopathies due to the herpes virus family. Varicella zoster virus (VZV) causes the majority of cases with other Herpes viruses and mixed infections involved as well. PORN afflicts patients who are severely immunocompromised, most often those infected with human immunodeficiency virus (HIV). This disease is characterized by its rapid onset, distinctive pattern of outer retinal opacification, and is universally bilateral. The absence of inflammation and relative sparing of retinal vasculature serves to differentiate PORN from acute retinal necrosis (ARN). The visual prognosis is extremely grim with 66 % of patients developing no light perception vision (NLP) even with prompt and aggressive antiviral therapy.

Clinical Presentation

Progressive outer retinal necrosis (PORN) was first described in 1990 by Forster et al. [36] as a rapidly progressive, bilateral retinal necrosis occurring in severely immunocompromised patients infected with HIV. The characteristic features of the disorder include absence of anterior chamber or vitreous inflammation, sparing of retinal vessels with perivascular clearing in a setting of choroiditis. This will rapidly evolve to an outer retinal opacification resulting in the "cracked mud" appearance characteristic of PORN. This pattern and degree of underlying immune dysfunction differentiate PORN from ARN.

In cases of PORN, patients typically present with complaints of a rapid, painless decrease in vision with an early afferent pupillary defect in the affected eye due to early optic nerve involvement. Optic nerve involvement often precedes retinal changes. Classic signs of inflammation are generally absent due to severe immune system dysfunction. There is little or no anterior chamber inflammation or vitritis. Retinal examination shows multifocal, white lesions deep in the retina or choroid which rapidly progress to a confluent full thickness retinal necrosis showing the characteristic cracked mud pattern. Though clinically these appear as outer retinal lesions, histopathological analysis suggests the inner retina may be a primary site of injury [37]. Many patients have bilateral disease at presentation [38], and those with unilateral disease typically progress to bilateral involvement quickly. Antecedent history or evidence of a herpes infection may or may not occur and is not necessary for the diagnosis. There is no gender predilection for PORN, and rare cases have been reported in the pediatric literature indicating this retinitis may affect all age groups.

PCR testing for PORN, like ARN, has assisted in diagnostic confirmation and clarification on the underlying organism. Overwhelmingly, varicella zoster virus is identified from ocular fluid in patients with active PORN.

Patients are severely immunocompromised and nearly all have AIDS; a few exceptional cases have occurred in patients following allogenic bone marrow transplantation [39–41] or undergoing aggressive chemotherapy for metastatic cancer [39]. The degree of underlying immune dysfunction is high regardless of the underlying etiology. Case reports prior to the HAART era indicated that patients with PORN typically have a CD4 count of <50cells/mm3) [42–44].

The visual prognosis is exceptionally poor in these patients with most failing to achieve better than counting fingers (CF) vision [45]. However, there has been improvement in visual outcomes reported in the intravitreal antiviral era with a decreased number of eyes losing all light perception (13 %) [45] compared with the initial case series reported by Engstrom et al. [42] where 90 % of patients degraded to no light perception (NLP) vision.

Treatment Options

PORN is a difficult to treat effectively. Even implementing immediate and aggressive treatment with systemic and intravitreal antiviral agents, the visual prognosis remains extremely poor. Given the relative rarity of this disorder, coupled with the advent of the highly active antiretroviral therapy (HAART) era rendering severe immunocompromised state less common, there is no clear consensus on treatment. There are no definitive treatment guidelines nor prospective case controlled series to guide optimal therapy. Most treatment paradigms originate from small case series in the peer-reviewed literature. These, combined with data from series of ARN patients, suggest combination therapy with multiple systemic antivirals and intravitreal injections (e.g., Foscarnet) as the most rational therapeutic approach.

Most patients are hospitalized for intravenous antiviral treatment due to the severity of this disease, rapid progression of vision loss, degree of systemic immunosuppression and frequent medical comorbidities. Induction therapy with intravenous (IV) medications, typically acyclovir (10 mg/kg every 8 h), Gancyclovir (5 mg/kg twice daily) or IV Foscarnet (90 mg/kg twice daily) alone or in combination will serve as the initial systemic treatment [43, 44, 46–49]. IV therapy is transitioned to oral maintenance therapy with Valacyclovir after 3–5 days [50, 51].

Intravitreal injections are commonly used as adjuvant therapy at the time of diagnosis, and there is steadily increasing evidence indicating these injections are a key element of the treatment approach [38, 46, 51, 52]. In spite of this trend, the outcome of therapy remains universally discouraging.

The rate of detachment is quite high in patients with PORN, with occurrence rates reported at >85 % [45]. Patients on HAART are less likely to detach than those who were not [45]. Like ARN, these detachments have proven difficult to repair due to the combined mechanism of traction and retinal breaks which require a combination of pars plana vitrectomy, silicone oil tamponade, and endolaser to offer an anatomically acceptable outcome.

Patients with HIV and PORN most commonly have CD4 counts of <50; initiation or reinstitution of HAART is critical for effective treatment. As the immune system is reconstituted, intravitreal injections, and systemic antivirals are gradually tapered off using clinical exam and CD4 counts to help guide these decisions. Again, no clear guidelines exist for reducing antivirals. There likely is a threshold CD4 count at which the immune system is able to effectively control the virus, but the threshold remains unclear at this time [51].

Summary

In summary, the herpes virus family are ubiquitous in the population and can manifest as a wide spectrum of eye disease involving both the anterior and posterior segment. Presentation often depends on the virus isolate and the immune status of the patient involved. Diagnosis can be established rapidly due to the availability of PCR and the ease and safety of performing in office anterior or vitreous taps to obtain specimens. This should allow for an expedited diagnosis in patients with atypical clinical presentations. However, it is important to maintain a high clinical suspicion for herpes virus associated disorders to efficiently diagnose and effectively treat these conditions.

References

1. Thygeson P, Hogan MJ, Kimura SJ. Observations on uveitis associated with viral disease. Trans Am Ophthalmol Soc. 1957;55:333.
2. O'Connor GF. Recurrent herpes simplex uveitis in humans. Surv Ophthalmol. 1976;21:165–70.
3. Jap A, Chee S. Viral Anterior Uveitis. Curr Opin Ophthal. 2011;22(6):483–8.
4. Sungur GK, Hazirolan D, Yalvac IS, et al. Incidence and prognosis of ocular hypertension secondary to viral uveitis. Int Ophthalmol. 2010;30:191–4.
5. Tugal-Tutkun I, Otük-Yasar B, Altinkurt E. Clinical features and prognosis of herpetic anterior uveitis: a retrospective study of 111 cases. Int Ophthalmol. 2010;30:559–65.
6. Barron BA, Gee L, Hauck WW, et al. Herpetic eye disease study: a controlled trial of oral acyclovir for herpes simplex stromal keratitis. Ophthalmology. 1994;101:1871–82.
7. Wilhelmus KR, Gee L, Hauck WW, Kurinij N, Dawson CR, Jones DB, Barron BA, Kaufman HE, Sugar J, Hyndiuk RA, Laibson PR. Herpetic eye disease study: a controlled trial of topical corticosteroids for herpes simplex stromal keratitis. Ophthalmology. 1994;101(12):1883–96.
8. Van Roois J, Rigneveld W, Remeijer L, et al. Effect of oral acyclovir after penetrating keratoplasty for herpetic keratitis: a placebo-controlled multicenter trial. Ophthalmology. 2003;110:1916–9.
9. Rapauno C, Azari A. What's Ahead in Cornea. Medscape. December 9th 2013.
10. Virus VZ. Herpes zoster overview: natural history and incidence. J Am Osteopath Assoc. 2009;109(2): S2–6.
11. Hope-Simpson RE. The nature of herpes zoster: a long-term study and a new hypothesis. Proc R Soc Med. 1965;58:9–20.
12. Yamamoto S, Pavan-Langston D, Tada R, et al. Possible role of herpes simplex virus in the origin of Posner-Schlossman syndrome. Am J Ophthalmol. 1995;119:796–8.
13. Anwar Z, Galor A, Albini TA, Miller D, Perez V, Davis JL. The diagnostic utility of anterior chamber paracentesis with polymerase chain reaction in anterioruveitis. Am J Ophthalmol. 2013;155 (5):781–6.
14. Urayama A, Yamada N, Sasaki T, et al. Unilateral acute uveitis with retinal periarteritis and detachment. Jpn J Clin Ophthalmol. 1971;25:607.
15. Culbertson WW, Blumenkranz MS, Haines H, Gass DM, Mitchell KB, Norton EW. The acute retinal necrosis syndrome. Part 2: histopathology and etiology. Ophthalmology. 1982;89(12):1317–25.
16. Young NJ, Bird AC. Bilateral acute retinal necrosis. Br J Ophthalmol. 1978;62(9):581–90.
17. Sternberg P, Knox DL, Finkelstein D, Green WR, Murphy RP, Patz A. Acute retinal necrosis syndrome. Retina. 1982;2(3):145–51.
18. Fisher JP, Lewis ML, Blumenkranz M, Culbertson WW, Flynn HW Jr, Clarkson JG, Gass JD, Norton EW. The acute retinal necrosis syndrome. Part 1: Clinical manifestations. Ophthalmology. 1982;89(12):1309–16.
19. Holland GN. Standard diagnostic criteria for the acute retinal necrosis syndrome. Executive committee of the American Uveitis society. Am J Ophthalmol. 1994;117(5):663–7.
20. Sugita S, Shimizu N, Watanabe K, Mizukami M, Morio T, Sugamoto Y, Mochizuki M. Use of multiplex PCR and real-time PCR to detect human herpes virus genome in ocular fluids of patients with uveitis. Br J Ophthalmol. 2008;92(7):928–32.
21. Sugita S, Ogawa M, Shimizu N, Morio T, Ohguro N, Nakai K, Maruyama K, Nagata K, Takeda A, Usui Y, Sonoda KH, Takeuchi M, Mochizuki M. Use of a comprehensive polymerase chain reaction system for diagnosis of ocular infectious diseases. Ophthalmology. 2013;120(9):1761–8.
22. Tran TH, Rozenberg F, Cassoux N, Rao NA, LeHoang P. Bodaghi B Polymerase chain reaction

analysis of aqueous humour samples in necrotising retinitis. Br J Ophthalmol. 2003;87(1):79–83.
23. Wensing B, de Groot-Mijnes JD, Rothova A. Necrotizing and nonnecrotizing variants of herpetic uveitis with posterior segment involvement. Arch Ophthalmol. 2011;129(4):403–8.
24. Tibbetts MD, Shah CP, Young LH, Duker JS, Maguire JI, Morley MG. Treatment of acute retinal necrosis. Ophthalmology. 2010;117(4):818–24.
25. Palay DA, Sternberg P, Davis J, Lewis H, Holland GN, Mieler WF, Jabs DA, Drews C. Decrease in the risk of bilateral acute retinal necrosis by acyclovir therapy. Am J Ophthalmol. 1991;112(3):250–5.
26. Aizman A, Johnson MW, Elner SG. Treatment of acute retinal necrosis syndrome with oral antiviral medications. Ophthalmology. 2007;114:307–12.
27. Aslanides IM, Giavedoni LR, Altomare F, Detorakis ET, Kymionis GD, Pallikaris IG. Oral valacyclovir in the treatment of acute retinal necrosis syndrome. Retina. 2002;22:352–4.
28. Emerson GG, Smith JR, Wilson DJ, Rosenbaum JT, Flaxel CJ. Primary treatment of acute retinal necrosis with oral antiviral therapy. Ophthalmology. 2006;113:2259–61.
29. Figueroa MS, Garabito I, Gutierrez C, Fortun J. Famciclovir for the treatment of acute retinal necrosis (ARN) syndrome. Am J Ophthalmol. 1997;123:255–7.
30. Garner HR, Latkany P. Oral drugs for viral retinitis Ophthalmology. 2007;114:2368.
31. Huynh TH, Johnson MW, Comer GM, Fish DN. Vitreous penetration of orally administered valacyclovir. Am J Ophthalmol. 2008;145:682–8.
32. Luu KK, Scott IU, Chaudhry NA, Verm A, Davis JL. Intravitreal antiviral injections as adjunctive therapy in the management of immunocompetent patients with necrotizing herpetic retinopathy. Am J Ophthalmol. 2000;129(6):811–3.
33. Flaxel CJ, Yeh S, Lauer AK. Combination systemic and intravitreal antiviral therapy in the management of acute retinal necrosis syndrome (an American Ophthalmological Society thesis). Trans Am Ophthalmol Soc. 2013;111:133–44.
34. Wong R, Pavesio CE, Laidlaw DA, Williamson TH, Graham EM, Stanford MR. Acute retinal necrosis: the effects of intravitreal foscarnet and virus type on outcome. Ophthalmology. 2010;117(3):556–60.
35. Lau CH, Missotten T, Salzmann J. Lightman S. Acute retinal necrosis features, management, and outcomes Ophthalmology. 2007;114:756–62.
36. Forster D, Dugel P, Frangieh G, Liggett P, Rao N. Rapidly progressive outer retinal necrosis in the acquired immunodeficiency syndrome. Am J Ophthalmol. 1990;110(4):341–8.
37. Gore DM, Gore SK, Visser L. Progressive outer retinal necrosis: outcomes in the intravitreal era. Arch ophthalmol. 2012;130(6):700–6.
38. Scott I, Luu K, Davis J. Intravitreal antivirals in the management of patients with acquired immunodeficiency syndrome with progressive outer retinal necrosis. Arch Ophthalmol. 2002;120(9):1219–22.
39. Lewis JM, Nagae Y, Tano Y. Progressive outer retinal necrosis after bone marrow transplantation. Am J Ophthalmol. 1996;122(6):892–5.
40. Kalpoe JS, van Dehn CE, Bollemeijer JG, Vaessen N, Claas EC, Barge RM, Willemze R, Kroes AC, Beersma MF. Varicella zoster virus (VZV)- related progressive outer retinal necrosis (PORN) after allogenic stem cell transplantation. Bone Marrow Transplant. 2005;36(5):467–9.
41. Khot A, Dignan F, Taylor S, Potter M, Cubitt D, Treleaven JG. Another case of PORN (bilateral progressive outer retinal necrosis) after allogeneic stem celltransplantation. Bone Marrow Transplant. 2006;37(1):113–4.
42. Engstrom RE Jr, Holland GN, Margolis TP, Muccioli C, Lindley JI, Belfort R Jr, Holland SP, Johnston WH, Wolitz RA, Kreiger AE. The progressive outer retinal necrosis syndrome. A variant of necrotizing herpetic retinopathy in patients with AIDS, Ophthalmology. 1994;101(9):1488–502.
43. Moorthy RS, Weinberg DV, Teich SA, Berger BB, Minturn JT, Kumar S, Rao NA, Fowell SM, Loose IA, Jampol LM. Management of varicella zoster virus retinitis in AIDS. Br J Ophthalmol. 1997;81(3):189–94.
44. Ormerod LD, Larkin JA, Margo CA, Pavan PR, Menosky MM, Haight DO, Nadler JP, Yangco BG, Friedman SM, Schwartz R, Sinnott JT. Rapidly progressive herpetic retinal necrosis: a blinding disease characteristic of advanced AIDS. Clin Infect Dis. 1998;26(1):34–45.
45. Gore DM, Gore SK, Visser L. Progressive outer retinal necrosis: outcomes in the intravitreal era. Archives of ophthalmology. 2012;130(6):700–6.
46. Blair MP, Goldstein DA, Shapiro MJ. Optical coherence tomography of progressive outer retinal necrosis. Retina. 2007;27(9):1313–4.
47. Galindez OA, Sabates NR, Whitacre MM, Sabates FN. Rapidly progressive outer retinal necrosis caused by varicella zoster virus in a patient infected with human immunodeficiency virus. Clin Infect Dis. 1996;22(1):149–51.
48. Kuppermann BD, Quiceno JI, Wiley C, Hesselink J, Hamilton R, Keefe K, Garcia R, Freeman WR. Clinical and histopathologic study of varicella zoster virus retinitis in patients with the acquired immunodeficiency syndrome. Am J Ophthalmol. 1994;118 (5):589–600.
49. Morley MG, Duker JS, Zacks C. Successful treatment of rapidly progressive outer retinal necrosis in the acquired immunodeficiency syndrome. Am J Ophthalmol. 1994;117(2):264–5.

50. Peck R, Gimple SK, Gregory DW, Youree B. Progressive outer retinal necrosis in a 73-year-old man: treatment with valganciclovir. AIDS. 2003;17 (7):1110–1.
51. Yin P, Kurup S, Fischer S, Rhee H, Bymes G, Levy-Clarke G, Buggage R, Nussenblatt R, Mican J, Wright M. Progressive outer retinal necrosis in the era of highly active antiretroviral therapy: Successful management with intravitreal injections and monitoring with quantitative PCR. J Clin Virol. 2007;38 (3):254–9 Epub 2007 Feb 5.
52. Roig-Melo E, Macky T, Heredia-Elizondo M, Alfaro D. Progressive outer retinal necrosis syndrome: successful treatment with a new combination of antiviral drugs. Eur J Ophthalmol. 2001;11 (2):200–2.

Human Immunodeficiency Virus

7

Nathan Scott

Introduction

Human Immunodeficiency Virus (HIV) causes an infection that is spread through certain body fluids and attacks the body's immune system. Specifically, the virus infects and destroys T Cells (CD4 + T cells) that the body uses to fight off infections. Despite advances in treatment, HIV remains an epidemic that has tremendous human, social, and economic impact around the world. According to the CDC, approximately 36.9 million people in the world were living with HIV at the end of 2014—17.1 %, or over 6.3 million, of whom did not know they were infected [1]. The CDC estimates nearly 2 million new infections a year.

The disease is characterized by an early stage (which may or may not occur in everyone), a latency stage, and progression to advanced disease or AIDS (acquired immunodeficiency syndrome). The early stage includes flu-like symptoms—fever, chills, rash, night sweats, muscles aches, sore throat, fatigue, swollen lymph nodes, and/or mouth ulcers—and can last anywhere from a few days to weeks. The latency stage, where viral replication is low, may have little to no symptoms at all. Finally, advanced infection, or AIDS, occurs when CD4 + cell count is below 200 cells per microliter and is exemplified by rapid weight loss, fever or profuse night sweats, fatigue, prolonged lymph node swelling, diarrhea, mouth/anus/genital sores, memory loss, depression, and/or red to purple blotches under the skin, mouth, nose, or eyelids. Ocular manifestations can occur at any stage of the disease; but most commonly occurs in advanced AIDS (CD4 + <50 cells per microliter).

Ocular Manifestations

Ocular manifestations can occur in up to 70–80 % of untreated HIV infected persons—more than half of which are associated with uveitis [2]. However, the prevalence of HIV-associated uveitis in the HIV or AIDS population is not known. Regardless, it is important to note that uveitis can occur in any stage of HIV infection and is caused by a number of distinct etiologies. Importantly, the characteristics of the uveal involvement reflect the pathology of the inciting disease process. The most common conditions causing uveitis in HIV infected persons are opportunistic infections (Cytomegalovirus [1, 3], Herpes zoster ophthalmicus, toxoplasmosis, etc.), but can also occur with ocular neoplasms associated with HIV, inflammation secondary to the

N. Scott (✉)
Massachuetts General Hospital, 55 Fruit Street, Boston, MA 02114, USA
e-mail: nathan.scott0434@gmail.com

G.N. Papaliodis (ed.), *Uveitis*,
DOI 10.1007/978-3-319-09126-6_7

HIV infection itself, HIV drug toxicity, or paradoxically, inflammatory dysregulation during the recovery of the immune system from HIV therapy (Immune Recovery Uveitis, IRU).

Anterior, posterior, and panuveitis have all been described in association with the various conditions causing uveitis in HIV. Anterior uveitis is typically seen with herpetic infections (Varicella Zoster Virus and Herpes Simplex Virus). It occurs with any CD4 + count and is commonly unilateral. It can often be associated with concurrent dermatitis, blepharoconjunctivitis, keratitis, or encephalitis. Patients can have decreased corneal sensation, elevated intraocular pressure, or patchy/sectoral iris atrophy [4, 5]. HIV drug toxicities also typically manifest with anterior uveitis. In particular, Cidofovir and Rifabutin, cause dose related inflammation when CD4 + count is less than 50 cells per microliter. The two drugs have subtle differences in that Cidofovir is granulomatous, associated with synechiae, can cause hypotony, and is more common in eyes with inactive CMV retinints; while Rifabutin is nongranulomatous, can be associated with hypopyon and is more common with concurrent antifungals and/or protease inhibitor use [6–9].

Posterior segment disease is the most common form of uveitis in HIV [10]. Necrotizing herpetic retinitis (CMV, VZV, HSV), occurs with CD4 + counts of less than 50 cells per microliter. CMV, the most prevalent opportunistic infection, presents with one or two active foci of retinitis and vitreous inflammation [11]. VZV and HSV retinitis (less than 5 % of HIV + patients) present more rapidly and with confluent areas of retinitis [12]. Toxoplasmic retinochoroiditis (~10 % of HIV + patients), occurs with CD4 + counts less than 250 cells per microliter. It typically presents with a single focus of retinitis adjacent to chorioretinal scars and is often unilateral [13]. Intraocular lymphoma can cause vitritis, retinitis, or retinal vasculitis with insidious onset in patients with CD4 + counts less than 50 cells per microliter [14]. Immune recovery uveitis, or paradoxical inflammation with reconstitution of CD4 + counts during therapy, most often occurs in eyes with inactive CMV retinitis. Inflammation of the vitreous is typical, but can involve the anterior chamber as well. Complications that have been described include macular edema, epiretinal membrane formation, vitreomacular traction syndrome, retinal neovascularization, and cataract [15–17]. Uveitis that is caused directly by inflammation of the virus itself also occurs at CD4 + counts less than 50 cells per microliter. Distinctly, it is typically moderate and examination reveals a lack of active retinitis [18].

Isolated choroiditis is most commonly seen with two types of infections: Pneumocystis carinii choroiditis and Cryptococcal choroiditis. Pneumocystis is typically bilateral, has multifocal choroid lesions, is associated with some vitreous inflammation but there is limited retinal hemorrhage. Cryptococcal infection presents similarly, but is associated with retinal hemorrhage and can have meningeal involvement.

Laboratory Testing

Laboratory tests used to identify the cause of uveitis in HIV + patients should complement the history and physical exam. After a thorough history is obtained to identify exposures and past medical events, followed by a physical exam that characterizes the laterality, severity, and anatomic structures involved in the disease process, CD4 + count can narrow the differential. If infectious processes are highest on the differential, serologic, or vitreous sampling is typically available (PCR, antibody analysis, culture, etc.). Neoplastic etiologies require biopsy and histologic analysis, while drug toxicities and IRU require an astute clinician to recognize the possibility of these complications. It is also important to evaluate for the causes of uveitis in HIV negative patients, especially if a patient presents with adequate CD4 + reconstitution. Specifically, sarcoidosis (10–20 % of all uveitis in adults) is screened for with a chest X-ray and serum angiotensin-converting enzyme. Syphilis and TB should also be tested for using serum antibody analysis and the Mantoux test, respectively.

Treatment

Treatment of uveitis in HIV + patients is specific to the etiology of the inciting disease process. The mainstay of therapy for both opportunistic infections and direct viral inflammation is maintaining immune reconstitution. This is achieved by ensuring adequate anti-retroviral therapy. However, targeted antimicrobial and/or antiviral therapies should be initiated as soon as possible if uveitis is identified in patients with low CD4 + counts. Antineoplastic therapy should be guided by histopathologic evaluation. If drug toxicity remains high on the differential, anti-retroviral regiments can be altered to discontinue/replace uveitis-associated medications while maintaining adequate anti-retroviral coverage—an infectious disease specialist should direct this management.

IRU therapy remains a challenge because the pathophysiology is not completely understood. The anterior chamber is treated with topical corticosteroids, but may also be observed overtime without treatment in mild cases. More severe infections are treated with systemic corticosteroids, but clinicians must be careful because HIV + patients are immunocompromised due to their underlying disease process. Further insults may lead to more severe infections. Intravitreal corticosteroids are also used in IRU, however appropriate risk assessment must take place prior to initiating therapy. Risks include glaucoma, reactivation of retinitis, cataracts, and/or recurrence of CMV retinitis. To this end, all corticosteroid management should be accompanied by empiric anti-CMV therapy [19].

Finally, recent studies have shown that complications of severe uvetitis (i.e., macular edema) can be effectively treated using intraocular methotrexate and anti-VEGF agents [20].

Conclusion

Human immunodeficiency virus/acquired immunodeficiency syndrome (HIV/AIDS) is an infectious disease process that not only limits the body's ability to ward off infection, but also compromises innate inflammatory regulation. Ophthalmic disease can manifest in a number of ways in HIV + patients, most commonly during opportunistic infection. Nearly half of the ophthalmic manifestations in HIV can be associated with uveitis. Diagnosis is established after a thorough history is obtained to identify exposures and past medical events, followed by a physical exam that characterizes the laterality, severity, and anatomic structures involved in the disease process, and ultimately serologic, tissue, or vitreous sampling (PCR, antibody analysis, culture, etc.). The inciting disease process defines treatment—antimicrobials, antivirals, antineoplastic, and corticosteroids are the mainstays of therapy.

References

1. CDC website. https://www.aids.gov/hiv-aids-basics/hiv-aids-101/global-statistics/index.html.
2. Cunningham ET Jr, Margolis TP. Ocular manifestations of HIV infection. N Engl J Med. 1998;339:236–44.
3. Jacobson MA. Treatment of cytomegalovirus retinitis in patients with the acquired immunodeficiency syndrome. N Engl J Med. 1997;337:105–14.
4. Cunningham ET Jr, Margolis TP. Ocular manifestations of HIV infection. N Engl J Med. 1998;339:236–44.
5. Margolis TP, Milner MS, Shama A, Hodge W, Seiff S. Herpes zoster ophthalmicus in patients with human immunodeficiency virus infection. Am J Ophthalmol. 1998;125(3):285–91.
6. Nichols CW. Mycobacterium avium complex infection, rifabutin, and uveitis—is there a connection? Clin Infect Dis. 1996;22(Suppl 1):S43–7.
7. Davis JL, Taskintuna I, Freeman WR, Weinberg DV, Feuer WJ, Leonard RE. Iritis and hypotony after treatment with intravenous cidofovir for cytomegalovirus retinitis. Arch Ophthalmol. 1997;115(6):733–7.
8. Akler ME, Johnson DW, Burman WJ, Johnson SC. Anterior uveitis and hypotony after intravenous cidofovir for the treatment of cytomegalovirus retinitis. Ophthalmology. 1998;105(4):651–7.
9. Ambati J, Wynne KB, Angerame MC, et al. Anterior uveitis associated with intravenous cidofovir use in patients with cytomegalovirus retinitis. Br J Ophthalmol. 1999;83:1153–8.
10. Cunningham ET Jr, Margolis TP. Ocular manifestations of HIV infection. N Engl J Med. 1998;339:236–44.

11. Jacobson MA. Treatment of cytomegalovirus retinitis in patients with the acquired immunodeficiency syndrome. N Engl J Med. 1997;337(2):105–14.
12. Margolis TP, Milner MS, Shama A, et al. Herpes zoster ophthalmicus in patients with human immunodeficiency virus infection. Am J Ophthalmol. 1998;125:285–91.
13. Holland GN, Engstrom RE Jr, Glasgow BJ, et al. Ocular toxoplasmosis in patients with the acquired immunodeficiency syndrome. Am J Ophthalmol. 1988;106(6):653–67.
14. Rivero ME, Kuppermann BD, Wiley CA, Garcia CR, Smith MD, Dreilinger A, Freeman WR. Acquired immunodeficiency syndrome–related intraocular B-cell lymphoma. Arch Ophthalmol. 1999;117 (5):616–22.
15. Zegans ME, Walton RC, Holland GN, et al. Transient vitreous inflammatory reactions associated with combination antiretroviral therapy in patients with AIDS and cytomegalovirus retinitis. Am J Ophthalmol. 1998;125:292–300.
16. Karavellas MP, Lowder CY, Macdonald C, et al. Immune recovery vitritis associated with inactive cytomegalovirus retinitis: a new syndrome. Arch Ophthalmol. 1998;116:169–75.
17. Karavellas MP, Plummer DJ, Macdonald JC, et al. Incidence of immune recovery vitritis in cytomegalovirus retinitis patients following institution of successful highly active antiretroviral therapy. J Infect Dis. 1999;179:697–700.
18. Rosberger DF, Heinemann MH, Friedberg DN, et al. Uveitis associated with human immunodeficiency virus infection. Am J Ophthalmol. 1998;125:301–5.
19. Holland GN. AIDS and ophthalmology: the first quarter century. Am J Ophthalmol. 2008;145 (3):397–408.
20. Modorati G, Miserocchi E. Intravitreal injection therapy in the treatment of noninfectious uveitis. Dev Opthalmol. 2012;51:110–21.

Measles

8

Milka C. Nova

Introduction

Measles (also called rubeola) is a single-stranded RNA virus of the genus *Morbilivirus* in the *Paramyxoviridae* family [1]. Humans and apes are the only natural host, and the disease can be contracted congenitally or acquired. The virus is highly contagious via aerosolized droplets and can cause the development of a generalized rash lasting greater than 3 days, fever greater than 101, cough, coryza, severe diarrhea, encephalitis, and pneumonia. Measles can be a fatal illness in young children. Due to the high vaccination rates in the United States, measles has not been widespread for over a decade, but it remains a significant cause of mortality worldwide among children younger than 5 years old responsible for more than 100,000 deaths annually [2]. Even in the US, 5–8 % of the population remains unvaccinated [3] due to religious convictions, parental apathy, misinformation, and contraindications.

M.C. Nova (✉)
Immunology Uveitis Service, MEEI,
243 Charles Street, Boston, MA 02114, USA
e-mail: Milka_Nova@meei.harvard.edu

G.N. Papaliodis (ed.), *Uveitis*,
DOI 10.1007/978-3-319-09126-6_8

Epidemiology

The number of measles cases has declined in United States as a result of a highly effective vaccine available since 1963 and a nationwide vaccination program implemented in 1965 [4]. Due to the low incidence of measles in adults, congenital measles rates have similarly plummeted since the advent of the vaccine.

Clinical Presentation

The clinical manifestations of acquired measles include fever greater than 101, conjunctivitis, cough, sore throat, coryza, small spots with white center on an erythematous base on the buccal mucosa (Koplik spots), and a characteristic red, blotchy maculopapular rash, beginning on the face and then becoming generalized [1].

The signs and symptoms typically ensue approximately 10–14 days after exposure to the virus. Patients develop fever and malaise, followed by cough, coryza, and conjunctivitis. As these symptoms intensify, Koplik spots develop in the buccal mucosa which is pathognomonic for measles. These consist of blue-white dots ~1 mm in diameter surrounded by an erythematous base. As the Koplik spots fade, the maculopapular rash develops.

The most dreaded and serious complication of measles is central nervous system involvement with acute encephalitis. Although this occurs in approximately 0.1 % of cases, the mortality can be as high as 20 %. Of those who survive, 20–50 % suffer from permanent neurologic damage. Subacute sclerosing panencephalitis (SSPE) is rare chronic, progressive encephalitis that affects primarily children and young adults caused by a persistent infection with measles virus.

An ocular manifestation of acquired measles includes a papillary, non-purulent conjunctivitis that is typically mild [5]. The conjunctivitis may be associated with the development of pseudomembranes. Epithelial keratitis (present in 76 % of patients) is the most common ocular manifestation of acquired measles [6]. Koplik spots on the conjunctiva (also called Hirschberg spots) are rarely present. There may be a transient, mild anterior uveitis during the acute phase of illness which may accompany the other anterior segment findings [7]. Measles retinopathy has rarely been described manifested by diffuse retinal edema, scattered retinal hemorrhages, and macular edema.

Congenital measles infection manifests as cardiomyopathy, pyloric stenosis, hearing dysfunction, vertebral anomalies, cleft lip, and palate. The ocular manifestations include cataract, optic nerve head drusen, and bilateral diffuse pigmentary retinopathy involving both posterior pole and retinal periphery.

Cataracts are the second most common ocular complication affecting approximately 15 % of children [5].

Diagnosis

Congenital measles is diagnosed by the history of maternal infection and by the presence of congenital anomalies (as described above). Acquired measles may be diagnosed via serologic testing demonstrating measles specific IgM. Additionally, PCR of samples obtained from nasopharynx, conjunctiva, lymphoid tissues, respiratory mucous membrane, urine, and blood may identify measles RNA.

Treatment

Measles is a self-limited disease and supportive treatment is usually adequate. In pregnant women, children under age one, and immunocompromised individual, infection may be prevented with prophylactic treatment of immune globulin. The ocular manifestations are treated symptomatically with antibiotics to prevent secondary infections in patient with keratitis or conjunctivitis. In rare cases of acute measles retinopathy, systemic corticosteroids should be considered.

Conclusion

Measles is a highly contagious infection caused by a single-stranded RNA virus of the genus *Morbillivirus* in the *Paramyxoviridae* family. The virus may be transmitted congenitally or acquired via aerosolization of nasopharyngeal secretions to the respiratory mucous membrane of the respiratory tract or through the conjunctiva. The disease is typically self-limited and only requires supportive treatment. The ocular manifestation is treated symptomatically with antibiotics to prevent secondary infections in patients with keratitis or conjunctivitis. In the rare case of acute measles retinopathy, systemic corticosteroids may also be considered.

References

1. Kasper D, Fauci A, Hauser S, Longo D, Jameson JL, Loscalzo J. Harrison's principles of internal medicine. McGraw-Hill Education; 2015. Vol. 15, pp. 1295–9.
2. Fiebelkorn AP, Goodson JL. Measles (Rubeola) infectious diseases related to travel. Center for disease control website. 2015 (10 Sept 2015).

3. Hinman AR, Eddings DL, Kirby CD, et al. Progress in measles elimination. JAMA. 1982;247:1592–5.
4. Centers for Disease Control and Prevention: Measles-United States, 1990. MMWR. 1991;40: 369–72.
5. Nussenblatt RB, Whitcup SM. Other viral diseases. Uveitis fundamentals and clinical practice. 3rd ed. USA: Elsevier; 2004; Vol. 12, p. 212.
6. Fedukowicz HB. Measles. External infections of the eye. 2nd ed. New York: Appleton-Century-Crofts; 1978, pp. 214–6.
7. Bowling B. Kanski's clinical ophthalmology: a systematic approach. Uveitis. 8th ed. USA: Elsevier; 2016; Vol. 11, p. 443.

9 Pneumocystis Jiroveci

George N. Papaliodis

Introduction

Pneumocystis jiroveci (previously *Pneumocystis carinii*) is an opportunistic infection typically limited to the lungs. The organism is a fungus of low virulence that is likely spread through the air. A healthy immune system is able to control and prevent significant disease. Patients who are immunosuppressed (secondary to Human Immunodeficiency Virus, malignancy, chemotherapy, and iatrogenic secondary to steroids and other immunosuppressive agents) can develop a severe and potentially lethal pneumonia (the mortality rate is between 5–40 % even with treatment). Extrapulmonary manifestations of *Pneumocystis* are rare but can involve the liver, bone marrow, lymph nodes, and eyes. The ocular manifestations may be discovered incidentally and typically manifest as subretinal/choroidal yellow to white plaque like lesions.

G.N. Papaliodis (✉)
Department of Ophthalmology, Harvard Medical School, Massachusetts Eye and Ear Infirmary, 243 Charles Street, Boston, MA 02114, USA
e-mail: George_Papaliodis@meei.harvard.edu

G.N. Papaliodis (ed.), *Uveitis*,
DOI 10.1007/978-3-319-09126-6_9

Epidemiology

It has been estimated that in the pre-highly active anti-retroviral therapy (HAART) era, the incidence of *Pneumocystis* associated pneumonia occurred in 70–80 % of patients with HIV, and *Pneumocystis* associated choroiditis was diagnosed in approximately 1 % of HIV patients with CD4 counts less than 200 [1]. The choroidal involvement was more commonly diagnosed in those who were on prophylactic therapy with aerosolized pentamidine (presumably inhaled prophylaxis was inadequate to prevent disseminated disease). In one case series by Shami et al., 76 % of the cases were bilateral [2]. Since the advent of HAART therapy and routine prophylaxis with Trimethoprim/Sulfamethoxazole (TMP/SMX), the rates of *Pneumocystis* and associated choroiditis have plummeted.

Clinical Manifestations

The typical exam findings of ocular pneumocystosis are unifocal or multifocal (ranging from 2 to 50) yellow-white flat choroidal lesions predominantly involving the posterior pole. Few patients have visual symptoms despite having extensive choroidal lesions [3]. Fluorescein angiography of the lesions demonstrates early hypofluorescence and homogenous late staining

[2]. There is generally no inflammation of the anterior chamber or vitreous.

Diagnosis

The diagnosis is often presumptive by identifying the characteristic fundus findings (yellow-white flat choroidal lesions) in patients with CD4 counts less than 200 or other high-risk criteria (chronic immunosuppression, malignancy, etc.). Although rarely performed due to risk of retinal complications, the diagnosis can be confirmed via chorioretinal biopsy demonstrating the characteristic cysts on toluidine blue or silver staining. More recently, quantitative polymerase chain reaction (qPCR) testing on bronchoalveolar lavage (BAL) specimens has been used to detect *Pneumocystis* DNA [4]. If validated, this type of testing may similarly be used on vitreous specimens.

Treatment

Pneumocystis choroidopathy requires systemic treatment as the ocular findings are a manifestation of disseminated infection. While officially classified as a fungal organism, *P. jiroveci* does not respond to antifungal therapy. The treatment of choice is TMP/SMX (dosing is TMP 15 mg/kg/day given for 21 days). Secondary agents include Pentamidine, Dapsone, and Atovaquone.

Conclusion

P. jiroveci is a rare disseminated opportunistic fungal infection that can manifest as choroidal infiltrates. The advent of HAART and prophylactic use of TMP/SMX has markedly reduced the incidence of this condition.

References

1. Goldberg DE, Smithen LM, Angelilli A, Freeman WR. HIV-associated retinopathy in the HAART era. Retina. 2005;25(5):633.
2. Shami MJ, Freeman WR, Friedberg D, Siderides E, Listhaus A, Ai E. A multicenter study of Pneumocystis choroidopathy. Am J Ophthalmol. 1991;112:15–22.
3. Foster RE, Lowder CY, Meisler DM, Huang SS, Longworth DL. Presumed Pneumocystis carinii choroiditis. Unifocal presentation, regression with intravenous pentamidine, and choroiditis recurrence. Ophthalmology. 1991;98(9):1360–5.
4. Fan LC1, Lu HW, Cheng KB, Li HP, Xu JF. Evaluation of PCR in bronchoalveolar lavage fluid for diagnosis of *Pneumocystis jirovecii* pneumonia: a bivariate meta-analysis and systematic review. PLoS One. 2013;8(9):e73099.

Presumed Ocular Histoplasmosis Syndrome

10

Lindsay Grotting

Introduction

Histoplasmosis is caused when airborne spores of the fungus *Histoplasma capsulatum* are inhaled. The lungs are the primary infection site. Unless it occurs in immunocompromised patients in whom it may mimic tuberculosis, systemic histoplasmosis often displays very mild symptoms and may even be asymptomatic. Usually occurring in children, it causes fever and malaise similar to the common cold or flu. However, despite these mild symptoms with initial infection, it can cause profound vision loss years later [1].

Presumed ocular histoplasmosis (POHS) is a choroidopathy, typically characterized by atrophic chorioretinal scars, peripapillary atrophy, and the absence of vitritis. POHS may or may not be associated with choroidal neovascularization (CNV), the primary reason for decreased vision in these patients. Rarely, histoplasmosis also can cause a histoplasmic endophthalmitis or a solitary histoplasmic chorioretinal granuloma [2]. The endophthalmitis form usually occurs in patients with disseminated histoplasmosis, and it lacks the classic lesions seen in POHS [3]. The solitary granuloma, also known as a histoplasmoma, may mimic toxocariasis and is usually seen in immunocompromised individuals.

Etiology

Over the past years, the exact origin of the disease has been debated. The most common theory is that POHS is caused by the yeast form of *H. capsulatum.* This has been demonstrated mostly by epidemiological studies. Hence the term *presumed. Histoplasma capsulatum* is a dimorphic fungus found in the soil, usually near the Ohio and Mississippi River Valleys. The fungus is strongly resistant to temperature and humidity extremes. Bird feathers of chickens, pigeons, and blackbirds carry the fungus. Bird and bat excretions have also been found to harbor the fungus. Infection occurs when the yeast is inhaled.

Reid et al. first described POHS in 1942 when a patient dying of disseminated histoplasmosis was described to have certain ocular findings [4]. Subsequently, Krause and Hopkins described a patient with atrophic chorioretinal lesions associated with a positive histoplasmin skin test and a chest X-ray showing lung nodules [5]. Later, Woods and Whalen reported a case series, describing patients with ocular lesions and

L. Grotting (✉)
Department of Ophthalmology, Massachusetts Eye and Ear Infirmary, 243 Charles St., Boston, MA 02114, USA
e-mail: lindsay.grotting@gmail.com

G.N. Papaliodis (ed.), *Uveitis*,
DOI 10.1007/978-3-319-09126-6_10

macular cysts [6]. All of these patients were noted to live in an area endemic for *H. capsulatum* and showed evidence of prior systemic infection with histoplasmosis such as calcified lung nodules. All of the patients had a positive histoplasmin skin antigen test, signifying a strong correlation between POHS and *H. capsulatum*.

However, other evidence in the literature refutes such a definite relationship [7]. The failure to actually isolate the fungus from the eye as well as negative histoplasmin skin antigen tests in patients with classic eye findings point toward the possibility of another causative organism. While a few papers do report the isolation of *H. capsulatum* in the eye, most of these patients suffered from disseminated histoplasmosis and lacked the classic ocular findings of POHS. Another study from the Netherlands reported a series of patients demonstrating clinical signs of POHS that all had negative histoplasmin skin antigen tests [8]. Furthermore, some patients reported in the literature with classic POHS findings denied any previous habitation or travel to an endemic area [9].

HLA haplotypes DRw2 and B7 have also been connected to POHS, suggesting that POHS represents an inflammatory reaction triggered against certain organisms, one of these being *H. capsulatum.* HLA-B7 has been associated in patients with disciform scarring. HLA-DRw2 was detected in 81 % of patients with disciform scarring and 62 % of patients with peripheral histo spots [10–12].

Epidemiology

POHS is most commonly found in patients living in the Ohio and Mississippi River Valley. This area is comprised of the following states: Arkansas, Kentucky, Missouri, Tennessee, West Virginia, Alabama, Illinois, Indiana, Iowa, Kansas, Louisiana, Maryland, Mississippi, Nebraska, Ohio, Oklahoma, Texas, and Virginia. This region is also known as the "Histo Belt". In these areas, which are endemic for *H. capsulatum,* around 60–90 % of the adult population have a positive histoplasmin skin antigen test. However, only 1.5 % of patients who test positive for histoplasmin actually demonstrate clinical signs of POHS [13]. Outside the United States, it is found in Central and South America, a small region in Italy, South Africa, and Southeast Asia.

Histopathology

POHS chorioretinal lesions demonstrate no fungal characteristics when examined with light microscopy. Rather, these lesions exhibit different stages of inflammatory activity, such as mixed populations of inflammatory cells with loss of retinal pigment epithelium as well as adhesions between outer retinal and choroidal lesions. Focal aggregations of lymphocytes without disruption of Bruch's membrane may be seen [14–16]. These findings also support that POHS is not caused by an active fungal infection but by an autoimmune response to a specific antigen.

Pathophysiology

The yeast is usually inhaled in the microconidia form (<5 μm in size). It then spreads hematogenously as evidenced by foci of the organism found in the liver and the spleen. When the antigen spreads to the uveal tract, focal choroidal granulomas may result, causing an inflammatory reaction in the choroid. This subsequently leads to a chorioretinal atrophic scar. There may be residual antigen within these scars resulting in a low-grade inflammation that prompts CNV to develop. Also hypothesized is that the infection sensitizes ocular proteins or that the fungal elements are similar in structure to those in the eye, inciting an immune response against the choroid [17].

POHS is able to be replicated in an animal model. Rabbits injected with intracarotid injections of yeast exhibited signs of choroiditis within one to two days in the eye on the side that was injected. Seven to twenty days later, the fellow eye developed lesions without vitreous inflammation similar to those seen in humans with POHS. No yeast organisms were able to be isolated in the healed granulomas after several weeks [18].

At one point, it was thought that histoplasmin skin testing might lead to the reactivation of old macular scars. However, a number of case series failed to demonstrate a clear relationship between the skin test and reactivation.

Risk Factors

Travel to or habitation in the Ohio and Mississippi River Valley is the main factor predisposing patients to POHS. Various activities that may increase inhalation of the fungus include spelunking, bulldozing, cleaning chicken coops, and raking. Patients usually present with symptoms of CNV during the second to fifth decades of life. The age may vary since patients without CNV are usually found to have POHS incidentally on a routine examination. There is no gender predilection. Patients are usually healthy individuals. Only 0.7 % of POHS patients are black, and patients with POHS and CNV tend to be Caucasian [19].

Diagnosis

History

If no CNV is present, POHS is asymptomatic. CNV is what usually brings the patient to medical attention. If CNV is present, patients will report painless vision loss, central scotoma, blurred central vision, and/or metamorphopsia. All patients should be asked details about where they have lived and traveled.

Physical Exam

POHS is a clinical diagnosis. Both eyes should be examined thoroughly because findings are bilateral in up to 60 % of cases [20]. Careful slit lamp and biomicroscopy should be performed

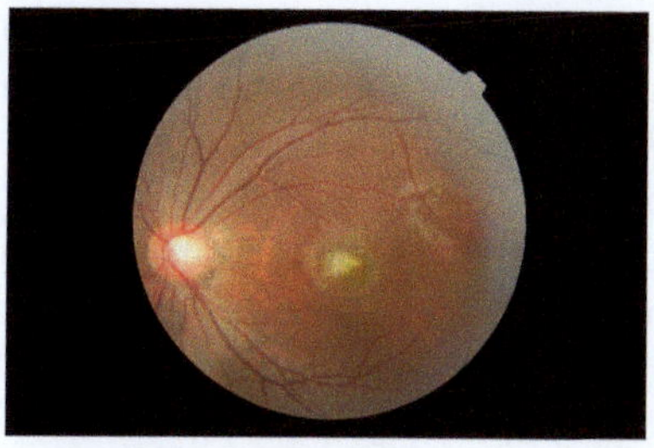

Fig. 10.1 Color fundus photograph of a patient with peripapillary atrophy and macular choroidal neovascular membrane secondary to POHS. There was no vitritis on physical exam

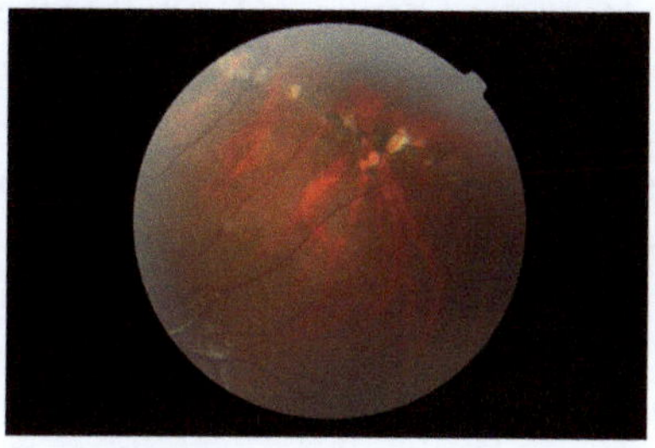

Fig. 10.2 Peripheral retina of patient in Fig. 10.1 demonstrating chorioretinal scarring

while looking for the three classic signs of POHS (see Figs. 10.1 and 10.2):

1. Multiple white atrophic chorioretinal scars (also known as histo spots)
2. Peripapillary atrophy
3. Absence of vitritis

Histo spots are discrete, focal; atrophic choroidal scars found in the posterior pole and the peripheral retina. They appear to be "punched out" of the inner choroid with central pigmentation, ring of pigmentation, or diffuse pigmentation. They may indicate former areas of subclinical CNV that have regressed spontaneously. Linear streaks that are parallel to the ora serrata may be found in around 5 % of patients [21]. These streaks may simply be the coalescence of small linear histo spots. The scars may remain stable but in some patients, they have been documented to grow in size or number [22, 23].

Peripapillary atrophy is more commonly associated with macular scars. About a third of patients with peripheral histo spots will have peripapillary chorioretinal scars versus over two-thirds of patients with macular scarring. The peripapillary atrophy may represent a ring of granulomas that formed during the active stage of the disease [20, 24].

POHS may only be diagnosed in the absence of vitreous cells or anterior inflammation. Pigmented cells should not be confused with inflammatory cells. The lack of cells may be attributed to patients presenting after the active inflammatory stage has passed. Another theory is that since POHS is mainly a choriodopathy, the cells do not reach the vitreous.

These classic POHS findings may or may not be associated with CNV. Active disciform lesions may look like a green-gray subretinal lacy discoloration with surrounding pigment, usually in the macula. It may be related to chorioretinal scars that have a break in Bruch's membrane. CNV usually occurs at the edge of an old scar. A scar in the macula or peripapillary region appears more predisposed to progressing to CNV. However, CNV can also form in the macula where there was previously no scar. If advanced, CNV appears as a white disciform scar with fibrovascular tissue. Rarely, as with age-related macular degeneration, CNV may result in vitreous hemorrhage due to a break in the retina [25].

Diagnostic Procedures

POHS is usually a clinical diagnosis, but fluorescein angiography (FA) can assist in the diagnosis. In areas of chorioretinal atrophy, staining and window defects versus late leakage can be seen with CNV. Defects in the retinal pigment epithelium and patchy loss of the choriocapillaris can be seen. Krill et al. described histo lesions as being hypofluorescent initially but then acquiring a more hyperfluorescent appearance late in the disease [26]. FA can be useful in locating areas of neovascularization if laser treatment is employed for CNV.

The histoplasmin skin antigen test can help determine if the patient has been exposed to *H. capsulatum*. However, since up to two-thirds of patients in endemic areas have a positive skin test, this testing is not routinely performed if the clinical findings are classic.

Differential Diagnosis

Diseases causing granulomas such as tuberculosis, coccidiomycosis, cryptococcosis, and sarcoidosis, should be considered. Careful examination for vitreous inflammation can help distinguish POHS from these other diseases.

Other causes of chorioretinitis must also be considered, including multifocal chorioretinitis, serpiginous choroiditis, birdshot chorioretinopathy, multiple evanescent white dot syndrome, acute multifocal placoid pigment epitheliopathy, toxoplasmosis, toxocariasis, rubella, Vogt-Koyanagi-Harada syndrome, and Behçet syndrome. Most commonly, multifocal choroiditis may be confused with POHS, but again, the absence of vitreous cells in POHS is the key distinguishing feature [27]. PIC lesions may also appear very similar to the chorioretinal scars of POHS, but the PIC scars tend to be small and confined to the posterior pole [28].

Management

Indications

POHS without CNV is monitored with biomicroscopy and the Amsler grid. Since there is no solid evidence of the organism being present in the eye, antifungal treatment such as amphotericin B is not beneficial [29, 30]. When CNV develops in the macula, it is treated similarly as age-related macular degeneration. Peripapillary CNV may be monitored unless it causes prolonged serous or hemorrhagic detachment close to the fovea.

Laser Therapy

The Macular Photocoagulation Study (MPS) evaluated laser photocoagulation for extrafoveal (>200 μm from the center of the foveal avascular zone), juxtafoveal (1–200 μm from the center of the foveal avascular zone), and peripapillary CNV. The MPS found that untreated eyes had 3.6 times the risk of laser treated eyes of losing six or more lines of visual acuity. However, the major complication of this treatment was a permanent scotoma from the laser, limiting its use for subfoveal lesions. Furthermore, 26 % of extrafoveal CNV and 33 % of juxtafoveal CNV recurred at the border of the treatment scar [31, 32].

The Verteporfin for Ocular Histoplasmosis Study examined the use of photodynamic therapy. This looked at photodynamic therapy for subfoveal CNV. The study found that 45 % of patients experienced improved vision, 18 % lost vision, and 9 % of patients suffered severe vision loss at the 2-year follow up. No serious adverse side effects were reported [33, 34].

Surgery

Submacular surgery has been explored for the treatment of subfoveal CNV. Thomas and Kaplan first described techniques to remove subfoveal CNV in POHS patients [35]. Using a small retinotomy with the creation of a neurosensory retinal detachment allowed access to the fibrovascular membrane. There was a significant improvement in their patients without recurrence of CNV. However, these dramatic findings were not duplicated by subsequent studies that employed a larger population and longer follow up. It has been speculated that surgery to remove membranes in POHS patients is more successful than surgery in patients with age-related macular degeneration, because POHS CNV lesions are not as deeply located. The retinal pigment epithelium may also recover and proliferate better given this more superficial location and the fact that most patients are younger than those with age-related macular degeneration. However, as with any vitreoretinal surgery, the risks include cataract, retinal detachment, and lesion recurrence [36–38].

Steroids

In 1977, Schlaegel et al. recommended high dose oral corticosteroids for acute exacerbations of macular CNV. With the advent of anti-VEGF treatment, this practice is not commonly used [39].

Anti-VEGF Agents

Most recently, anti-vascular endothelial growth factor (anti-VEGF) agents such as bevacizumab and ranibizumab have been used in patients with POHS given the success of these treatments for age-related macular degeneration. A recent retrospective study of POHS-associated CNV found that the average visual acuity improved from 20/53 to 20/26 in 54 eyes treated over a 26-month period. The average number of injections was 4.5 over one year [40]. Anti-VEGF agents are now considered first line treatment for patients with POHS and CNV. Risks of anti-VEGF injections include endophthalmitis, subconjunctival hemorrhage, cataract formation, retinal tears, and increased intraocular pressure [41].

Prognosis

Patient with histo spots in one eye have an 8–24 % chance of developing CNV in the fellow eye over 3 years [31, 32]. Complications of CNV include disciform scarring, resulting in loss of central vision. The visual acuity has been reported to be about 20/200 in about half of patients untreated. Spontaneous recovery has been reported but may have been secondary to the development of eccentric vision [42]. However, when CNV is identified early, anti-VEGF treatments can maintain good visual acuity. Patients should be counseled appropriately on their risk of developing macular disease [43].

Prevention

There is no current primary prevention. Patients with clinical signs of POHS should be screened for CNV with routine dilated fundoscopic exams. Patients should monitor disease activity at home with the Amsler grid.

Conclusion

POHS is a choroidopathy, typically characterized by atrophic chorioretinal scars, peripapillary atrophy, and the absence of vitritis. The ocular manifestations are presumably secondary to a complex and poorly defined interaction between the fungal organism *H. capsulatum* and the host immune response. Patients without CNV require monitoring without treatment. When CNV develops in the macula, intraocular anti-VEGF agents are the preferred option for therapy.

References

1. Nussenblatt RB, Whitcup SM, Palestine AG. Ocular histoplasmosis. In Nussenblatt RB et al., editors. Uveitis: fundamentals and clinical practice, 2nd ed. St. Louis: Mosby; 1996.
2. Craig EL, Svie T. *Histoplasma capsulatum* in human ocular tissue. Arch Ophthalmol. 1974;91:285–9.
3. Goldstein BG, Buettuer H. Histoplasmic endophthalmitis: a clinical correlation. Arch Ophthalmol. 1983;101:774.
4. Reid JD, Schere JH, Herbut PA, Irving H. Systemic histoplasmosis diagnosed before death and produced experimentally in guinea pigs. J Lab Clin Med. 1942;27:219–23.
5. Krause AC, Hopkins WG. Ocular manifestations of histoplasmosis. Am J Ophthalmol. 1951;34:564–6.
6. Woods AC, Wahlen HE. The probable role of benign histoplasmosis in the etiology of granulomatous uveitis. Am J Ophthalmol. 1960;49:205–20.
7. Prasad AG, Van Gelder RN. Presumed ocular histoplasmosis syndrome. Curr Opin Ophthalmol. 2005;16:364–8.
8. Ongkosuwito JV, Kortbeek LM, Van der Lelij A, Molicka E, Kijlstra A, de Smet MD, Suttorp-Schulten MS. Aetiological study of the presumed ocular histoplasmosis syndrome in the Netherlands. Br J Ophthalmol. 1999;83:535–9.
9. Braunstein RA, Rusen DA, Bird AC. Ocular histoplasmosis syndrome in the United Kingdom. Br J Ophthalmol. 1974;58:893.
10. Braley RE, Meredith TA, Aaberg TM, Koethe SM, Witkowski JA. The prevalence of HLA-B7 in presumed ocular histoplasmosis. Am J Ophthalmol. 1978;85:859.
11. Meredith TA, Smith RP, Braley RE, Witkowski JA, Koethe SM. The prevalence of HLA-B7 and presumed ocular histoplasmosis in patients with peripheral atrophic scars. Am J Ophthalmol. 1978;86:325.
12. Meredith TA, Smith RE, Dueqesnoy RJ. Association of HLA-DR2 antigen with presumed ocular histoplasmosis. Am J Ophthalmol. 1980;89:70.
13. Hawkins BS, Alexander J, Schachat AP. Ocular histoplasmosis. In: Ryan SJ, Schahchat AP, editors. Retina. Missouri: Mosby; 2001.
14. Ryan SJ. Histopathologic correlates of presumed ocular histoplasmosis. Int Ophthalmol Clin. 1975;15:125.
15. Check IJ, Diddle KR, Jay WM, Merker R, Hunter RL. Lymphocyte stimulation by yeast phase *Histoplasma capsulatum* in presumed ocular histoplasmosis syndrome. Am J Ophthalmol. 1979;87:311.
16. Khalil MK. Histopathology of presumed ocular histoplasmosis. Am J Ophthalmol. 1982;94:369–76.
17. Kaplan HJ, Waldrep JC. Immunological basis of presumed ocular histoplasmosis. Int Ophthalmol Clin. 1983;23(2):19–31.
18. Smith RE, O'Connor GR, Halde CJ, Scalarone MA, Easterbrook WM. Clinical course in rabbits after experimental induction of ocular histoplasmosis. Am J Ophthalmol. 1973;76:284.
19. Baskin MA, Jampol LM, Huamonte FU, Rabb MF, Vygantas CM, Wyhinny G. Macular lesions in blacks with the presumed ocular histoplasmosis syndrome. Am J Ophtahlmol. 1980;89:77–83.
20. Smith RE, Ganley JP, Knox DL. Presumed ocular histoplasmosis II. Patterns of periperal and peripapillary scarring in persons with nonmacular disease. Arch Ophthalmol. 1972;87:251–7.
21. Fountain JA, Schlaegel TF. Linear streaks of the equator in the presumed ocular histoplasmosis syndrome. Arch Ophthalmol. 1981;99:246–8.
22. Schlaegel TF. The natural history of histo spots in the disc and macular area. Int Ophthal Clin. 1975;15:19.

23. Lewis ML, Van Newkirk MR, Gass JD. Follow-up study of presumed ocular histoplasmosis syndrome. Ophthalmology. 1980;87:390.
24. Schlaegel TF, Kenney D. Changes around the optic nerve head in presumed ocular histoplasmosis. Am J Ophthalmol. 1966;62:454–8.
25. Kranias G. Vitreous hemorrhage secondary to presumed ocular histoplasmosis syndrome. Ann Ophthalmol. 1985;17:295.
26. Krill AE, Christi MI, Klien BA, Newell FW, Potts AM. Multifocal inner choroiditis. Trans Am Acad Ophthalmol Otolaryngol. 1969;73:222.
27. Dreyer RF, Gass JDM. Multifocal choroiditis and panuveitis: a syndrome that mimics ocular histoplasmosis. Arch Ophthalmol. 1984;102:1776.
28. Deutsch T, Tessler H. Inflammatory pseudo histoplasmosis. Ann Ophthalmol. 1985;17:461.
29. Giles CL, Falls HF. Further evaluation of amphotericin-B therapy in presumptive histoplasmosis chorioretinitis. Am J Ophthalmol. 1961;51: 588–98.
30. Oliver A, Ciulla TA, Comer GM. New and classic insights into presumed ocular histoplasmosis syndrome and its treatment. Curr Opin Ophthalmol. 2005;16:160–5.
31. Macular Photocoagulation Study Group. Argon laser photocoagulaion for ocular histoplasmosis: results of a randomized clinical trial. Arch Ophthalmol. 1987;105:1499–507.
32. Macular Photocoagulation Study Group. Laser photocoagulation for juxtafoveal choroidal neovascularization: five-year results form randomized clinical trials. Arch Ophthalmol. 1991;109:1109–14.
33. Sickenberg M, Schmidt-Erfurth U, Miller JW, Pournaras CJ, Zografos L, Piguet B, Donati G, Laqua H, Barbazetto I, Gragoudas ES, Lane AM, Birngruber R, van den Bergh H, Strong HA, Manjuris U, Gray T, Fsadni M, Bressler NM. A preliminary study of photodynamic therapy using verteprorfin for choroidal neovascularization in pathologic myopia, ocular histoplasmosis syndrome, angioid streaks, and idiopathic causes. Arch Ophthalmol. 2000;118:327.
34. Rosenfeld PJ, Saperstein DA, Bressler NM, Reaves TA, Sickenberg M, Rosa RH Jr, Sternberg P Jr, Aaberg TM Sr, Aaberg TM Jr. Photodynamic therapy with verteporfin in ocular histoplasmosis: uncontrolled, open-label 2-year study. Ophthalmology. 2004;111:1725–33.
35. Thomas M, Kaplan H. Surgical removal of subfoveal neovascularization in the presumed ocular histoplasmosis syndrome. Am J Ophthalmol. 1991;111:1.
36. Hawkins BS, Bressler NM, Bressler SB, Davidorf FH, Hoskins JC, Marsh MJ, Miskala PH, Redford M, Sternberg P Jr, Thomas MA, Toth CA. Surgical removal vs observation for subfoveal choroidal neovascularization, either associated with the ocular histoplasmosis syndrome or idiopathic: I. Ophthalmic findings from a randomized clinical trial: submacular surgery trials (SST) group H trial: SST report no. 9. Arch Ophthalmol. 2004;122:1597–611.
37. Berger A, Conway M, Del Priore LV, Walker RS, Pollack JS, Kaplan HJ. Submacular surgery for subfoveal choroidal neovascular membranes in patients with presumed ocular histoplasmosis. Arch Ophthalmol. 1997;115:991.
38. Holekamp N, Thomas M, Dickinson J, Valluri S. Surgical removal of choroidal neovascularization in presumed ocular histoplasmosis. Ophthalmology. 1997;104:22.
39. Schlaegel TF. Treatment of the POHS. In: Schlaegel TF, editor. Ocular histoplasmosis. New York: Grune and Stratton; 1977.
40. Nielsen JS, Fick TA, Saggau DD, Barnes CH. Intravitreal anti-vascular endothelial growth factor therapy for choroidal neovascularization secondary to ocular histoplasmosis syndrome. Retina. 2012;32:468–72.
41. Adan A, Navarro M, Casaroli-Marano RP, Ortiz S, Molina JJ. Intravitreal bevacizumab as initial treatment for choroidal neovascularization associated with presumed ocular histoplasmosis syndrome. Graefes Arch Clin Exp Ophthalmol. 2007;245:1873.
42. Singerman LJ, Wong BA, Smith S. Spontaneous visual improvement in the first affected eye of patients with bilateral disciform scars. Retina. 1985;5:135.
43. Hawkins BS, Ganley JP. Risk of visual impairment attributable to ocular histoplasmosis. Arch Ophthalmol. 1994;112:655–66.

Rubella

11

George N. Papaliodis

Introduction

Rubella, also called German measles, is an acute exanthematous disease spread by droplet transmission. The virus is comprised of single-stranded RNA that is highly contagious. Since the advent of vaccination programs, the incidence of outbreaks of rubella has plummeted worldwide. By 2004, the US Centers for Disease Control (CDC) declared that rubella had been eliminated in the United States [1]. There are two distinct clinical syndromes that involve the eye: congenital and acquired. The classic triad of congenital rubella includes hearing impairment, ocular anomalies, and congenital heart disease. Acquired rubella typically manifests as a mild febrile illness with associated maculopapular rash that initially appears on the face and then spreads to involve the whole body within 24 h. The ocular manifestations of acquired rubella can include conjunctivitis, keratitis, uveitis, and retinitis. There is an association between rubella virus with Fuchs heterochromic iridocyclitis (please see chapter in this book).

Epidemiology

Before the advent of widespread vaccination programs, outbreaks of rubella usually occurred every 6–9 years in the United States mostly affecting children ages 5–9. Since the introduction of the rubella vaccine in 1969, occurrences are rare in those countries with high vaccination rates. By 2002, rubella vaccines were available worldwide and by 2006, 123 of 212 countries had national immunization programs (~58 %) [2]. The CDC declared the rubella virus was eliminated from the US in 2004 [1].

Clinical Manifestations

The clinical manifestations of rubella are differentiated based on the mode of exposure to the virus. Congenital rubella syndrome can occur in a developing fetus of a pregnant woman who has contracted the rubella virus usually in the first trimester. If the infection occurs within the first month of conception, the infant has a 43 % chance of being affected [3]. The classic triad of congenital rubella syndrome includes hearing impairment (58–80 %), ocular anomalies (43–78 %), and congenital heart disease (30–50 %) [4]. Cognitive impairment is also a common associated complication. The ocular manifestations include pigmentary retinopathy (aka "salt

G.N. Papaliodis (✉)
Department of Ophthalmology, Harvard Medical School, Massachusetts Eye and Ear Infirmary, Boston, MA 02114, USA
e-mail: George_Papaliodis@meei.harvard.edu

G.N. Papaliodis (ed.), *Uveitis*,
DOI 10.1007/978-3-319-09126-6_11

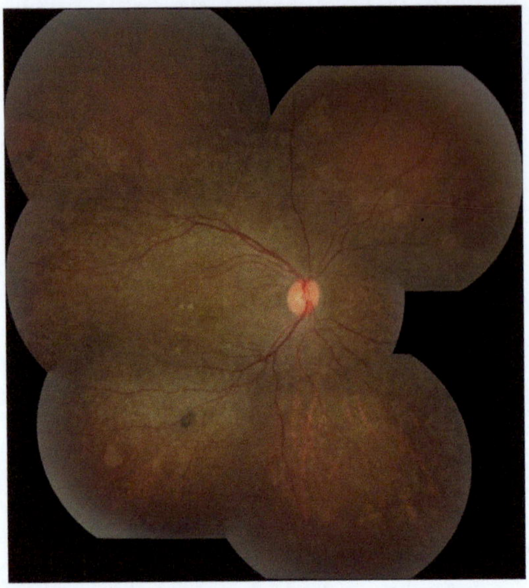

Fig. 11.1 Fundus photograph montage of a patient with pigmentary retinopathy secondary to congenital rubella syndrome

and pepper" retinopathy—see Fig. 11.1), cataract, strabismus, and glaucoma. Pigmentary retinopathy is the most common ophthalmic complication of the syndrome (reported in 9–88 % of patients with ocular involvement) [5].

Acquired rubella manifests as a maculopapular rash and mild systemic symptoms including fever and lymphadenopathy. The incubation period for the virus is 14–18 days, and infected individuals may shed virus and are potentially contagious for 1–2 weeks before the onset of classic symptoms. Arthritis and arthralgias occur in approximately 70 % of teenagers and adult females; this complication rarely develops in children and adult males [1]. The most common ocular manifestation is conjunctivitis which is present in 70 % of patients. Other ocular sequelae include epithelial keratitis and retinitis. There has been growing evidence to support a causal association with chronic rubella virus infection and Fuchs heterochromic iridocyclitis. This has been proposed due to the presence of rubella-specific intraocular antibody production in the anterior chamber of patients with Fuchs [6].

Diagnosis

The diagnosis of congenital rubella is established via the presence of maternal rubella infection and congenital anomalies. Serologic data can confirm the diagnosis via the detection of rubella-specific IgM antibodies in the infant or cord blood. The diagnosis of acquired rubella can be established by a fourfold increase in rubella-specific IgG titers obtained 1–2 weeks apart or the new appearance of rubella-specific IgM.

Treatment

Treatment for those afflicted with rubella virus is typically supportive care: there is no specific therapy. For women in the first 20 weeks of pregnancy with exposure to the virus, immune globulin may be administered to prevent both maternal and fetal infection. For those with acquired rubella, no treatment is indicated for the conjunctivitis or keratitis as these are self-limited. The uncommon manifestation of rubella retinitis responds well to systemic steroids. The treatment for Fuchs heterochromic iridocyclitis is detailed in the respective chapter of this text.

Conclusion

Rubella is an exceedingly rare acute infection spread via droplet transmission that has been eradicated in the United States per the CDC due to effective vaccination programs. The congenitally acquired variant of this disease can induce significant harm to the fetus including hearing loss and pigmentary retinopathy. The acquired form generally poses little risk to ocular structures.

References

1. Atkinson W, Wolfe S, Hamborsky J. Centers for disease control and prevention epidemiology and prevention of vaccine-preventable diseases, Pink Book, Washington. DC: Public Health Foundation; 2011.

2. Reef SE, Cochi SL. The evidence for the elimination of rubella and congenital rubella syndrome in the United States: a public health achievement. Clin Infect Dis. 2006;43(Supplement 3):S123–5.
3. Freij BJ, South MA, Sever JL. Maternal rubella and the congenital rubella syndrome. Clin Perinatolo. 1988;15(2):247–57.
4. Oster ME, Riehle-Colarusso T, Correa A. An update on cardiovascular malformations in congenital rubella syndrome. Birth Defects Res Part A: Clin Mol Teratolo. 2010;88(1):1–8.
5. Givens KT, Lee DA, Jones T, Lustrup DM. Congenital rubella syndrome: ophthalmic manifestations and associated systemic disorders. Br J Ophthalmol. 1993;77:358–63.
6. de Groot-Mijnes JD, De Visser L, Rothova A, Schuller M, van Loon AM, Weersink AJ. Rubella virus is associated with Fuchs heterochromic iridocyclitis. Am J Ophthalmol. 2006;141(1):212–4.

Syphilis

12

Miriam B. Barshak and Marlene L. Durand

Introduction/Clinical Features

Uveitis is the most common manifestation of ocular syphilis and may present as anterior, intermediate, posterior, or panuveitis. Posterior segment involvement (especially chorioretinitis) and panuveitis are the most common presentations of syphilitic uveitis [1].

Syphilitic anterior uveitis (see Fig. 12.1) is granulomatous in two thirds of patients [2] and bilateral in half. Interstitial keratitis, iris nodules, dilated iris vessels, and iris atrophy may also be seen. The most common form of posterior uveitis is multifocal chorioretinitis, but other manifestations include focal chorioretinitis (see Fig. 12.2), pseudoretinitis pigmentosa, retinal necrosis, neuroretinitis, optic neuritis (see Fig. 12.3), and acute zonal occult outer retinopathy. A pale optic nerve head from prior syphilitic optic neuritis may mimic glaucomatous optic atrophy. Chorioretinitis was the type of uveitis seen in 15 of 20 patients with syphilitic posterior uveitis in one review [1]. A specific type of focal chorioretinitis, acute posterior placoid chorioretinitis, has been described in syphilis and is characterized by large, often solitary yellow lesions that are typically in the macula [3]. Retinal vasculitis may occur in ocular syphilis, and branch retinal vein occlusions have been described [4].

Uveitis may occur in either congenital or acquired syphilis. Typical ocular findings in congenital disease include interstitial keratitis and so-called *salt-and-pepper* fundi. Interstitial keratitis does not usually occur until the patient is a teenager or young adult. It may be accompanied by anterior uveitis. The patient may have no other stigmata of congenital syphilis, but other possible features include prematurity, low birth weight, nonimmune hydrops fetalis, placental and umbilical cord abnormalities, fever, hepatomegaly, failure to thrive, rhinitis, maculopapular rash, vesicular rash (pemphigus syphiliticus), condyloma lata, jaundice, and hematologic, musculoskeletal, neurologic, pulmonary, and/or renal disease.

In acquired syphilis, uveitis may occur in secondary or tertiary syphilis. The chancre of primary syphilis, a painless lesion that develops at the inoculation site (usually genital area) an average of 3 weeks after inoculation, may have been unnoticed by the patient. The chancre lasts 3–6 weeks then spontaneously resolves.

M.B. Barshak (✉) · M.L. Durand
Department of Medicine, Massachusetts General Hospital, Harvard Medical School, Massachusetts Eye and Ear Infirmary, 55 Fruit Street, Boston, MA 02114, USA
e-mail: mbarshak@partners.org

M.L. Durand
e-mail: mdurand@mgh.harvard.edu

G.N. Papaliodis (ed.), *Uveitis*,
DOI 10.1007/978-3-319-09126-6_12

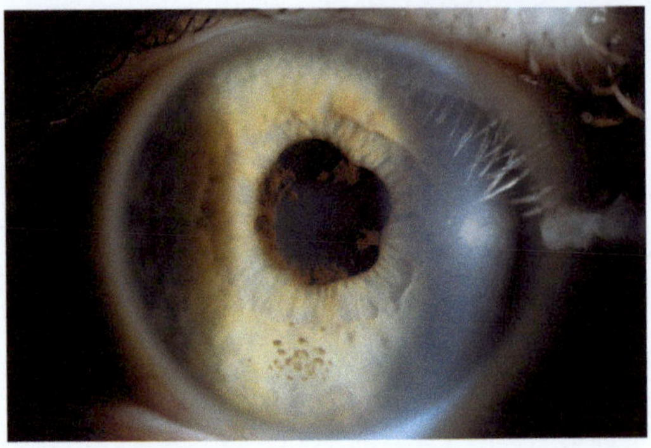

Fig. 12.1 Slit lamp photograph of a patient with syphilitic iritis, pigmented/granulomatous keratic precipitates, and posterior synechiae

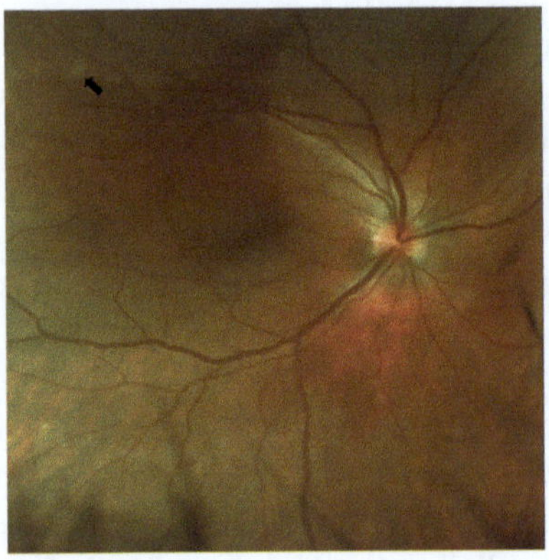

Fig. 12.2 Focal chorioretinitis (*arrow*) in a patient with ocular syphilis

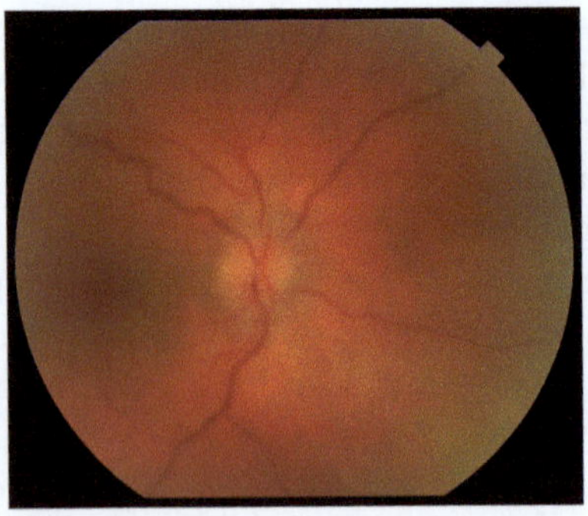

Fig. 12.3 Optic nerve swelling and vitritis in a patient with ocular syphilis

Secondary syphilis typically begins 2–8 weeks after the chancre, but this period is variable. With ocular manifestations that occur during secondary syphilis, eye symptoms are often acute. In older reports, the most common ocular finding in secondary syphilis was iritis, which accounted for more than 70 % of eye findings [4]. More recent reports suggest that posterior segment inflammation predominates; these reports include larger numbers of patients with concomitant HIV infection and low CD4 cell counts, which may predispose to more aggressive and posteriorly-located disease [5, 6]. Other manifestations of secondary syphilis may include fever, rash (classically involving the palms and soles—see Fig. 12.4), swollen lymph glands, sore throat, patchy hair loss, headaches, weight loss, muscle aches, and fatigue.

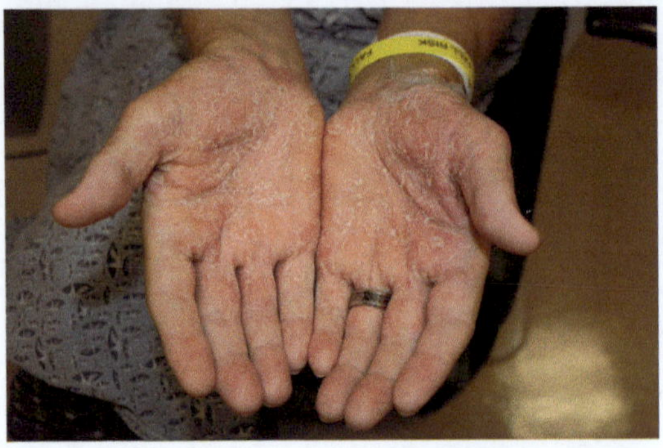

Fig. 12.4 Syphilitic rash involving the palms in a patient with secondary syphilis and uveitis (Photograph courtesy of Dr. George Papaliodis)

In contrast, when ocular syphilis develops in tertiary disease, patients often have slowly progressive decrease in vision as their only symptom. The eye findings are protean and include all of the above-listed findings. In contrast to patients with secondary disease, patients with tertiary disease often are middle-aged or older. They often have no knowledge of prior exposure to syphilis, which likely occurred decades earlier. The diagnosis may be missed if only nontreponemal tests are checked, because these tests are often negative in tertiary syphilis. In a series of 50 patients with a reactive treponemal test [absorbed fluorescent treponemal antibody (FTA-ABS)] and eye findings consistent with active or inactive ocular syphilis (e.g., chorioretinitis, optic atrophy, iritis, interstitial keratitis), the average age was 59, and the VDRL was reactive in only 24 % [7].

Epidemiology

The rates of primary and secondary syphilis in the United States dropped by 90 % from 1990 to 2000, then increased from 2001 to 2014; the majority of these diagnoses were in men who have sex with men (MSM) [8]. Although the peak incidence of all cases of primary and secondary syphilis occurs in ages 15–30, this infection is seen in older adults as well—about 5 % of cases occur in adults age 55 and older [9]. Therefore, any patient who presents with eye findings compatible with ocular syphilis should be screened for this treatable condition.

Diagnostic Evaluation

Diagnosis of ocular syphilis typically relies on a compatible history, examination, and positive serologic tests for syphilis. Nontreponemal tests (VDRL, RPR) are not specific for syphilis but yield a titer that can be used to assess for timing of infection and follow response to treatment, particularly in secondary syphilis. As noted above, these tests are less helpful in tertiary disease, as they may revert to negative over time even in patients who have not undergone treatment for syphilis. Treponemal tests (e.g., FTA-ABS) confirm the diagnosis of syphilis but do not revert to negative after treatment. False-positive FTA-ABS may occur in approximately 5 % of cases (e.g., from Lyme disease or rheumatologic conditions), thus all reactive FTA-ABS tests should be confirmed with another specific test such as TPPA (T. pallidum particle agglutination).

All patients with ocular syphilis should be tested for HIV as these infections share common modes of transmission. In a study of 24 patients treated for ocular syphilis between 1998 and 2006, 11 patients were found to be HIV positive, and this was a new diagnosis in seven [10]. HIV-positive patients are more likely than HIV-negative patients to have acute, bilateral uveitis with more extensive eye involvement (vitreous, retina, and optic nerve involvement simultaneously) [4, 11].

All patients with presumed ocular syphilis should undergo lumbar puncture to obtain baseline CSF studies, but antibiotic treatment should not be delayed if a lumbar puncture cannot be performed promptly or if the patient declines the procedure. Concomitant neurosyphilis may be present in up to 40 % of patients with ocular syphilis [7]. Importantly, a normal CSF examination does not exclude ocular syphilis, as ocular syphilis is frequently present without evidence of neurosyphilis. Patients with HIV have a higher rate of concurrent ocular syphilis and neurosyphilis [4, 12].

Treatment and Monitoring

Treatment of ocular syphilis is the same as for neurosyphilis, with penicillin G (3–4 mU IV q 4 h or continuous infusion) for 10–14 days [13]. Because the duration of treatment is shorter for neurosyphilis than for latent syphilis, the CDC notes that IM benzathine penicillin 2.4 mU once weekly for 3 weeks may be given at the end of the IV penicillin course in order to treat any latent treponemes in the periphery (note that benzathine penicillin does not cross the blood brain barrier). Patients with penicillin allergy should be desensitized to penicillin, although the 2015 CDC guidelines note that "Limited data suggest that ceftriaxone 2 g daily either IM or IV for 10–14 days can be used as an alternative treatment for patients with neurosyphilis" and penicillin allergy [13]. Patients starting treatment for syphilis should be advised to anticipate the Jarisch–Herxheimer reaction, an acute febrile syndrome that may be accompanied by headache, myalgias, rigors, sweating, and hypotension. This syndrome occurs in approximately 30 % of patients; patients with early stages of syphilis and a high (≥1:32) RPR titer have an increased risk, while patients previously treated with penicillin for syphilis have a reduced risk [14]. This syndrome typically occurs within the first 24 h after treatment begins. Antipyretics can alleviate the symptoms, which often self-resolve within 12–24 h. The value of corticosteroids in preventing Jarisch-Herxheimer has not been proven, but patients with worsening vision after penicillin therapy of ocular syphilis have improved with institution of corticosteroids [15], and there may be benefit to treating the inflammatory component of uveitis with prednisone initially.

For patients with a reactive RPR at diagnosis, posttreatment monitoring includes measurement of RPR titers at 3 and 6 months posttreatment, then every 6 months for up to 2 years or until the serology reverts to nonreactive. Titers typically decrease fourfold within a year, and then continue to fall, but serologic responses to treatment are variable, particularly among patients with HIV. If baseline CSF was abnormal, then repeat CSF studies are recommended every 6 months until the cell count has normalized. Changes in CSF VDRL and protein concentrations are slower to resolve. Retreatment should be considered if the CSF cell count has not decreased by 6 months or if the CSF cell count or protein is not normal by 2 years.

Prognosis

Most patients with syphilitic uveitis have a good visual prognosis, and with prompt diagnosis and treatment may return to normal vision. However, irreversible visual loss may occur if diagnosis and antibiotic therapy are delayed, especially in patients with panuveitis or posterior uveitis. For all patients, early diagnosis and treatment as well as careful follow-up after treatment are critical, as even with the standard regimens, the relapse or reinfection rate for ocular syphilis may be as high as 14–25 % [16, 17]. In one case series, 3 of 12 patients with HIV and ocular syphilis required retreatment within 1.5 years [17].

References

1. Villanueva AV, Sahouri MJ, Ormerod LD, Puklin JE, Reyes MP. Posterior uveitis in patients with positive serology for syphilis. Clin Infect Dis. 2000;30 (3):479–85.
2. Barile GR, Flynn TE. Syphilis exposure in patients with uveitis. Ophthalmology. 1997;104(10):1605–9.
3. Eandi CM, Neri P, Adelman RA, Yannuzzi LA, Cunningham ET Jr. Acute syphilitic posterior placoid chorioretinitis: report of a case series and comprehensive review of the literature. Retina. 2012;32 (9):1915–41.
4. Becerra LI, Ksiazek SM, Savino PJ, et al. Syphilitic uveitis in human immunodeficiency virus-infected and noninfected patients. Ophthalmology. 1989;96 (12):1727–30.
5. Butler NJ, Smith JR. Ocular syphilis in HIV-positive individuals. Clin Exp Ophthalmol. 2010;38(9):829–30.
6. Tucker JD, Li JZ, Robbins GK, et al. Ocular syphilis among HIV-infected patients: a systematic analysis of the literature. Sex Transm Infect. 2011;87(1):4–8.
7. Spoor TC, Ramocki JM, Nesi FA, Sorscher M. Ocular syphilis 1986. Prevalence of FTA-ABS reactivity and cerebrospinal fluid findings. J Clin Neuroophthalmol. Dec 1987;7(4):191–195, 196–197.
8. http://www.cdc.gov/std/tg2015/. Accessed 15 Sept 2016.
9. 2015 Sexually Transmitted Diseases Surveillance. Centers for Disease Control Website. http://www.cdc.gov/std/stats14/syphilis.htm. Accessed 15 Sept 2016.
10. Kunkel J, Schurmann D, Pleyer U, et al. Ocular syphilis–indicator of previously unknown HIV-infection. J Infect. 2009;58(1):32–6.
11. Ormerod LD, Puklin JE, Sobel JD. Syphilitic posterior uveitis: correlative findings and significance. Clin Infect Dis. 2001;32(12):1661–73.
12. Levy JH, Liss RA, Maguire AM. Neurosyphilis and ocular syphilis in patients with concurrent human immunodeficiency virus infection. Retina. 1989;9 (3):175–80.
13. 2015 STD Treatment Guidelines. Centers for Disease Control Website. http://www.cdc.gov/std/tg2015/syphilis.htm. Accessed 15 Sept 2016.
14. Yang CJ, Lee NY, Lin YH, et al. Jarisch-Herxheimer reaction after penicillin therapy among patients with syphilis in the era of the hiv infection epidemic: incidence and risk factors. Clin Infect Dis. Oct 15;51 (8):976–979.
15. Fathilah J, Choo MM. The Jarisch-Herxheimer reaction in ocular syphilis. Med J Malaysia. 2003;58(3):437–9.
16. Browning DJ. Posterior segment manifestations of active ocular syphilis, their response to a neurosyphilis regimen of penicillin therapy, and the influence of human immunodeficiency virus status on response. Ophthalmology. 2000;107(11):2015–23.
17. Li JZ, Tucker JD, Lobo AM, et al. Ocular syphilis among HIV-infected individuals. Clin Infect Dis. 2010;51(4):468–71.

13 Ocular Toxocariasis

Sonia Utley and George N. Papaliodis

Introduction

Toxocariasis is an infection caused by the parasitic roundworms commonly found in the intestines of dogs (*Toxocara canis*) and cats (*Toxocara cati*). A US study in 1996 demonstrated that 30 % of dogs younger than 6 months deposit Toxocara eggs in their feces; each worm releases 200,000 eggs per day. Once released in the stool, the eggs require 2–4 weeks to develop and become infectious. *Toxocara* embryonic eggs have a tough shell which lengthens their viability once in the stool. If these eggs are subsequently ingested, larvae hatch in the small intestine, then continue through the intestinal wall, entering the bloodstream and migrating to muscles, lungs, liver, central nervous system, and the eyes. Often the infections are asymptomatic however the two most common syndromes are systemic toxocariasis (visceral larva migrans) and ocular toxocariasis (ocular larva migrans). The severity of the organ damage depends upon the parasite load, site of larval migration, and the host's inflammatory response. Visceral larva migrans occurs mostly in children who are at a higher risk of infection due to exposure to the eggs in sandboxes and dirt on outdoor playgrounds. Ocular larva migrans can occur even if only a single larva reaches the eye [1].

Epidemiology

Approximately 13.9 % of the US population have antibodies to Toxocara implying that millions of people have been exposed to the organism [2]. Ocular toxocariasis accounts for 1–2 % of all uveitis in children throughout the world [3]. The organism is not specific to any region of the world or US but occurs at substantially higher rates in Asia and in areas of the US with higher levels of poverty [4]. The increased prevalence of ocular toxocariasis in Asia is generally thought to be caused by food habits and traditional dishes specific to many Asian cultures. Specifically in Korea 80.8 % of ocular toxocariasis patients reported having eaten raw cow liver [5]. The higher levels of ocular toxocariasis in poverty-ridden communities in the US are associated with animal interactions, specifically stray cats and dogs, along with a higher number of pets living in less sterile environments enabling easier transmission of toxocariasis to humans [6, 7].

S. Utley (✉)
Ocular Immunology and Uveitis Service, Massachusetts Eye and Ear Infirmary, Boston, MA, USA
e-mail: sclucc@gmail.com

G.N. Papaliodis
Department of Ophthalmology, Harvard Medical School, Massachusetts Eye and Ear Infirmary, 243 Charles Street, Boston, MA 02114, USA
e-mail: George_Papaliodis@meei.harvard.edu

G.N. Papaliodis (ed.), *Uveitis*,
DOI 10.1007/978-3-319-09126-6_13

Clinical Manifestations

Toxocariasis manifests as two general syndromes: systemic toxocariasis and ocular toxocariasis. Systemic toxocariasis (visceral larva migrans) is typically seen in young children and can be asymptomatic. The severity of the symptoms is dictated by the age of the patient, quantity of larva ingested, distribution of the larva in the body, and host response. The condition can be mild but may be associated with a varied range of symptoms including cough, wheezing, abdominal pain, fever, and fatigue. In more severe cases, patients can develop hepatitis, pneumonitis, and encephalitis [8]. Ocular involvement is usually not present in cases of systemic toxocariasis, and conversely systemic toxocariasis is rarely seen in cases of ocular toxocariasis.

Ocular toxocariasis manifests as granulomatous uveitis commonly involving the posterior pole or in the periphery as the most commonly affected ocular tissue is the retina. Posterior pole toxocariasis lesions are typically white or gray, round, and elevated. The degree of intraocular inflammation can vary from scant to robust depending upon the number of larvae present. The infection alone can result in direct retinal injury but secondary complications from the inflammatory response can similarly induce severe vision loss. The major causes of decreased vision have been attributed to vitreous traction, endophthalmitis, macular involving lesions, retinal detachment, and papillitis [9, 10].

Diagnosis

The diagnosis of toxocariasis is based on the clinical manifestations and supportive serologic testing. The sensitivity and specificity of the serum ELISA assay is approximately 90 % [9]. A more sensitive assay is the detection of Toxocara antibodies in the aqueous humor (calculation of a Goldmann-Witmer coefficient) [4].

Treatment

The paradigm for the treatment of infectious ocular inflammatory disease often combines appropriate antimicrobial therapy with corticosteroids to reduce the propensity for tissue injury from the associated immune response. In patients with ocular toxocariasis, the focus has been directed predominantly toward the destructive inflammatory reaction, and corticosteroids have been the mainstay of treatment administered locally and systemically (alone and in conjunction with systemic antihelminthic agents). There are case reports and limited trials demonstrating efficacy of thiabendazole (25 mg/kg twice daily for 5 days) and albendazole (100–200 mg twice daily for 5 days) in the treatment of ocular toxocariasis [11, 12].

Surgical procedures have also been employed to treat associated complications of the disease including pars plana vitrectomy, retinal cryopexy, and photocoagulation.

Conclusion

Ocular toxocariasis is a common worldwide infection caused by the roundworms *T. canis* and less commonly *T. cati*. The ocular manifestations may include granulomatous uveitis, endophthalmitis, retinal granulomas, intermediate uveitis, vitreous traction, papillitis, and tractional retinal detachment. The diagnosis is established with the appropriate clinical findings and confirmed via serum ELISA or aqueous humor aspirate for detection of *Toxocara* antibodies. The predominant modality for treatment is local and systemic corticosteroids administered alone and in conjunction with appropriate antihelminthic treatment.

References

1. Stewart JM, Cubillan LD, Cunningham ET Jr. Prevalence, clinical features, and causes of vision loss among patients with ocular toxocariasis. Retina. 2005;25(8):1005–13.

2. Lee AC, Schantz PM, Kazacos KR, Montgomery SP, Bowman DD. Epidemiologic and zoonotic aspects of ascarid infections in dogs and cats. Trends Parasitol. 2010 Apr;26(4):155–61. Epub 19 Feb 2010.
3. Hotez PJ. Neglected infections of poverty in the United States of America. PLoS Negl Trop Dis. 2008;2(6):e256.
4. De Visser L, Rothova A, De Boer JH, Van Loon AM, Kerkhoff FT, Canninga-van Dijk MR, et al. Diagnosis of ocular toxocariasis by establishing intraocular antibody production. Am J Ophthalmol. 2007;145:369–74.
5. Ahn SJ, Woo SJ, Jin Y, Chang YS, Kim TW, Ahn J, Heo JW, Yu HG, Chung H, Park KH, Hong ST. Clinical features and course of ocular toxocariasis in adults. PLoS Negl Trop Dis. 2014;8:e2938.
6. Hotez PJ, Wilkins PP. Toxocariasis: America's most common neglected infection of poverty and a helminthiasis of global importance? PLoS Negl Trop Dis. 2009;3(3):e400.
7. Herrmann N, Glickman LT, Schantz PM, Weston MG, Domanski LM. Seroprevalence of zoonotic toxocariasis in the United States: 1971–1973. Am J Epidemiol. 1985;122(5):890–6.
8. Marx C, Lin J, Masruha MR, Rodrigues MG, da Rocha AJ, et al. Toxocariasis of the CNS simulating acute disseminated encephalomyelitis. Neurology. 2007;69(8):806–7.
9. Paola P. Ocular toxocariasis. Int J Med Sci. 2009;6 (3):129–30.
10. Hagler WS, Jarret H, Chang M. Rhegmatogenous retinal detachment following chorioretinal inflammatory disease. Am J Ophthalmol. 1978;86:373.
11. Woodhall D et al. Ocular toxocariasis: epidemiologic, anatomic, and therapeutic variations based on a survey of ophthalmic subspecialists. Ophthalmology. 2012 Jun;119(6) (PubMed.gov).
12. Stürchler D, Schubarth P, Gualzata M, Gottstein B, Oettli A. Thiabendazole vs. albendazole in treatment of toxocariasis: a clinical trial. Ann Trop Med Parasitol. 1989;83:473–8.

Ocular Toxoplasmosis

14

Jay Wang, Eleni Konstantinou and Demetrios G. Vavvas

Introduction

Toxoplasmosis is an infectious disease that is caused by *Toxoplasma gondii*, a protozoan parasite. The organism itself has a unique life cycle that involves cats in particular and can be transmitted to humans via direct contact with cat feces or contaminated soil, ingestion of raw or undercooked meat containing the organism, and vertical transmission from mother to fetus via the placenta. Toxoplasmosis is more common in South America and Central America than North America or Europe. The ocular manifestations can lead to severe visual loss with disease involving the macular and/or optic nerve.

J. Wang · E. Konstantinou · D.G. Vavvas (✉)
Department of Ophthalmology, Massachusetts Eye and Ear Infirmary, 243 Charles Street, Boston MA 02114, USA
e-mail: vavvas@meei.harvard.edu

J. Wang
e-mail: jay_wang@hms.harvard.edu

E. Konstantinou
e-mail: Eleni_Konstantinou@meei.harvard.edu

D.G. Vavvas
Department of Ophthalmology, Massachusetts Eye and Ear Infirmary, Massachusetts General Hospital, Boston, MA 02114, USA

G.N. Papaliodis (ed.), *Uveitis*,
DOI 10.1007/978-3-319-09126-6_14

Etiology

T. gondii is a ubiquitous protozoan obligate intracellular parasite of warm-blooded animals and is one of the most common parasitic infections of humans. Infection can result in encephalitis (predominantly in immunocompromised hosts), chorioretinitis in immunocompetent hosts, or congenital transmission if a pregnant woman becomes infected.

There are three infectious stages of *T. gondii*: the tachyzoites (in groups or clones, Tachy, from the Greek "fast"), the bradyzoites (in tissue cysts, brady, form the Greek for slow), and the sporozoites (in oocysts) [1]. These stages are linked in a complex life cycle (Fig. 14.1).

The only known definitive hosts for *T. gondii* are members of family Felidae (domestic cats and their relatives). Cats shed oocysts in their feces which may then be ingested by intermediate hosts in nature (including birds and rodents). Oocysts transform into tachyzoites shortly after ingestion, which then proliferate and can infect virtually any cell in the body. Bradyzoites, which are more slow growing than tachyzoites, are also present in tissue cysts in the brain and visceral organs, in particular the lungs, kidneys, and liver. An intact tissue cyst can persist for a long period of time (for the life of the host) without causing any inflammatory response.

There are three major routes of acquiring *T. gondii* infection: the first is via foodborne transmission, the second is from animal to human

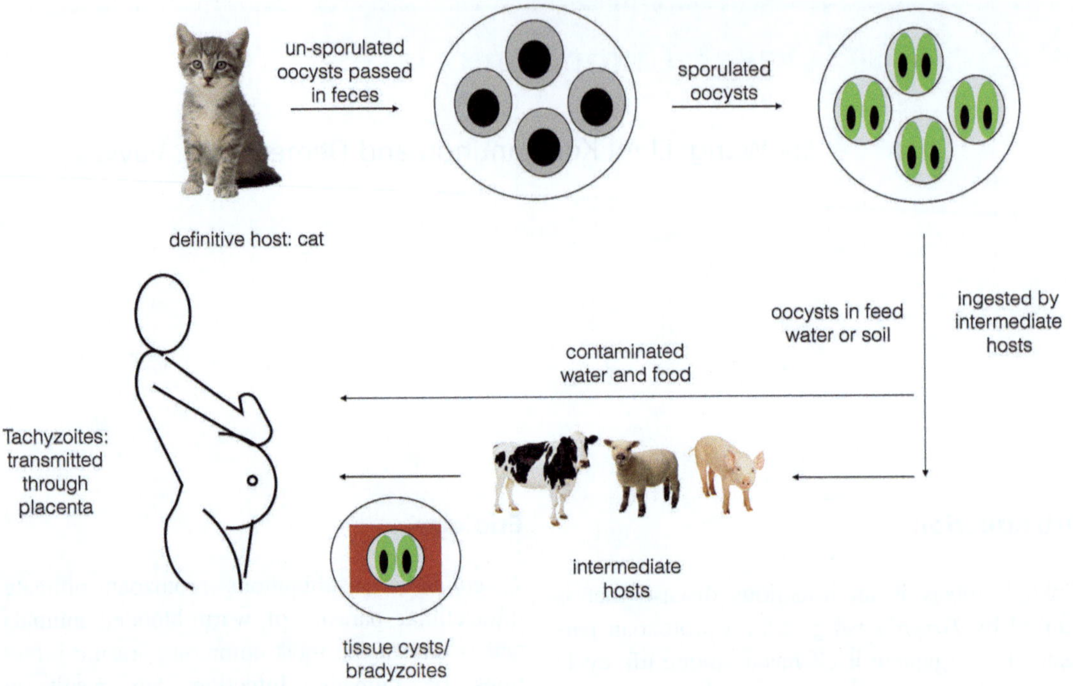

Fig. 14.1 *Toxoplasma gondii*, life cycle

(zoonotic transmission), and the third is from mother to fetus (congenital) transmission [1]. Foodborne transmission is most commonly caused by the ingestion of undercooked meat that contains encysted bradyzoites. The prevalence of *T. gondii* is higher in sheep than in horse or cattle. Thus, people eating raw or poorly cooked meat especially from goat or lamb may have a higher risk of acquiring infection. However, both humans and livestock can be infected by ingestion of soil that contains *T. gondii* oocysts as a result of either poorly washed fruit or vegetables or by drinking water that is contaminated with oocysts. Furthermore, *T. gondii* oocysts are shed from the feces of an infected cat into the environment or litter boxes. The latter may be a possible route of infection for pregnant women, which can lead to transmission of parasites to the fetus through the placenta. This condition is known as congenital toxoplasmosis and can cause serious medical problems for the fetus including chorioretinitis, intracranial calcifications, and hydrocephalous.

Less common routes of transmission have also described such as through organ transplantation or blood transfusion.

Epidemiology

Toxoplasmosis, and more specifically retinal toxoplasmosis, is one of the most serious and most important causes of posterior uveitis worldwide.

Recent studies demonstrate that the prevalence of ocular toxoplasmosis varies throughout the world. Those living in tropical areas such as South America, Central America, and Caribbean appear to be more susceptible to ocular toxoplasmosis, which may be related to the presence of more virulent genotypes of the parasites in these areas.

Seroprevalence in areas of South America have been reported to be as high as 73 %, while the seroprevalence in the United States ranges from 12 to 19 % [2]. Nevertheless, recent studies in the United States indicate that "toxoplasma is the most common infection in the States" [3]. The seroprevalence in Europe varies, higher in Southern Europe and lower in northern Europe (Sweden and Norway). There is evidence that ocular toxoplasmosis is increasing in Asia, Africa and Australia as well.

Clinical Presentation

Signs and Symptoms in the Immunocompetent Patient

The vast majority of acquired toxoplasma infections in immunocompetent hosts are subclinical and asymptomatic [4]. In some cases, lymphadenopathy may be the only presenting symptom [5]. However, ocular toxoplasmosis may be seen even in immunocompetent hosts and is caused by reactivation of the parasite after an initial self-resolving infection of the retina [6]. This is characterized by a chorioretinitis with a predilection for the posterior pole and presents with blurry vision and eye pain that may progress to blindness if involving the macula or region near the optic nerve. Importantly, ocular toxoplasmosis can be due to reactivation of a congenitally acquired infection as well as an acute acquired infection as an adult [7]. There is a documented lag time of several years from initial infection to ocular manifestation [8]. Presentation is typically unilateral when the infection is acquired as an adult, but can be bilateral if the infection was acquired congenitally or in early childhood.

Signs and Symptoms in the Immunocompromised Patient

When the host is immunocompromised, reactivation of the latent parasite or acute infection is more systemic and severe. In patients with HIV, toxoplasmosis becomes a real concern when the CD4 count drops below 100 cells/microliter [9]. Cases of ocular toxoplasmosis have also been reported in organ or bone marrow transplantation patients on chronic immunosuppressive regimens [10–12]. The symptoms and signs of ocular toxoplasmosis in immunosuppressed patients include decreased vision and eye pain. However, the eye disease may be more severe, especially in elderly patients [13]. While bilateral disease is overall rare, there have been multiple reports of bilateral involvement in immunocompromised patients [10–12].

Cerebral involvement characterized by brain abscesses is the most common manifestation of toxoplasmosis in the immunocompromised patient and induces symptoms including headache, confusion, fever, focal neurological deficits, and seizures [9]. In one study, 50 % of patients with cerebral toxoplasmosis also had ocular toxoplasmosis, and 63 % of patients with ocular toxoplasmosis also had cerebral lesions [14]. Pneumonitis also occurs commonly presenting with nonproductive cough and dyspnea [15]. Toxoplasma may also affect other organs, including the liver, heart, musculoskeletal system, and the gastrointestinal tract. Widely disseminated toxoplasmosis has also been reported to lead to septic shock [14].

Congenital Toxoplasmosis

Congenital toxoplasmosis occurs when the mother becomes infected with the parasite during pregnancy, and the infection is passed to the fetus via the placenta. The mother can be either asymptomatic or can develop a "mononucleosis like" syndrome. Transmission by breastfeeding has not been demonstrated. Fetal infection in the first trimester has been associated with increased severity of disease [16], and can lead to still birth or result in central nervous system involvement, such as intracranial calcification and hydrocephalous. Most cases of congenital toxoplasmosis are actually subclinical, but even in this subset, retinal scars are often present, and recurrent reactivation of the parasite may occur later in life [17]. When infection is symptomatic, disease usually occurs in the neonatal period and first few months of life. The eye is involved in approximately 85 % of cases [18], with bilateral disease occurring in a majority of cases with ocular involvement, with reports ranging from 65 to 85 % [19–21]. In addition to chorioretinitis, other findings such as retinal detachment, nystagmus, microphthalmia, strabismus, and cataract have been reported [20].

Extraocular manifestations of congenital toxoplasmosis include hydrocephalus, intracranial calcifications, seizures, jaundice, lymphadenopathy, hepatosplenomegaly, pneumonitis, and fever. However, the classic triad of chorioretinitis, hydrocephalus, and intracranial calcifications occurs in fewer than 10 % of clinically apparent infections [22].

Fundoscopic Exam

Typical Presentation

The typical presentation of an acute episode of ocular toxoplasmosis in immunocompetent patients is unilateral chorioretinitis characterized by a focal necrotizing fluffy whitish lesion in the retina with surrounding edema (Figs. 14.2 and 14.6). The degree of vitritis can be severe enough to be described as a "headlight in the fog" via indirect ophthalmoscopy. The retina is the primary site of inflammation which may spread to the choroid and sclera. Over the course of 2–4 months in immunocompetent patients, this lesion results in scar formation. These scars are often variably pigmented with an area of central atrophy where the sclera is often visible (Fig. 14.3).

Often, the disease recurs at the outer regions of old retinal scars, known as "satellite" lesions (Fig. 14.4). These active lesions are frequently adjacent to old scars, suggesting previous infection, either acquired or congenital infection. Vitreous inflammation may be present as well, and can be either localized or diffuse. In severe cases, the view of the underlying retina may be obscured, and the inflammation can even spread to the anterior segment. In as many as 30 % of cases, the intraocular pressure may be elevated [23]. Other conditions can have similar ocular manifestations to toxoplasmosis and should be considered [24] (see Table 14.1).

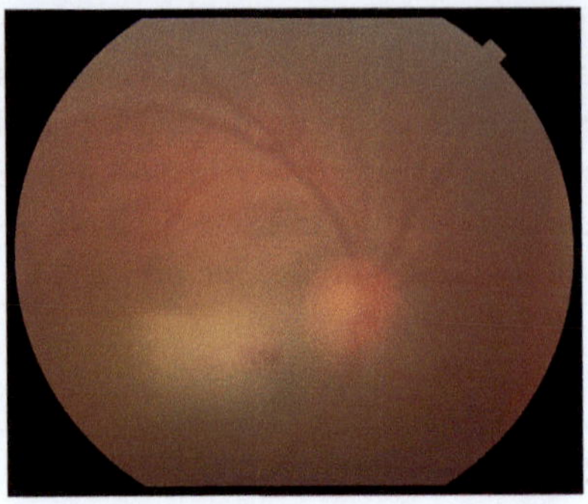

Fig. 14.2 Fundus photograph of a patient with ocular toxoplasmosis showing the typical focal necrotizing fluffy whitish lesion in the macula with dense vitritis

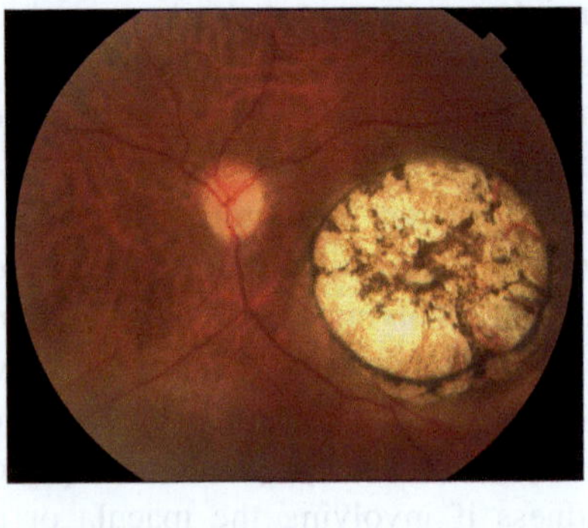

Fig. 14.3 Fundus photograph of a patient with ocular toxoplasmosis showing a macular retinal scar suggestive of prior infectious episode

Atypical Presentation

Immunocompromised patients (especially HIV-positive patients with CD4 count below 100 cells/microliter, patients on chronic immunosuppression or corticosteroids, and elderly patients) can have more severe presentations of ocular toxoplasmosis. The areas of retinal necrosis are often more extensive, multifocal, and present bilaterally. In some cases, the presentation can appear similar to acute retinal necrosis. In immunocompromised patients, the disease is more aggressive, and

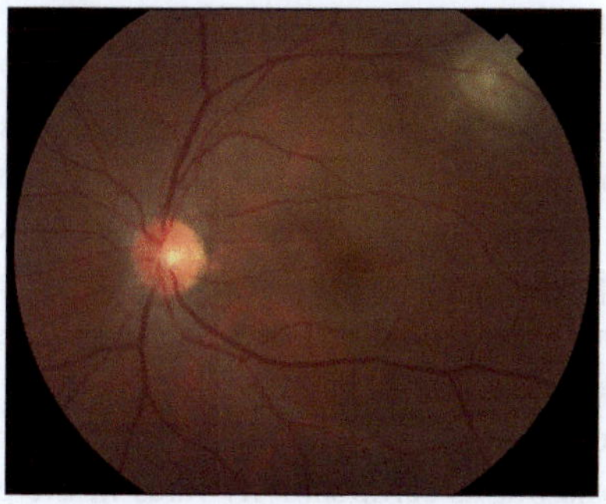

Fig. 14.4 Fundus photograph demonstrating larger toxoplasmic lesion and associated smaller satellite lesions

complications including retinal detachment, endophthalmitis, and even orbital cellulitis may occur without prompt treatment [25].

In less typical cases, ocular toxoplasmosis presents as punctate outer retinal lesions. These are characterized by multiple gray-white lesions that are associated with little to no vitreous inflammation [26]. This is because the inflammation involves deeper layers of the retina and the retinal pigment epithelium as has been demonstrated by optical coherence tomography (OCT) [27], although early one the inner retina is affected (Fig. 14.6).

Other atypical presentations of ocular toxoplasmosis include neuroretinitis characterized by optic nerve edema and a macular stellate exudate, typically presenting with rapid loss of vision. Retinal vasculitis is a common finding (see Figs. 14.5 and 14.6), typically affecting vessels in the same quadrant as the chorioretinitis, manifesting as sheathing of the vessels. Rarely, this can lead to vascular occlusion and subsequent infarction of the retina [28]. Retinal and subretinal neovascularization have also been observed as a result of retinal vasculitis in ocular toxoplasmosis. Retinal detachment, usually rhegmatogenous or tractional, may occur in approximately 5 % of cases [29]. Scleritis has been described as a manifestation of ocular toxoplasmosis but is quite rare [30].

Table 14.1 Differential diagnosis of acquired toxoplasmosis

Infectious
Bacterial
Syphilis
Tuberculosis
Bartonellosis (neuroretinitis, focal retinitis, angiomatous lesions)
Lyme disease
Endogenous endophthalmitis
Others
Viral
Acute retinal necrosis/necrotizing herpetic neuropathy
Cytomegalovirus retinitis
Progressive outer retinal necrosis
Others
Fungal
Candidiasis (especially endogenous endophthalmitis)
Aspergillosis
Others
Parasitic
Diffuse unilateral subacute neuroretinitis
Toxocariasis
Others
Noninfectious
Associated with systemic disease
Behçet's disease
Sarcoidosis
Others
Focal disease
Serpiginous/ampiginous choroiditis and others
Multifocal choroiditis and panuveitis
Punctate inner choroidopathy
Multiple evanescent white dots syndrome
Unilateral acute idiopathic maculopathy
Others
Neoplastic
Primary vitreoretinal lymphoma
Others

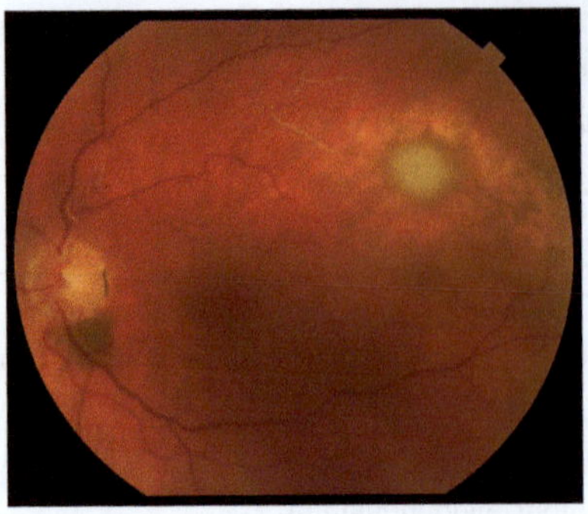

Fig. 14.5 Fundus photograph demonstrating an active toxoplasmic lesion with associated retinal vasculitis

Congenital Toxoplasmosis Ocular Manifestations

The typical whitish retinal lesions seen in adults are also seen in children with congenital toxoplasmosis. However, the more typical finding on fundoscopy is a wagon wheel-shaped scar in the retina [20]. It is comprised of a central area of variable pigmentation surrounded by a ring of pigment. These lesions commonly involve the macula. Other ocular manifestations of congenital toxoplasmosis include cataract, nystagmus, strabismus, and microphthalmia [20]. In a recent largest observational series of infected newborns from France showed that of 2361 suspected consecutive pregnancies, 485 live-born children were infected and 30 % of them developed ocular manifestation over the follow-up time (median 10.5 years of follow-up). Seventy percent of the children had only one eye affected and 80 % of those lesions caused no vision loss. The initial lesion was detected during the first 2 weeks of life in only 5 % and overall detection of first lesion occurred at a median age of 4.2 years (range: 35 days to 20.7 years). Incidence of retinochoroiditis increased steadily over time with a cumulative estimated probability at 18 years of close to 50 % [31]. There are other potential infectious conditions that can mimic congenital toxoplasmosis which should also be excluded (see Table 14.2).

Diagnosis

The diagnosis of ocular toxoplasmosis is most often made by clinical findings based on the characteristic focal necrotizing chorioretinitis with or without accompanying retinal scars and other sequelae such as vitritis, neuroretinitis, retinal vasculitis, and anterior segment inflammation [24].

Serology can be supportive in making the diagnosis but as seropositivity rates in the general population are high (approximately 25 % of the patients in the United States are seropositive [32]), the presence of positive IgG antibody testing may not necessarily be diagnostic. Conversely, the absence of IgG antibodies can effectively exclude the disease even in immunocompromised patients [33]. In addition, low IgG avidity suggests primary infection while high IgG avidity suggests reactivation [34]. Seropositivity for immunoglobulin M (IgM) supports primary infection [35].

In atypical or uncertain cases, additional tests on ocular fluids may be performed to further support the diagnosis. In these cases, sampling of the aqueous humor can be helpful. The presence of anti-toxoplasma IgG antibodies in the aqueous humor supports active infection. Furthermore, the Goldmann-Witmer (GW) coefficient can be used to increase both sensitivity and specificity [36]. This metric is the ratio of intraocular anti-toxoplasma IgG to total intraocular IgG and serum anti-toxoplasma IgG to total serum IgG. A high coefficient of 3 or greater suggests active ocular infection [37, 38].

More recently, polymerase chain reaction (PCR) analysis of either the aqueous humor or vitreous humor can aid in the diagnosis, particularly in immunosuppressed patients where serology may be less sensitive. In addition, PCR has the advantage of requiring a smaller volume of fluid. PCR is highly specific and sensitivities vary from 15 to 100 % depending on the study [39]. Sampling from the vitreous humor as opposed to aqueous humor may increase sensitivity [39, 40]. If the diagnosis remains uncertain, a diagnostic para plans vitrectomy (PPV) with or without chorioretinal biopsy may be performed to obtain tissue for analysis [39].

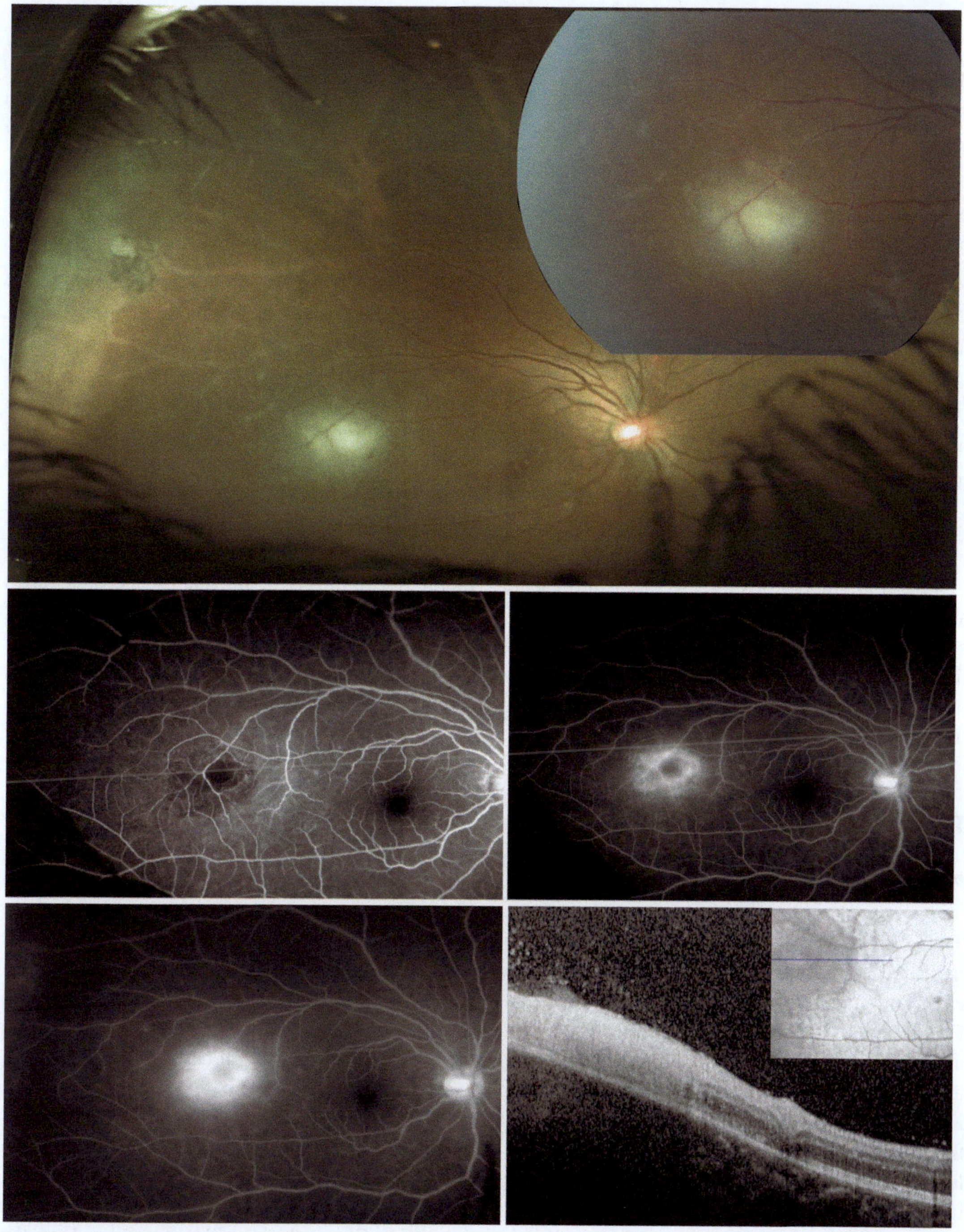

Fig. 14.6 Fundus photograph, fluorescein angiogram and spectral domain OCT demonstrating a fresh new active toxoplasmic lesion with associated retinal vasculitis and overlying mild vitreous debris/inflammation

Table 14.2 Differential diagnosis of congenital toxoplasmosis

Infectious
Rubella
CMV
Herpes
Syphilis
West Nile virus
Acute lymphocytic choriomeningitis
Noninfectious
Retinochoroidal colobomata
Persistent hyperplastic vitreous
Neoplastic
Retinoblastoma
Retinocytoma

Imaging modalities such as fluorescein angiography and OCT may aid in further characterizing retinal lesions and other accompanying findings such as vascular leakage, occlusion, macular edema, or choroidal neovascularization but they add little diagnostic value in most cases.

Treatment

Pharmacologic

Treatment of ocular toxoplasmosis is not always indicated as the disease is self-limiting in many cases and may involve the periphery of the retina. For smaller, peripheral retinal lesions (in the absence of macular or optic nerve involvement) and with minimal effect on visual acuity in immunocompetent patients, observation is often the treatment advised. However, if the retinal lesions encroach upon the macula or optic nerve, if there is considerable vitritis or other complication, anti-toxoplasmic treatment is warranted.

Treatment should always be initiated in immunocompromised patients or in cases of congenital toxoplasmosis.

The standard treatment of ocular toxoplasmosis has been the "triple therapy" comprised of the antiparasitic drugs sulfadiazine and pyrimethamine, and a corticosteroid such as prednisone. A typical triple therapy regimen consists of oral sulfadiazine (2–4 g loading dose, followed by 1 g 4 times per day), oral pyrimethamine (75–100 mg loading dose, followed by 25–50 mg/day), and prednisone (20–40 mg/day started at least 24–48 h after initiation of anti-toxo therapy) for 4–6 weeks depending on the response to treatment. As pyrimethamine can suppress the bone marrow, periodic complete blood counts should be monitored, and patients should receive supplementation with folinic acid (5–7.5 mg/day or 15 mg 3×/week). Corticosteroids should be started only after initiation of anti-toxoplasmic therapy and tapered off either before or synchronously with termination of antimicrobial therapy. The timing of starting the steroids varies from concurrent to 24 h later, with the authors of this chapter starting steroids concurrently.

Other alternative regimens have been studied, including the addition of clindamycin (300 mg 4 times a day) to triple therapy [41], intravitreal clindamycin (1 mg) with and without dexamethasone (400 μg) [42, 43], azithromycin (250–500 mg/day) with pyrimethamine (100 mg loading dose, followed by 50 mg/day) [44], and trimethoprim–sulfamethoxazole (TMP–SMX) (160/800 mg twice/day) with prednisolone (1 mg/kg starting from the third day after anti-toxoplasmosis therapy) [45]. These therapies have all been found to be comparable to the classic triple therapy in small randomized trials and allow for flexibility in cases of drug allergies or intolerable side effects.

Atovaquone (750 mg every 6 h) is an infrequently used anti-toxoplasmosis agent that has the potential advantage of being active against the bradyzoite form of the organism (at least in vitro). Given this profile, it may reduce the potential for recurrences, although this has not been studied extensively in a randomized controlled trial [46, 47]. There is however evidence that TMP–SMX (160/800 mg) administered every 2–3 days significantly reduces recurrence of ocular toxoplasmosis and can be considered for secondary prevention in patients with frequent recurrence of the disease [48].

During pregnancy, maternal infection should be treated with spiramycin (500 mg qid) to reduce the risk of vertical transmission [49]. However, if fetal infection is confirmed by amniotic fluid PCR, sulfadiazine, pyrimethamine, and folinic acid at the standard doses should be administered. A more recent study by Valentini et al. showed that spiramycin (administered from diagnosis to delivery) along with TMP–SMX (sulfamethoxazole 800 mg plus trimethoprim 160 mg twice daily) administered from the start of the second trimester and suspended one week prior to child birth was more effective in reducing vertical transmission. [50].

Despite clinical practices, a Cochrane review found no evidence to support antibiotic treatment in ocular toxoplasmosis, citing lack of reported long-term visual outcomes and poor methodological studies [51]. There is also scant evidence to support the superiority of one antimicrobial regimen over another. A recent review of the current treatments of toxoplasmic retinochoroiditis by Harrell and Carvounis corroborated the conflicting evidence in the literature regarding the effectiveness of systemic antibiotics and the lack of demonstrated superiority of any single regimen [52]. Though corticosteroids are widely used in conjunction with anti-toxoplasmic medications, there is lack of evidence from randomized controlled trials to support their use [53, 54]. These studies underscore the need for further randomized controlled trials to guide treatment of the disease (see Table 14.3 for summary of therapies).

Surgical Management

In rare patients with recalcitrant disease, laser photocoagulation and cryotherapy have been used to treat retinal lesions. However, there is no clear evidence to support use of these procedures; the efficacy is unclear and recurrence may still occur outside the treated area [54]. Additionally, complications such as vitreous hemorrhage, intra-retinal hemorrhage, and retinal detachment may occur with these interventions.

Prognosis

The prognosis of ocular toxoplasmosis depends on numerous factors, including age, immune status, size and location of lesion, macular involvement, and secondary complications, such as cataract, secondary glaucoma, cystoid macular edema, choroidal neovascularization, retinal detachment, neuroretinitis, or retinal vascular occlusion are present. Logically, the most important factor seems to follow the rule of real estate investing: location, location, location. Severe inflammation involving the macula and/or optic nerve herald worse visual outcomes.

Recurrences occur commonly resulting from rupture of toxoplasma cysts, ranging from 14 to 79 % depending on the study [55–58]. One early study found that 41 % of patients with acquired ocular toxoplasmosis were left with visual acuities of 20/100 or worse unilaterally [59], and another study cited final visual acuities of less than 20/200 in 61 % of patients [56]. These studies likely suffer from selection bias. Most long-term follow-up studies of patients with congenital toxoplasmosis found that the visual prognosis is generally good, with approximately 6–25 % of patients having visual acuity of 20/200 or worse in one eye [55, 60–62. In general, visual impairment only occurs when the retinal lesion involves the macula. Rarely are both macula affected, and thus severe bilateral visual impairment was infrequently seen in these studies.

Duration of the infection and activity prior to treatment are very important factors in prognosis of visual outcome. Thus a prompt referral and a rapid targeted treatment could potentially improve visual prognosis.

Table 14.3 Toxoplasmosis therapies

Toxoplasmosis therapies	Regimen	Notes
Observation	If small peripheral without significant vitritis. Observe q 4–5 days for the first 2–3 weeks. Then bi-weekly until resolution. Usually total time 1–2 months.	Non-macula, non-optic nerve cases and no significant vitritis
TMP-SMX twice a day	Trimethoprim-sulfamethoxazole (TMP-SMX) (160/800 mg twice/day). Can add prednisolone (1 mg/kg starting from the third day of therapy) [45]	Affordable
Atovaquone	Atovaquone (750 mg every 6 h) +/− prednisone 1 mg/kg daily [46, 47]	Expensive. Theoretical benefit in reducing bradyzoites
Triple	Oral sulfadiazine (2–4 g loading dose, followed by 1 g 4 times a day), oral pyrimethamine (75–100 mg loading dose, followed by 25–50 mg/day) total for 2–3 weeks. [41]	Thrombocytopenia, leukopenia, rashes, and fever
Clindamycin and sulfadiazine	Clindamycin (300 mg qid), sulfadiazine (1 g qid), +/− prednisone (60 mg, then taper)	Not widely used
Clindamycin plus triple	Clindamyçin (300 mg four times a day) to triple therapy [41]	Increased side effects
Intravitreal clindamycin	Intravitreal clindamycin (1 mg) with dexamethasone (400 µg) [42, 43]. May repeat q 1–2 weeks as needed	Minimally invasive
Azithromycin and Pyrimethamine	Azithromycin (250–500 mg/day) with pyrimethamine (100 mg loading dose, followed by 50 mg/day) [44]	Less side effects than sulfadiazine/pyrimethamine combination
Azithromycin	500 mg PO daily 4–6 weeks course +/− steroid [44]	Not much experience with this regime [44]
Recurrence prevention	Trimethoprim-sulfamethoxazole (TMP-SMX) 160/800 mg every 2–3 days for a year [48]	Level I evidence [48]
In pregancy	• Spiramycin alone 3 × 106 IU (3 × 106 international unit = 870mg) four times daily until delivery (protocol abbreviation: Spy) • Pyrimethamine 25mg per day (50mg for first dose), sulfadiazine 0.75 g per day (1.5 g for first dose), prescribed from 16 weeks of gestation onwards and continued until delivery. Spiramycin was given if TP was diagnosed before 16 weeks gestation (protocol abbreviation: Pyr/Sul) and • Spiramycin (3 × 106 IU four times daily), administered from diagnosis to delivery, and TMP-SMX 160/800 twice a day, plus folinic acid, 4 mg per day, administered from the 14th week of gestation and suspended a week before the child birth (protocol abbreviation: Sp/C [50]	Spiramycin and TMP-SMX tend to have better efficacy [50]

Prevention

Preventing an infection in a susceptible population like pregnant women and immunocompromised patients is very important, especially by educating these people to avoid contact with cats or cat litters and consumption of undercooked meats in endemic areas. Pre-pregnancy screening accompanied by serial titers along with appropriate counseling in women with initial negative titers may minimize cases of congenital toxoplasmosis.

Conclusion

Toxoplasmosis is caused by the obligate intracellular protozoan *T. gondii*. The organism can be transmitted via multiple vectors including foodborne transmission, zoonotic transmission, and congenital transmission. Ocular toxoplasmosis is the most common cause of posterior uveitis in the world accounting for over 80 % of the cases (depending upon series and region of the world). There is no clear consensus regarding the most effective treatment although most patients who are treated receive either Pyrimethamine/Sulfadiazine or trimethoprim/sulfamethoxazole with or without oral Prednisone.

References

1. Weiss LM, Kim K. *Toxoplasma gondii*, the model apicompleaxan: perspectives and methods. 2007; Chapter 1–2.
2. Petersen E, Kijlstra A, Stanford M. Epidemiology of ocular toxoplasmosis. Ocul Immunol Inflamm. 2012;20(2):68–75.
3. Jones JL, Holland GN. Annual burden of ocular toxoplasmosis in the US. Am J Trop Med Hyg. 2010;82(3):464–5.
4. Remington JS. Toxoplasmosis in the adult. Bull N Y Acad Med. 1974;50(2):211–27.
5. McCabe RE, Brooks RG, Dorfman RF, Remington JS. Clinical spectrum in 107 cases of toxoplasmic lymphadenopathy. Rev Infect Dis. 1987;9(4):754–74.
6. Montoya JG, Remington JS. Toxoplasmic chorioretinitis in the setting of acute acquired toxoplasmosis. Clin Infect Dis. 1996;23(2):277–82.
7. Silveira C, Belfort R, Burnier M, Nussenblatt R. Acquired toxoplasmic infection as the cause of toxoplasmic retinochoroiditis in families. Am J Ophthalmol. 1988;106(3):362–4.
8. Silveira C, Belfort R, Muccioli C, et al. A follow-up study of *Toxoplasma gondii* infection in southern Brazil. Am J Ophthalmol. 2001;131(3):351–4.
9. Renold C, Sugar A, Chave JP, et al. Toxoplasma encephalitis in patients with the acquired immunodeficiency syndrome. Medicine (Baltimore). 1992;71(4):224–39.
10. Pauleikhoff D, Messmer E, Beelen DW, Foerster M, Wessing A. Bone-marrow transplantation and toxoplasmic retinochoroiditis. Graefes Arch Clin Exp Ophthalmol. 1987;225(3):239–43.
11. Chung H, Kim JG, Choi SH, Lee SY, Yoon YH. Bilateral toxoplasma retinochoroiditis simulating cytomegalovirus retinitis in an allogeneic bone marrow transplant patient. Korean J Ophthalmol. 2008;22(3):197–200.
12. Palkovacs EM, Correa Z, Augsburger JJ, Eagle RC. Acquired toxoplasmic retinitis in an immunosuppressed patient: diagnosis by transvitreal fine-needle aspiration biopsy. Graefes Arch Clin Exp Ophthalmol. 2008;246(10):1495–7.
13. Smith JR, Cunningham ET. Atypical presentations of ocular toxoplasmosis. Curr Opin Ophthalmol. 2002;13(6):387–92.
14. Rabaud C, May T, Amiel C, et al. Extracerebral toxoplasmosis in patients infected with HIV. A French National Survey. Medicine (Baltimore). 1994;73(6):306–14.
15. Rabaud C, May T, Lucet JC, Leport C, Ambroise-Thomas P, Canton P. Pulmonary toxoplasmosis in patients infected with human immunodeficiency virus: a French National Survey. Clin Infect Dis. 1996;23(6):1249–54.
16. Dunn D, Wallon M, Peyron F, Petersen E, Peckham C, Gilbert R. Mother-to-child transmission of toxoplasmosis: risk estimates for clinical counselling. Lancet. 1999;353(9167):1829–33.
17. Guerina NG, Hsu HW, Meissner HC, et al. Neonatal serologic screening and early treatment for congenital *Toxoplasma gondii* infection. The New England Regional Toxoplasma Working Group. N Engl J Med. 1994;330(26):1858–63.
18. Couvreur J, Desmonts G. Congenital and maternal toxoplasmosis: review of 300 cases. JAMA. 1963;183(11):201.
19. Vasconcelos-Santos DV, Machado Azevedo DO, Campos WR, et al. Congenital toxoplasmosis in southeastern Brazil: results of early ophthalmologic examination of a large cohort of neonates. Ophthalmology. 2009;116(11):2199–205.e1.
20. Melamed J, Eckert GU, Spadoni VS, Lago EG, Uberti F. Ocular manifestations of congenital toxoplasmosis. Eye (Lond). 2010;24(4):528–34.
21. Wilson CB, Remington JS, Stagno S, Reynolds DW. Development of adverse sequelae in children born with subclinical congenital Toxoplasma infection. Pediatrics. 1980;66(5):767–74.
22. Tamma P. Toxoplasmosis. Pediatr Rev. 2007;28(12):470–1.
23. Dodds EM, Holland GN, Stanford MR, et al. Intraocular inflammation associated with ocular toxoplasmosis: relationships at initial examination. Am J Ophthalmol. 2008;146(6):856–65.e2.
24. Vasconcelos-Santos DV, Dodds EM, Oréfice F. Review for disease of the year: differential diagnosis of ocular toxoplasmosis. Ocul Immunol Inflamm. 2011;19(3):171–9.

25. Moorthy RS, Smith RE, Rao NA. Progressive ocular toxoplasmosis in patients with acquired immunodeficiency syndrome. Am J Ophthalmol. 1993;115 (6):742–7.
26. Doft BH, Gass JDM. Punctate outer retinal toxoplasmosis. Arch Ophthalmol. 1985;103(9):1332–6.
27. De Souza EC, Casella AMB. Clinical and tomographic features of macular punctate outer retinal toxoplasmosis. Arch Ophthalmol. 2009;127(10):1390–4.
28. Theodossiadis P, Kokolakis S, Ladas I, Kollia AC, Chatzoulis D, Theodossiadis G. Retinal vascular involvement in acute toxoplasmic retinochoroiditis. Int Ophthalmol. 1995;19(1):19–24.
29. Bosch-Driessen LH, Karimi S, Stilma JS, Rothova A. Retinal detachment in ocular toxoplasmosis. Ophthalmology. 2000;107(1):36–40.
30. Schuman JS, Weinberg RS, Ferry AP, Guerry RK. Toxoplasmic scleritis. Ophthalmology. 1988;95 (10):1399–403.
31. Wallon M, et al. Ophthalmic outcomes of congenital toxoplasmosis followed until adolescence. Pediatrics. 2014;133:e601–8.
32. Jones JL. *Toxoplasma gondii* Infection in the United States: seroprevalence and risk factors. Am J Epidemiol. 2001;154(4):357–65.
33. Zufferey J, Sugar A, Rudaz P, Bille J, Glauser MP, Chave JP. Prevalence of latent toxoplasmosis and serological diagnosis of active infection in HIV-positive patients. Eur J Clin Microbiol Infect Dis. 1993;12(8):591–5.
34. Suresh S, Nor-Masniwati S, Nor-Idahriani MN, Wan-Hazabbah W-H, Zeehaida M, Zunaina E. Serological IgG avidity test for ocular toxoplasmosis. Clin Ophthalmol. 2012;6:147–50.
35. Papadia M, Aldigeri R, Herbort CP. The role of serology in active ocular toxoplasmosis. Int Ophthalmol. 2011;31(6):461–5.
36. Witmer R. Clinical implications of aqueous humor studies in uveitis. Am J Ophthalmol. 1978;86(1):39–44.
37. De Boer JH, Verhagen C, Bruinenberg M, et al. Serologic and polymerase chain reaction analysis of intraocular fluids in the diagnosis of infectious uveitis. Am J Ophthalmol. 1996;121(6):650–8.
38. Baarsma GS, Luyendijk L, Kijlstra A, et al. Analysis of local antibody production in the vitreous humor of patients with severe uveitis. Am J Ophthalmol. 1991;112(2):147–50.
39. Moshfeghi DM, Dodds EM, Couto CA, et al. Diagnostic approaches to severe, atypical toxoplasmosis mimicking acute retinal necrosis. Ophthalmology. 2004;111(4):716–25.
40. Montoya JG, Parmley S, Liesenfeld O, Jaffe GJ, Remington JS. Use of the polymerase chain reaction for diagnosis of ocular toxoplasmosis. Ophthalmology. 1999;106(8):1554–63.
41. Lam S, Tessler HH. Quadruple therapy for ocular toxoplasmosis. Can J Ophthalmol. 1993;28(2):58–61.
42. Baharivand N, Mahdavifard A, Fouladi RF. Intravitreal clindamycin plus dexamethasone versus classic oral therapy in toxoplasmic retinochoroiditis: a prospective randomized clinical trial. Int Ophthalmol. 2013;33(1):39–46.
43. Soheilian M, Ramezani A, Azimzadeh A, et al. Randomized trial of intravitreal clindamycin and dexamethasone versus pyrimethamine, sulfadiazine, and prednisolone in treatment of ocular toxoplasmosis. Ophthalmology. 2011;118(1):134–41.
44. Bosch-Driessen LH, Verbraak FD, Suttorp-Schulten MS, et al. A prospective, randomized trial of pyrimethamine and azithromycin vs pyrimethamine and sulfadiazine for the treatment of ocular toxoplasmosis. Am J Ophthalmol. 2002;134(1):34–40.
45. Soheilian M, Sadoughi M-M, Ghajarnia M, et al. Prospective randomized trial of trimethoprim/sulfamethoxazole versus pyrimethamine and sulfadiazine in the treatment of ocular toxoplasmosis. Ophthalmology. 2005;112(11):1876–82.
46. Winterhalter S, Severing K, Stammen J, Maier AK, Godehardt E, Joussen AM. Does atovaquone prolong the disease-free interval of toxoplasmic retinochoroiditis? Graefes Arch Clin Exp Ophthalmol. 2010;248(8):1187–92.
47. Pearson PA, Piracha AR, Sen HA, Jaffe GJ. Atovaquone for the treatment of toxoplasma retinochoroiditis in immunocompetent patients. Ophthalmology. 1999;106(1):148–53.
48. Silveira C, Belfort R, Muccioli C, et al. The effect of long-term intermittent trimethoprim/ sulfamethoxazole treatment on recurrences of toxoplasmic retinochoroiditis. Am J Ophthalmol. 2002;134(1):41–6.
49. Paquet C, Yudin MH. Toxoplasmosis in pregnancy: prevention, screening, and treatment. J Obstet Gynaecol Can. 2013;35(1):78–9.
50. Valentini P, Buonsenso D, Barone G, Serranti D, Calzedda R, Ceccarelli M, Speziale D, Ricci R, Masini L. Spiramycin/cotrimoxazole versus pyrimethamine/sulfonamide and spiramycin alone for the treatment of toxoplasmosis in pregnancy. J Perinatol. 2015;35(2):90–4. doi:10.1038/jp.2014.161 Epub 2014 Sep 11.
51. Gilbert RE, Harden M, Stanford M. Antibiotics versus control for toxoplasma retinochoroiditis. In: The Cochrane Collaboration, ed. Chichester, UK: John Wiley & Sons, Ltd; 2002.
52. Harrell M, Carvounis PE. Current treatment of toxoplasma retinochoroiditis: an evidence-based review. J Ophthalmol. 2014;2014:273506.
53. Jasper S, Vedula SS, John SS, Horo S, Sepah YJ, Nguyen QD. Corticosteroids as adjuvant therapy for ocular toxoplasmosis. In: Nguyen QD, editor. The Cochrane Collaboration. Chichester, UK: John Wiley & Sons, Ltd; 2013.
54. Kim SJ, Scott IU, Brown GC, et al. Interventions for toxoplasma retinochoroiditis: a report by the American Academy of Ophthalmology. Ophthalmology. 2013;120(2):371–8.
55. Wallon M, Garweg JG, Abrahamowicz M, et al. Ophthalmic outcomes of congenital toxoplasmosis followed until adolescence. Pediatrics. 2014;133(3):e601–8.

56. Atmaca LS, Simsek T, Batioglu F. Clinical features and prognosis in ocular toxoplasmosis. Jpn J Ophthalmol. 2004;48(4).
57. Kianersi F, Naderi Beni A, Naderi Beni Z. Clinical manifestation and prognosis of active ocular toxoplasmosis in Iran. Int Ophthalmol. 2012;32(6):539–45.
58. Bosch-Driessen LE, Berendschot TTJ, Ongkosuwito JV, Rothova A. Ocular toxoplasmosis. Ophthalmology. 2002;109(5):869–78.
59. Friedmann CT, Knox DL. Variations in recurrent active toxoplasmic retinochoroiditis. Arch Ophthalmol. 1969;81(4):481–93.
60. Wallon M, Kodjikian L, Binquet C, et al. Long-term ocular prognosis in 327 children with congenital toxoplasmosis. Pediatrics. 2004;113 (6):1567–72.
61. Berrébi A, Assouline C, Bessières M-H, et al. Long-term outcome of children with congenital toxoplasmosis. Am J Obstet Gynecol. 2010;203 (6):552.e1–6.
62. Faucher B, Garcia-Meric P, Franck J, et al. Long-term ocular outcome in congenital toxoplasmosis: a prospective cohort of treated children. J Infect. 2012;64(1):104–9.

Tuberculosis

15

Soumyava Basu and Narsing A. Rao

Introduction

Ocular tuberculosis (TB) is a common cause of infectious uveitis in TB-endemic countries, and is being increasingly reported from non-endemic countries. The diagnosis of ocular TB poses two major challenges to treating physicians: multiple clinical manifestations of the disease that overlap with other forms of uveitis, and absence of definitive diagnosis based on detection of the pathogen in majority of cases. Despite these challenges, there have been advances in our understanding of clinical manifestations and diagnostic criteria for ocular TB, in the last two decades.

Epidemiology

TB is a major global health problem. In 2012, there were 8.6 million new TB cases and 1.3 million TB deaths, worldwide [1]. In addition, one-third of the world population is infected with latent *Mycobacterium tuberculosis* infection. About 5–10 % of such infected persons are known to develop active TB disease at some time in their lives [2]. The problem has been largely controlled in developed nations during the last century, though it continues to persist in the foreign-born who migrated to developed nations from TB-endemic countries and HIV-infected population. Importantly, the decline in prevalence of extrapulmonary TB in the developed nations has been much slower than pulmonary TB [3].

Majority of reports on ocular TB during the last two decades have been from high-endemic countries like India and other Asian countries, where it accounted from 0.6 to 20 % of all uveitis cases [4, 5]. The difference in prevalence rates reflects evolution in diagnostic criteria, and recognition of varied clinical manifestations of ocular TB. Additionally, in recent years, there have been several reports from low endemic countries, most of which are related to the foreign-born population [6–8].

Clinical Manifestations

Ocular TB has protean manifestations that encompass nearly every tissue in the eye (Table 15.1). They range from anterior and intermediate uveitis to various forms of posterior

S. Basu
Retina-Vitreous and Uvea Service, L V Prasad Eye Institute, Bhubaneswar 751024, Odisha, India
e-mail: eyetalk@gmail.com

N.A. Rao (✉)
Department of Ophthalmology, The Keck School of Medicine, USC Eye Institute, University of Southern California, Los Angeles, CA 90033, USA
e-mail: NRao@doheny.org

G.N. Papaliodis (ed.), *Uveitis*,
DOI 10.1007/978-3-319-09126-6_15

and panuveitis, keratitis, necrotizing, or non-necrotizing scleritis, sclerouveitis, orbital inflammation, optic neuropathy, and endophthalmitis [9].

Anterior Uveitis

This is typically granulomatous though the non-granulomatous form has also been described. Granulomatous uveitis is identified by presence of mutton-fat keratic precipitates and iris nodules (Koeppe and Busacca) and may be associated with broad posterior synechiae (Fig. 15.1).

Intermediate Uveitis

TB can account for nearly half the cases of intermediate uveitis in high-endemic countries [10]. It presents as chronic, low-grade inflammation associated with vitritis, and 'snowballs' in vitreous cavity. 'Snow-banking' is less commonly seen. Long-standing disease may lead to cystoid macular edema, complicated cataract, elevated intraocular pressure, epiretinal membrane, and peripheral retinal neovascularization.

Posterior and Panuveitis

The most common manifestations of tubercular posterior uveitis in ophthalmic practice are retinal vasculitis and multifocal serpiginoid choroiditis. Different manifestations of posterior uveitis may co-exist in the same or opposite eye (Fig. 15.2). The posterior uveitis can be accompanied by generalized intraocular inflammation (panuveitis), anterior, and intermediate uveitis.

Retinal Vasculitis

Tubercular retinal vasculitis typically involves the retinal veins, i.e., it causes retinal periphlebitis. It has two distinguishing features that can help in making a clinical diagnosis in high-endemic countries: presence of healed or active choroiditis patches usually overlying blood vessels and large areas of capillary non-perfusion (on fluorescein angiography) in segments drained by the involved veins (Figs. 15.3a, b and 15.4). Common complications include macular edema, retinal neovascularization, vitreous hemorrhage, and tractional retinal detachment.

Eales' disease is a related form of retinal periphlebitis, associated with recurrent vitreous hemorrhage. Polymerase chain reaction (PCR)-based analysis of ocular tissue samples from Eales' disease patients has linked this condition to TB [11].

Infectious Multifocal Serpiginoid Choroiditis (MSC)

This is a chronic recurrent inflammation of the retinal pigment epithelium and inner choroid that shows central healing and active margins progressing in an ameboid fashion (Fig. 15.5a, b).

Table 15.1 Clinical manifestations of ocular tuberculosis

Anterior uveitis	Granulomatous
	Non-granulomatous
Intermediate uveitis	
Posterior and panuveitis	Retinal vasculitis
	Multifocal serpiginoid choroiditis
	Choroidal tubercles/tuberculoma
	Subretinal abscess
Tubercular optic neuropathy	Papillitis
	Neuroretinitis
	Optic nerve granuloma
Endophthalmitis and panophthalmitis	

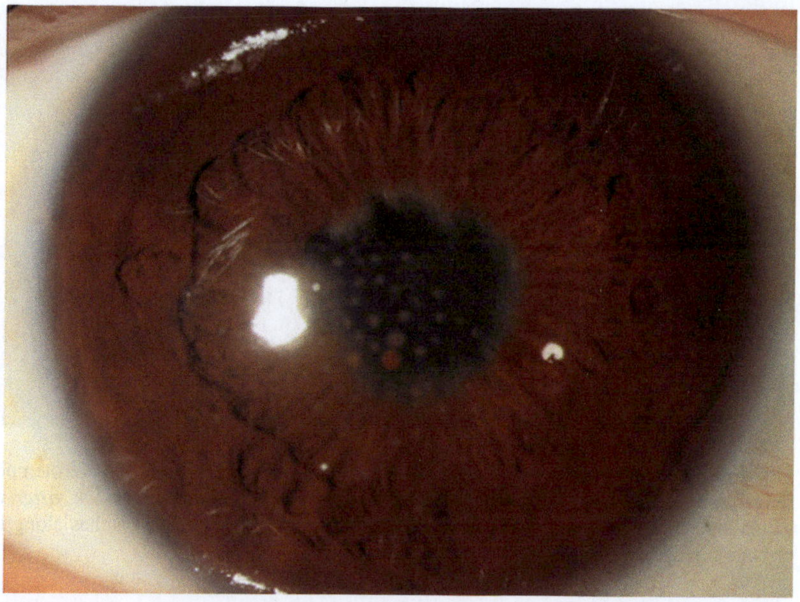

Fig. 15.1 Tuberculous anterior uveitis showing 'mutton-fat' keratic precipitates and broad posterior synechiae

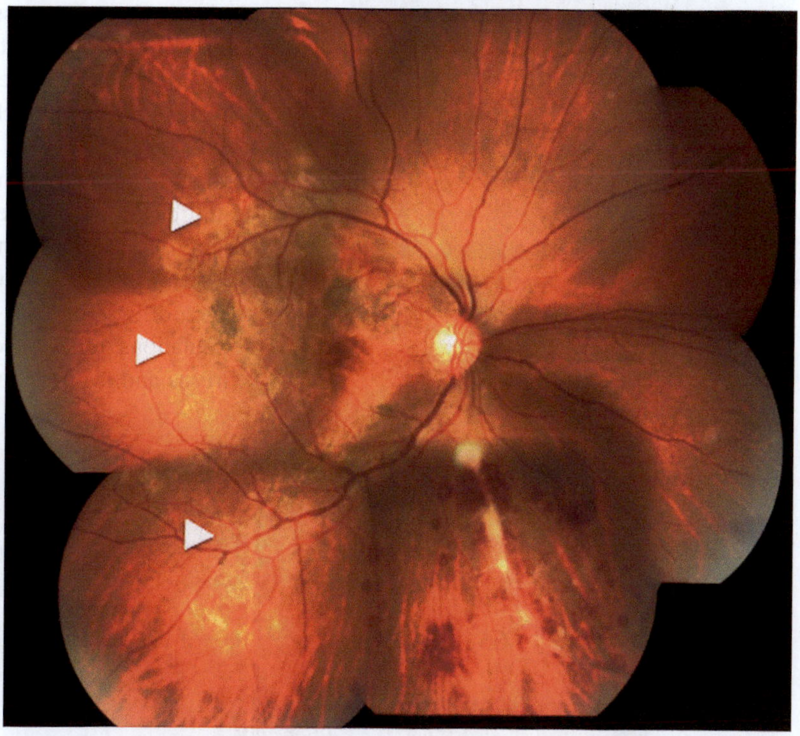

Fig. 15.2 Fundus photograph of right eye showing multifocal serpiginoid choroiditis (*arrowheads*) associated with retinal vasculitis and hemorrhages along inferonasal quadrant

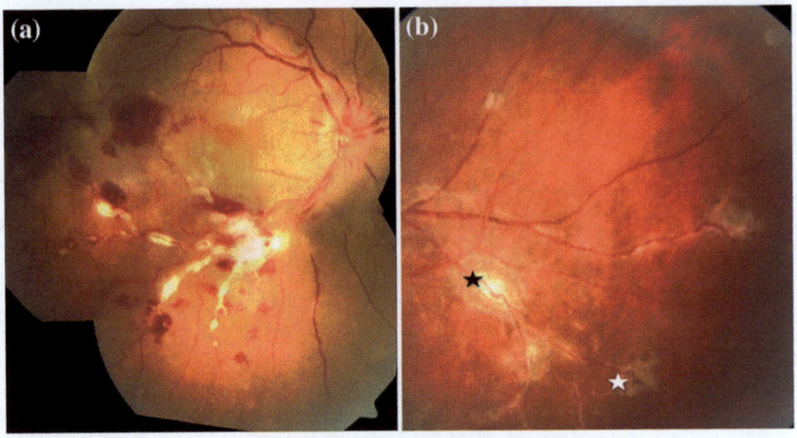

Fig. 15.3 **a** Fundus photograph of right eye showing retinal periphlebitis associated with massive perivascular exudation, in the inferotemporal quadrant. Retinal hemorrhages and macular edema are also seen. **b** Fundus photograph of inferotemporal quadrant of left eye showing active (*black asterix*) and healed (*white asterix*) choroiditis patches along blood vessels

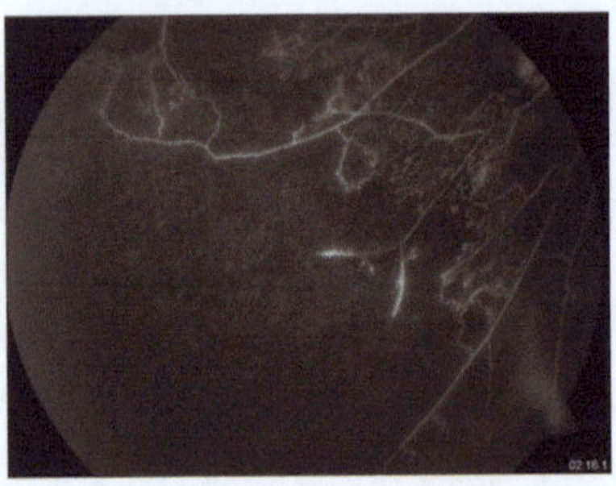

Fig. 15.4 Fluorescein angiogram of inferotemporal quadrant of an eye with retinal vasculitis showing extensive areas of capillary non-perfusion and early retinal neovascularization

Three patterns have been described: multifocal lesions that progress to confluent, diffuse choroiditis, lesions that are diffuse at presentation and a mixed variety (between opposite eyes) [12].

The following characteristics distinguish MSC from classical serpiginous choroiditis: endemic population/travel to endemic area, multifocality, presence of vitritis, lesions originating at macular, dense pigmentation at center of lesions, and immunological/radiological evidence of systemic TB [13]. In TB non-endemic populations, other infective etiologies like herpes viruses and syphilis can present with features of

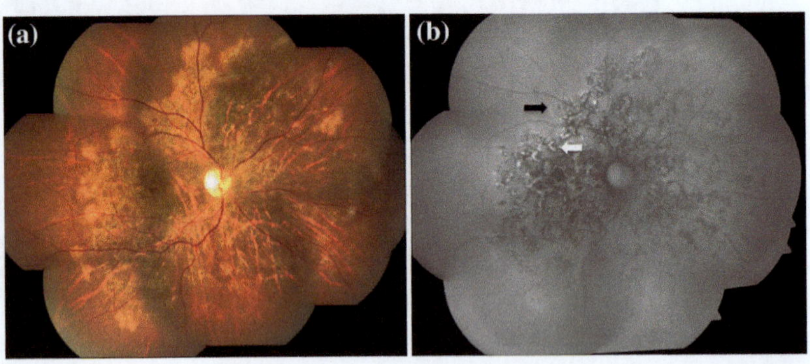

Fig. 15.5 **a** Fundus photograph of right eye showing large confluent area of serpiginoid choroiditis with central healing and active temporal margins **b** fundus autofluorescence of the same eye showing ill-defined halo of hyperfluorescence (*black arrow*) corresponding to the active lesions and dark ring of hypofluorescence (*white arrow*) appearing around early healing lesions. Multiple skip lesions along the nasal quadrants are also seen

MSC. However, in some the infectious agent cannot be detected even after extensive investigations including qPCR and retina-choroidal biopsy. Such cases remain as idiopathic.

Choroidal Tubercles/Tuberculoma

These may be solitary or multiple and are typically associated with active pulmonary/extrapulmonary TB. As such, they are more likely to be encountered in general hospitals than in ophthalmic practice. The lesions heal into atrophic patches with variable pigmentation. Occasionally, the tubercle may grow into a large solitary mass that is then called a *tuberculoma*, that need to be distinguished from neoplastic lesions; benign, or malignant (Fig. 15.6).

Subretinal Abscess

These are large yellowish subretinal lesions that occur due to liquefaction of caseous material in large tuberculous granulomas. They usually respond well to antituberculous therapy (ATT), healing with atrophy and variable pigmentation.

Tubercular Optic Neuritis

Theses may range from papillitis and neuroretinitis to optic nerve granuloma [14]. They are usually associated with some form of uveitis. Most cases recover well after appropriate therapy.

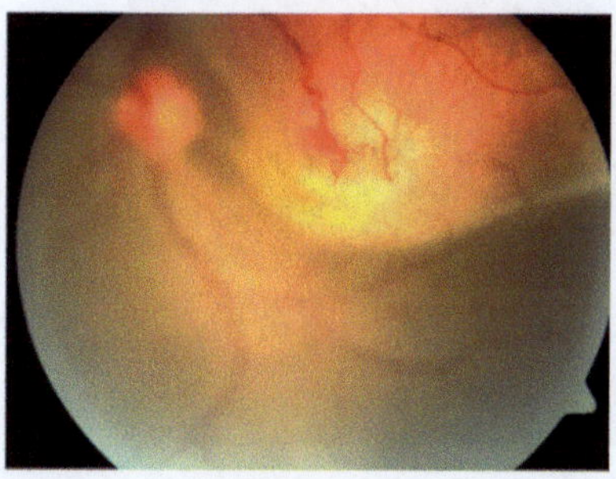

Fig. 15.6 Fundus photograph of left eye showing large mass lesion in superotemporal quadrant extending on to the macula. An area of retinal angiomatous proliferation is seen at the apex of the lesion

Endophthalmitis and Panophthalmitis

These present acutely with hypopyon and dense vitritis. Subretinal or choroidal abscess can be present that may burst into the vitreous cavity. Unlike the previously mentioned clinical manifestations, acid-fast bacilli may be demonstrated in aqueous or vitreous samples in such cases.

Pathogenesis

The pathogenesis of ocular TB in the form of intraocular inflammation/uveitis has long been debated. The identification of *M. tuberculosis* in enucleated eyes and amplification of mycobacterial DNA from ocular fluid samples suggest that this condition results from an inflammatory response to the bacteria in ocular tissues [15, 16]. Animal models have shown that mycobacteria are disseminated to the eye from pulmonary foci, as in other cases of extrapulmonary TB [17]. It has been suggested that mycobacteria remain sequestered in the RPE in a dormant form for long periods and on their activation they lead to recurrent inflammation [18]. Most recently, it has been shown that RPE cells are better able to control growth of *M. tuberculosis* than macrophages, which helps them survive longer in the presence of infection [19].

However, ocular TB is also paucibacillary, as noted in a large series of 42 patients with histopathologically proven ocular TB [20]. Thus the organism is rarely found in ocular tissues. This has led many authors to believe that ocular TB results from immune reaction to tubercular antigens released from extraocular foci. Such a phenomenon is not seen in any other form of TB and has not been validated for ocular TB.

Ocular Imaging

Although ocular TB is a clinical diagnosis in the majority of patients, imaging studies can be helpful in assessing disease activity, and evaluating associated complications of intraocular inflammation.

Fundus Photography

Serial fundus photography can be very useful in documenting disease progression as well as identifying small lesions that may be missed on routine examination.

Fluorescein Angiography

It is most useful in patients with retinal vasculitis in demonstrating areas of capillary non-perfusion and associated neovascularization (Fig. 15.4) [9]. In MSC, active margins show initial hypofluorescence and late hyperfluorescence while healed areas show transmission hyperfluorescence or blocked hypofluorescence depending on RPE atrophy or proliferation. It can also help in the diagnosis choroidal neovascular membranes that may complicate MSC.

Fundus Autofluorescence

It has emerged as a quick imaging tool for monitoring the course of MFC lesions [21]. Typically, acute lesions show an ill-defined halo of hyperautofluorescence. With healing, a dark outer rim of hypoautofluorescence appears, that progressively increases to occupy the entire lesion.

Optical Coherence Tomography (OCT)

It also shows characteristic changes in MFC lesions [22]. In spectral-domain optical coherence tomography (OCT), acute lesions show hyperreflective areas in outer retina and RPE with no back-scattering from inner choroid (Fig. 15.7). As the lesions heal, choroidal reflectance increases and the outer retina/RPE shows transition from hyperreflectivity to knob-like elevations and finally atrophy. OCT is also useful in documenting macular pathology like cystoid macular edema and epiretinal membranes.

Ultrasonography and Ultrasound Biomicroscopy

In hazy media, ultrasonography can help in differentiating tuberculomas and subretinal abscesses (moderate to low internal reflectivity) from intraocular tumors, while ultrasound biomicroscopy can help in studying the pars plana for ciliary body atrophy or presence of a granuloma [9].

Laboratory Investigations

These are directed at obtaining immunological/radiological evidence of systemic TB as well as direct evidence of *M. tuberculosis* in ocular

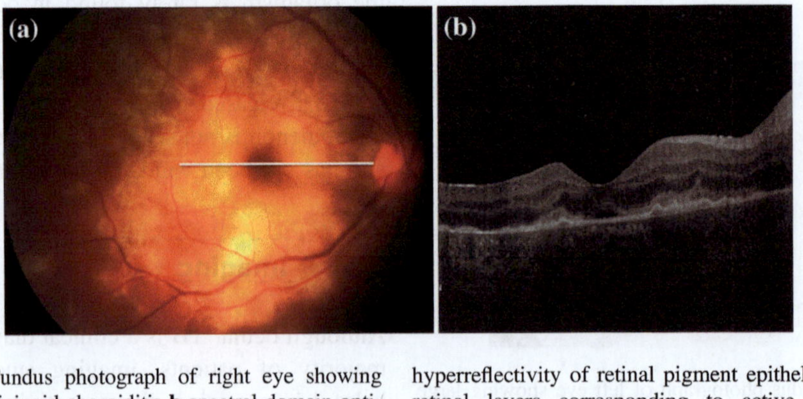

Fig. 15.7 **a** Fundus photograph of right eye showing multifocal serpiginoid choroiditis **b** spectral-domain optical coherence tomography of same eye showing hyperreflectivity of retinal pigment epithelium and outer retinal layers corresponding to active lesions, with minimum back scattering from underlying choroid

fluids. Additional tests are required to rule out other infectious and noninfectious entities that have overlapping features with those in a given patient, and for confirming immune competence in the patient.

Immunological Tests

Two tests are available for immunological diagnosis of mycobacterial infection: the purified protein derivative (PPD) or Mantoux skin test, and the interferon-gamma release assays (IGRA). There has been much debate over the superiority of one test over the other in diagnosis of ocular TB. As per the Centers for Disease Control and Prevention, the sensitivity of IGRA is 'statistically similar to that of PPD for detecting infection in persons with untreated culture-confirmed TB' [23]. Importantly, neither test can distinguish between active and latent TB.

PPD Skin Test

The CDC guidelines suggest intradermal injection of 5 tuberculin units on forearm and measuring size of induration 48–72 h after injection [24]. The test is reported positive if the size is ≥15 mm in non-endemic population, ≥10 mm in TB-endemic population and ≥5 mm in immune deficient patients, those having chest radiographic signs of healed TB and those having recent contact with active TB. Prior BCG vaccination in childhood usually has minimal residual effect after 10 years of age, and is not a contraindication for PPD skin test.

IGRA

Two types of IGRA are commercially available: QuantiFERON-Gold-in-Tube (Cellestis Inc, Australia) and T-SPOT.TB (Oxford Immunotech, UK). Recent reports suggest that QFT is superior to T-SPOT test for diagnosis of TB uveitis [25]. In general, IGRAs have the advantage of higher specificity than PPD in patients exposed to environmental mycobacteria, and recent BCG vaccination, or in detection of latent TB in patients with sarcoidosis. However, they are significantly more expensive [26].

Radiological Tests

Routine chest radiography can reveal evidence of healed or active pulmonary TB anywhere in the lung fields. Mediastinal or paratracheal lymphadenopathy may also be present but is not diagnostic of TB. High resolution computed tomography (HRCT) of thorax may have increased sensitivity for the detection of pulmonary or mediastinal TB [27]. Recently, positron emission tomography (PET)/CT scan has been used to demonstrate metabolic activity in mediastinal lymph nodes that were not detected on CT scan of thorax [28].

Definitive Evidence of *M. Tuberculosis* in Ocular Tissues

Detection of mycobacteria by microscopy or culture requires high bacillary load (microscopy > culture), which is almost never found in ocular fluids that are accessible for evaluation. Mycobacteria from ocular tissues are generally reported in cases of endophthalmitis/panophthalmitis or in enucleated eyes.

PCR-based assays have recently emerged as a promising approach for definitive diagnosis of ocular TB in large number of cases [29]. New innovations like multi-target PCR (multiple gene targets including IS6110, MPB64 and Protein B) have helped in achieving greater than 70 % positivity rates in clinically suspected cases of ocular TB [30]. It is important for ocular fluid samples being tested to have cellular reaction since *M. tuberculosis* is an intra-cellular organism. Application of real-time PCR can help in differentiating true mycobacterial infection of the eye from false positive cases especially in TB-endemic populations.

Approach to Diagnosis

The majority of cases of ocular TB are diagnosed on the basis of clinical signs, ancillary tests (immunological and radiological), and exclusion of other uveitic entities.

In high-endemic regions, the following clinical signs were found to be predictive of

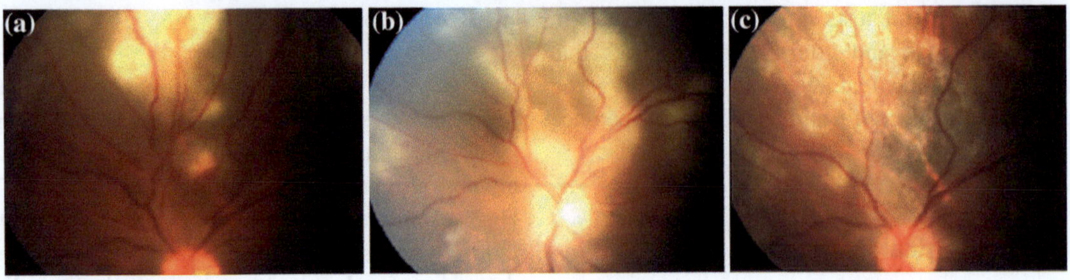

Fig. 15.8 Fundus photographs of left eye showing active choroiditis lesions in superior quadrant **a** that increased in size after one week of anti-TB therapy **b** and resolved completely on escalation of corticosteroid therapy and continuation of anti-TB therapy **c**

tubercular uveitis: broad based posterior synechiae, retinal vasculitis with or without choroiditis, and serpiginous-like choroiditis, though other clinical presentations are not uncommon [31]. The key to diagnosis lies in exclusion of other uveitic entities—infectious and noninfectious that may have similar clinical presentation in the given geographic region. In low-endemic areas, the most important factors in diagnosis are the origin of the patient from TB-endemic country and presence of immune-deficiency like HIV infection, health-care workers, homeless people, and those incarcerated. Recent reports suggest that a large majority of ocular TB patients in these non-endemic countries had either migrated from, or had traveled to high-endemic countries [6–8].

Systemic evidence of TB (immunological and radiological) is not essential for the diagnosis of ocular TB. In 42 cases of histopathologically proven cases of ocular TB, 40 % of tested patients had negative TST and 57 % had normal chest radiograph [20]. In another series of 80 PCR positive patients, 44 % patients had negative PPD skin test, and 83 % had normal chest radiograms [30]. It is likely that with further refinements in PCR technique, more patients without systemic evidence of TB will be diagnosed as ocular TB.

Treatment

Treatment of ocular TB is based on a combination of antituberculosis treatment (ATT) commonly composed of four drugs and anti-inflammatory therapy (usually corticosteroids). ATT has been shown to reduce the rate of recurrent inflammation from 46 to 16 %, in patients with clinically suspected ocular TB [32]. ATT should be given for a minimum of 6 months in total—2 months of four-drug therapy (isoniazid 5 mg/kg daily, rifampicin 450 mg daily, pyrazinamide 30 mg/kg daily and ethambutol 15 mg/kg daily) followed by a 4-month continuation phase of isoniazid and rifampicin. Many authors have suggested a longer duration for the continuation phase, citing slow response to the drug in intraocular tuberculosis. It was found that those receiving > 9 months ATT were significantly less likely to develop recurrence compared to those not receiving ATT [33]. However, the reduction in recurrence compared to other ATT durations (<6 months, 6–9 months) was not statistically significant. Patients on ATT need to be monitored for ocular and systemic toxicities both by the ophthalmologist and internist with expertise in the management of systemic tuberculosis. Systemic issues that arise are primarily from the drug related hepatotoxicity. Ocular toxicities include optic neuropathy (ethambutol, especially if used >15 mg/day for >2 months, and rarely, isoniazid) and anterior uveitis (rifabutin). Concomitant corticosteroid therapy is vital to control the inflammatory tissue damage caused by delayed type hypersensitivity to *M. tuberculosis*. The mode of corticosteroid therapy (topical, periocular, intraocular, or systemic) depends upon the degree and primary site of inflammation.

Paradoxical worsening of ocular inflammation is occasionally seen after initiation of ATT for ocular TB [34]. Such paradoxical worsening usually occurs in the initial 4–6 weeks after initiation of ATT and needs to be differentiated from various causes of treatment failure like drug resistance, reinfection or missed diagnosis. It responds well to continuance or escalation of corticosteroids (Fig. 15.8).

Besides ATT and corticosteroids, various forms of ancillary therapy may be required for management of complications of ocular TB. These include laser photocoagulation and/or anti-vascular endothelial growth factor therapy for retinal or disk neovascularization in retinal vasculitis, pars plana vitrectomy for tractional retinal detachment or epiretinal membrane, and surgery for complicated cataracts and glaucoma.

References

1. http://www.who.int/tb/publications/global_report/gtbr13_main_text.pdf?ua=1. Accessed 24 Feb 14.
2. http://www.cdc.gov/tb/publications/factsheets/general/LTBIandActiveTB.pdf. Accessed 24 Feb 14.
3. Peto HM, Pratt RH, Harrington TA, et al. Epidemiology of extrapulmonary tuberculosis in the United States, 1993–2006. Clin Infect Dis. 2009;49(9):1350–7.
4. Biswas J, Narain S, Das D, Ganesh SK. Pattern of uveitis in a referral uveitis clinic in India. Int Ophthalmol. 1996–1997;20(4):223–8.
5. Singh R, Gupta V, Gupta A. Pattern of uveitis in a referral eye clinic in north India. Indian J Ophthalmol. 2004;52(2):121–5.
6. Gan WL, Jones NP. Serpiginous-like choroiditis as a marker for tuberculosis in a non-endemic area. Br J Ophthalmol. 2013;97(5):644–7.
7. La Distia Nora R, van Velthoven ME, Ten Dam-van Loon NH, et al. Clinical manifestations of patients with intraocular inflammation and positive QuantiFERON-TB Gold in-tube test in a country nonendemic for tuberculosis. Am J Ophthalmol. 2013;pii:S0002-9394(13)00736-8. doi:10.1016/j.ajo.2013.11.013. [Epub ahead of print].
8. Hong BK, Khanamiri HN, Bababeygy SR, Rao NA. The utility of routine tuberculosis screening in county hospital patients with uveitis. Br J Ophthalmol. 2014. doi:10.1136/bjophthalmol-2013-303937. [Epub ahead of print].
9. Gupta V, Gupta A, Rao NA. Intra-ocular tuberculosis—an update. Surv Ophthalmol. 2007;52:561–87.
10. Parchand S, Tandan M, Gupta V, Gupta A. Intermediate uveitis in the Indian population. J Ophthalmic Inflamm Infect. 2011;1(2):65–70.
11. Madhavan HN, Therese KL, Gunisha P, et al. Polymerase chain reaction for detection of *Mycobacterium tuberculosis* in epiretinal membrane in Eales' disease. Invest Ophthalmol Vis Sci. 2000;41(3):822–5.
12. Gupta V, Gupta A, Arora S, et al. Presumed tubercular serpiginouslike choroiditis: clinical presentations and management. Ophthalmology. 2003;110(9):1744–9.
13. Nazari Khanamiri H, Rao NA. Serpiginous choroiditis and infectious multifocal serpiginoid choroiditis. Surv Ophthalmol. 2013;58(3):203–32.
14. Davis EJ, Rathinam SR, Okada AA, et al. Clinical spectrum of tuberculous optic neuropathy. J Ophthalmic Inflamm Infect. 2012;2(4):183–9.
15. Biswas J, Madhavan HN, Gopal L, Badrinath SS. Intraocular tuberculosis. Clinicopathologic study of five cases. Retina. 1995;15(6):461–8.
16. Gupta V, Arora S, Gupta A, et al. Management of presumed intraocular tuberculosis: possible role of the polymerase chain reaction. Acta Ophthalmol Scand. 1998;76(6):679–82.
17. Rao NA, Albini TA, Kumaradas M, et al. Experimental ocular tuberculosis in guinea pigs. Arch Ophthalmol. 2009;127(9):1162–6.
18. Rao NA, Saraswathy S, Smith RE. Tuberculous uveitis: distribution of *Mycobacterium tuberculosis* in the retinal pigment epithelium. Arch Ophthalmol. 2006;124(12):1777–9.
19. Nazari H, Karakousis PC, Rao NA. Replication of *Mycobacterium tuberculosis* in retinal pigment epithelium. JAMA Ophthalmol. 2014. doi:10.1001/jamaophthalmol.2014.270. [Epub ahead of print].
20. Wroblewski KJ, Hidayat AA, Neafie RC, et al. Ocular tuberculosis: a clinicopathologic and molecular study. Ophthalmology. 2011;118:772–7.
21. Gupta A, Bansal R, Gupta V, Sharma A. Fundus autofluorescence in serpiginous-like choroiditis. Retina. 2012;32(4):814–25.
22. Bansal R, Kulkarni P, Gupta A, et al. High-resolution spectral domain optical coherence tomography and fundus autofluorescence correlation in tubercular serpiginous-like choroiditis. J Ophthalmic Inflamm Infect. 2011;1(4):157–63.
23. Mazurek GH, Jereb J, Vernon A, et al. Updated guidelines for using interferon gamma release assays to detect *Mycobacterium tuberculosis* infection—United States, 2010. MMWR Recomm Rep 2010;59(RR-5):1–25.
24. American Thoracic Society. Targeted tuberculin testing and treatment of latent tuberculosis infection. MMWR Recomm Rep 2000;49:1e51 (A).
25. Ang M, Wong WL, Kiew SY, et al. Prospective head-to-head study comparing two commercial interferon-gamma release assays for the diagnosis of tuberculous uveitis. Am J Ophthalmol. 2014; pii:S0002-9394(14)00061-0. doi:10.1016/j.ajo.2014.01.031. [Epub ahead of print].
26. Albini TA, Karakousis PC, Rao NA. Interferon-gamma release assays in the diagnosis of tuberculous uveitis. Am J Ophthalmol. 2008;146(4):486–8.

27. Ganesh SK, Roopleen, Biswas J, Veena N. Role of high-resolution computerized tomography (HRCT) of the chest in granulomatous uveitis: a tertiary uveitis clinic experience from India. Ocul Immunol Inflamm. 2011;19(1):51–7.
28. Doycheva D, Pfannenberg C, Hetzel J, et al. Presumed tuberculosis-induced retinal vasculitis, diagnosed with positron emission tomography (18F-FDG-PET/CT), aspiration biopsy, and culture. Ocul Immunol Inflamm. 2010;18(3):194–9.
29. Sharma K, Gupta V, Bansal R, et al. Novel multi-targeted polymerase chain reaction for diagnosis of presumed tubercular uveitis. J Ophthalmic Inflamm Infect. 2013;3(1):25.
30. Balne PK, Modi RR, Choudhury N, et al. Factors influencing polymerase chain reaction outcomes in patients with clinically suspected ocular tuberculosis. J Ophthalmic Inflamm Infect. 2014;25;4(1):10. [Epub ahead of print].
31. Gupta A, Bansal R, Gupta V, et al. Ocular signs predictive of tubercular uveitis. Am J Ophthalmol. 2010;149:562–70.
32. Bansal R, Gupta A, Gupta V, et al. Role of anti-tubercular therapy in uveitis associated with latent tuberculosis. Am J Ophthalmol. 2008;146(5):772–9.
33. Ang M, Hedayatfar A, Wong W, Chee SP. Duration of anti-tubercular therapy in uveitis associated with latent tuberculosis: a case-control study. Br J Ophthalmol. 2012;96(3):332–6.
34. Basu S, Nayak S, Padhi TR, Das T. Progressive ocular inflammation following anti-tubercular therapy for presumed ocular tuberculosis in a high-endemic setting. Eye. 2013;27(5):657–62.

16 Whipple's Disease

George N. Papaliodis

Introduction

Whipple's disease is a rare systemic disorder caused by the Gram positive bacterium *Tropheryma whippelii* (*T. whippelii*). Although the initial report was characterized by a malabsorption syndrome involving the small intestine, this malady can affect the joints, central nervous system, cardiovascular system, and eyes. The ocular manifestations are similarly uncommon (approximately 5 % of patients with Whipple's disease will have ocular involvement) but can include vitritis, retinal vasculitis, choroiditis, ophthalmoplegia, and keratitis [1].

Epidemiology

The first case report of this entity in the medical literature was in 1895, but this was not recognized as a specific disease until George Hoyt Whipple described a patient with diarrhea secondary to malabsorption, weight loss, migratory polyarthritis, and mesenteric lymphadenopathy in 1907 [2]. The disorder is exceptionally rare with fewer than 1000 cases reported world-wide. The condition appears to be associated with human leukocyte antigen HLA-B27 haplotype [3] and is more common in white males (male to female ratio approximately 8–9:1).

Clinical Manifestations

The clinical manifestations of the disease are presumed to be caused by infiltration of various body tissues by the Gram positive bacterium *T. whippelii*. The disease is characterized by a chronic diarrhea secondary to malabsorption and polyarthritis. Approximately 90 % of those with the disorder have unintentional weight loss. Seronegative arthritis has been reported in 90 % of patients and may precede other systemic symptoms. The ocular inflammation can present as vitritis, retinal vasculitis, retinitis, retinal hemorrhages, choroiditis, optic atrophy, and keratitis [1]. In a retrospective series of patients with central nervous system Whipple's disease, manifestations included: delirium (17 %), cognitive impairment/memory dysfunction (61 %), hypersomnia (17 %), abnormal movements, e.g. myoclonus (39 %), cerebral ataxia (11 %), seizure/status epilepticus (17 %), ophthalmoplegia (17 %) [4]. Up to 33 % of patients will develop cardiac involvement including systolic

G.N. Papaliodis (✉)
Department of Ophthalmology, Harvard Medical School, Massachusetts Eye and Ear Infirmary, Boston, MA 02114, USA
e-mail: George_Papaliodis@meei.harvard.edu

G.N. Papaliodis (ed.), *Uveitis*,
DOI 10.1007/978-3-319-09126-6_16

murmurs, congestive heart failure, and conduction abnormalities.

Diagnosis

The diagnosis of Whipple's disease is established by tissue biopsy (often from the small bowel as this is the most commonly involved site) demonstrating periodic acid-Schiff (PAS) positive macrophages in the lamina propria. Polymerse chain reaction of blood, saliva, and ocular fluids is highly sensitive for the detection of the organism but not highly specific; thus the interpretation of a positive test in a healthy patient may not necessarily be diagnostic of pathology [5].

Treatment

The mainstay of treatment for Whipple's disease is protracted antibiotic therapy. Numerous antibiotic regimens have demonstrated efficacy including: penicillin, erythromycin, ampicillin, chloramphenicol, tetracycline, and trimethoprim-sulfamethoxazole [1]. Given the rare incidence of this disorder, it is impossible to determine which regimen is superior nor the appropriate duration of therapy. Several investigators suggest treatment with 14 days of intravenous penicillin followed by one year of trimethoprim-sulfamethoxazole (one double strength BID for 12 months) [1]. The associated intraocular inflammation can be treated with topical, regional, or systemic corticosteroids.

Conclusion

Whipple's disease is a rare systemic disorder caused by the organism *T. whippelii* more commonly manifesting as a malabsorptive diarrhea and migratory oligoarthritis. Ocular involvement has been documented in approximately 5 % of patients. Historically Whipple's disease had a poor prognosis with nearly 100 % mortality after one year in patients who were untreated. Current treat regimens with protracted antibiotics (1 year of therapy) are highly successful.

References

1. Dobbins WO III. Whipple's disease. Springfield, IL: Charles C Thomas; 1987. p. 242.
2. Whipple GH. A hitherto undescribed disease characterized anatomically by deposits of fat and fatty acids in the intestinal and mesenteric lymphatic tissues. Bull Johns Hopkins Hosp. 1907;18:382–91.
3. Dobbins WO III. HLA antigens in Whipple's disease. Arthritis Rheum. 1987;30(1):102–5.
4. Compain C, Sacre K, Puéchal X, Klein I, Vital-Durand D, Houeto JL, et al. Central nervous system involvement in Whipple disease: clinical study of 18 patients and long-term follow-up. Medicine (Baltimore). 2013;92(6):324–30.
5. Schneider T, Moos V, Loddenkemper C, Marth T, Fenollar F, Raoult D. Whipple's disease: new aspects of pathogenesis and treatment. Lancet Infect Dis. 2008;8(3):179–90.

Part III
Causes-Inflammatory Uveitis

Adamantiades-Behçet's Disease

17

Alice Lorch and Lucia Sobrin

Introduction

Adamantiades-Behçet's Disease (ABD) was first described in the fifth century CE by Hippocrates of Kos, who noted the association of oral and genital ulcers with eye and skin lesions. This association was again published in 1930 by the Greek ophthalmologist Benediktos Adamantiades and then in 1937 by Turkish dermatologist Hulusi Behçet, after whom the disease was named [1]. ABD is a chronic, relapsing, multisystem inflammatory vasculitis that commonly involves the eyes.

Epidemiology

ABD is most common between latitudes 30 and 45 N from the Mediterranean to the Far East, and as such has been called the "Silk Road Disease" in reference to old commercial routes in this area [1, 2]. Estimates of prevalence are variable but thought to be 7.6–420/100,000 in the Middle East (such as Turkey and Greece) and 7.3–30.5/100,000 in the Far East (such as Japan). Rates of the disease are much lower in other parts of Europe and in the United States and negligible in African or American Indian peoples [2]. The Human Leukocyte Antigen (HLA)-B51 allele has been identified consistently as a risk factor for the disease, although only 62 % of ABD patients carry HLA-B51 [2, 21].

The disease typically presents in young adults of their third or fourth decade [3]. Diagnosis in childhood is rare, with presentations before the age of 16 accounting for only 3–5.3 % of cases [1]. Although most ABD cases occur spontaneously, some pediatric cases have been identified in pedigrees that appear to have autosomal recessive inheritance patterns, suggesting a stronger genetic component of the disease in pediatric versus adult patients [2]. Presentation after 40 years of age is uncommon and is characterized in the literature as "late-onset." These patients more commonly have anterior rather than posterior uveitis and as such have a more favorable prognosis [4]. There is no evidence for gender predominance. However, genital and skin lesions are more frequent in women while ocular lesions, vascular involvement and neurologic disease are more frequent in men [1].

A. Lorch (✉) · L. Sobrin
Department of Opthalmology, Harvard Medical School, Massachusetts Eye and Ear Infirmary, Boston, MA 02114, USA
e-mail: alice_lorch@meei.harvard.edu

L. Sobrin
e-mail: lucia_sobrin@meei.harvard.edu

G.N. Papaliodis (ed.), *Uveitis*,
DOI 10.1007/978-3-319-09126-6_17

Pathogenesis

ABD is a vasculitis affecting small- and medium-sized vessels. The systemic inflammation in ABD is thought to be due to dysregulation of the immune system but the exact etiology of this is unknown. This dysregulation involves both innate and adaptive immune processes, demonstrated by neutrophil, natural killer cell, and T lymphocyte hyperactivity with proinflammatory cytokine production [2].

ABD can be classified as a polygenic disease where both genetic susceptibility and environmental factors contribute to development of disease. Despite a clear association, there have been no studies that have explained the role of HLA-B51 in the pathogenesis of ABD. HLA-A2601 has recently been identified as an additional susceptibility allele candidate for ocular ABD in Japan [2].

The interplay between environmental and genetic risk factors is highlighted by the observation that people who are from an area endemic for the disease and have emigrated have significantly lower risk of the disease. This risk reduction has been demonstrated among Japanese living in Hawaii and mainland United States as well as Turks living in Germany [1]. The specific environmental triggers are unknown. Exposure to *Streptococcus sanguinis* is one risk factor that has been explored. Patients with ABD have been found to be colonized with *S. sanguinis*, an oral flora. Delayed-type hypersensitivity to this microbe may play a role in aphthous ulceration in patients with underlying genetic predisposition [5, 6]. A high serum antibody titer against *S. sanguinis* in patients with ABD has been reported and inoculation of this microbe into experimental mice has been reported to cause iridocyclitis [7].

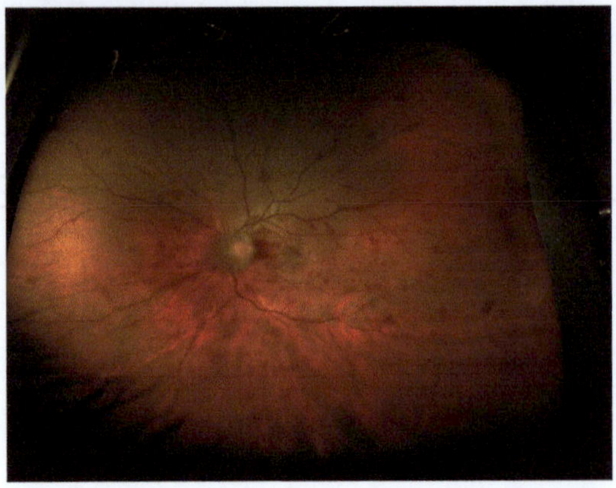

Fig. 17.1 46-year-old woman with ABD. Color photograph of the left eye showing vitreous infiltrates overlying an edematous optic nerve and scattered intraretinal hemorrhages consistent with posterior uveitis and retinal vasculitis. Photographs courtesy of Dr. George Papaliodis

Clinical Presentation and Diagnosis

Patients can experience a six- to ten-year prodrome with relapsing or chronic malaise, fever, or sore throat prior to diagnosis [8]. Ocular disease is the first presentation in only 10–20 % of cases and characterized by nongranulomatous uveitis attacks of sudden onset followed by spontaneous resolution [1]. Uveitis is usually bilateral but can be unilateral as a presenting episode, and sterile hypopyon is common [9]. Posterior uveitis is found in 30–53 % of patients and panuveitis in 44–80 % of patients. Of the patients with posterior involvement, retinal perivasculitis is most common, with diffuse retinal hemorrhages (Fig. 17.1) and retinitis (Fig. 17.2) also being frequently seen [1]. When vitritis resolves, white pearl-like precipitates can form on the inferior retina [1].

The most common ocular complications include macular edema, intraocular pressure rise, cataracts, and optic atrophy. Less commonly, patients develop branch retinal vein occlusions (Fig. 17.3), iris atrophy, macular degeneration with pigment epithelial changes, epiretinal membrane formation, and retinal neovascularization. Neovascularization can result in vitreous hemorrhage or tractional retinal detachment [1]. Fluorescein angiography (FA) can be used to monitor vasculitis as well as look for neovascularization. Peripheral retinal capillary leakage on FA can be seen in asymptomatic patients and can indicate inadequate therapeutic response.

As a multisystem vasculitis, ABD causes symptoms throughout the body. Patients often

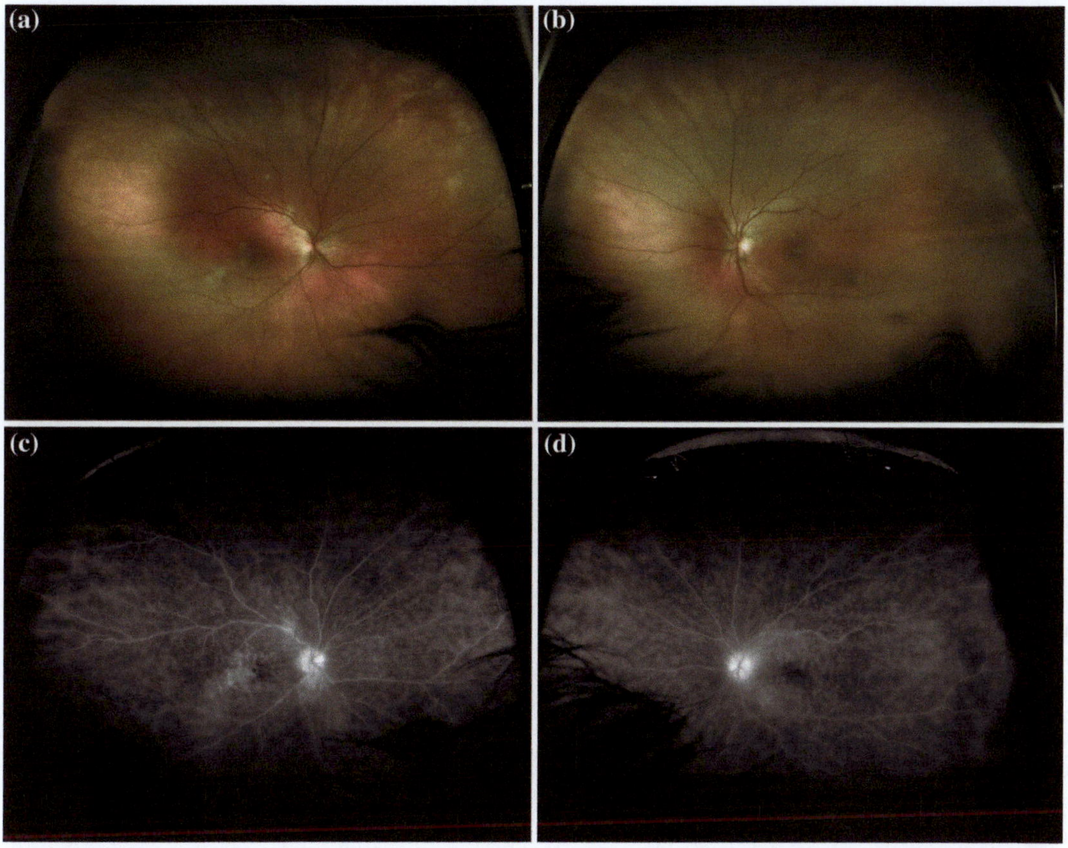

Fig. 17.2 29-year-old woman with ABD. **a** Color photograph of the right eye shows multifocal retinal whitening along the inferior arcade and near the fovea and mild disc edema. **b** Color photograph of the left eye shows mild disc edema. Late-frame fluorescein angiography of the right **c** and left **d** eyes shows diffuse vascular leakage consistent with vasculitis and optic disc leakage. Photographs courtesy of Dr. Ann-Marie Lobo

have oral aphthous ulcers; these are painful, last up to 14 days and present an average of seven and a half years prior to diagnosis [1]. These ulcers are covered by white to yellow pseudomembranes, surrounded by an erythematous halo, and occur on mucous membranes [11]. Genital ulcers are also common. These ulcers have sharp borders with a fibrin-covered floor and surrounding erythema. They most commonly occur on the scrotum and inguinal area in men and vulva and inguinal area in women [11]. Two common skin manifestations are erythema nodosum and pseudofolliculitis. Patients will classically have a positive pathergy test, which is the formation of an indurated erythematous papule 24–48 h after intracutaneous prick with a needle on the forearm [1]. Patients can have transient arthralgias, neurologic symptoms ranging from hemiparesis to behavioral changes, vascular thrombosis, and GI symptoms including colitis or ulceration. Cardiac angina or infarction, pulmonary manifestations, epididymitis, orchitis, and renal manifestations are rare but have been reported [1].

Formal diagnosis is based on two sets of guidelines: the International Study Group Classification from 1990 and the revised criteria by the Behcet's Disease Research Committee of Japan from 2003 [7, 10]. The International Study Group Classification is used in most countries in the world. Because a subset of patients with ABD will have ocular involvement as their initial manifestation of disease, ophthalmologists should be aware of these diagnostic guidelines

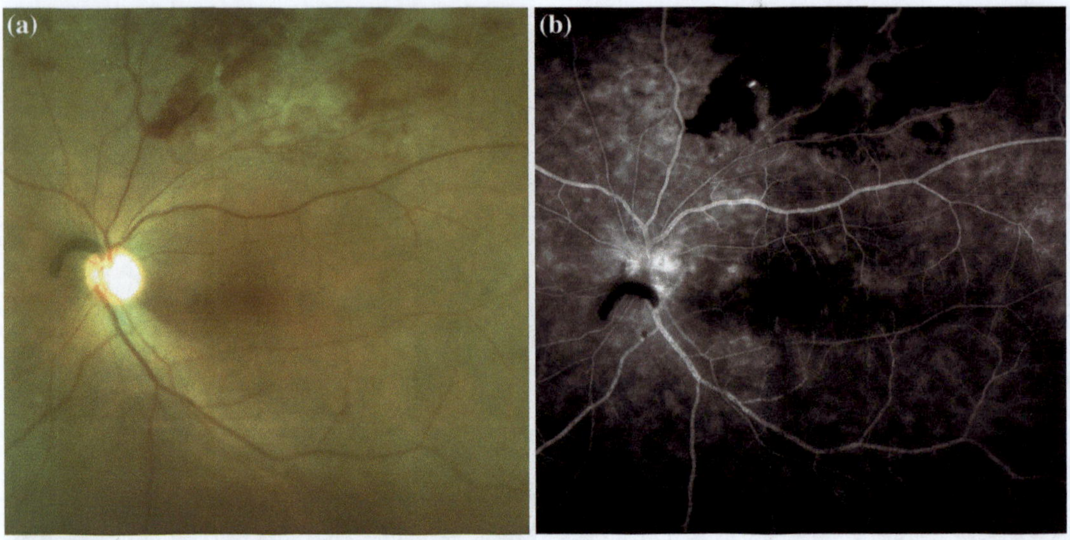

Fig. 17.3 32-year-old man with ABD. **a** Color photograph of the left eye shows intraretinal hemorrhage superotemporally consistent with a branch retinal vein occlusion. **b** Late fluorescein angiography frame shows some leakage from the retinal vessels and blockage from hemorrhage in the area of the vein occlusion. Photographs courtesy of Dr. George Papaliodis

and ask uveitis patients about systemic symptoms of ABD. Patients with suggestive systemic symptoms should be referred to a rheumatologist for formal diagnosis. HLA-B51 testing is indicated when there are systemic symptoms suggestive of ABD. In this context, a positive HLA-B51 result can help fulfill diagnostic criteria for the disease. Since a significant proportion of patients with ABD do not have the HLA-B51 allele, a negative result does not necessarily exclude the diagnosis.

The International Behcet's Study Group Classification (IBSGC) requires the presence of recurrent (at least three times in a one-year period) oral ulcers to make a diagnosis, with at least two of the following: recurrent genital ulcers, skin lesions, eye lesions, or a positive pathergy test (Table 17.1) [3]. This classification has been validated in several populations and is 91 % sensitive and 96 % specific [11].

The Japanese Criteria (JC) classifies recurrent aphthous ulcers on the oral mucosa, skin lesions, eye lesions, and genital ulcers as main symptoms. It classifies arthritis, gastrointestinal lesions characterized by ileocecal ulcers, epidydimitis, vascular lesions, and central nervous system symptoms as additional symptoms. A "complete" diagnosis requires four main symptoms. An "incomplete" diagnosis requires three main symptoms, or two main with two additional symptoms, or a typical ocular lesion with a main symptom, or a typical ocular lesion with two additional symptoms. These revised criteria also allow laboratory and clinical testing to contribute to the diagnosis. They include pathergy testing and prick testing for sensitivity to dead *Streptococci* (Table 17.2) [7].

Differential Diagnosis

There is no pathognomonic finding for ABD and the diagnosis is based on a combination of signs and symptoms. The differential diagnosis for uveitis secondary to ABD includes uveitis associated with reactive arthritis, which can also present with anterior uveitis and oral ulcers. However, the uveitis in reactive arthritis is generally unilateral and rarely posterior. Arthralgias, skin disease, and uveitis can be found in sarcoidosis, and this diagnosis can be explored with chest imaging for hilar adenopathy and serum

Table 17.1 International study group criteria (1990)

Must have	Plus two of the following
Recurring oral ulceration	Eye lesions
	Skin lesions
	Recurring genital ulceration
	Positive pathergy test

Table 17.2 Japanese revised criteria (2003)

A	
Major symptoms	Recurrent oral ulceration
	Skin lesions
	Eye lesions
	Genital ulcers
Additional symptoms	Arthritis without deformity
	Epididymitis
	Gastrointestinal lesions represented by ileocecal ulceration
	Vascular lesions
	Neuronal lesions
Clinical laboratory data (contributing to	Positive pathergy test
diagnosis but not essential)	Positive prick test for *Streptococci*
	Increased ESR, CRP, neutrophilia in peripheral blood, increased complement activity
	Positive for HLA-B51
	Pathological findings (skin biopsy)
B	
Complete type	Four major symptoms
Incomplete type	Three of the main four symptoms OR
	Two main symptoms and two additional symptoms OR
	Typical ocular lesion and another main symptoms OR
	Typical ocular lesion and two additional symptoms
ABD suspected	Some main symptoms, but not meeting criteria for incomplete
	Additional symptom becomes recurrent or severe

testing for elevated angiotensin-converting enzyme and lysozyme levels. The areas of peripheral retinitis in ABD can mimic those seen in acute retinal necrosis [12]. Other entities that have overlapping signs and symptoms with ABD and should be considered in the appropriate clinical contexts are tuberculosis (including Eales disease), syphilis, systemic vasculitides such as lupus erythematosus, toxoplasma retinochoroiditis, and intraocular lymphoma [9].

Treatment

Treatment of ABD can be challenging due to the chronic and relapsing nature of the disease. Topical steroids can be used for isolated anterior uveitis [9]. For posterior involvement, systemic immunomodulation is often necessary. Systemic corticosteroids can be used for rapid control of inflammation initially but are not an optimal choice for long-term control of this chronic disease. A variety of steroid-sparing immunomodulators have had success in ABD. Conventional agents such as azathioprine (2.5 mg/kg/day) and cyclosporine (2–5 mg/kg/day) can be effective and are part of the European League Against Rheumatism (EULAR) recommendations for ABD treatment [13]. Risk of infections, liver toxicity, and renal toxicity, among other potential side effects, need to be explained to patients and monitored for with serologies. Interferon-alpha (3–6 million units subcutaneously, three times weekly) has also been extensively used in ABD patients with success [12, 14, 15]. Interferon-alpha side effects including flu-like symptoms and significant depression need to be discussed thoroughly prior to initiation of therapy.

Biologic agents, particularly those targeted against tumor necrosis factor-alpha (TNF-alpha), have had significant success in the treatment of ABD [16]. Patients with intraocular inflammation due to ABD have increased TNF-alpha in their serum and aqueous fluid [13]. Of the anti-TNF-alpha agents, infliximab, a chimeric monoclonal antibody to TNF-alpha given intravenously, has been most extensively studied and shown success in decreasing the frequency of ocular attacks in chronic management [17]. Adalimumab is a monoclonal human antibody to TNF-alpha administered subcutaneously and has shown similar effectiveness in case series [13, 18]. Of note, an important potential side effect of TNF-alpha inhibition is the reactivation of tuberculosis and/or viral hepatitis so patients should be screened for these conditions before therapy initiation. Rituximab, a chimeric monoclonal antibody that binds to CD20 on B cells, is also being considered for treatment but as of yet has limited evidence to support its use [13, 19].

Colchicine, which inhibits neutrophil and endothelial cell adhesion molecules, has been used as an adjunct to other anti-inflammatory treatments in the past to inhibit inflammation in ABD. However, a recent study showed no significant difference in frequency of attack or best-corrected visual acuity when colchicine with infliximab was compared to the use of infliximab alone, and this medication is employed in decreasing frequency by specialists [20].

Prognosis

Vision loss in ABD can be progressive due to recurrent attacks of inflammation. Repeated inflammation and occlusive vasculitis can result in retinal atrophy and gliosis with optic atrophy [3]. On FA, disc neovascularization, macular window defects, and macular ischemia are all associated with a poor visual prognosis. On ocular coherence tomography, decreased foveal thickness, and interruption of the ellipsoid layer indicate irreversible macular damage and as such are also associated with poor visual function. An International Collaborative Study in 2007 showed that 23 % of patients with ocular inflammation from ABD had equal to or worse than 20/200 vision [21]. Although historically the recurrent inflammation of ABD has led to poor visual outcomes, vision can be preserved with prompt initiation of immunomodulatory therapy. With an increase in the available treatment options, particularly the anti-TNF-alpha agents, permanent vision loss is now avoidable in most cases of ABD [22].

References

1. Khairallah M, Accorinti M, Muccioli C, Kahloun R, Kempen J. Epidemiology of Behcet disease. Ocular Immunol Inflamm. 2012;20(5):324–35.
2. Piga M, Mathieu A. Genetic susceptibility to Behcet's disease: role of genes belonging to the MHC region. Rheumatology. 2011;50:299–310.
3. Tugal-Tutkun I. Imaging in the diagnosis and management of Behcet disease. Int Ophthalmol Clin. 2012;52(4):183–90.
4. Hazirolan D, Sungur G, Duman S. Demographic, clinical and ocular features in patients with late-onset Behcet disease. Ocular Immunol Inflamm. 2012;20 (2):119–24.
5. Emmi G, Silvestri E, Squatrito D, et al. Behcet's syndrome pathophysiology and potential therapeutic targets. Intern Emerg Med. 2014;9:257–65.
6. Kaneko F, Togashi A, Saito S, et al. Behcet's disease (Adamantiades-Behcet's disease). Clin Dev Immunol. 2011;. doi:10.1155/2011/681956.

7. Suzuki Kurokawa M, Suzuki N. Behcet's disease. Clin Exp Med. 2004;3:10–20.
8. Chajek T, Fainaru M. Behcet's disease: report of 41 cases and a review of the literature. Medicine. 1975;54:179.
9. Wakefield D, Cunningham E, Tugal-Tutkun I, Khairallah M, Ohno S, Zierhut M. Controversies in Behcet disease. Ocular Immunol Inflamm. 2012;21 (1):6–11.
10. Lee S, Bang D, Lee E, Sohn S. Behcet's diseases: a guide to its clinical understanding. Germany: Springer-Verlag, Berlin Heidelberg; 2001.
11. Mat C, Yurdakul S, Sevim A, Ozyazgan Y, Tuzun Y. Behcet's syndrome: facts and controversies. Clin Dermatol. 2013;31:352–61.
12. Balansard B, Bodaghi B, Cassoux N, et al. Necrotising retinopathies simulating acute retinal necrosis syndrome. Br J Ophthalmol. 2005;89(1):96–101.
13. Hatemi G, Silman A, Band D, et al. EULAR recommendations for the management of Behcet disease. Ann Rheum Dis. 2008;67:1656–62.
14. Deuter CM, Zierhut M, Mohle A, Vonthein R, Stobiger N, Kotter I. Long-term remission after cessation of interferon-alpha treatment in patients with severe uveitis due to Behcet's disease. Arthritis Rheum. 2010;62(9):2796–805.
15. Benitah N, Sobrin L, Papaliodis G. The use of biologic agents in the treatment of ocular manifestations of Behcet's disease. Semin Ophthalmol. 2011;26(4–5):295–303.
16. Levy-Clarke G, Jabs D, Read R, et al. Expert panel recommendations for the use of anti-tumor necrosis factor biologic agents in patients with ocular inflammatory disorders. Ophthalmology. 2014;121:785–96.
17. Keino H, Okada AA, Watanabe T, Taki W. Decreased ocular inflammatory attacks and background retinal and disc vascular leakage in patients with Behcet's disease on infliximab therapy. Br J Ophthalmol. 2011;95(9):1245–50.
18. Mushtaq B, Saeed T, Situnayake RD, Murray PI. Adalimumab for sight-threatening uveitis in Behcet's disease. Eye. 2007;21(6):824–5.
19. Davatchi F, Shams H, Rezaipoor M, et al. Rituximab in intractable ocular lesions of Behcet's disease; randomized single-blind control study (pilot study). Int J Rheum Dis. 2010;13(3):246–52.
20. Takeuchi M, Asukata Y, Kawagoe T, Ito N, Nishide T, Mizuki N. Infliximab monotherapy versus infliximab and colchicine combination therapy in patients with Behcet's disease. Ocular Immunol Inflamm. 2012;20(3):193–7.
21. Kitaichi N, Miyazaki A, Stanford M, Chames H, Iwata D, Ohno S. Ocular features of Behcet's disease: an international collaborative study. Br J Ophthalmol. 2007;91:1579–82.
22. Tabbara K, Al-Hemidan A. Infliximab effects compared to conventional therapy in the management of retinal vasculitis in Behcet's disease. Am J Ophthalmol. 2008;146:845–50.

Acute Posterior Multifocal Placoid Pigment Epitheliopathy/Serpiginous Choroiditis

18

Stephanie M. Llop

Acute Posterior Multifocal Placoid Pigment Epitheliopathy: Introduction

Acute posterior multifocal placoid pigment epitheliopathy was first described by J. Donald M. Gass, MD in 1968 [1]. It is a rare entity that is typically present in young adults, who develop sudden vision loss, mostly bilateral, with associated central or paracentral scotoma. It has no sex predilection and may be preceded by a viral illness. On fundus examination, APMPPE is characterized by scattered, flat, multifocal, creamy white or yellow subretinal plaques at the level of the Retinal Pigment Epithelium (RPE), throughout the posterior pole and extending into the equator. It is believed that APMPPE likely occurs secondary to a type IV (delayed-type) hypersensitivity reaction, and has been reported to be associated with adenovirus, mumps, tuberculosis, dengue fever among other infectious diseases [2–5]. Tubuloinsterstitial Nephritis and Uveitis (TINU) syndrome, multiple brain and spinal cord infarctions have also been associated with the condition [6, 7].

S.M. Llop (✉)
Department of Uveitis, Massachusetts Eye and Ear Infirmary, 243 Charles St, Boston, MA 02114, USA
e-mail: Stephanie.llopsantiago@upr.edu

G.N. Papaliodis (ed.), *Uveitis*,
DOI 10.1007/978-3-319-09126-6_18

Clinical Manifestations

Presenting symptoms may include photophobia, decreased vision, paracentral scotoma, or metamorphopsia. Patients may complain of headache, malaise, fever, or upper respiratory symptoms prior to developing the visual problems. Visual acuity may range from 20/20 to counting fingers at the onset of the disease. On physical exam, patients may have mild anterior uveitis, keratic precipitates, and vitritis. The placoid lesions are usually less than one disk-diameter in size and are mostly limited to the posterior pole. Acute lesions fade and are replaced by various degrees of RPE atrophy and hyperpigmentation [2]. The presence of serous retinal detachments, optic neuritis, and vein occlusions have all been reported [8, 9].

Testing

Fluorescein Angiography (FA) reveals early hypofluorescence due to lesions masking the choroidal fluorescence, and late staining of the lesions that gradually become apparent and progressively increase throughout the study [10].

The Fundus Autofluorescence (FAF) in APMPEE shows in the acute phase, central hyperautofluorescence within the lesions surrounded by a narrow, but fairly uniform, zone of decreased autofluorescence. The resolving lesions have a light halo surrounding altered pigmentation on fundus exam, and are seen in FAF as a central portion displaying increased autofluorescence, surrounded by a hypoautofluorescent strip that corresponds to the halo seen on ophthalmoscopy [11].

Indocyanine Green (ICG) angiography demonstrates widespread choroidal hypofluorescence of the active and healed lesions; these choroidal abnormalities are more numerous than the overlying lesions [12]. This supports the hypothesis that the main cause of these lesions may represent some type of choroidal vascular occlusion.

Optical Coherence Tomography (OCT) findings in the acute phase of APMPPE include increased reflectance of the external retinal layers (outer plexiform layer up to the level of RPE) with sparing of the inner retinal layers and no evidence of retinal thickening. Later in the disease, the OCT scans of the same areas in the retina may demonstrate a normal appearance with complete resolution of the previous hyper-reflectance of the outer retinal layers [13].

Treatment

No treatment is generally recommended; in a published article, close to 90 % of the eyes without foveal involvement at presentation, had visual acuity of 20/25 or better. The visual prognosis of the disease is strongly affected by the presence of initial foveal involvement [14]. A recurrent course of the disease has been documented in various reports [15].

Serpiginous Choroiditis: Introduction

Serpiginous choroiditis is a rare asymmetric bilateral condition that affects healthy patients, and is marked by chronic and progressive inflammation of the inner half of the choroid and RPE. It was described in 1932 by Junius and affects people in the second to sixth decade of life with most studies reporting a higher prevalence in men than women. The disease constitutes less than 5 % of posterior uveitides in retrospective epidemiologic series in inflammatory eye disorders. There is no familial predisposition and most cases are not associated with systemic disease. Recurrence is very common and may occur weeks to years after the initial event.

Clinical Manifestations

Patients typically present with blurry vision, photopsias, metamorphopsia, paracentral scotomas, and visual field loss. Anterior segment of the eye is typically normal with no inflammatory cells or flare in the anterior chamber, although there are case reports with these findings. On funduscopy, the pattern of chorioretinal scaring represents a peripapillary serpiginous or geographic pattern in about 80 % of cases [16]. The active disease begins with ill-defined patches of grayish or creamy yellow sub-retinal infiltrates originating in the peripapillary region and progress in an irregular serpentine fashion centrifugally. The overlying retina is usually edematous and serous detachments can occur. Active lesions resolve over 6–8 weeks, leaving an area of atrophy of choriocapillaris and RPE (see Fig. 18.1). Patients could have multiple lesions in different stages of evolution, and recurrences usually occur at the borders of previous atrophic scars. In chronic cases, chorioretinal atrophy, subretinal fibrosis, and RPE pigment clumping

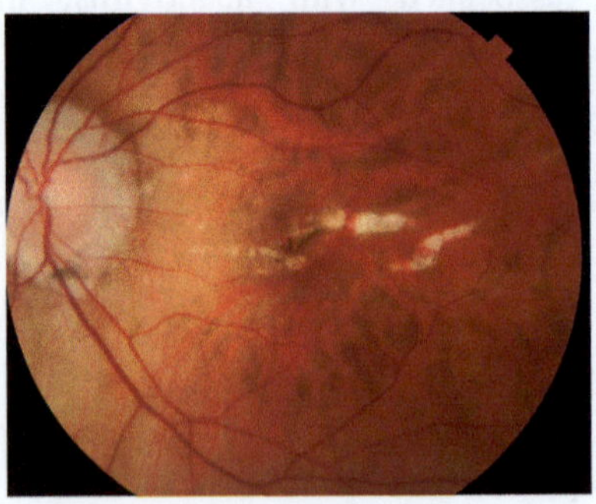

Fig. 18.1 53-year-old male with serpiginous choroiditis involving the macula. The acute creamy lesions resolved leaving a region of chorioretinal atrophy

may be seen. The disease can be insidious with many patients presenting with no symptoms until the macula is involved. These patients have a worse visual prognosis due to foveal involvement and higher risk of choroidal neovascularization (13–35 %) [16].

Causes

Pathogenesis of this condition remains unknown despite many studies attempting to identify infectious or autoimmune etiologies. An autoimmune etiology has been proposed and supported by the presence of anterior uveitis, vitritis, and the resolution of lesions when treated with corticosteroids and other anti-inflammatory agents. A vasculopathy has also been suggested but most patients do not manifest systemic vascular abnormalities. An association with tuberculosis exposure and herpes viruses has also been considered as potential predisposing factors but this remains to be proven.

Testing

On FA, serpiginous choroiditis demonstrates early hypofluorescence secondary to the atrophy of choriocapillaris and progressive hyperfluorescence at the margin of the lesions. The active lesions, usually at the borders of old lesions, block fluorescein early and show diffuse staining and leakage progressively in the later frames.

In the acute stage of serpiginous choroiditis, the lesions show an ill-defined halo of increased (Fundus Autofluorescence) FAF giving a diffuse, amorphous appearance.

ICG angiography is characterized by geographically confluent or patchy hypofluorescent areas with irregular shapes and indistinct borders beginning from early to the late phase and either remain hypofluorescent or become isofluorescent in the late phase. ICG can be helpful in disclosing active subclinical lesions [17].

Visual fields demonstrate absolute and/or relative scotomatas corresponding to the geographic lesion and as lesions resolve, scotomas can become less dense. The role of OCT is complementary to the other modalities of testing mentioned above.

Treatment

The natural history of the condition is one of multiple recurrences and progressive scarring that can eventually involve the posterior pole and the fovea with poor visual outcome. Often, when patient have symptoms, the lesions are already in the fovea and at this stage, usually there is significant scarring and high risk of permanent vision loss. The role of any successful treatment is to control the active lesions rapidly and prevent further recurrences and subsequent progression of the disease.

The use of corticosteroids can be effective in controlling the active lesions but they have no effect on the prevention of recurrences, hence it does not alter the natural course of the disease and the final visual outcome. Cyclosporine has been used with mixed results. In one series with seven patients, the treating physician used oral cyclosporine (3–5 mg/kg/day) for a duration of 1.3–5 years (median 3 years). No patient in this series had significant vision loss, and six of the seven achieved remission and were able to stop medications without recurrence [18]. Combination therapy consisting of cyclosporine, azathioprine, and prednisolone has also been described. This combination of agents induced rapid control of ocular inflammation and promoted visual recovery, but some patients had a relapse upon tapering the medications and others required protracted duration of therapy to maintain quiescence.

The efficacy of antimetabolites (methotrexate, mycophenolate mofetil, and azathioprine) in serpiginous choroiditis has been documented in multiple case series. Similarly, alkylating agents such as cyclophosphamide and chlorambucil are effective in rapidly controlling the inflammation and inducing drug-free remission. Without large multicenter trials, it is difficult to determine the best treatment strategy for these patients [16].

Relentless Placoid Chorioretinitis

A related entity described as Relentless Placoid Chorioretinitis (RPC) (also known as ampiginous choroiditis) shares typical findings of both APMPPE and serpiginous choroiditis but with an atypical distribution of retinal lesions and different progression of the disease. On exam, patients have bilateral posterior creamy white lesions at the level of the RPE that are usually smaller in size (half disk area) compared to APMPPE, and have involvement anterior and posterior to the equator. Eventually, the lesions may become numerous (>50 lesions) and can be active in both eyes synchronously [19]. The clinical course of RPC tends to be prolonged with persistent lesions that evolve and may recur. Due to the scarcity of cases, the most effective treatment is unknown but prognosis is generally favorable with immunosuppressive strategies (as detailed in the management of serpiginous).

Conclusion

APMPPE and serpiginous choroiditis are inflammatory diseases of the choroid that are categorized under the "white dot syndromes." Both conditions usually present bilaterally and have a predilection for young, healthy adults. They have characteristic funduscopic findings at the level of the RPE and choriocapillaris. The lesions of APMPPE are subretinal, creamy-yellow or white, and mostly involve the posterior pole. Serpiginous choroiditis has a pattern of lesions that typically follow a serpiginous (snake-like) or pseudopodial fashion extending from the optic disk. The FA pattern of APMPPE characteristically shows early hypofluorescence and late staining of the lesions; serpiginous also demonstrates early hypofluorescence with late hyperfluorescence at the borders of the lesions. The exact pathophysiology of both conditions remains unknown.

APMPPE is usually self-limited with improvement of visual acuity and no need for treatment. Serpiginous may have an insidious onset with some patients noticing vision loss due to macular involvement resulting in poor prognosis and higher risk of developing CNVM. For this reason, treatment of serpiginous should be aggressive and may involve the use of systemic immunomodulatory therapy. Finally, a related entity has been described and the terms "relentless placoid chorioretinitis" and "ampiginous" have been used for this condition, which has characteristics of both APMPPE and serpiginous. The hallmark of this disorder is the presence of numerous lesions that are smaller and extend anterior and posterior to the equator.

References

1. Gass JD. Acute posterior multifocal placoid pigment epitheliopathy. Arch Ophthalmol. 1965;80(2):177–85.
2. Crawford CM, Igboeli O. Review article: a review of the inflammatory chorioretinopathies: the white dot syndromes. ISRN Inflamm. 2013;783190.
3. Azar P Jr, Gohd RS, Waltman D, et al. Acute posterior multifocal placoid pigment epitheliopathy associated with an adenovirus type 5 infection. Am J Ophthalmol. 1975;80(6):1003–5.
4. Borruat FX, Piguet B, Herbort CP. Acute posterior multifocal placoid pigment epitheliopathy following mumps. Ocul Immunol Inflamm. 1998;6(3):189–93.
5. Goldhardt R, Patel H, Davis JL. Acute posterior multifocal placoid pigment epitheliopathy following dengue fever: a new association for an old disease. Ocul Immunol Inflamm. 2016;22:1–5.
6. Lee AR, Sharma S, Mahmoud TH. Tubulointerstitial nephritis and uveitis syndrome with a primary presentation of acute posterior multifocal placoid pigment epitheliopathy. Retin Cases Brief Rep. 2016.
7. Castro P, Costa A, Abreu P, et al. Acute posterior multifocal placoid pigment epitheliopathy presenting with multiple brain and spinal cord infarctions. J Neurol Sci. 2016;15(361):26–8.
8. Bird AC, Hamilton AM. Placoid pigment epitheliopathy. Presenting with bilateral serous retinal detachment. Br J Ophthalmol. 1972;56(12):881–6.
9. Allee SD, Marks SJ. Acute posterior multifocal placoid pigment epitheliopathy with bilateral central retinal vein occlusion. Am J Ophthalmol. 1998;126(2):309–12.
10. Fitzpatrick PJ, Robertson DM. Acute posterior multifocal placoid pigment epitheliopathy. Arch Ophthalmol. 1973;89(5):373–6.
11. Spaide RF. Autofluorescence imaging of acute posterior multifocal placoid pigment epitheliopathy. Retina. 2006;26(4):479–82.

12. Park D, Schatz H, McDonald HR, et al. Indocyanine green angiography of acute multifocal posterior placoid pigment epitheliopathy. Ophthalmology. 1995;102(12):1877–83.
13. Souka AA, Hillenkamp J, Gora F, et al. Correlation between optical coherence tomography and autofluorescence in acute posterior multifocal placoid pigment epitheliopathy. Graefes Arch Clin Exp Ophthalmol. 2006;244(10):1219–23.
14. Fiore T, Iaccheri B, Androudi S, et al. Acute posterior multifocal pigment epitheliopathy: outcome and visual prognosis. Retina. 2009;29(7):994–1001.
15. Cohen LM, Munk MR, Goldstein DA, et al. Acute, posterior multifocal placoid pigment epitheliopathy: a case of 11 recurrences over 15 years. Retin Cases Brief Rep. 2015;9(3):226–30.
16. Lim WK, Buggage RR, Nussenblatt RB. Serpiginous Choroiditis. Surv Ophthalmol. 2005;50(3):231–44.
17. Bansal R, Gupta A, Gupta V. Imaging in the diagnosis and management of serpiginous choroiditis. Int Ophthalmol Clin. 2012;52(4):229–36.
18. Araujo AA, Wells AP, Dick Ad, et al. Early treatment with cyclosporine in serpiginous choroidopathy maintains remission and good visual outcome. Br J Ophthalmol. 2000;84:979–82.
19. Jampol LM, Mirza RG. Relentless Placoid Chorioretinitis. Int Ophthalmol Clin. 2012;52(4):237–42.

Ankylosing Spondylitis

19

Mark Dacey

Introduction

Ankylosing spondylitis (AS) is a chronic systemic inflammatory disease of the spine and sacroiliac joints with potentially debilitating manifestations. Its etymology stems from two Greek words: "ankylos", meaning joint stiffening, and "spondylo", meaning vertebra [1]. AS is one of the seronegative spondyloarthropathies, which are covered in significant detail in the chapter on HLA-B27. AS is characterized by spinal inflammation and several potential extra-articular manifestations. The most common extra-articular manifestation of AS is acute anterior uveitis (AAU), with a pooled prevalence of 25.8 % of AS patients in a recent meta-analysis [2], while AS is also the most common extraocular manifestation of anterior uveitis [3].

History

AS has been identified in a wide variety of primates dating back to the Mesozoic era of the dinosaurs 200–70 million years ago [4], with human involvement documented as early as ancient Egypt through studies of Egyptian mummies [5]. Galen distinguished spondylitis from rheumatoid arthritis in the second century A. D [6]. The modern literature of AS stems from 1559, when Realdo Colombo first described two skeletons with typical AS manifestations [7]. More extensive clinical descriptions began to appear in the mid-1800s from von Bechterew (Russia) [8], Strumpell (Germany) [9] and Marie (France) [10], with the terms Bechterew's and Marie–Strumpell disease evolving from their classic descriptions of AS.

Epidemiology

Age onset for AS occurs between 15 and 40 years of age in 90 % of patients [11] with a worldwide prevalence of AS of approximately 0.9 % [12]. AS accounts for 4–5 % of all cases of chronic low back pain. AS is most common in Caucasian patients from Northern European countries and is least common in patients of Afro-Caribbean descent, reflecting the associated prevalence of the HLA-B27 gene in the Caucasian population [13]. Males are diagnosed with AS three times more commonly than women; however, many rheumatologists believe this discrepancy is due to the disease being more mild in women with typically less severe spinal changes [14]. The spine and pelvis are most commonly affected in men,

M. Dacey (✉)
Colorado Retina Associates, P.C, 8101 E. Lowry Blvd., Ste 210, Denver, CO 80230, USA
e-mail: mdacey@retinacolorado.com

G.N. Papaliodis (ed.), *Uveitis*,
DOI 10.1007/978-3-319-09126-6_19

with some involvement of the chest wall, hips, shoulders, and feet. In contrast, women have less severe involvement of the spine, with more symptoms in the knees, wrists, ankles, hips, and pelvis [15]. Patients with ankylosing spondylitis who have peripheral arthritis also have a higher prevalence of uveitis [16].

Ankylosing spondylitis is associated with a number of extra-articular manifestations in addition to AAU, including psoriasis (10–25 %), inflammatory bowel disease (5–10 %), and cardiovascular abnormalities, including conduction disturbances and aortic insufficiency (1–10 %). The risk of atherosclerotic events in AS patients is doubled. Pulmonary complications are rare and include apical pulmonary fibrosis and rigidity of the chest wall [17].

Genetics

HLA-B27 is strongly associated with both AS and acute anterior uveitis 95 % of patients with AS are HLA-B27 positive, representing the strongest genetic link with any disease which has been encountered in the field of rheumatology [18]. Patients who are HLA-B27 positive have a 5–6 % chance of developing ankylosing spondylitis, while patients who are HLA-B27 positive and have a first-degree relative with AS have a 10–20 % change of developing the disease [19]. There is a fivefold to 16-fold increase in having ankylosing spondylitis if a first-degree relative has the disease [20]. The observed frequency of the concurrence of AAU and AS was 0.4 % in the HLA-B27 positive population and 0.02 % in the HLA-B27 negative population [21]. Patients with late onset of disease (after age 40) tend to be HLA-B27 negative (13 % vs. 5 %) [22].

Recently, several additional genes, including IL23R and ERAP1, have also been identified as being associated with ankylosing spondylitis [23]. These genes may account for some cases of AS in HLA-B27 negative patients.

Pathophysiology

The pathogenesis of AS is poorly understood. Immune mediated mechanisms are suggested by inflammatory histology, raised serum levels of IgA and acute phase reactants, and the close relationship between HLA-B27 and AS. No single agent or event has been identified as the cause of the disease, but the interrelationship between AS, reactive arthritis, and inflammatory bowel disease suggests that enteric bacteria may play a part [24]. In a similar vein, frequent GI infections have been identified as a risk factor for the development of AS, [25] in addition to classic risk factors of HLA-B27 positivity, family history of AS, and male sex. The role of T-cells, macrophages, and proinflammatory cytokines (TNF-alpha, et al.) will be discussed in the treatment section.

The classic pathologic lesion in AS is an enthesopathy, inflammation at the insertion of the ligaments and capsules into bones, which lead to a progressive ossification of the sacroiliac (SI) joints and the intravertebral discs [26].

Clinical Manifestations

The initial manifestation of AS is most commonly dull deep pain in the lower lumbar or gluteal regions upon awakening. Symptoms tend to improve with activity and worsen with subsequent inactivity. Bone tenderness may accompany stiffness over time. Arthritis in the hips and shoulders may occur early in the course of the disease in 20–25 % of patients, while neck pain and stiffness are more characteristic of advanced disease. Findings on physical examination include loss of spinal mobility, pain upon direct palpation of the sacroiliac joints, and marked dorsocervical kyphosis with loss of lumbar lordosis. The classic "bamboo spine" finding is seen in advanced disease once fusion of the vertebral body has occurred. Clinical signs can be wide-ranging, from mild stiffness to a fused spine, with any combination of hip involvement and peripheral arthritis. A pre-spondylitic phase of 5–10 years has been described, during which progressive structural damage occurs; an average delay in diagnosis of 8.9 years in AS patients has been reported [27].

Diagnosis

The modified New York criteria [28] (Table 19.1) details the diagnostic criteria for anklyosing spondylitis and includes both clinical and radiological criteria. The anterior uveitis typically associated with AS is recurrent, non-granulomatous, alternating, and acute.

Imaging

X-ray films of the SI joints are the gold standard for diagnosis of AS (Fig. 19.1), with radiographic evidence of sacroiliitis required for diagnosis based on the modified New York criteria. Figure 19.2 demonstrates the "bamboo spine" with fusion of multiple vertebral bodies. However, plain films can significantly lag behind symptoms [29] and consequently other imaging modalities have utilized in recent years [30]. Recent studies have shown that MRI has the highest sensitivity and specificity of all imaging techniques for SI joint inflammation [31], with T1 with gadolinium or fat-suppressed T2 images being the most effective in visualization of inflammatory features.

Table 19.1 Modified New York criteria for ankylosing spondylitis

Radiological criterion	Clinical criteria
Grade ≥2 bilateral sacroillitis on X-ray OR Grade 3 or 4 unilateral sacroillitis on X-ray	Low back stiffness/pain for >3 months which improves with exercise Limitation of lumbar spine movement in both frontal and sagittal planes Limitation of chest expansion relative to normal values for sex and age

Diagnosis requires the radiological criterion and at least one clinical criterion

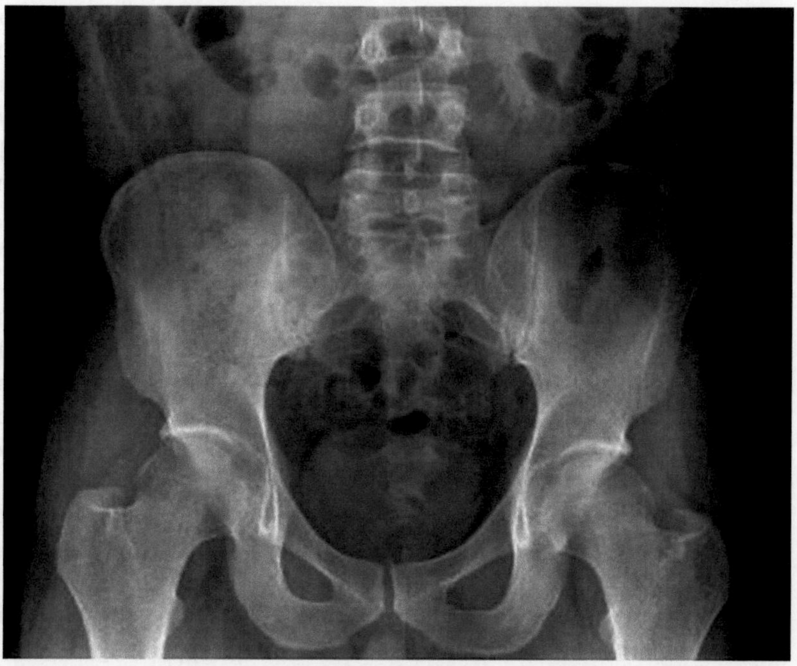

Fig. 19.1 Late stage sacroiliitis with extensive sclerosis and early ankyloses

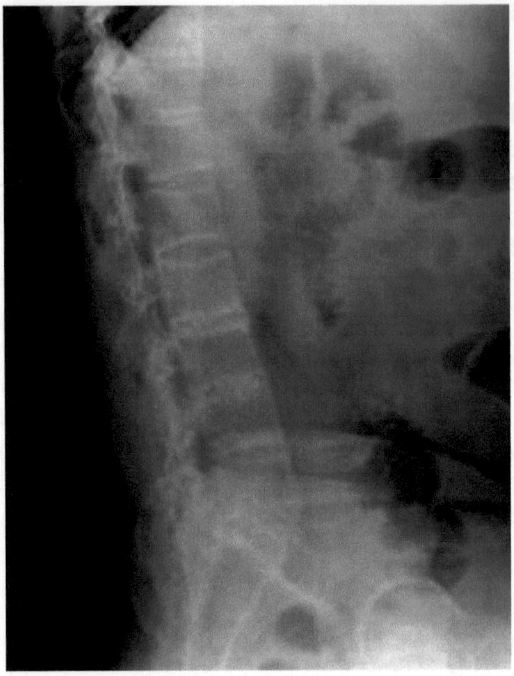

Fig. 19.2 Lateral lumbar X-ray demonstrating bridging syndesmophytes and the classic "bamboo spine" appearance in later stages of ankylosing spondylitis

Ocular Manifestations

Acute anterior uveitis (AAU) is the most common ophthalmologic manifestation of AS. Presenting symptoms include pain, redness, photophobia, and blurred vision. Exam findings include ciliary flush, conjunctival hyperemia, nongranulomatous keratic precipitates, anterior chamber cell/flare, and posterior synechiae. HLA-B27 AAU is frequently associated with formation of a hypopyon. The majority of cases are isolated to the anterior chamber, but posterior segment involvement has been reported in 17.4 % of patients with HLA-B27 uveitis, most commonly presenting with vitritis (93.1 %), papillitis (82.7 %), retinal vasculitis (24.1 %), and pars plana exudates (6.8 %) [32].

Scleritis is also associated with AS, in 0.34–0.93 % of patients with AS [33]. Scleritis typically presents after many years of active AS and tends to present most frequently as mild–moderate diffuse anterior scleritis [34].

Treatment

Acute treatment of AAU is typically with a course of topical corticosteroids and cycloplegic eyedrops, though more severe cases may require additional agents. Topical Prednisolone 1 % has been used for decades with excellent efficacy. Recently, topical Difluprednate 0.05 % (Durezol) has been shown to be at least as effective at @4x/day dosing as topical Prednisolone 1 % at 8x/day dosing [35]. Cycloplegic agents including Atropine 1 %, Homatropine 5 %, Isopto Hyoscine 0.25 %, and Cyclopentolate 1 % are effective in treating posterior synechiae, reducing pain and photosensitivity.

Periocular steroid injections of triamcinolone (40 mg/1 mL), administered either into sub-Tenon's space or trans-septal into the peribulbar space are effective for more severe flares that fail to respond to topical therapy. A course of oral Prednisone can be employed for patients with severe disease, particularly those with posterior segment involvement.

Various non-pharmacologic therapeutic options have been attempted in AS, including exercise, massage, and hydrotherapy, which may be effective for early disease or as an adjunct to pharmacologic therapy in those predominantly with joint manifestations.

NSAIDs have been the first-line therapy for the treatment of AS since their introduction in the 1950s, with superior outcomes with the use of COX-2 inhibitors [36]. Superior outcomes have also been noted with continuous, rather than intermittent, use of NSAIDs in AS [37]. Similarly, NSAIDs have been shown to be effective in the treatment of AAU, reducing the average number of flares from 2.84 to 0.53 per patient over a 2 year period in a recent study [38].

For patients with chronic or frequently recurrent AAU, steroid-sparing agents have been recommended by numerous expert panels [39] as the standard of care. Methotrexate has shown excellent efficacy in the treatment of recurrent uveitis [40] and is often employed as a steroid-sparing entity in this disease. However, the results for MTX with AS have been generally disappointing, with a recent Cochrane review stating there is not enough evidence to support any benefit of MTX in the treatment of AS [41]. This report was focused on arthritic manifestations and joint destruction; ocular manifestations of ankylosing spondylitis were not assessed by this review. Sulfasalazine has also been evaluated for the treatment of AS and found to be ineffective in a recent meta-analysis [42].

Biologic therapies have shown excellent promise in both the treatment of AS and uveitis. TNF-alpha is expressed in high amounts at the site of inflammation in AS [43] and TNF-alpha inhibitors have shown efficacy in the treatment of AS. These include Adalimumab (Humira), Etanercept (Enbrel), Infliximab (Remicade), Golimumab (Simponi), and Certolizumab Pegol (Cimzia). All five of these medications have been approved by the FDA for treatment of ankylosing spondylitis and are frequently used in patients whose disease has progressed despite NSAID therapy.

However, these medications have shown variable results in the treatment of uveitis. Etanercept, in particular, has been shown to be ineffective in the treatment of uveitis [44] and has been suggested to even induce uveitis in some patients [45]. Infliximab, conversely, has been demonstrated to be effective for several forms of uveitis [46], including a large retrospective review of patients with birdshot retinochoroidopathy [47]. Adalimumab received FDA approval in July 2016 for the treatment of noninfectious intermediate, posterior and panuveitis, the first biologic to be approved for uveitis. This was the result of a multinational phase 3 trial that demonstrated lower risk of uveitic flares in patients treated with Adalimumab [48]. Golimumab and Certolizumab Pegol have more limited data, with a small case series supporting the use of Golimumab in JIA-associated uveitis [49].

In patients with both uveitis and arthritis from ankylosing spondylitis, selection of an appropriate chronic anti-inflammatory therapy can be effective in ameliorating disease manifestations. Often this approach requires coordination between the ophthalmologist and rheumatologist. Based on available data, NSAIDs and TNF-alpha inhibitors are drug classes which have excellent evidence of efficacy and safety for both uveitis and arthritis associated with AS.

References

1. What is Ankylosing Spondylitis? Online publication. National Institute of Arthritis and Musculoskeletal and Skin Disease, National Institutes of Health, Bethesda, MD.
2. Stolwijk C, van Tubergen A, Castillo-Ortiz JD, Boonen A. Prevalence of extra-articular manifestations in patients with ankylosing spondyolitis: a systematic review and meta-analayis. Ann Rheum Dis. doi:10.1136/annrheumdis-2013-203582.
3. Brewerton DA, Caffrey M, Hart FD, et al. Ankylosing spondylitis and HLA-B27. Lancet. 1973;1:904.
4. Zorab PA. The historical and prehistorical background of ankylosing spondylitis. Proc R Soc Med. 1961;54(5):415–20.
5. Ruffer MA. Studies of the paleopathophysiology of Egypt. Chicago: University of Chicago Press; 1921.
6. Dieppe P. Did Galen describe rheumatoid arthritis? Ann Rheum Dis. 1988;47(1):84–7.
7. Colombo MR. De Re Anatomica. Venice, 1559.
8. Bechterew W. Steifigkeit der wirbelsaule und ihre verkrummung als besondere erkrankungsform. Neurol Centralbl. 1893;12:426–34.
9. Strümpell A. Bemerkungen über chronisch-ankylosierende Entzündung der wirbelsoule und der huftergelenks. Deutsch Nervenheilk. 1897;11:338–42.
10. Marie P. Sur la spondylose rhizomelique. Rev Med. 1898;18:285–315.
11. Feldtkeller E. Age at disease onset and delayed diagnosis of spondyloarthropathies. Rheumatol. 1999;58:21–30.
12. Firestein GS, Budd RC, Gabreil SE, McInnes IB, O'Dell JR. Kelly's textbook of rheumatology, 9th edn. 75, 1202–1220.e5. Copyright © 2013.
13. Ankylosing Spondylitis—Profession reference for doctors—Patient UK. Patient UK. Retrieved 22 Dec 2013.
14. Arthritis Research Campaign—Ankylosing Spondylitis Case History. Arthritis Research Campaign. 2009. Retrieved 25 Aug 2009.
15. Jimenez-Balderas FJ, Mintz G. Ankylosing spondylitis: clinical course in women and men. J Rheumatol. 1993;20:2069–72.
16. Singh G, Lawrence A, Agarwal V, Misra R, Aggarwal A. Higher prevalence of extra-articular manifestations in ankylosing spondylitis with peripheral arthritis. J Clin Rheumatol. 2008;14(5):264–6.
17. Van der Horst-Bruinsma IE, Nurmohamed MT. Management and evaluation of extra-articular manifestations in spondyloarthritis. Ther Adv Musculoskel Dis. 2012;4(6):413–22.
18. Khan M. HLA-B27 and its subtypes in world populations. Curr Opin Rheumatol. 1995;7:263–9.

19. Braun J, Bollow M, Remlinger G, et al. Prevalence of spondyloarthropathies in HLA-B27 positive and negative blood donors. Arthritis Rheum. 1998;41:58–67.
20. Baron M, Zendel I. HLA-B27 testing in AS: an analysis of the pre-testing assumptions. J Rheumatol. 1989;16:631–4.
21. Linssen A, Rothova A, Valkenburg HA, Dekker-Saeys AJ, Luyendiik L, Kijlstra A, Feltkamp TE. The lifetime cumulative incidence of acute anterior uveitis in a normal population and its relation to ankylosing spondylitis and histocompatibility antigen HLA-B27. Invest Ophthalmol Vis Sci. 1991;32(9):2568–78.
22. Feldtkerr E, Khan M, Hejde D, Linden S, Braun J. Age of disease onset and diagnosis delay in HLA-B27 negative vs positive patients with ankylosing spondylitis. Rheumatol Int. 2003;23 (2):61–66.
23. Lee Y, Choi S, Ji J, Song G. Associations between ERAP1 polymorphisms and ankylosing spondylitis susceptibility: a meta-analysis. Inflamm Res. 2011;60 (11):999–1003.
24. Brophy S, Pavy S, Lewis P, Taylor G, Bradbury L, Robertson D, et al. Inflammatory eye, skin, and bowel disease in spondyloarthritis: genetic, phenotypic, and environmental factors. J Rheumatol. 2001;28:2667–73.
25. Chou CT. Factors affecting the pathogenesis of ankylosing spondylitis. Chin Med J (Engl). 2001;114:212–3.
26. Resnick D. Niwayama G: Ankylosing spondylitis. Diagnosis of bone and joint disorders. Philadelphia: WB Saunders; 1988. p. p1103.
27. Khan MA. Ankylosing spondylitis: introductory comments on its diagnosis and treatment. Ann Rheum Dis. 2002;61:iii3–iii7.
28. Van der Linden S, Valkenburg H, Cats A. Evaluation of diagnostic criteria for ankylosing spondylitis. a proposal for modification of the New York criteria. Arthritis Rheum. 1984;27:361–8.
29. Huerta-Sil G, Casasola-Vargas J, Londono J, et al. Low grade radiographic sacroiliitis as prognostic factor in patients with undifferentiated spondyloarthritis fulfilling diagnostic criteria for ankylosing spondylitis throughout follow up. Ann Rheum Dis. 2006;65:642–6.
30. Klauser A, Bollow M, Calin A, et al. Workshop report: Clinical diagnosis and imaging of sacroiliitis, Innsbruck, Austria, October 9, 2003. J Rheumatol. 2004;31:2041–7.
31. Oostveen J, Prevo R, den Boer J, van de Laar M. Early detection of sacroiliitis on magnetic resonance imaging and subsequent development of sacroiliitis on plain radiography. A prospective, longitudinal study. J Rheumatol. 1999;26:1953–8.
32. Rodriguez A, Akova YA, Pedroza-Seres M, Foster CS. Posterior segment ocular manifestations in patients with HLA_B27-associated uveitis. Ophthalmology. 1994;101(7):1267–74.
33. de la Maza MS, Jabbur NS, Foster CS. Severity of scleritis and episcleritis. Ophthalmology. 1994; 101:389.
34. Foster CS, de la Maza MS. The sclera. New York: Springer; 1994.
35. Foster CS, Davanzo R, Flynn TE, McLeod K, Vogel R, Crockett RS. Durezol (Difluprednate Ophthalmic Emulsion 0.05 %) compared with Pred Forte 1 % ophthalmic suspension in the treatment of endogenous anterior uveitis. J Ocul Pharacol Ther. 2010;26(5):475–83.
36. Maksymowych WP. Update on the treatment of ankylosing spondylitis. Ther Clin Risk Manag. 2007;3(6):1125–33.
37. Wanders A, Heijde DV, Landewe R, Beheir JM, Calin A, Olivieri I, Zeidler H, Dougados M. Nonsteroid anti-inflammatory drugs reduce radiographic progression in patients with ankylosing spondylitis: a randomized clinical trial. Arthritis Rheum. 2005;52 (6):1756–65.
38. Fiorelli VM, Bhat P, Foster CS. Nonsteroidal anti-inflammatory therapy and recurrent acute anterior uveitis. Ocul Immunol Inflamm. 2010;18 (2):116–20.
39. Jabs DA, Rosenbaum JT, Foster CS, Holland GN, Jaffe GJ, Louie JS, Nussenblatt RB, Stiehm ER, Tessler H, Van Gelder RN, Whitcup SM, Yocum D. Guidelines for the use of immunosuppressive drugs in patients with ocular inflammatory disorders: recommendations of an expert panels. Am J Ophthalmol. 130(4):492–513.
40. Samson CM, Waheed N, Baltatzis S, Foster CS. Methotrexate therapy for chronic noninfectious uveitis; Analysis of a case series of 160 patients. Ophthalmology. 108(6):1134–1139.
41. Chen J, Veras MM, Liu C, Lin J. Methotrexate for ankylosing spondylitis. Cochrane Database Syst Rev. 2013;28:2.
42. Chen J, Liu C. Review Is sulfasalazine effective in ankylosing spondylitis? A systematic review of randomized controlled trials. J Rheumatol. 2006;33 (4):722–31.
43. Zou JX, Braun J, Sieper J. Immunological basis for the use of TNF-blocking agents in ankylosing spondylitis and immunological changes during treatment. Clin Exp Rheumatol 2002;20 (Suppl. 28).
44. Foster CS, Tufail F, Waheed N, Chu D, Miserocchi E, Baltatzis S, Vredeveld C. Efficacy of Etanercept in preventing relapse of uveitis controlled by Methotrexate. Arch Ophthalmol. 2003;121(4):437–40.
45. Taban M, Dupps WJ, Mandell B, Perez VL. Etanercept (enbrel)-associated inflammatory eye disease: case report and review of the literature. Ocular Immunology and Inflammation. 2006;14(3):145–50.
46. Suhler EB, Smith JR, Wertheim MS, Lauer AK, Kurz DE, Pickard TD, Rosenbaum JT. A prospective trial of infliximab therapy for refractory uveitis. Arch Ophthalmol. 2005;123(7):903–12.

47. Artornsombudh P, Gevorgyan O, Payal A, Siddique S, Foster CS. Infliximab treatment of patients with birdshot retinochoroidopathy. Ophthalmology. 120(3);588–592.
48. Jaffe G, Dick AD, Brezin AP, Nguyen QD, Thorne JE, Kestelyn P, et al. Adalimumab in patients with active noninfectious uveitis. N Engl J Med 2016; 375(10): 932–43.
49. William M, Faez S, Papaliodis G, Lobo AM. Golimumab for the treatment of refractory juvenile idiopathic arthritis-associated uveitis. J Ophthal Inflamm Infect. 2012;2:231.

Birdshot Retinochoroidopathy

20

Eduardo Uchiyama

Introduction

Birdshot retinochoroidopathy (BSRC), also known as Birdshot chorioretinopathy, is a relatively uncommon bilateral, chronic, idiopathic, inflammatory condition that affects predominantly the posterior segment of the eye with involvement of retinal and choroidal structures. This condition was first reported in 1941 by Franceschetti and Babel [1] and later described by Ryan and Maumenee in 1980 who named it Birdshot retinochoroidopathy [2] and Gass in 1981 who called it vitiliginous chorioretinitis [3]. This condition is characterized by mild anterior chamber inflammation, vitritis, retinal vasculitis, and the presence of multiple distinctive, hypopigmented fundus lesions and it is strongly associated with human leukocyte antigen (HLA) A29 [4]. Blurred vision and floaters are the most common presenting complaints [4]. Loss of vision is caused by chronic cystoid macular edema (CME) and/or diffuse retinal dysfunction [5, 6]. The diseases progresses very slowly and its effects on vision may not be reflected in Snellen visual acuity until late in the disease process [4].

E. Uchiyama (✉)
Retina Group of Florida, 6333 N. Federal Hwy, Suite 300, Fort Lauderdale, FL 33308, USA
e-mail: uchiyamamd@gmail.com

G.N. Papaliodis (ed.), *Uveitis*,
DOI 10.1007/978-3-319-09126-6_20

Etiology

The etiology and pathogenesis of BSRC remains unknown to date but the high association with the HLA-A29 suggests an immune process in genetically predisposed individuals [7, 8].

The association between BSRC and the HLA-A29 allele is the strongest link between an HLA class I antigen and a disease [9]. The HLA-A29 allele is present in as many as 7 % of Caucasian individuals but more than 95 % of reported BSRC patients have been HLA-A29-positive [4]. Given the high frequency of the HLA-A29 allele in Caucasians (7 %), other triggering factors may play a role [10]. The presence of the HLA-A29 allele alone does not establish the diagnosis of BSRC [4].

The large majority of patients with BSRC do not have any family history of uveitis [10]. Familial forms of BSRC are rare and do not justify systematic examination of relatives of affected patients [11]. There is one report of monozygotic twins with BSRC [12].

Epidemiology

BSRC is an uncommon cause of uveitis, representing about 1.2–2.9 % of patients with posterior uveitis [13, 14]. It affects mostly middle-aged individual with a mean age of presentation of 53 years but there are cases reported with ages between 15 and 79 years old [4, 15]. There is a slight female predominance (54 %) [4], and there does not appear to be any significant difference in clinical presentation between genders [16]. The disease is more common in Caucasians with only few case reports of more pigmented races being affected [15, 17].

Clinical Manifestations and Diagnosis

BSRC may have heterogeneous presentations which may correspond to different stages or forms of the disease [10].

Some series have suggested systemic associations including cardiovascular disease [18], vitiligo [3], hearing loss [19], etc. There are no confirmed systemic disorders associated with BSRC, and the disease usually affects otherwise healthy individuals [4].

Patients usually present with different complaints including blurred vision, photosensitivity, photopsias, floaters, and nyctalopia. The symptoms are usually bilateral, but they can be asymmetric.

The classic clinical findings as described by Ryan and Maumenee in their original report [2] include: quiet and non painful eyes, minimal to no anterior chamber inflammation, vitritis with no snowbanking, retinal vascular leakage (Fig. 20.2) with CME and disc leakage, and presence of multiple deep cream-colored lesions located in the posterior fundus (Fig. 20.1).

A newer criterion for research purposes has been published and includes supportive findings such as the presence of HLA-A29 positivity [19]. It also considers keratic precipitates, posterior synechiae, or the presence of other causes of multifocal choroiditis as exclusion criteria [20].

HLA-A29 positivity is not required for the diagnosis of BSRC, but given the high correlation, one should consider revisiting the diagnosis if the test is negative [21].

Imaging modalities and ancillary tests are helpful in the diagnosis of BSRC. Fluorescein angiography (FA) is used to evaluate retinal vascular leakage and associated CME and disc leakage. Indocyanine green angiography (ICG) demonstrates the presence of multiple hypocyanescent lesions (Fig. 20.3) that are smaller and do not correspond with the lesions seen clinically. Ocular coherence tomography (OCT) testing is useful in the evaluation of CME and also to assess changes in the outer retinal layers consistent with damage to the photoreceptors due to long-standing disease. Electroretinography (ERG) [6] and Goldmann visual field testing [22] demonstrate abnormalities in long-standing disease due to global retinal dysfunction.

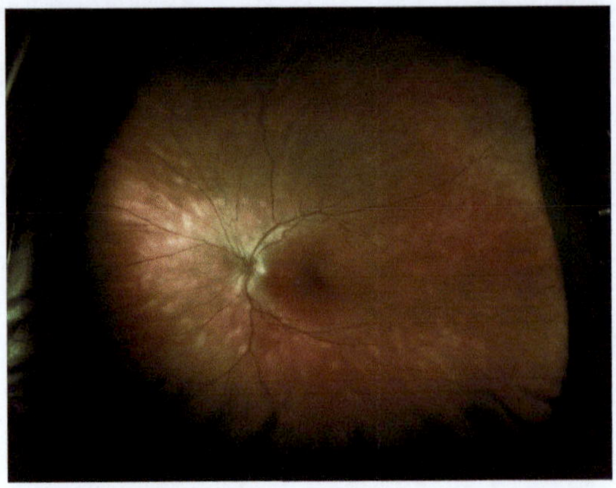

Fig. 20.1 Characteristic multiple deep cream-colored lesions in a patient with BSRC

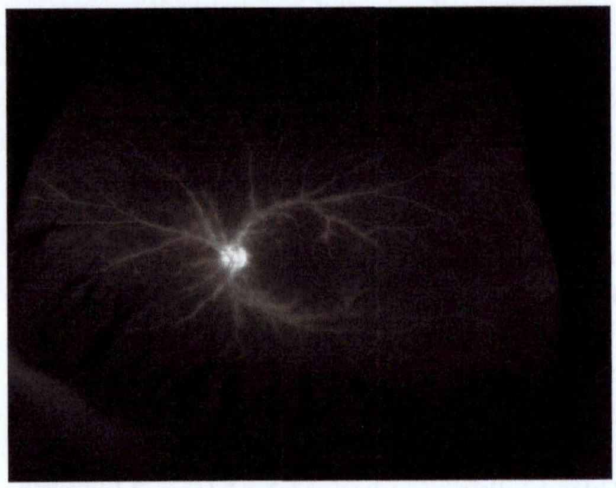

Fig. 20.2 Fluorescein angiography demonstrating retinal vasculitis in a patient with BSRC

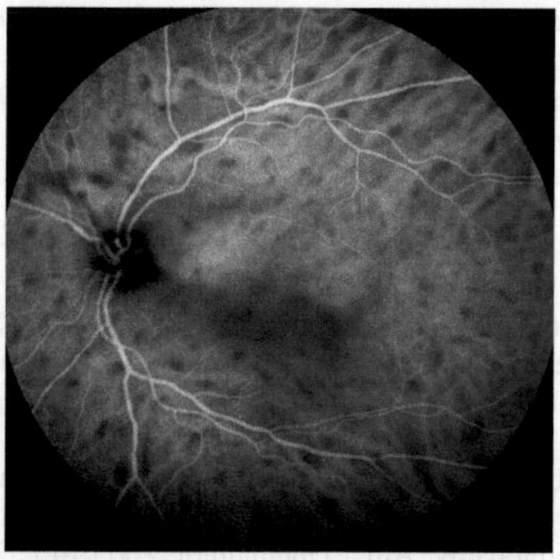

Fig. 20.3 ICG angiography in a BSRC patient demonstrating hypocyanescent lesions

Differential Diagnosis

The clinical features of BSRC are very distinct as the disease involves both the retina and choroid. These findings can be subtle early in the disease and the diagnosis more difficult to establish. Conditions that can be considered in the differential diagnosis of BSRC are sarcoidosis [23], syphilis, tuberculosis, intraocular lymphoma [24], multifocal choroiditis, and other "white dot syndromes" [25]. Demographics, systemic symptoms, ancillary testing, blood work, and sometimes surgery (i.e., diagnostic vitrectomy), are useful in differentiating these conditions from BSRC.

Treatment

Multiple different treatment approaches have been utilized in the management of BSRC but there is no consensus regarding the ideal treatment. Many patients can develop a chronic course leading to vision loss if effective treatment is not started. A small fraction of patients may develop a self-limiting disease but this is uncommon.

Historically, treatment was reserved for patients that developed macular edema but this approach does not take into account loss of vision due to global retinal dysfunction [5].

BSRC responds well to systemic or periocular/intravitreal steroids but in most cases, the disease progresses after steroid taper or discontinuation. Steroids are used acutely and during exacerbations but are usually not enough to maintain control of the disease. It has been reported that more than 50 % of patients treated with steroid monotherapy may experience deterioration in visual acuity over time [26].

A uveitis expert panel published guidelines for the use and monitoring of immunosuppressive drugs in ocular inflammatory diseases in 2000. They suggested that patients with BSRC and other posterior uveitides may benefit from the use of immunosuppressive drugs as they appear to have a poor long-term outcome from steroid therapy alone [27].

Different immunomodulatory therapy (IMT) agents have been reported to control the progression of this disease including antimetabolites, cyclosporine [26], TNF alpha blockers [28], intravenous immunoglobulin [29], etc.

Ideally, the management of a patient with noninfectious uveitis should be based on a step-up or stepladder approach, consisting of intensification of treatment guided by disease severity [30]. One strategy when dealing with BSRC is to start systemic or periocular/intravitreal steroids acutely and discuss the likely need for further therapy. If IMT is initiated, antimetabolites such as mycophenolate or methotrexate are good first line agents [31]. If the disease continues to be active and/or steroids are unable to be tapered, cyclosporine can be added as adjuvant therapy [32]. In patients with persistent inflammation despite the use of these drugs, the transition to a TNF alpha inhibitor [28] or the use of an intravitreal steroid implant such as the fluocinolone acetonide intravitreal implant should be considered [33].

Monitoring of Disease Activity

Multiple imaging modalities and ancillary tests are utilized to follow course and response to treatment of patients with BSRC. FA is used to follow resolution of vascular and disc leakage and CME. ICG can demonstrate involution of choroidal lesions. OCT is useful to evaluate macular changes such as CME or the developing of subretinal fluid associated with choroidal neovascularization. Progressive global retinal dysfunction can be measured by electroretinography (ERG) [6] or by Goldmann visual field testing [22]. Goldmann testing is preferred over Humphreys automated perimetry as it test a broader field and is likely more sensitive to earlier peripheral retinal changes [22].

Annual ERGs can help monitor stability or progression in patient with BSRC [6]. ERG in association with other ancillary testings is a useful tool to establish efficacy of treatment [6].

Prognosis

This disease is often characterized by multiple relapses or chronically active, smoldering inflammation resulting in loss of useful vision in one or both eyes in 40 % of patients [2]. BSRC is a slowly progressive disease with profound dysfunction of vision that may not be reflected in Snellen visual acuity [4]. Loss of visual field defects is due to global retinal dysfunction and loss of central vision is due to CME, or less common CNV.

Conclusion

BSRC is an uncommon, chronic ocular inflammatory condition involving the posterior segment of the eye linked to the presence of the HLA-A29 antigen which is found in 95 % of patients with the disease. Regional and systemic corticosteroids are an effective initial treatment modality, but most patients will require therapy with systemic immunomodulatory therapy to control the disease and prevent loss of vision.

References

1. Franceschetti A, Babel J. La choriorétinite en taches de bougie, manifestation de la maladie de Besnier-Boeck. Ophthalmologica. 1949;118:701–10.
2. Ryan SJ, Maumenee AE. Birdshot retinochoroidopathy. Am J Ophthalmol. 1980;89:31–45.
3. Gass JD. Vitiliginous chorioretinitis. Arch Ophthalmol. 1981;99:1778–87.
4. Shah KH, Levinson RD, Yu F, Goldhardt R, Gordon LK, Gonzales CR, Heckenlively JR, Kappel PJ, Holland GN. Birdshot chorioretinopathy. Surv Ophthalmol. 2005;50:519–41.
5. Rothova A, Berendschot TT, Probst K, van Kooij B, Baarsma GS. Birdshot chorioretinopathy: long-term manifestations and visual prognosis. Ophthalmology. 2004;111:954–9.
6. Sobrin L, Lam BL, Liu M, Feuer WJ, Davis JL. Electroretinographic monitoring in birdshot chorioretinopathy. Am J Ophthalmol. 2005;140:52–64.
7. Vitale AT. Birdshot Retinochoridopathy. In: Foster CS, Vitale AT, editors. Diagnosis and treatment of uveitis. 2nd ed. New Delhi: Jaypee Brothers Medical Publishers; 2013. p. 982–1004.
8. Wee R, Papaliodis G. Genetics of birdshot chorioretinopathy. Semin Ophthalmol. 2008;23:53–7.
9. Nussenblatt RB, Mittal KK, Ryan S, Green WR, Maumenee AE. Birdshot retinochoroidopathy associated with HLA-A29 antigen and immune responsiveness to retinal S-antigen. Am J Ophthalmol. 1982;94:147–58.
10. Monnet D, Brézin AP. Birdshot chorioretinopathy. Curr Opin Ophthalmol. 2006;17:545–50.
11. Trinh L, Bodaghi B, Fardeau C, Monin C, Labetoulle M, Soubrane G, Lehoang P. Clinical features, treatment methods, and evolution of birdshot chorioretinopathy in 5 different families. Am J Ophthalmol. 2009;147:1042–7.
12. Fich M, Rosenberg T. Birdshot retinochoroidopathy in monozygotic twins. Acta Ophthalmol (Copenh). 1992;70:693–97.
13. Henderly DE, Genstler AJ, Smith RE, Rao NA. Changing patterns of uveitis. Am J Ophthalmol. 1987;103:131–6.
14. Rodriguez A, Calonge M, Pedroza-Seres M, Akova YA, Messmer EM, D'Amico DJ, Foster CS. Referral patterns of uveitis in a tertiary eye care center. Arch Ophthalmol. 1996;114:593–9.
15. Gasch AT, Smith JA, Whitcup SM. Birdshot retinochoroidopathy. Br J Ophthalmol. 1999;83:241–9.
16. Faia LJ. Gender differences in Birdshot Chorioretinopathy and the white dot syndromes: do they exist? J Ophthalmol. 2014;2014:146768.
17. Barondes MJ, Fastenberg DM, Schwartz PL, Rosen DA. Peripheral retinal neovascularization in birdshot retinochoroidopathy. Ann Ophthalmol. 1989;21:306–8.
18. Priem HA, Oosterhuis JA. Birdshot chorioretinopathy: clinical characteristics and evolution. Br J Ophthalmol. 1988;72:646–59.
19. Heaton JM, Mill RP. Sensorineural hearing loss associated with birdshot retinochoroidopathy. Arch Otolaryngol Head Neck Surg. 1993;119:680–1.
20. Levinson RD, Brezin A, Rothova A, Accorinti M, Holland GN. Research criteria for the diagnosis of

birdshot chorioretinopathy: results of an international consensus conference. Am J Ophthalmol. 2006;141:185–7.
21. Jones N. Birdshot retinochoroidopathy. In: Jones N, editor. Uveitis. 2nd ed. London: JP Medical Ltd; 2013. p. 325–6.
22. Thorne JE, Jabs DA, Kedhar SR, Peters GB, Dunn JP. Loss of visual field among patients with birdshot chorioretinopathy. Am J Ophthalmol. 2008;145:23–8.
23. Vrabec TR, Augsburger JJ, Fischer DH, Belmont JB, Tashayyod D, Israel HL. Taches de bougie. Ophthalmology. 1995;102:1712–21.
24. Miserocchi E, Modorati G, De Benedetto U, Colucci A, Bandello F. Birdshot retinochoroidopathy masquerading as intraocular lymphoma. Ocul Immunol Inflamm. 2012;20:306–8.
25. Opremcak EM. Uveitis: a clinical manual for ocular inflammation. New York: Springer; 1995.
26. Vitale AT, Rodriguez A, Foster CS. Low-dose cyclosporine therapy in the treatment of birdshot retinochoroidopathy. Ophthalmology. 1994;101:822–31.
27. Jabs DA, Rosenbaum JT, Foster CS, Holland GN, Jaffe GJ, Louie JS, Nussenblatt RB, Stiehm ER, Tessler H, Van Gelder RN, Whitcup SM, Yocum D. Guidelines for the use of immunosuppressive drugs in patients with ocular inflammatory disorders: recommendations of an expert panel. Am J Ophthalmol. 2000;130:492–513.
28. Artornsombudh P, Gevorgyan O, Payal A, Siddique SS, Foster CS. Infliximab treatment of patients with birdshot retinochoroidopathy. Ophthalmology. 2013;120:588–92.
29. LeHoang P, Cassoux N, George F, Kullmann N, Kazatchkine MD. Intravenous immunoglobulin (IVIg) for the treatment of birdshot retinochoroidopathy. Ocul Immunol Inflamm. 2000;8:49–57.
30. Uchiyama E, Papaliodis GN, Lobo AM, Sobrin L. Side-effects of anti-inflammatory therapy in uveitis. Semin Ophthalmol. 2014;29:456-67.
31. Becker MD, Wertheim MS, Smith JR, Rosenbaum JT. Long-term follow-up of patients with birdshot retinochoroidopathy treated with systemic immunosuppression. Ocul Immunol Inflamm. 2005;13:289–93.
32. Cervantes-Castañeda RA, Gonzalez-Gonzalez LA, Cordero-Coma M, Yilmaz T, Foster CS. Combined therapy of cyclosporine A and mycophenolate mofetil for the treatment of birdshot retinochoroidopathy: a 12-month follow-up. Br J Ophthalmol. 2013;97:637–43.
33. Rush RB, Goldstein DA, Callanan DG, Meghpara B, Feuer WJ, Davis JL. Outcomes of birdshot chorioretinopathy treated with an intravitreal sustained-release fluocinolone acetonide-containing device. Am J Ophthalmol. 2011;151:630–6.

21 Cogan Syndrome

Victoria Chang

Introduction

Cogan syndrome (CS) is a rare systemic inflammatory disease that is characterized by Ménière-like vestibuloauditory symptoms (tinnitus, vertigo, and hearing loss) and acute ocular inflammation [1, 2].

Historical Perspective

A case of non-syphilitic interstitial keratitis (IK) associated with dizziness and hearing loss was first described in 1934 by Mogan and Baumgartner [3]. However, the syndrome went unrecognized for over a decade until it was characterized in a case series published by Cogan [1]. The definition of Cogan syndrome (CS) was further expanded in 1980 by Haynes et al. to include "typical" and "atypical" forms of the disease [2].

Due to its obscurity, most reports of CS have consisted of individual case reports and several case series. However, advances in modern medicine have led to a deeper understanding of the underlying pathogenesis resulting in innovative treatments for this potentially devastating disease.

Epidemiology

Due to its variable presentation, rarity, and clinical overlap with other autoimmune disorders, CS is commonly misdiagnosed. Thus, the true prevalence of CS is likely under-represented in the literature. CS predominantly affects young- to middle-aged Caucasian adults in the second through fourth decades of life [4–8]. Though uncommon in young children, the age of disease onset reportedly spans from 2.5 to 60 years [9–11]. 80 % of patients present between the ages of 14 and 47 years [7]. Although there is no gender predilection in adults, males are found to be twice as likely to be affected than females in the pediatric population [12]. CS is thought to be nonhereditary [13].

Pathogenesis

The etiology of CS is thought to be secondary to an autoimmune process. The existence of an infectious precipitant (viral, bacterial, or even fungal) causing an immune hypersensitivity reaction in the pathogenesis of CS has been postulated.

V. Chang (✉)
Department of Ophthalmology, Harvard Medical School, Massachusetts Eye and Ear Infirmary, 243 Charles Street, Boston, MA 02114, USA
e-mail: Victoria_Chang@meei.harvard.edu

G.N. Papaliodis (ed.), *Uveitis*,
DOI 10.1007/978-3-319-09126-6_21

Infectious

Evidence for a single causative organism in the pathogenesis of CS, such as consistent serological detection or clinical improvement after treatment with antimicrobials alone, has not been found. However, 23–69 % of CS patients report symptoms of a preceding upper respiratory infection (URI), typically with sinusitis or otitis media [2, 5, 7, 12, 14–16].

An increased incidence of chlamydia infections associated with CS has been reported in the literature. However, the vast majority of those infected with chlamydia do not go on to develop immune- mediated eye, ear, or vascular damage [5]. Chlamydia is associated with cardiovascular injury, as it has been recovered from atherosclerotic plaques [13]. Chlamydia is also a known cause of myocarditis, endocarditis, and valvular heart disease [13, 17]. *Chlamydophila psittaci* and *Chlamydophila pneumonia* have both been isolated from the sera of CS patients [13, 14, 17, 18]. *Chlamydia trachomatis* has been implicated in a number of chronic human infections, including those related to the eye and ear. In Haynes' study, 9 out of 13 patients had positive anti-chlamydia IgG titers, but only four had positive IgM titers to *C. trachomatis* [2]. Despite these findings, attempts to isolate chlamydia directly from ocular biopsy specimens have not been successful [7, 19]. Other bacteria that have been associated with CS include borrelia, tuberculosis, and yersinia [12, 13, 18, 20].

Viruses that have been associated with CS include herpes, reovirus, mumps, measles, rubella, influenza A and B, parainfluenza, poliovirus, parvovirus, coxackievirus, and respiratory syncytial virus [2, 7, 18]. It is believed that a viral trigger may initiate an autoimmune hypersensitivity reaction via antigenic mimicry, the exposure of hidden epitopes, or the release of the cytokine cascade [2, 18]. Previous attempts to isolate viruses in CS patients have not yielded positive results [7]. However, Lunardi et al. found homology between density enhanced protein tyrosine phosphatase-1 (DEP-1/CD148), a transmembrane protein located on the endothelial cells and sensorineural epithelium of the inner ear, and reovirus III major core protein λ1, which lends credence to the hypothesis of a viral precipitant in the pathogenesis of the disease [21].

Autoimmune

CS is thought to be an autoimmune process due to clinical improvement after steroid and other immunosuppressant treatments; its association with other autoimmune disorders; and the detection of antibodies against the cornea and inner ear tissues in the sera of patients [4, 12, 18, 22]. Other rheumatologic diseases that have been found in association with CS include inflammatory bowel disease (IBD), rheumatoid arthritis (RA), idiopathic juvenile arthritis (IJA), thrombocytopenic purpura, HLA-B27 positive spondyloarthropathies, sarcoidosis, Grave's disease, and polyarteritis nodosum (PAN) [4, 12, 18, 22]. Detection of antiphospholipid antibodies (APA), antineutrophil cytoplasmic antibodies (ANCA), and antigens of the human leukocyte antigen system (HLA) A9, Bw17, Bw35, Cw4 have been reported in the literature [12, 15]. Perhaps the strongest evidence for an underlying autoimmune process came from Lunardi and colleagues' breakthrough paper published in 2002: Purified IgG from the sera of eight CS patients was exposed to a random peptide library [21]. All the sera sampled recognized an autoantigen, coined the "Cogan peptide," which was found to be analogous to DEP-1/CD148, reovirus III major core protein λ1, laminin, SSA/Ro, and connexin 26 (an inner ear gap junction protein responsible for electrolyte balance, and has been implicated in the pathogenesis of congenital deafness) [21]. To confirm that DEP-1/CD148 was indeed the Cogan peptide, Balb/c mice were injected with DEP-1/CD148, and subsequently developed CS-like symptoms including hearing loss, IK, and systemic vasculitis [21].

Other Associated Factors

In addition to preceding infections, retrospective reviews have found increased incidence of malignancy (B-cell lymphoma, gastric mucosa associated lymphoid tissue lymphoma, melanoma, ovarian cancer), vaccinations, pregnancy, and coexisting inflammatory disorders in association with CS [2, 7, 8, 23, 24]. However, the significance of these findings is unclear. Interestingly, Gluth and colleagues found CS patients were twice as likely to be smokers [8]. The association between smoking and CS is only speculative, and a clear link has not yet been established.

In addition, there have been reports of CS exacerbations during pregnancy and the postpartum period, suggesting a possible association with hormonal changes [24]. In one series, 10 % of typical CS and 5 % of atypical CS patients were found to be pregnant [2]. Thus, basic lab work, an ophthalmic exam, hearing and vestibular evaluation, and close follow-up are indicated in both the pre- and postpartum periods and during pregnancy in CS patients [24, 25]. Treatment with low-dose steroids can usually be safely administered in pregnant women [24].

Diagnosis

CS is commonly misdiagnosed due to its variable presentation, nonspecific constitutional symptoms, staggered appearance of clinical manifestations, and lack of diagnostic laboratory or radiological testing [26]. CS can also mimic other systemic inflammatory diseases. Only 5 % of patients initially present with the classic clinical triad of IK, sensorineural hearing loss (SNHL), and vestibular dysfunction [27]. 85 % of patients, however, will develop all three manifestations within 2 years [27]. In one series, the average delay between initial presentation and diagnosis was 10 months for typical CS, and 34.6 months for atypical CS [22].

The diagnosis of CS is mainly clinical and based on ocular and vestibuloauditory symptoms. Since it is considered a diagnosis of exclusion, one must retain a high degree of clinical suspicion to correctly identify CS patients.

It is important to note that the separation of typical and atypical CS is a clinical distinction and not based on differing underlying pathophysiology [2]. Furthermore, the classification of CS into subsets can be a challenge. There is often a staggered development of symptoms, which may blur boundaries between what is considered “typical” or “atypical” CS [8]. Some have even suggested such categorization has become outdated despite being widely used in the literature today [19].

Diagnostic Criteria

Typical CS

The definition of “typical CS” encompasses the original criteria set forth by D.G. Cogan in 1945. It is defined by typical Ménière’s-like vestibuloauditory dysfunction (vertigo, tinnitus, hearing loss) and non-syphilitic interstitial keratitis [1, 2] (see Fig. 21.1). The ocular and vestibuloauditory symptoms must occur within 2 years of each other [2]. The presentation of both symptoms typically occurs concomitantly within 1–6 months [23, 28]. Other ocular findings that may be present include iritis and subconjunctival hemorrhage [2]. Approximately 70–80 % of CS patients present as “typical” [8, 10].

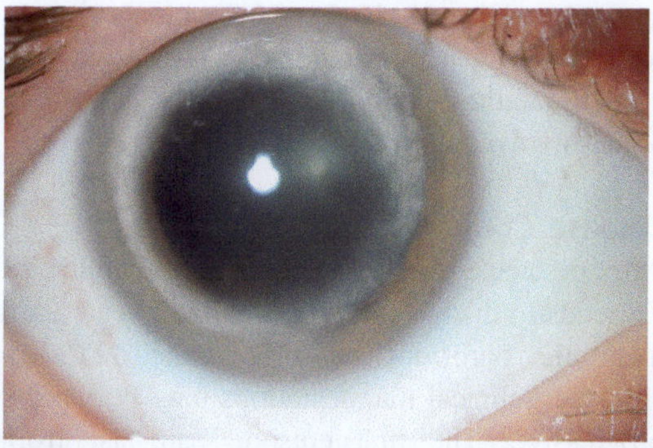

Fig. 21.1 Slit lamp photograph of patient with Cogan’s syndrome demonstrating interstitial keratitis

Atypical CS

"Atypical CS" refers to the presence of ocular inflammation such as scleritis, episcleritis, vitritis, retinitis, choroiditis; acute angle closure glaucoma; orbital pseudotumor; retinal artery or vein occlusion; retinal hemorrhages; papilledema, exophthalmos; oculomotor palsy; ptosis; endophthalmitis; and/or tendonitis in addition to vestibuloauditory symptoms [2, 4, 10, 22, 29, 30]. "Atypical" CS may also refer to patients who present with the typical vestibuloauditory symptoms but without IK; non "Ménière-like" (ataxia, oscillopsia) vestibuloauditory symptoms; or, ocular and otolaryngologic symptoms that occur more than 2 years apart [2]. In one review, the average delay between eye and ear symptoms in atypical CS was 27.1 months [22].

These labels have clinical relevance since atypical CS has been associated with an increased incidence of vasculitis and coexisting inflammatory disorders [2, 8, 22]. According to Haynes et al., aortic insufficiency is more common in typical CS, and systemic vasculitis is more common in atypical CS [2, 31]. Thus, typical CS should not be thought to be only isolated to eye and ear symptoms [31].

Clinical Presentation

Adults

Patients typically manifest with either ocular or vestibuloauditory involvement on initial presentation. In adults, 25–50 % of CS patients present with ocular manifestations, 32–36 % with vestibuloauditory symptoms, and 5 % with both organ involvement [7, 8, 32, 33].

Disease Course

After the acute onset of symptoms, the course of CS tends to fluctuate during the first 2 years until a chronic "burnt out" phase is reached [22, 34]. However, clinical manifestations may be rapidly progressive. The first episode can last from weeks to months, and subsequent exacerbations may be triggered by infection, hormonal changes, or even LASIK surgery [22, 24, 26, 30]. In one review, 13 % of patients had single relapses, 62 % had more than one relapse, and only 22 % had no documented relapses [8]. Two patients in the same series had persistently active symptoms without remission [8].

Eye Findings

Patients often present with generalized bilateral eye discomfort, redness, photophobia, tearing, and blurred vision. In the majority of cases, these complaints are secondary to IK, but may also be attributable, in part, to conjunctivitis, episcleritis, scleritis, iridocyclitis, choroiditis, and/or retinitis. In one study, the most common ocular findings were IK (100 %), episcleritis and scleritis (23 %), iritis (23 %), and conjunctivitis (15 %) [2]. 23 % of patients have more than one site of inflammation [8]. Other ocular complaints include oscillopsia, diplopia, and amaurosis fugax [7, 12, 35].

IK is classically described as bilateral peripheral granular infiltration of the anterior- to mid-corneal stroma that may be followed by neovascularization and permanent stromal haze [1, 22]. The IK associated with CS typically presents suddenly, fluctuates daily, and is patchy in distribution [30]. The severity of keratopathy tends to be related to the degree of corneal neovascularization [36]. There have been rare case reports documenting severe lipid keratopathy as a consequence of chronic inflammation in CS, necessitating corneal transplantation [37].

As previously described, the ocular inflammation in atypical CS may affect the anterior and posterior segments of the eye, and the surrounding extraocular and periorbital tissues. Of note, cases of bilateral close angle glaucoma have been described, with an incidence of 5 % in one series [8]. Other causes of significant visual sequelae include corneal ulceration, retinal vasculitis, synechie, central retinal artery occlusion (CRAO), central retinal vein occlusion (CRVO), posterior scleritis, choroidal detachments, cataracts, cystoid macular edema, papillitis, and retinal hemangiomas [7, 12, 35, 38–40].

Ear Findings

The majority of CS patients will develop vestibuloauditory symptoms at some point during their clinical course, and SNHL is the most common otolaryngologic complaint [8, 10]. The SNHL in CS is typically bilateral (although it may start unilaterally), and can be strikingly asymmetric in presentation. Characteristically, there is decreased perception of the highest and lowest frequencies [18]. Bilateral auricular chondritis and ear pain have also been reported in association with CS [10, 23, 41].

Approximately 50 % of patients suffering from CS will develop permanent and bilateral SNHL within 3 months of presentation [4, 7, 42]. Furthermore, episodes of hearing loss may recur up to 13 years after the initial onset despite chronic immunosuppressive therapy [4, 43]. For these reasons, it is imperative that systemic immunosuppression be started as early as possible to minimize the risk of this devastating consequence.

Vestibular complaints included vertigo (90 %), tinnitus (80 %), ataxia (53 %), and oscillopsia (25 %) [8]. Other commonly reported symptoms include nausea, vomiting, and nystagmus. It is common for vestibular symptoms to precede SNHL in CS [12].

Systemic Manifestations

Approximately 50–72 % of CS patients experience systemic manifestations; and, 12–33 % of patients develop vasculitis [8, 10, 39, 44–46]. Vascular inflammation can lead to end-organ ischemia, and may result in a number of neurological, musculoskeletal, gastrointestinal, and even mucocutaneous complications [46]. The overlap of CS with other inflammatory conditions suggests CS may encompass a wider phenotype than previously thought [47]. For instance, there have been reports of chondritis, sinusitis, auricular perichondritis, and ANCA glomerulonephritis in association with CS, suggesting possible clinical overlap with Wegener's granulomatosis, relapsing polychondritis, and tubulointerstitial nephritis and uveitis syndrome (TINU) [14, 22, 47]. The most devastating clinical complications of CS include deafness, blindness (permanent visual loss less than 20/200), aortic insufficiency, vasculitis, and even death [7].

Grasland et al. [22] divided the systemic manifestations of CS into nine distinct categories as follows:

(1) In CS, approximately, 50 % of patients complain of vague constitutional symptoms including headaches, fever, fatigue, and weight loss, which are suggestive of an underlying active vasculitis [4, 7, 8].
(2) One-third of patients complain of musculoskeletal symptoms including arthritis, arthralgias, and myalgias [7].
(3) Cardiovascular symptoms: 10–17 % of CS sufferers develop cardiac complications [7, 22, 48]. It typically takes about 7 months (3 weeks to 8 years) before the development of vasculitis after disease onset [7]. Vasculitis associated with CS can affect the aorta, coronary arteries, mesenteric arteries, femoral vessels, and the renal vasculature [21, 48]. Consequently, CS may result in aortitis, symptomatic extremity claudication, mesenteric arteritis, or renal artery stenosis [18, 20, 49]. Other significant cardiac findings that have been reported include pericarditis, left ventricular hypertrophy, myocardial infarction, myocarditis, and arrhythmia [12, 22].
Aortitis resulting in aortic valve or mitral valve insufficiency, aortic aneurysms, first-degree atrioventricular (AV) block, and aortic dilatation is a significant cause of morbidity and mortality in CS patient [12, 50]. Signs of aortitis include lack of radial pulse, aortic regurgitation, and congestive heart failure (CHF) [4]. In one series, aortitis was reported in 10–12 % of cases [2, 8]. Risks associated with increased risk of aortic rupture include rapidly enlarging aneurysm, symptomatic aortitis, and the use of steroids prior to vascular grafting [20].

40 % of those with cardiac involvement will have coronary artery involvement either by coronary ostia occlusion or vasculitis [28]. Approximately 15 % of AR patients will require surgical valvular repair [5].

(4) Approximately 13–33 % of CS patients experience gastrointestinal signs and symptoms including abdominal pain due to mesenteric ischemia, hepatosplenomegaly, diarrhea, hepatitis, esophagitis, melena, liver steatosis, and intestinal perforation [2, 7, 22, 42, 51].

(5) Up to 29 % of patients with CS develop neurological symptoms such as peripheral neuropathy, cerebellar involvement, seizures, cranial nerve palsies (temporary facial palsy), trigeminal neuralgia, cerebral vasculitis, aseptic meningitis, hemiparesis, myelopathies, cerebral aneurysm, encephalitis, cavernous sinus thrombosis, cerebral vascular accident (CVA), and transient ischemic attacks (TIA) [2, 7, 8, 21, 22, 43, 52]. Psychosis has rarely been reported in association with CS [8]. Secondary hypothyroidism has been detected in a patient with CS, with reversal of pituitary swelling and improved thyroid hormone levels after treatment with immunosuppression [53].

(6) 10 % of CS patients have skin and mucous membrane manifestations, which encompass rashes, purpura, vitiligo, oral and genital ulcers, nodules, and pyoderma gangrenosum (PG) [4, 7, 22, 54, 55].

(7) Urogenital symptoms include orchitis and testicular pain due to testicular artery vasculitis.

(8) Renal manifestations such as ANCA-positive glomerulonephritis and renal failure with associated flank pain, proteinuria, abnormal renal function testing, and systemic hypertension have been reported [7, 13, 15, 44, 56].

(9) Lymphadenopathy [21, 22].

Pediatric

In pediatric CS, ocular and vestibuloauditory symptoms are the predominant presenting symptoms [12]. In one series, two-thirds of patients had evidence of IK [12]. Compared to adults, IK in children may be more diffuse, and likely to involve the central cornea [36, 57]. For these reasons, pediatric CS may result in devastating visual consequences, such as amblyopia.

The largest series of pediatric CS reported included 23 children with a mean age of 11.4 years: 47.8 % experienced constitutional symptoms (fever, weight loss, arthralgias, myalgias, and headaches); 91.3 % had ocular symptoms (interstitial keratitis, episcleritis/conjunctivitis, uveitis); 39.1 % had vestibular symptoms (vertigo, nausea/vomiting, dizziness), 65.2 % had auditory involvement (SNHL, tinnitus, and deafness), 17.3 % experienced cardiac valve complications, and 13 % had skin manifestations [12]. The majority of patients (69.6 %) experienced permanent complications from the disease including SNHL, vestibular dysfunction, ocular sequelae, and cardiac valve damage [12].

Pathology

CS is a primary vasculitis (involving both veins and arteries), which is characterized by inflammation of endothelial cells causing vessel occlusion, tissue ischemia and necrosis, which can ultimately lead to end organ damage [51]. Pathologically, CS vasculitis can involve large (similar to Takayasu's arteritis), medium, (similar to polyarteritis nodosa), and small arteries [20].

Eye

The first description of corneal histopathology in CS was published in 1961 [58]. Thickening of the corneal epithelium; neovascularization, lymphocytic and plasma cells infiltration; crystalline lipids, and hyalinization of the optic nerve have been described in CS patients [2, 4, 7, 15, 26]. A conjunctiva biopsy from a suspected case of IK revealed plasma cell and monocyte infiltration [2].

Ear

SNHL is attributable to lymphocytic and plasma cell infiltration resulting in degeneration and atrophy of cells in the semicircular canals, spiral ligament of the cochlea, organ of Corti, utricle, saccule, and proximal portion of the eight cranial nerve [7, 12, 18, 21, 59]. Endolymphatic hydrops of the temporal bone and osteogensis of the round window membrane secondary to chronic inflammation have also been detected on histological exam [7, 41, 60]. The role of vasculitis in hearing loss is debatable. Pathological samples have not shown evidence of vasculitis, but rather chronic inflammatory changes [18].

Cardiovascular and Other Vessels

Grossly, dilatation of the aorta and narrowing of the coronary ostia near the aortic valve have been found on autopsies [33, 39]. Fibrinoid necrosis, degradation of the elastic lamellae, and fibromyxoid changes of the aorta can result in deformation and aneurysms of the aorta and aortic valve leaflets [7, 39, 61]. Thickening and inflammatory cell infiltration of the pericardium, myocardium, and endocardium have been described, with resultant fibrosis and infarction of the involved tissues [2, 7].

Inflammation of the vessels of the kidneys, dura, brain, mesentery, bowel, skin, and muscles resulting have also been reported [7, 39, 43].

Other Organs

Skin biopsies from CS patients have shown vasculitis, leukocytic evasion, ulceration, and fibrosis [7, 8, 22]. Lymph node biopsies have shown granulomatous inflammation with nonspecific inflammatory hyperplasia [7]. Pathologic findings of abdominal organs in CS patients have included hepatic granulomas, bile duct proliferation, glomerulonephritis, renal cortical infarction, caseating necrosis of the spleen, and inflammation of the lamina propria and submucosa of the bowel [7]. In the brain, hemosiderin deposit in the subarachnoid, cerebral petechiae and edema, and gliosis of the occipital lobe have been reported [7].

Differential Diagnosis

Infectious

The corneal manifestations of congenital syphilis tend to be significantly more severe than CS [19]. Congenital syphilis can cause bilateral, progressive IK, with significant posterior corneal scarring, edema, and neovascularization in the presence of other luetic stigmata (skin, dental, skeletal) [1, 30]. Hearing loss may also be associated, but vestibular function is typically not affected, unlike CS [1, 19, 30].

Other infectious etiologies that may present with similar symptoms as CS include tuberculosis, chlamydia, *Borrelia burgdorferi*, and certain viruses. Tuberculosis rarely causes IK; however, when it occurs, there is usually minimal corneal infiltration with mild neovascularization [1]. Associated hearing loss can result from treatment with streptomycin [2, 30]. The chlamydia species, in particular, have been investigated for its possible role in the pathogenesis of CS. It is a known infectious cause of ocular, otolaryngologic, and cardiovascular complications in humans [2, 13]. Lyme disease, caused by the spirochete *Borrelia burgdoreferi*, can cause skin changes (erythema migrans, borrelia lymphocytoma, achrodermatitis chronica atrophicans), carditis (resulting in conduction abnormalities), neurological symptoms (aseptic meningitis and peripheral nerve palsies), arthritis, and, rarely, ocular manifestations (conjunctivitis, episcleritis, keratitis, endophthalmitis) that may mimic CS [62]. HSV/VZV can cause hearing loss due to involvement of CN VIII, as it can become strangulated in the auditory canal due to mass effect from swelling [30]. Herpetic viruses can also cause corneal lesions, but they are usually dendritic in appearance. Mumps and rubella may affect the ear and can rarely cause IK [7]. Viral labyrinthitis is a common cause of unilateral inner ear dysfunction, associated with vertigo, nausea, and vomiting [63].

Inflammatory

Inflammatory causes of both vestibuloauditory and ocular symptoms include PAN, granulomatosis with polyangiitis (GPA, formerly known as Wegener granulomatosis), temporal arteritis, Bechet's disease, Grave's disease, lupus, and relapsing polychondritis [7, 18]. Relapsing polychondritis is a systemic inflammatory disorder affecting cartilaginous tissues of the body, which may result in auricular collapse, ear pain, otitis media, SNHL, and vestibular dysfunction [64]. Associated ocular manifestations of relapsing polychondritis include episcleritis, scleritis, corneal infiltrates, peripheral ulcerative keratitis, iridocyclitis, and rarely, posterior segment involvement [65]. Takayasu's arteritis, like CS, affects large vessels [13]. Underlying granulomatous inflammation of the aorta in Takayasu's arteritis may lead to nonspecific constitutional symptoms, claudication of the extremities, aorta aneurysms, coronary artery ischemia, and renal artery stenosis [66]. However, unlike CS, Takaysu's arteritis rarely affects the eyes and ears [13]. Sarcoidosis characteristically affects the lungs, heart, skin, eye, and lymph nodes, but seldomly results in vestibuloauditory symptoms [26].

Vogt– Koyanagi–Harada (VLH) disease is a systemic process that targets melanin-containing tissue that can result in meningitis, decreased vision, and hearing loss [31]. However, the ocular inflammatory manifestations (iritis, choroiditis, and retinal detachments) in VKH tend to be much more severe compared to CS [19]. VKH patients also present with poliosis and vitiligo, which is not typical of CS [67].

Drugs/Toxins

Aminoglycosides, antimalarials (quinine), diuretics, salicylates, heavy metals can all cause hearing loss [7, 26]. Streptomycin can cause Ménière-like vestibular symptoms. 3-methyl-1-pentyn-3-yl-acid phthalate (Whipcide) is used for whip worm treatment, and can induce CS-like symptoms such as IK and hearing loss [2, 19]. Symptoms tend to wane after drug discontinuation [19].

Other

Symptoms of Meniere's disease include vertigo, hearing loss, tinnitus, and aural fullness [8, 10, 52]. CS can present very similarly to Ménière's disease; however, there are certain key differences. The symptoms in CS tend to be bilateral, more acute on onset, rapidly progressive, and chronic in duration [41]. Whereas in Ménière's disease, symptoms tend to be unilateral, last for only minutes to hours at a time, and result in more mild vestibuloauditory dysfunction compared to CS [8, 10, 52].

Diagnostic Approach

Laboratory Data

Laboratory data is typically not helpful in the diagnosis of CS [5]. Nonspecific markers of inflammation include leukocytosis (36–70 %), thrombocytosis (12–33 %), elevated erythrocyte sedimentation rate (ESR, 25–100 %) and C-reactive protein (CRP, 33 %), anemia (15–39 %), and abnormal liver enzymes (16 %) [2, 7, 8, 14, 55]. In the assessment of suspected CS patients, basic laboratory assessment includes a complete blood count (CBC); complete metabolic panel; urine analysis; ESR/CRP levels, and, treponemic pallidum and chlamydia titers. In cases of positive chlamydia titers, treatment should be initiated with azithromycin or doxycycline [14]. In endemic areas, Lyme disease serology should also be obtained. Surveillance of

ESR and CRP levels may be helpful in monitoring disease activity in CS patients [14, 29].

Given CS's association with other inflammatory disorders, additional testing should be performed based on clinical presentation and suspicion. Other inflammatory markers that may be elevated include antiphospholipid antibodies (APA), anti-DNA antibodies myeloperoxidase (MPO), proteinase 3 (PR3), antineutrophil cytoplasmic antibodies (ANCA), and rheumatoid factor (RF) [6, 14]. However, these non- specific antibodies are not consistently elevated in CS patients. For instance, in one series, less than 11 % of patients had positive APA, ANCA, or RF levels [8]. Several studies have reported detection of antibodies against heat shock protein 70 in CS patients, but they are not routinely obtained in clinical practice [33]. Decreased albumin, IgG, and complement levels have been reported, along with increased IgA, IgM, and haptoglobin levels in association with chronic inflammation [7, 22]. In cases complicated by meningoencephalitis, cerebrospinal fluid (CSF) may shows pleocytosis, lymphocytosis, or increased protein levels [52].

Imaging

Chest X-Ray

In one series, 40 out of 51 had normal chest X-rays, while 11 had non-diagnostic findings [8].

Neuroimaging

Acute, progressive hearing loss should be evaluated with a magnetic resonance imaging (MRI) to rule out a cerebellopontine lesion, such as an acoustic neuroma [18]. In CS, an MRI with gadolinium may show vasculitis-related white matter changes; labyrinthitis-related enhancement; and, calcification or narrowing of the cochlea, vestibular nerve, semicircular canal, and/or vestibule [13, 22, 31, 33, 68, 69].

Computer tomographic scanning may be used to detect areas of infarction, but is typically found to be normal in CS patients [22].

Other Testing

Positron emission tomography (PET) has increasingly played a larger role in the diagnosis of vasculitides, as other modalities may be unable to detect the true extent of systemic inflammation (e.g., MRI, biopsy, ultrasound) [46]. Inflammed cells increase expression of glucose transporters, and thus accumulate more 2-doxy-2-[18F]fluoro-D-glucose (F18-FDG), which is helpful in detecting areas of vasculitis [46]. PET/CT can also be used to follow the course of systemic vasculitides, and thus dictate treatment [46].

Cardiac evaluation should be done to rule out evidence of arrhythmias, aortitis, ischemic heart disease, and valvular damage [18]. Electrocardiogram (EKG) and echocardiography are indicated once the diagnosis of CS is suspected, and should be repeated routinely to monitor disease progression once cardiac damage is detected. If there is evidence of ischemia, then coronary angiography should be performed [18].

Pure tone audiometry, caloric testing, and electronystagmography should be done to evaluate vestibular function, quantify hearing loss, and to follow the disease course in CS [26, 33].

A thorough ocular evaluation at the slit lamp is essential to determine the extent of ocular involvement, and periodic follow-up by an ophthalmologist is critical for good visual prognosis.

Treatment

There are no double-blind, randomized, placebo controlled trials comparing different immunosuppression regimens in the treatment of CS. Therapy is mostly based on individual cases, case series, and the management of similar inflammatory diseases. A multidisciplinary team approach with the expertise of an ophthalmologist, an otolaryngologist, a rheumatologist, and specialists from other medical disciplines as warranted by clinical presentation, is paramount in the management of CS [18].

Medical

Corticosteroids

Most patients respond favorably to steroids and dosing should be adjusted according to clinical response. In one series, 58 % had improvement of both ophthalmic and otolaryngologic symptoms after treatment [8]. The ocular manifestations of CS, in particular, tend to be very responsive to steroid treatment, with improvements usually within one week of initiation [7]. For purely mild ocular symptoms, topical steroids can be used to control inflammation along with a cycloplegic. Adjuvant therapy with cool compresses, artificial tears, topical NSAIDS (flubiprofen), and oral NSAIDS (naproxen 200 mg BID) may be considered [70]. Subconjunctival triamcinolone may also be beneficial in the treatment of ocular inflammation.

High-dose systemic steroids are indicated in the presence of severe ocular inflammation, vestibuloauditory symptoms, and vasculitis, after ruling out infections causes [12]. Intravenous steroids are preferred for the initial treatment of vasculitis, especially during the first week of therapy [31]. Steroids should be started within 2 weeks of hearing loss to maximize the chances of recovery [2, 41]. However, even with treatment, hearing loss can be progressive and permanent, leading to deafness in half of CS patients [71]. Prolonged period without treatment can result in atrophy of inner ear structures, endolymphatic hydrops, and osteogenesis within the perilymphatic space due to chronic inflammation. Once these changes occur, they are usually permanent [13].

Prednisone is typically started at a dose of one to two mg/kg/day for 7–10 days. It is then tapered over the first 2–4 weeks if there is a good response; then, more slowly over the next 2–6 months [22]. If there is no clinical response within 2 weeks or a dose of ≤10 mg/day cannot be achieved; then, prednisone should be quickly tapered, and another immunosuppressive agent should be initiated [18]. Due to poor concentrations of steroids in the endolymph compared to plasma concentrations after systemic dosing of steroids, injections of intratympanic dexamethasone has been advocated by some if there is hearing loss [72]. The literature suggests that patients with SNHL may have a better prognosis with combination treatment (corticosteroid plus another immunosuppressant) compared to corticosteroids alone [12].

Other Immunosuppressive Therapies

Steroid-sparing agents that have been used with varying degrees of success in the treatment of CS include methotrexate (MTX, 15–25 mg/week), azathioprine (1.5–2.5 mg/kg/day), cyclophosphamide (1–3 mg/kg per day), mycophenolate mofetil (MMF, 750 mg–1 g twice a day), cyclosporin A (CsA, 1–5 mg/kg/day), tacrolimus (FK506, 0.1 mg/kg), and leflunomide (0.33 mg/kg/day) [12, 18, 33, 41, 73, 74]. Evidence of their clinical efficacy has been based mainly on single cases reports or small case series. The side effects of steroid-sparing agents can be considerable, and should be used with caution especially in the pediatric population.

In the treatment of CS, many consider methotrexate to be the steroid-sparing agent of choice [33, 41]. In a 12-month, open-label study involving patients with autoimmune hearing loss, all three CS patients saw improvement in their vestibuloauditory symptoms [75]. The addition of methotrexate to the treatment regimen may allow for reduced dosage of required prednisone. In one case, prednisone was even stopped and the patient remained in remission on methotrexate alone [22]. In the pediatric population, methotrexate is commonly used if there is a poor response to steroids or another medication is desired due to intolerable side effects [12]. Even with methotrexate, however, chronic treatment may be necessary to maintain disease remission.

Cyclophosphamide has been used in conjunction with prednisone to stabilize vasculitis, induce remission, and allow for eventual steroid taper [7, 76]. In one case, monthly pulse treatment with cyclophosphamide (700 mg) was used successfully to a patient off his chronic steroid regimen [76].

Mycophenolate mofetil (MMF) is a noncompetitive and reversible inhibitor of inosine monophosphate dehydrogenase, which is an enzyme required in the synthesis of purines; thus, targeting B and T lymphocytes which play a critical role in the pathogenesis of CS [77]. In one case of steroid-resistant pediatric CS, MMF (750 mg twice a day) was found to be effective in inducing and maintaining disease remission [11].

Tacrolimus inhibits CD-4T cell activation and proliferation, and may have fewer side effects compared to CsA [77]. Clinical improvement on only oral FK506 has been reported in treatment-resistant CS [74].

TNF-α blockers are a relatively new class of agents used in the treatment of CS. However, they have been used in the past to treat other inflammatory disorders such as RA, IBD, and resistant Takayasu's arteritis [18, 33]. TNF-α is a cytokine produced by macrophages, endothelial cells, lymphocytes, and fibroblasts during inflammation [18]. Infliximab, a chimeric monoclonal antibody, has been described as an effective therapeutic agent in improving hearing loss and maintaining remission in therapy-resistant cases [13]. In a review of ten CS patients treated with infliximab after previous failure with steroids, methotrexate, cyclophosphamide, and/or azathioprine, nine demonstrated overall improvement in ocular and vestibuloauditory symptoms [18]. Reports suggest infliximab is best used early in the disease course due to decreased efficacy in later stages [78, 79]. Tayer-Shifman et al. [18] have proposed using infliximab as first-line therapy in CS patients with severe eye inflammation, rapid hearing loss, or bilateral ear involvement.

Etanercept consists of two recombinant p75 TNF-α receptors linked to the Fc portion of human IgG1, and has been proven to be useful in the treatment of RA, AS, psoriasis, and psoriatic arthritis [77]. It has decreased efficacy, however, in the treatment of ocular inflammation [18]. In one small case series, etanercept did not stabilize hearing loss, but did result in improved word recognition [6, 13].

Rituximab is a chimeric human-mouse monoclonal antibody against CD20, a B-cell surface protein, which effectively depletes levels of circulating lymphocytes [13, 18]. It is FDA approved to use in conjunction with MTX for the treatment of RA. Additionally, it appears to be have good efficacy against ocular inflammation [18]. There is a single case report documenting clinical improvement in a CS patient with hearing loss after treatment with rituximab (500 mg for 4 weeks) [4, 57].

Of note, toclizumab, a humanized anti-IL 6 receptor antibody, was reported to improve the symptoms and quality of life of a 69-year-old CS patient with treatment-resistant disease [48]. Its role in the treatment of systemic vasculitides is still being investigated.

Surgical

Surgical intervention should not be performed until inflammation is controlled. In CS patients with significant hearing loss, cochlear implants have been enormously beneficial in rehabilitating some function with relatively low rates of complications [80, 81]. Due to cochlear ossification, gains in hearing after cochlear implantation may regress after surgery [80].

In the presence of significant lipid keratopathy due to long-standing ocular inflammation, corneal transplantation may be considered [30]. Patients who develop glaucoma secondary to CS may require trabeculectomy and long-term treatment with pressure-lowering medications [45].

Multiple aneurysms and significant valvular insufficiency resulting in heart failure, ischemic heart failure, and/or aortic rupture may require aortic stent grafting with or without valvular repair [20, 22, 50, 82, 83]. Approximately 14 % of patients with aortic regurgitation require surgical intervention [9].

Follow-Up

Systemic symptoms can occur years after initial presentation, thus regular follow-up is essential, especially in suspected pediatric cases [31]. If patients present only with vestibuloauditory symptoms, they should be carefully followed for a period of at least 2 years if there is any clinical suspicion of CS.

The aims of long-term management in CS are to screen for complications, appropriately manage immunosuppression therapy, and plan for surgical rehabilitation as indicated. Migliori et al. proposed a follow-up schedule for vestibuloauditory evaluation once the diagnosis of CS is made: monthly for the first 3 months after disease onset; then, every 3 months for the first 1–2 years; then, every 6 months during the third year; and, annually thereafter (assuming the patient is clinically stable) [52].

Prognosis

Due to increased association with systemic manifestations and other inflammatory disorders, patients with atypical CS are generally thought to have a worse prognosis compared to those with typical CS [4, 41, 49]. However, Pagnini et al. found that patients who presented with multi-organ involvement had better outcomes compared to those with single organ involvement (eyes or ears) likely due to accelerated time to presentation, proper medical evaluation, and diagnosis [12]. In one series, cardiac symptoms, abdominal complaints, weight loss, abnormal laboratory values (elevated ESR, anemia, leukocytosis, and thrombocytosis) were associated with worse clinical outcomes [7, 22]. However, delayed diagnosis and treatment is likely the strongest predictor for worse clinical outcomes in CS.

The most common cause of morbidity in CS is hearing loss, which may occur even with treatment [8, 21]. In Grasland's review, 54 % of typical CS and 37 % of atypical CS developed complete hearing loss bilaterally [22]. Vollertsen et al. reported 78 out of 156 ears progressed to deafness, (34 patients developed deafness bilaterally), with a median interval of three months after initial presentation [7]. Patients who have already suffered hearing damage at the time of treatment will likely fare worse, with decreased chance of recovering function despite aggressive immunosuppression [29].

Vision loss, on the other hand, is uncommon, and typically responds well to topical steroid treatment [8, 22]. In the largest retrospective series to date, only 8 out of 156 eyes (5.1 %) became blind [7]. In another more recent study, 82 % at their last visit had normal or near normal vision while only 10 % had permanent visual sequelae secondary to their disease [8].

CS has a mortality rate of 10 % [9, 41]. Causes of death include systemic vasculitis, cardiac complications (ruptured aortic aneurysms, myocardia infarction, cardiac failure), GI bleed, CVA, subarachnoid hemorrhage, and renal complications [7, 8, 22].

Conclusion

Cogan syndrome (CS) is a rare systemic inflammatory disease that is characterized by Ménière-like vestibuloauditory symptoms (tinnitus, vertigo, and hearing loss) and acute ocular inflammation [1, 2]. Aside from the effects on the sensory organs, the disease can manifest as a systemic vasculitis with a 10 % mortality rate. The most common treatments are high-dose corticosteroids. There are no double blinded, placebo controlled, randomized studies to assess the most effective treatments for the disease, but there are published case series/reports demonstrating efficacy with methotrexate, mycophenolate mofetil, cyclophosphamide, and more recently TNF alpha inhibitors.

References

1. Cogan DG. Syndrome of nonsyphilitic interstitial keratitis and vestibuloauditory symptoms. Arch Ophthalmol. 1945;33:144–9.
2. Haynes BF, Kaiser-Kupfer MI, Mason P, Fauci AS. Cogan syndrome: studies in thirteen patients, long-term follow-up, and a review of the literature. Medicine. 1980;59:426–41.
3. Mogan RF, Baumgartner CJ. Meniere's disease complicated by recurrent interstitial keratitis: excellent result following cervical ganglionectomy. West J Surg. 1934;42:628–31.
4. Kessel A, Vadasz Z, Toubi E. Autoimmun Rev. 2014;13:351–4.
5. Lee LY, Akhtar MM, Kirresh O, Gibson T. Interstitial keratitis and sensorineural hearing loss as a manifestation of rheumatoid arthritis: clinical lessons from a rare complication. BMJ Case Rep. 2012;2012.
6. Ghadban R, Couret M, Zenone T. Efficacy of infliximab in Cogan's syndrome. J Rheumatol. 2008;35:2456–8.

7. Vollertsen RS, McDonald TJ, Younge BR, et al. Cogan's syndrome: 18 cases and a review of the literature. Mayo Clin Proc. 1986;61:344–61.
8. Gluth MB, Baratz KH, Matteson EL, Driscoll CLW. Cogan syndrome: a retrospective review of 60 patients throughout a half century. Mayo Clin Proc. 2006;81:483–8.
9. Cundiff J, Kansal S, Kumar A, et al. Cogan's syndrome: a cause of progressive hearing deafness. Am J Otolaryngol. 2006;27:68–70.
10. Vasileiadis I, Stratoudaki R, Karakostas E. Int J Pediatr Otorhinolaryngol. 2012;76:601–5.
11. Hautefort C, Loundon N, Montchilova M, et al. Mycophenolate mofetil as a treatment of steroid dependent Cogan's syndrome in childhood. Int J Pediatr Otorhinolaryngol. 2009;73:1477–9.
12. Pagnini I, Zannin ME, Vittadello F, et al. Clinical features and outcome of Cogan syndrome. J Pediatr. 2012;160(303–307):e1.
13. Greco A, Gallo A, Fusconi M, et al. Autoimmun Rev. 2013;12:396–400.
14. Lepur D, Vranjican Z, Himbele J, et al. *Chlamydia pneumoniae* infection as a trigger for a Cogan's syndrome. J Infect. 2006;52:223–6.
15. Sugimoto K, Miyazawa T, Nishi H, et al. Childhood Cogan syndrome with aortitis and anti-neutrophil cytoplasmic antibody-associated glomerulonephritis. Pediatr Rheumatol. 2014;12:1–5.
16. Nolte KW, Hans VJ, Schattenfroh C, et al. Perineurial cells filled with collagen in "atypical" Cogan's syndrome. Acta Neuropathol. 2007;115:589–96.
17. Darougar S, John AC, Viswalingam M, et al. Isolation of *Chlamydia psittaci* from a patient with interstitial keratitis and uveitis associated with otological and cardiovascular lesions. Br J Ophthalmol. 1978;62:709–14.
18. Tayer-Shifman OE, Ilan O, Tovi H, Tal Y. Cogan's syndrome—clinical guidelines and novel therapeutic approaches. Clin Rev Allerg Immunol. 2014.
19. McCallum RM, Haynes BF. Ocular infection and immunity. In: Pepose JS, Holland GN, editors. Mosby year book. St. Louis, MO; 1996. p. 446–59.
20. Bisdas TE, Teebken OE, Wilhelmi M, et al. Surgical treatment of a thoracoabdominal aneurysm in Cogan's syndrome. ATS. 2009;88:1668–70.
21. Lunardi C, Bason C, Leandri M, et al. Autoantibodies to inner ear and endothelial antigens in Cogan's syndrome. Lancet. 2002;360:915–21.
22. Grasland A. Typical and atypical Cogan's syndrome: 32 cases and review of the literature. Rheumatology. 2004;43:1007–15.
23. Georgakopoulos CD, Makri OE, Exarchou AM, Pharmakakis N. Atypical Cogan's syndrome presenting as bilateral endogenous endophthalmitis. Clin Exp Optom. 2012;97:87–9.
24. Deliveliotou A, Moustakarias T, Argeitis J, et al. Successful full-term pregnancy in a woman with Cogan's syndrome: a case report. Clin Rheumatol. 2007;26:2181–3.
25. Currie C, Wax JR, Pinette MG, et al. Cogan's syndrome complicating pregnancy. J Matern Fetal Neonatal Med. 2014;22:928–30.
26. Singh P, Gupta M, Lehl SS, Singh K. Cogan's syndrome: achievement of complete resolution of auditory deficit with steroids. BMJ Case Rep. 2013;2013.
27. Best C, Thömke F, Hitzler W, Dieterich M. Immunol Lett. 2013;150:87–8.
28. Branislava I, Marijana T, Nemanja D, et al. Atypical Cogan's syndrome associated with coronary disease. Chin Med J Beijing. 2011;124:3192.
29. Pysden KS, Long V, Ferrie CD. Leeds teaching hospitals NHS trust. Cogan's syndrome: a rare cause of meningoencephalitis. J Child Neurol. 2009;24:753–7.
30. Tomita M, Chiba A, Inoue N, et al. Cogan syndrome presenting after uneventful laser in situ keratomileusis. J Cataract Refract Surg. 2013;39:1260–6.
31. Ndiaye IC, Rassi SJ, Wiener-Vacher SR. Cochleovestibular impairment in pediatric Cogan's syndrome. Pediatrics. 2002;109:E38.
32. Fricker M, Baumann A, Wermelinger F, et al. A novel therapeutic option in Cogan diseases? TNF-α blockers. Rheumatol Int. 2006;27:493–5.
33. Murphy G, Sullivan MO, Shanahan F, et al. Cogan's syndrome: present and future directions. Rheumatol Int. 2009;29:1117–21.
34. Podder S, Shepherd RC. Cogan's syndrome: a rare systemic vasculitis. Arch Dis Child. 1994;71:163–4.
35. Semeraro FF, Russo AA, Duse SS, et al. Retinal angiomatosis and cystoid macular oedema in Cogan's syndrome. Optom Vis Sci. 2011;88:E1262–6.
36. Martinez-Osorio H, Fuentes-Paez G, Calonge M. Severe keratopathy in paediatric Cogan's syndrome. Rheumatology. 2006;45:1576–7.
37. Zamir E, Pe'er J, Solomon A. Cogan syndrome with disfiguring lipid keratopathy. Arch Ophthalmol. 2004;122:1242–3.
38. Kondo Y, Ito S, Ohi Y, et al. Atypical Cogan's Syndrome with Aortitis. Intern Med. 2009;48:1093–7.
39. Albayram MS, Wityk R, Yousem DM, Zinreich SJ. The cerebral angiographic findings in Cogan syndrome. AJNR Am J Neuroradiol. 2001;22:751–4.
40. Yaginuma A, Sakai T, Kohno H, et al. A case of atypical Cogan's syndrome with posterior scleritis and uveitis. Jpn J Ophthalmol. 2009;53:659–61.
41. Baumann A, Helbling A, Oertle S, et al. Cogan's syndrome: clinical evolution of deafness and vertigo in three patients. Eur Arch Otorhinolaryngol. 2004;262:45–9.
42. Scharl M, Frei P, Fried M, et al. Association between Cogan's syndrome and inflammatory bowel disease: a case series. J Crohn's Colitis. 2011;5:64–8.
43. Antonios N, Silliman S. Cogan syndrome. Neurologist. 2012;18:55–63.
44. Udayaraj UP, Hand MF, Shilliday IR, Smith WG. Renal involvement in Cogan's syndrome. Nephrol Dial Transplant. 2004;19:2420–1.

45. Chen SI, Sahni J, Hart IK. Atypical Cogan's syndrome presenting with bilateral acute glaucoma. Eye (London, England). 2004;18:328–29.
46. Balink H, Bruyn GAW. The role of PET/CT in Cogan's syndrome. Clin Rheumatol. 2007;26: 2177–9.
47. Brogan K, Eleftheriou D, Rajput K, et al. Tubulointerstitial nephritis, uveitis, hearing loss and vestibular failure: TINU-atypical Cogan's overlap syndrome. Rheumatology. 2012;51:950–2.
48. Shibuya M, Fujio K, Morita K, et al. Successful treatment with tocilizumab in a case of Cogan's syndrome complicated with aortitis. Mod Rheumatol. 2012;23:577–81.
49. Azami A, Maleki N, Kalantar Hormozi M, Tavosi Z. Case report. Case Rep Med. 2014:1–4. Available at: http://www-ncbi-nlm-nih-gov.ezproxy.hsc.usf.edu/pmc/articles/PMC3970326/pdf/CRIM2014-830831.pdf.
50. Erb N, Sinha A, Slaney PL, Rowe IF. Acute atrioventricular node block requiring cardiac pacing in Cogan's syndrome. Rheumatology. 2003;42:1126–8.
51. Parra-García GD, Callejas-Rubio JL, Ríos-Fernández R, et al. Otolaryngologic manifestations of systemic vasculitis. Acta Otorrinolaringol (English Edition). 2012;63:303–10.
52. Migliori G, Battisti E, Pari M, et al. A shifty diagnosis: Cogan's syndrome. A case report and review of the literature. Acta Otorhinolaryngol Ital. 2009;29:108–13.
53. Kanatani M, Nakamura R, Kurokawa K, et al. Hypopituitarism associated with Cogan's syndrome; high-dose glucocorticoid therapy reverses pituitary swelling. Jpn J Med. 1991;30:164–9.
54. Van Doornum S, McColl G, Walter M, et al. Prolonged prodrome, systemic vasculitis, and deafness in Cogan's syndrome. Ann Rheum Dis. 2001;60:69–71.
55. Boulinguez S, Bernard P, Bedane C, et al. Pyoderma gangrenosum complicating Cogan's syndrome. Clin Exp Dermatol. 1998;23:286–9.
56. Lydon EJ, Barisoni L, Belmont HM. Cogan's syndrome and development of ANCA-associated renal vasculitis after lengthy disease remission. Clin Exp Rheumatol. 2009;27:S144–S144.
57. Orsoni JG, Zavota L, Vincenti V, et al. Cogan syndrome in children: early diagnosis and treatment is critical to prognosis. Am J Ophthalmol. 2004;137:757–8.
58. Pellistri I, Mora P, Ponzin D, et al. Cogan syndrome: confocal microscopy assessment of corneal damage. Eur J Ophthalmol. 2010;20:504–8.
59. Dua HS, Azuara-Blanco A. Corneal allograft rejection: risk factors, diagnosis, prevention, and treatment. Indian J Ophthalmol. 1999;47:3–9.
60. Son HJ, Ulualp SO. Course of auditory impairment in Cogan's syndrome. Am J Otolaryngol Head Neck Med Surg. 2009;30:65–8.
61. Gasparovic H, Djuric Z, Bosnic D, et al. Aortic root vasculitis associated with Cogan's syndrome. ATS. 2011;92:340–1.
62. Stanek G, Strle F. Lyme borreliosis. Lancet. 2003;362:1639–47.
63. Beyea JA, Agrawal SK, Parnes LS. Recent advances in viral inner ear disorders. Curr Opin Otolaryngol Head Neck Surg. 2012;20:404–8.
64. Sharma A, Gnanapandithan K, Sharma K, Sharma S. Relapsing polychondritis: a review. Clin Rheumatol. 2013;32:1575–83.
65. Yoo JH, Chodosh J, Dana R. Relapsing polychondritis: systemic and ocular manifestations, differential diagnosis, management, and prognosis. Semin Ophthalmol. 2011;26:261–9.
66. Keser G, Direskeneli H, Aksu K. Management of Takayasu arteritis: a systematic review. Rheumatology. 2014;53:793–801.
67. Sakata VM, da Silva FT, Hirata CE, et al. Autoimmun Rev. 2014;13:550–5.
68. Weyn T, Haine S, Conraads V. Cogan's syndrome with left main coronary artery occlusion. Cardiol J. 2009;16:573–6.
69. Fugate JE, Smith JH, Claassen DO. Bilateral cochlear enhancement in Cogan syndrome. Neurology. 2009;73:75.
70. Akpek EK, Uy HS, Christen W, et al. Severity of episcleritis and systemic disease association. Ophthalmology. 1999;106:729–31.
71. Inoue Y, Tomemori T, Suzuki S, et al. Low-dose oral methotrexate for the management of childhood Cogan's syndrome: a case report. Clin Rheumatol. 2007;26:2201–3.
72. Ying Y-LM, Hirsch BE. Atypical Cogan's syndrome: a case report. Am J Otolaryngol Head Neck Med Surg 2010;31:279–82.
73. Xie L, Cai Y, Bao X, Cao L. Leflunomide for the successful management of juvenile Cogan's syndrome. Clin Rheumatol. 2009;28:1453–5.
74. Roat MI, Thoft RA, Thomson AW, et al. Treatment of Cogan's syndrome with FK 506: a case report. Transpl Proc. 1991;23:3347.
75. Matteson EL, Fabry DA, Facer GW, et al. Open trial of methotrexate as treatment for autoimmune hearing loss. Arthritis Rheum. 2001;45:146–50.
76. Watanabe K, Nishimaki T, Yoshida M, et al. Atypical Cogan's syndrome successfully treated with corticosteroids and pulse cyclophosphamide therapy. Fukushima J Med Sci. 2000;46:49–54.
77. Nussenblatt RB, Whitcup SM. Uveitis. Elsevier Health Sciences; 2010.
78. Touma Z, Nawwar R, Hadi U, et al. The use of TNF-α blockers in Cogan's syndrome. Rheumatol Int. 2007;27:995–6.
79. Beccastrini E, Emmi G, Squatrito D, et al. Infliximab and Cogan's syndrome. Clin Otolaryngol. 2010;35:441–2.

80. Bovo R, Ciorba A, Trevisi P, et al. Cochlear implant in Cogan syndrome. Acta Otolaryngol. 2011;131:494–7.
81. Kontorinis G, Giourgas A, Neuburger J, et al. Long-term evaluation of Cochlear implantation in Cogan syndrome. ORL. 2010;72:275–9.
82. Su JW, Low AHL, Tay KH, et al. Recurrent aortic aneurysms following thoracic aortic stent-graft repair in a patient with Cogan syndrome. J Endovasc Surg. 2006;13:779–82.
83. Kim JS, Park JB, Joo JC, et al. A case of Cogan's syndrome with angina. Korean Circ J. 2010;40:680.

22 Fuchs Heterochromic Iridocyclitis

Parvathy Pillai

Introduction

Fuchs heterochromic iridocyclitis (FHI) is a low-grade, chronic uveitis. While it bears the name of Dr. Ernest Fuchs, he was not the first to describe this syndrome. In 1843, Lawrence published "A treatise on Disease of the Eye," in which he described an association between iris heterochromia and cataract development [2]. Almost 50 years later, in 1906, Fuchs published a case series of 38 patients, with heterochromia and iridocyclitis [3]. He further observed that most patients with this disorder presented with cataracts.

Epidemiology

Patients with FHI can range from age 20 to 60 years with no clear sex predilection. The mean age of presentation is 40. The incidence fluctuates between 2 and 7 %, but is thought to be frequently under reported due to its asymptomatic nature [4].

Etiology

FHI has an unclear etiology with suggestion of an infectious etiology. In Fuchs' original case series, he reported peripheral necrotizing chorioretinal scars in some, but not all, patients with this disorder. Since that time, there have been reports of an association between FHI and both *Toxoplasma gondii* and *Toxocara canis* [5, 6]. Schwab et al. conducted a review of 25 patients with FHI compared to 590 normal control patients. They found over 50 % of the FHI patients ($n = 13$) had chorioretinal scars, compared to only 4 % ($n = 24$) of the control population [7]. Most studies however report the prevalence of peripheral chorioretinal scars and FHI to be closer to 10 % [8, 9]. Mild cases of toxoplasmosis (especially if involving the far periphery of the retina) may mimic FHI by causing fine KP and anterior uveitis with minimal vitritis.

Recently, there has been investigation into an association between FHI and the rubella virus. Antibody to the rubella virus has been isolated from aqueous humor of patients with FHI [10, 11]. There may also be some evidence that the prevalence of FHI in the United States has decreased since the introduction of the rubella vaccination program in 1969 [12].

A theory that FHI is due to a neurogenic factor that causes iris hypopigmentation by

P. Pillai (✉)
Sinai Hospital of Baltimore, The Krieger Eye Institute, 2401 West Belvedere Avenue, Baltimore, MD 21215, USA
e-mail: ppillai18@gmail.com

G.N. Papaliodis (ed.), *Uveitis*,
DOI 10.1007/978-3-319-09126-6_22

reduced innervation, similar to the sympathetic denervation in congenital Horner syndrome, has been proposed but remains unsubstantiated.

Clinical Presentation

FHI is most often classified as a chronic anterior uveitis. Anterior segment manifestations such as low-grade iritis and iris heterochromia are considered as its most prominent features. The classic presentation is a patient with small, white keratic precipitates evenly distributed over the endothelium of a relatively uninflamed/white eye with mild anterior chamber cell. However, the disease can also affect multiple regions of the eye, such as the vitreous or even the optic nerve. Typical patients are young with vague visual complaints and no classic symptoms of anterior chamber inflammation, such as eye pain or redness [13]. They may complain of decreased vision due to cataract formation or floaters due to vitreous opacities.

On slit lamp exam, mild anterior chamber inflammation with minimal flare is typically found in the presence of a white eye with no ciliary injection. Microscopic studies have confirmed the presence of inflammatory cells in the iris stroma, anterior chamber, ciliary body, and sometimes even the trabecular meshwork [14]. The inflammation is persistent; although the degree can fluctuate over time, and is not responsive to topical corticosteroid therapy. Despite the chronic inflammation, posterior synechiae do not typically form. Another key feature is the presence of fine, nonpigmented stellate keratic precipitates that are diffusely distributed across the cornea. Stellate KP can also be seen in uveitis due to toxoplasmosis, herpes virus, and cytomegalovirus.

Historically, iris heterochromia was thought to be the key feature, although it is not required for the diagnosis. Heterochromia, seen in 75–90 % of patients, is due to gradual loss of anterior iris pigmentation. This loss causes an affected brown eye to appear lighter brown, while an affected blue eye appears darker due to exposure of the posterior pigment epithelium (see Fig. 22.1).

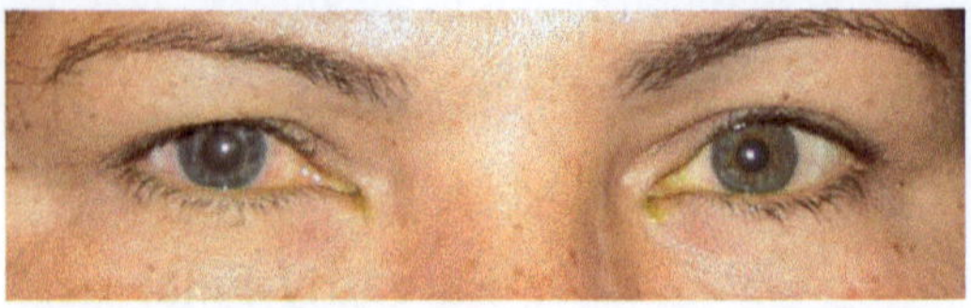

Fig. 22.1 Iris heterochromia (borrowed with permission from Dr. Teresa Chen, Glaucoma Service, Massachusetts Eye and Ear Infirmary)

Heterochromia can be difficult to observe in dark colored irides and up to 10–15 % of patients can have bilateral disease, and therefore no obvious heterochromia [15, 16]. More frequently, the careful observer can appreciate subtle diffuse iris atrophy. Blurring of the iris stroma due to pigment epithelial layer atrophy can be seen on slit lamp examination with loss of detail of the iris surface [17, 18]. The iris surface becomes smoother due to loss of rugae and crypts. The pupillary pigmentary ruff can also take on a "moth-eaten" appearance.

Posterior subcapsular cataracts are frequently seen in FHI, and the diagnosis should be suspected in a young patient with a unilateral cataract in the absence of trauma or steroid use. Vision loss from cataracts is often the chief complaint.

The posterior segment of the eye is largely unaffected, although low-grade vitritis and vitreous opacities can often be observed. In some cases, the degree of vitreous cell can be greater than what is observed in the anterior chamber. The vitreous cell may even coalesce into vitreous "snowballs." Despite posterior chamber inflammation, cystoid macular edema is rarely reported, except following cataract surgery. The occurrence of chorioretinal scars similar to those seen in ocular toxoplasmosis has been described in several case reports. These scars are typically small and peripheral, with no impact on visual acuity. Disc involvement is considered to be a rare complication. Recent studies using fluorescein angiography in FHI patients, however, demonstrated disc hyperfluorescence from 22 to 97 % of cases [19, 20].

In 1946, Amsler and colleagues reported an additional feature of FHI heterochromic iridocyclitis. During routine cataract surgery, they noted a small hemorrhage occurring during paracentesis creation [21]. Now known as the Amsler sign, this hemorrhage can lead to a hyphema. This bleeding has also been reported after minor trauma, gonioscopy, peribulbar anesthesia, and sometimes spontaneously [16]. Gonioscopy of FHI patients often reveals delicate, abnormal vessels bridging the anterior chamber angle. However, up to 1/3 of normal eyes can have similar vessels without an increased risk of bleeding [22]. Prominent blood vessels can be observed in the iris and are thought to be due to iris atrophy causing the vessels to appear more prominent.

Diagnosis

Currently there are no accepted diagnostic criteria or laboratory studies for FHI. Diagnosis is made through clinical history and physical examination. The classic triad of iridocyclitis, heterochromia, and cataract does not take into account the myriad of other findings that can be observed. Also, the differential diagnosis of iris heterochromia includes a variety of diseases from malignant melanoma to congenital Horner's syndrome (see Table 22.1). As mentioned previously, heterochromia can often be subtle, particularly in dark irides. Therefore, it is more useful to look for subtle changes on the iris surface. The absence of heterochromia and the presence of vitreous opacities can often lead to misdiagnosis. Studies have found that in more than 70 % of cases of misdiagnosed FHI, posterior uveitis was the initial diagnosis [23]. Vitreous involvement often leads the clinician away from a diagnosis of FHI. Cataract development typically occurs later in FHI, which limits its use diagnostically.

Low-grade iridocyclitis, diffuse small KP and vitreous opacities with a lack of posterior synechie or cystoid macular edema may be more useful diagnostic criteria than the classic triad. As FHI typically has a fairly benign course, making the correct diagnosis early can save a patient from unnecessary treatments.

Table 22.1 Differential of iris heterochromia

Malignant Melanoma of the iris
Congenital Horner's syndrome
Chronic anterior uveitis with iris atrophy
Prostaglandin use
Herpes simplex/zoster uveitis
Waardernburg's syndrome
Ocular melanosis
Possner-Schlossman syndrome
Neovascular glaucoma

Complications

Cataract formation is the primary cause of vision loss in patients with FHI. Incidence of cataracts range from 15 to 80 % in FHI and are often correlated to chronicity of disease. Cataracts are typically posterior subcapsular, as seen with other types of uveitis due to chronic inflammation and topical steroid use. Surgery itself is no more technically difficult than other routine cataract surgery, and postoperative complications are less frequent than with other types of uveitis. Surgical complications include hyphema, vitreous hemorrhage, vitreous opacification, and cystoid macular edema. Rates of postoperative CSME are less than with other types of uveitis but more than with age-related cataracts [24]. Rarely, posterior synechiae can form after surgery. Pars plana vitrectomy can be considered to treat visual significant vitreous opacification following cataract extraction.

The incidence of secondary glaucoma is also significantly higher in FHI patients; reported prevalence ranges from 10 to 59 % [25]. The etiology of glaucoma is unknown but is thought to be multifactorial in origin. Degenerative changes of the trabecular meshwork are the most common cause of secondary glaucoma. IOP elevation is often isolated and intermittent early in the disease course developing over time into true glaucoma. Initially, the IOP elevation can be managed medically, but filtering surgery is often needed. Due to a high incidence of bleb failure in trabeculectomy, glaucoma drainage implant devices are usually the preferred surgical option [26].

Treatment

FHI typically follows a benign course that does not warrant treatment. Common complications associated with uveitis, such as CME and posterior synechiae typically do not occur. Corticosteroids and other immunosuppressive medications have not been found to cure FHI or to improve visual outcomes. Short durations of topical corticosteroids can be helpful with IOP spikes or in the rare case of a patient who is experiencing symptoms due to increase in anterior chamber reaction. Long-term topical corticosteroid therapy can hasten cataract development and induce glaucoma in certain subsets of patients. Glaucoma is the most significant source of vision loss in these patients, and must be carefully managed. Most patients will fail medical treatment and require a glaucoma drainage implant. Cataracts can be safely removed in these patients with very good visual outcomes [27].

Conclusion

Fuchs heterochromic iridocyclitis (FHI) is type of low-grade chronic uveitis that makes up between 2 and 7 % of all cases of uveitis [1]. The majority of cases are unilateral and present with characteristic low-grade, asymptomatic iridocyclitis, iris heterochromia, and diffuse stellate keratic percipitates. While the etiology is unknown, there are several hypotheses linking the disorder to an infectious etiology, such as rubella or toxoplasmosis. Patients typically do not require treatment for their uveitis. The main source of vision loss is from cataracts and secondary glaucoma.

References

1. Wakefield D, Chang JH. Epidemiology of uveitis. Int Ophthalmol Clin. 2005;45(2):1–13.
2. Lawrence W. Changes in colour in the iris. In: Hays I, editor. A treatise on diseases of the eye. Philadelphia: Lea & Blanchard; 1843. p. 411–6.
3. Fuchs E. Über Komplicaationen der Heterochromie. Z Augenheilkd. 1906;15:191–212.
4. Gritz DC, Wong IG. Incidence and prevalence of Uveitis in Northern California, the Northern California epidemiology of Uveitis study. Ophthalmology. 2004;111:491–500.
5. Toledo de Abreu M, Belfort RJ, Hirata P. Fuchs' heterochromic cyclitis and ocular toxoplasmosis. Am J Ophthamol 1982;93:739–44.
6. Teyssot N, Cassoux N, Lehoang P, et al. Fuchs heterochromia and ocular toxocariasis. Am J Ophthalmol. 2005;139(5):915–6.
7. Schwab I. The epidemiologic association of Fuch's heterochromic iridocyclitis and ocular toxoplasmosis. Am J Ophthalmol. 1991;1:356–62.
8. La Hey E, et al. Fuch's heterochromic iridocyclitis is not associated with ocular toxoplasmosis. Arch Ophthalmol. 1992;110:806–11.
9. Saraux H, Laroche L, Le Hoang P. Secondary Fuch's heterochromic cyclitis: a new approach to an old disease. Ophthalmologica. 1985;190:193–8.
10. De Groot-Mijnes JD, de Visser L, Rothova A, et al. Rubella virus is associated with Fuchs' heterochromic iridocyclitis. Am J Ophthalmol. 2006;141:212–4.
11. Quentin CD, Reiber H. Fuchs' heterochromic cyclitis: rubella virus antibodies and genome in aqueous humor. Am J Ophthalmol. 2004;138:46–54.
12. Birnbaum AD, Tessler HH, Schultz KL, et al. Epidemiologic relationship between Fuchs' heterochromic iridocyclitis and the United States rubella vaccination program. Am J Ophthalmol. 2007;144 (3):424–8.
13. Norrsell K, Sjodell L. Fuchs' heterochromic uveitis: a longitudinal clinical study. Acta Ophthalmol. 2008;86(1):58–64.
14. Goldberg ME, Erozan YS, Duke JR, et al. Cytopathologic and histopathologic aspects of Fuchs' heterochromic iridocyclitis. Arch Ophthalmol. 1965;74:604–9.
15. Kimura SJ, Hogan MJ, Thygeson P. Fuchs' syndrome of heterochromic cyclitis. Arch Ophthalmol. 1955;54:179–86.
16. Kimura SJ. Fuchs' syndrome of heterochromic cyclitis in brown-eyes patients. Trans Am Ophthalmol Soc UK. 1978;76:76–89.
17. Liesegang TJ. Clinical features and prognosis in Fuchs' uveitis syndrome. Arch Ophthalmol. 1982;100:1622–6.

18. Jones NP. Fuchs' heterochromic uveitis: an update. Surv Ophthalmol. 1993;37:253–72.
19. Azis S, Arya B, Westcott M, Pavesio C. An investigation of the disc hyperfluourescence in Fuchs uveitis syndrome using optical coherence tomography imaging. Ocul Immunol Inflamm 2014; Epub.
20. Bouchenaki N, Herbort CP. Fluorescein angiographic findings and clinical features in Fuchs' uveitis. Int Ophthalmol. 2010;30(5):511–9.
21. Amsler M. New clinical aspects of the vegetative eye. Trans Ophthalmol Soc UK. 1948;68:45–74.
22. Henkind P. Angle vessels in normal eyes: a gonioscopic evaluation and anatomic correlation. Br J Ophthalmol. 1964;48:551–7.
23. Bouchenaki N, Herbort CP. Fuchs' uveitis: failure to associate vitritis and disc hyperfluorescence with disease is the major factor for misdiagnosis and diagnostic delay. Middle East Afr J Ophthalmol. 2009;16(4):239–44.
24. Smith RE, O'Connor R. Cataract extraction in Fuchs' syndrome. Arch Ophthalmol. 1974;91(39):41.
25. La Hey E, de Vries J, Langerhorst CT, et al. Treatment and prognosis of secondary glaucoma in Fuchs' heterochromic iridocyclitis. Am J Ophthalmol. 1993;116:327–40.
26. Da Mata A, Burk SE, Netland PA, et al. Management of uveitic glaucoma with Ahmed glaucoma valve implantation. Ophthalmology. 1999;106(11):2168–72.
27. Ram J, Kaushik S, Brar GS, et al. Phacoemulsification in patients with Fuchs' heterochromic uveitis. J Cataract Refract Surg. 2002;28:1372–878.

HLA-B27

23

Erik Letko

Introduction

The HLA-B27 gene is likely the most studied gene in the history of medicine. The oldest evidence of association between this gene and a systemic condition comes from the Middle Ages. In a recent report, a medieval skeleton with signs consistent with ankylosisng spondylitis (AS) was found to carry HLA-B27 gene [1]. A strong association of HLA-B27 with AS and other arthropathies was established in multiple epidemiologic studies in the 1960s and 1970s (Table 23.1). More recently, a number of other conditions including autoimmune and infectious diseases were linked to HLA-B27. Furthermore, identification of HLA-B27 subtypes helped understand pathogenic and in some cases protective role of the gene (Table 23.2). The mechanism of action of HLA-B27 in disease remains unknown. However, several pathogenic mechanisms have been proposed (Table 23.3; Fig. 23.1).

E. Letko (✉)
Deparment of Ophthalmology, Colorado Permanente Medical Group, 855 S Columbine St., Denver CO 80209, USA
e-mail: letkoerik@gmail.com

G.N. Papaliodis (ed.), *Uveitis*,
DOI 10.1007/978-3-319-09126-6_23

Epidemiology

The prevalence of HLA-B27 gene varies geographically by race and by ethnicity. The prevalence of the gene is relatively low around the equator and rises with increase in latitude. It varies from as high as 50 % in Haida Indians in the Pacific Northwest of the United States to 25 % in Eskimos, 20 % in Sardinians, 8 % in UK population, and 3 % in Southern Italy to as low as 0 % in Australian Aborigines [2]. In a 2009 study in the US, HLA-B27 was found in 7.5 % of non-Hispanic whites and 3.5 % among all other US races/ethnicities combined [3].

Acute anterior uveitis (AAU), the most common ocular condition associated with HLA-B27 gene, develops in 1 % of the gene carriers. Up to 55 % of all AAU cases are reported to carry HLA-B27 [4–6]. The association between AAU and HLA-B27 increases to 70 % in recurrent cases. Up to 30 % of patients with AS or reactive arthritis will experience at least one episode of AAU during their lifetime. Interestingly, AAU is more likely to be bilateral in females (31 % cases) compared to males (13 %). Acute episode of HLA-B27 associated uveitis is the most common cause of non-infectious hypopyon in Western countries, reported in as many as 31 % of cases with AAU.

A haplotype of HLA-B27 seems to play a significant role in the pathogenic mechanisms

Table 23.1 Musculoskeletal disease and HLA-B27

Ankylosing spondylitis
Reactive arthritis
Psoriatic arthropathy
Enteropathic arthropathy
Juvenile spondarthritis
Undifferentiated spondarthritis
Isolated peripheral enthesitis

and likelihood of disease development. Individuals with haplotype HLA-B2705 in Caucasians and American Indian descent have been found to be at higher risk for AAU [7, 8]. Other commonly associated haplotypes with AAU include HLA-B2704 in Asians and HLA-B2702 in Mediterranean populations. Conversely, haplotypes HLA-B2707 found in Cypriots and HLA-B2708 in Mestizos were found to be protective against AS and other diseases.

Clinical Presentation

Typical clinical symptoms of an acute episode of HLA-B27 associated anterior uveitis includes sudden onset of unilateral eye redness, pain, photophobia, and decreased vision. An external eye exam typically reveals conjunctival injection with or without ciliary flush that in more severe cases may be accompanied by scleritis. The slit lamp examination typically reveals non-granulomatous keratic precipitates, anterior chamber cells and flare and in some cases the presence of fibrin and/or hypopyon in the anterior chamber. Posterior synechiae and pigment on the corneal endothelium and anterior capsule might be present in cases with delayed onset of treatment of acute uveitis or in those with recurrent episodes.

The age at the time of a first episode of acute HLA-B27 associated anterior uveitis can vary greatly. According to one report that examined a cohort of 148 patients, the median age at onset of uveitis was 32 years and 5 % of these individuals were older than 55 years [9]. Although most patients will present with acute inflammation in one eye, bilateral simultaneous acute episodes were noted in 7 % of patients [10].

It is important to acknowledge the fact that approximately two thirds of patients with acute HLA-B27 uveitis will have an associated systemic disease and that half of these patients' systemic condition is diagnosed because of the ocular presentation [10]. It is also noteworthy that about a third of individuals have a family history of spondylarthropathy [10]. Taking a detailed clinical history and review of systems in every patient with AAU is essential since up to 60 % may have systemic involvement affecting one or more organ

Table 23.2 Extra-articular disease and HLA-B27

	Definite or probable association	Possible association
Ocular	• *Acute anterior uveitis (AAU)*	• *HSV recurrence after corneal graft*
Aural	• *Scieritis (anterior and posterior)*	• Sensorineural hearing loss
Pulmonary	• Upper lobe fibrosis	• Asbestosis, pleurisy, pleural abscess, bronchitis, pneumonia, pneumothorax, sarcoidosis
Cardiovascular	• Aortic regurgitation	
	• Cardiac conduction abnormalities	• Myelodysplastic syndrome
	• Aortitis, aortic aneurism, aortic dissection	• Agranulocytosis
Haematological	• Acute leukemia	• Childhood nephritic syndrome
Renal	• IgA nephropathy	• Autoimmune thyroiditis
Endocrine	• Inflammatory bowel disease	• Cushing's disease
Gastrointestinal	• Ulcerative colitis	• Osteoporosis
Bone	• Type II psoriasis	• Vitiligo
Skin	• Palmoplantar pustulosis	• Increased susceptibility to
Immune system	• Attenuation of viral infections	– Malaria
	– HIV, HCV, influenza, EBV, HSV-2	– Tuberculosis

Modified from: Rheumatology, 2010;49:621–631

systems. A referral to and collaboration with the appropriate specialist might be required to diagnose and treat the systemic condition.

Table 23.3 Proposed pathogenic mechanisms of action of HLA-B27

1. Thymic selection – Selection of arthritogenic T cells
2. Arthritogenic peptide – Cytotoxic T cell response to a peptide in joint
3. Antigen cross reactivity – HLA class II restricted T cells stimulated by bacteria may cross react with HLA-B27 derived peptide presented by host cells
4. Unique biological properties – May predispose to disease development
5. Altered self – Unpaired cysteine residue at position 67
6. Interaction with microbial superantigens – Although not usual for HLA class I antigens
7. Molecular mimicry (antibody cross reactivity) – Cross-reactive antibody response between portion of HLA-B27 and bacterial epitope
8. Receptor hypothesis – Bacteria use HLA-B27 to enter the cell
9. HLA-B27 misfolding – Leads to pro-inflammatory cytokine production

Treatment and Management

The main treatment for an acute episode of HLA-B27 associate uveitis consists of frequent application of topical corticosteroid drops. Dilating drops are used to prevent posterior synechiae formation and reduce photophobia. Most patients respond favorably to this regimen and their uveitis resolves within 4–6 weeks while the corticosteroids are gradually tapered.

Individuals with more severe inflammation (e.g., hypopyon, severe fibrinous anterior chamber reaction, significant vitreous involvement, macular edema) or a prolonged episode of uveitis may require additional corticosteroids delivered systemically (oral or intravenous) and/or locally (periocular injection).

Patients who continue to have frequent episodes of anterior uveitis may benefit from steroid sparing immunomodulatory therapy in order to prevent visual complications which typically result from active inflammation and steroid induced side effects such as cataracts and glaucoma [11]. Oral non-steroidal anti-inflammatory drugs (NSAIDs) may reduce the frequency of the attacks and can be considered as first line of

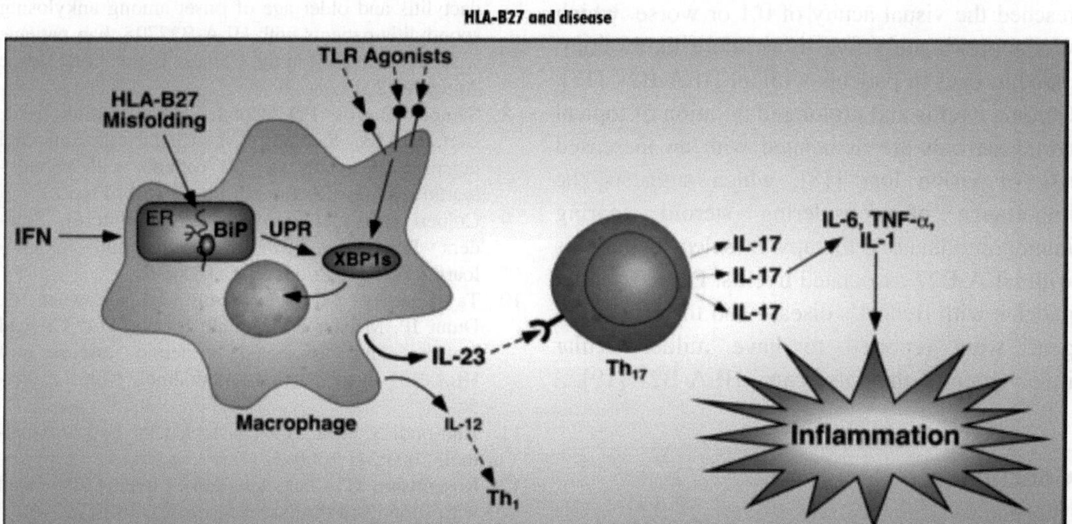

From: Prion, 2009; 3(1):15-26. Legend: IFN – interferon, ER- endoplasmic reticulum, BiP – chaperone BiP, UPR – unfolded protein response, XBP1s – X-box binding protein 1, TLR – Toll like receptor, IL – interleukin, Th – T cell helper, TNF – tumor necrosis factor.

Fig. 23.1 Mechanism of action mediated by HLA-B27 misfolding. From Prion [1: 15–26]

steroid sparing therapy [12, 13]. Immunosuppressive agents such as methotrexate, azathioprine or mycophenolate mofetil or biologics agents such as TNF-α antagonists should be considered as second line treatment options in those who fail systemic NSAIDs or have a contraindication [14].

Complications

Ocular complications can include the development of cataract, posterior synechiae, increased intraocular pressure, and cystoid macular edema [15]. Approximately 13 % of patients were reported to develop CME; vitreous cells represent an increased risk for CME development [16].

Prognosis

The long-term prognosis for vision in patients with HLA-B27 associated uveitis is generally favorable. In one case series, none of the patients had bilateral visual acuity of less than 0.5 develop after follow-up of 10 years [15]. However, according to another report 11 % of eyes with HLA-B27 associated anterior uveitis reached the visual acuity of 0.1 or worse, which was approximately five times more likely compared to eyes in patients without HLA-B27 [17]. Chronic uveitis and prolonged duration of topical corticosteroids are associated with an increased risk of vision loss [18], which suggests the importance of considering steroid sparing immunomodulatory therapy in selected patients with HLA-B27 associated uveitis. Paradoxically, patients with Behcet's disease and the HLA-B51 gene were reported to have milder ocular involvement if they also carry HLA-B27 [19].

Conclusion

HLA-B27 is a common gene found in 7.5 % of non-Hispanic Caucasians in the United States. The mechanism of action of the gene and ability to incite inflammation remain unknown. The most common ocular manifestation of HLA-B27 is AAU. The initial treatment of choice is aggressive topical steroids. For those with chronic inflammation, frequently recurring inflammation or an inability to taper off topical steroids, steroid sparing immunomodulatory therapy should be considered.

References

1. Haak W, Gruber P, Rühli FJ, et al. Molecular evidence of HLA-B27 in a historical case of ankylosing spondylitis. Arthritis Rheum. 2005;52:3318–9.
2. Khan AK. A worldwide overview: the epidemiology of HLA-B27 and associated spondyloarthritides. In: Calin A, Taurog JD, editors. The spondylarthritides. Oxford: Oxford University Press; 1998. p. 17–26.
3. Reveille JD, Hirsch R, Dillon CF, Carroll MD, Weisman MH. The prevalence of HLA-B27 in the US: data from the US National Health and Nutrition Examination Survey, 2009. Arthritis Rheum. 2012;64(5):1407–11. doi:10.1002/art.33503.
4. Brewerton DA, Caffrey M, Nichols A, et al. Acute anterior uveitis and HLA-B27. Lancet. 1973:994–6.
5. Feltkamp TE. Ophthalmological significance of HLA associated uveitis. Eye. 1990:839–44.
6. Mapstone R, Woodrow JC. HLA-B27 and acute anterior uveitis. Br J Ophthalmol. 1975:270–5.
7. Qi J, Li Q, Lin Z, et al. Higher risk of uveitis and dactylitis and older age of onset among ankylosing spondylitis patients with HLA-B*2705 than patients with HLA-B*2704 in the Chinese population. Tissue Antigens. 2013:380–6.
8. Sampaio-Barros PD, Conde RA, Bonfiglioli R, Bértolo MB, Samara AM. Characterization and outcome of uveitis in 350 patients with spondyloarthropathies. Rheumatol Int. 2006:1143–6.
9. Colbert RA, DeLay ML, Layh-Schmitt G, Sowders DP. HLA-B27 misfolding and spondyloarthropathies. Prion. 2009;3:15–26.
10. Tay-Kearney ML, Schwamm BL, Lowder C, Dunn JP, Meister DM, Vitale S, Jabs DA. Clinical features and associated systemic diseases of HLA-B27 uveitis. Am J Ophthalmol. 1996;121:46–56.
11. Androudi S, et al. Graefes Arch Clin Exp Ophthalmol. 2003;241:1000–5.
12. Rosenbaum JT. Characteriztion of uveitis associated with spondyloarthritis. J Rheumatol. 1989:792–6.
13. Fiorelli VM, Bhat P, Foster CS. Nonsteroidal anti-inflammatory therapy and recurrent acute anterior uveitis. Ocul Immunol Inflamm. 2010:116–20.
14. Heldmann F, Dybowski F, Saracbasi-Zender E, et al. Update on biologic therapy in the management of

axial spondyloarthritis. Curr Rheumatol Rep. 2010: 225–31.
15. Braakenburg AM1, de Valk HW, de Boer J, Rothova A. Human leukocyte antigen-B27-associated uveitis: long-term follow-up and gender differences. Am J Ophthalmol. 2008;145:472–9.
16. Uy et al. Ocul Immunol Inflamm. 2001;9:177–83.
17. Power WJ, Rodriguez A, Pedroza-Seres M, Foster CS. Outcomes in anterior uveitis associated with the HLA-B27 haplotype. Ophthalmology. 1998;105:1646–51.
18. Loh RA, Acharya NR: Incidence rates and risk factors for ocular complications and vision loss in HLA-B27 associated uveitis. Am J Ophthalmol. 2010:534–42.
19. Ahn JK, Park YG. Human leukocyte antigen B27 and B51 double-positive Behcet uveitis. Arch Ophthalmol. 2007;104:705–8.

Inflammatory Bowel Disease

24

Durga S. Borkar and Nicholas J. Butler

Introduction

Inflammatory bowel disease (IBD), comprised mainly of Crohn's disease and ulcerative colitis, is a chronic, inflammatory gastrointestinal disease of unknown etiology. The incidence of IBD peaks in early adulthood, although this trend is more evident in women [1]. Although the exact pathogenesis of IBD is unknown, environmental factors (microbial, dietary, allergic, et al.) and genetic susceptibility appear necessary for the development of the disease [2]. Further, the reduction of antigenic challenges early in life may play a role, as such exposures appear critical for the development of immune tolerance [3, 4]. Accordingly, IBD is most prevalent in the increasingly sterile environment of developed countries [3, 4]. However, the incidence of IBD is on the rise in developing countries, such as India, as demographic changes occur toward more relative affluence and sanitation and other public health measures improve [3].

While Crohn's disease and ulcerative colitis are considered separate disease entities, patients often have common presenting symptoms, such as abdominal pain, diarrhea, hematochezia, and urgency [2]. Systemic symptoms, including fever, weight loss, and joint pain, are common [5]. A detailed history inquiring about these symptoms should be taken when approaching any patient with uveitis. Heightening the role of the ophthalmologist in assisting with diagnosis and management in these individuals, the ocular manifestations and complaints may precede the diagnosis of IBD on occasion.

In addition to the primary gastrointestinal manifestations, IBD is associated with several extraintestinal complications. Most commonly, these include arthritis, aphthous stomatitis, erythema nodosum, ankylosing spondylitis, psoriasis, pyoderma gangrenosum, primary sclerosing cholangitis, and uveitis [6, 7]. These extraintestinal manifestations may precede the gastrointestinal disease by years and some, including uveitis, have a course that may run independent of the gastrointestinal disease activity [6].

Ocular Manifestations of IBD

The prevalence of ocular complications in patients with IBD varies considerably, likely based upon differences in reporting and classification [2, 8]. When examining IBD patients prospectively for related eye disease, either symptomatic or silent,

D.S. Borkar · N.J. Butler (✉)
Department of Ophthalmology, Veterans Affairs Boston Healthcare System, 150 South Huntington Avenue, Jamaica Plain Campus, C8-11, Jamaica Plain, MA 02130, USA
e-mail: nicholas.butler4@va.gov

G.N. Papaliodis (ed.), *Uveitis*,
DOI 10.1007/978-3-319-09126-6_24

more than 40 % will have evidence of an ocular complication [9]. Approximately half of these complications are merely dry eye, which appears to be more prevalent among IBD patients as seen with numerous other autoimmune diseases [10]. Episcleritis is the most common non-dry eye-related ocular manifestation, affecting up to 30 % [2]. However, in many studies, uveitis is the most commonly reported ocular manifestation, presumably because episcleritis is often self-limited and not necessitating treatment [2]. The spectrum of eye disease though is broad. Other ocular manifestations of IBD include conjunctivitis, keratitis with or without peripheral ulceration, scleritis, episcleritis, scleromalacia perforans, retinitis, optic neuritis, orbital myositis, ocular myasthenia gravis, retinal artery occlusion, and retinal detachment [11–21]. In some cases, these ocular manifestations can occur concurrently with uveitis.

Epidemiology and Spectrum of Uveitis in IBD

The reported occurrence of uveitis in patients with IBD varies, generally in the range of 2–12 % [6, 22–25], but may be significantly less common in pediatric patients with IBD [26]. Crohn's disease appears to carry a higher risk of uveitis as compared to ulcerative colitis, more than 1.6-fold in a large, prospective cohort study [6]; however, the data regarding a differential incidence between the two subtypes of IBD are conflicting [27]. This relationship is further obfuscated by the fact that colonic or ileocolonic involvement in Crohn's disease patients appears to increase the risk of ocular inflammation (uveitis, episcleritis, and scleritis) by more than eightfold [5, 28]. Women with IBD have a higher incidence of uveitis [25, 29]. Additionally, there is a strong link between sacroiliac joint abnormalities, arthritis, HLA-B27 positivity, ANCA positivity, and the development of uveitis in IBD patients [22, 25, 29, 30]. Other genetic risk factors have been identified; ulcerative colitis patients with the HLA-DRB1*0103 allele more frequently suffer from associated uveitis and arthritis [31]. These associations, particularly HLA-B27 positivity, can be particularly important since ocular disease course and treatment response can vary based on the presence of this genetic profile [32].

While there is a strong association between IBD and uveitis, there is discordance between the severity of bowel disease and uveitis [22, 25]. Uveitis can occur during active gastrointestinal flares or during periods of remission [28, 33]. In some cases, uveitis may precede the diagnosis of IBD by several years [28, 34–36].

As for most uveitides of other causes, a careful assessment of ocular symptoms can help predict the location of uveitis that will be found on ocular examination. Redness, photophobia, pain, and decreased vision suggest an anterior uveitis, while decreased vision with floaters often indicates intermediate pathology. Although rare, scotomata could be suggestive of posterior involvement.

Overall, the most common type of uveitis associated with IBD is an acute, recurrent anterior uveitis, often bilateral [29]. This presentation accounts for more than 60 % of IBD-associated uveitis [37]. Typically, this is a nongranulomatous, low-grade inflammation although there have been reports of granulomatous uveitis as well as hypopyon associated with IBD [28, 38, 39]. Less commonly, patients with an anterior presentation may have a monophasic episode of nonrecurrent anterior uveitis, but this is estimated to occur in roughly ten percent of patients with IBD-associated uveitis [37]. In comparison to the uveitis associated with ankylosing spondylitis, a disease closely related to and often difficult to differentiate from IBD, the uveitis associated with IBD is more likely to be bilateral, posterior, insidious in onset, and chronic [29].

While anterior uveitis accounts for a majority of IBD-associated uveitis, up to 10–30 % percent of IBD patients with uveitis have posterior or panuveitis, sometimes mimicking other disease entities [37]. Many of these patients will have an associated retinal vasculitis [8]. Rarely, intermediate uveitis with snowbanks has been observed [34]. Multifocal choroiditis has been described in Crohn's disease; similarly, numerous cases of choroidal inflammation with associated serous retinal detachments have been reported [8, 21, 23, 40]. Acute multifocal placoid pigment epitheliopathy has been described [41]. Additionally, ulcerative colitis has been associated with subretinal fibrosis and uveitis syndrome in one report [42]. Although these cases are rare, they illustrate the broad spectrum of uveitis, including posterior uveitis, which can be associated with IBD.

In most instances, ocular symptoms prompt presentation to an ophthalmologist for evaluation and treatment of uveitis. As a result, there are currently no screening guidelines for uveitis in patients with IBD [43]. More so, ophthalmic symptoms in patients with IBD have a low positive predictive value for identifying true ocular inflammatory disease (uveitis, scleritis, keratitis, et al.) [44]. However, it is possible that subclinical anterior uveitis may be more common than originally believed, particularly in children. Multiple prospective case series have described an asymptomatic anterior uveitis in pediatric patients with IBD, particularly Crohn's disease [45–47]. Asymptomatic anterior uveitis was seen in 6.2–16.7 % of patients with Crohn's disease in these cohorts [45, 47]. In many cases, inflammation was transient and subsided without treatment, suggesting that routine screening for uveitis among pediatric IBD patients is likely unnecessary.

Management

When considering treatment for uveitis associated with IBD, the ophthalmologist must inquire about the activity of the underlying gastrointestinal disease and any concurrent, systemic anti-inflammatory therapy. If the patient has active bowel disease currently not under treatment, the management plan should be coordinated with the patient's primary gastroenterologist and/or rheumatologist in order to find a regimen that minimizes risk and optimizes benefit in controlling inflammation in both organ systems.

As with other autoimmune or autoinflammatory uveitides with or without systemic association, most uveitis specialists employ a step-up approach to treatment, commencing with less potent and ideally, less risk laden, medications first and saving more efficacious, and potentially more toxic, therapies for nonresponders. At the same time, initial management of IBD-associated uveitis is guided by the location of inflammation. Since most patients present with anterior uveitis, many will respond to topical corticosteroids and cycloplegics alone. Occasionally, local steroid injections may be needed. Depending on the course of the anterior uveitis (acute recurrent, acute monophasic, or chronic), the ophthalmologist can determine whether or not the topical steroid can be tapered to discontinuation or maintained at an infrequent, suppressive dose. However, the course of IBD-associated anterior uveitis may recur with excessive frequency or a chronic anterior uveitis may not be controllable with low-dose topical steroid. As a result, patients may require oral steroid therapy with subsequent transition to immunosuppressive treatment, if unable to taper the oral steroids to 5 mg of prednisone (or equivalent) or less daily or if prolonged steroid treatment leads to a significant number of intolerable side effects. This is more common in patients with HLA-B27 positivity [32]. Patients presenting with posterior uveitis generally require initial treatment with oral steroids and often will need to transition to steroid-sparing agents when the course of uveitis is persistent.

Several options are available for steroid-sparing immunosuppressive therapy for IBD-associated uveitis. In keeping with the step-up approach, the most common drugs initially employed are antimetabolites, namely methotrexate, azathioprine, and mycophenolate mofetil. Methotrexate and azathioprine, specifically, have demonstrated effectiveness in suppressing uveitis in the setting of IBD, though the data are limited [32, 48]. Extrapolating from an 82 % success rate in suppressing noninfectious uveitis and other ocular inflammation, mycophenolate mofetil is similarly routinely used [49]. Currently, there are no studies comparing the relative efficacy of these medications for uveitis associated with IBD.

Less commonly, T cell inhibitors, such as cyclosporine and tacrolimus, have been used as steroid-sparing treatment for uveitis in IBD patients, although the side effect profile, namely nephrotoxicity and hypertension, can limit the tolerability of these medications [8, 32]. These may be combined with an antimetabolite for refractory uveitis or used as monotherapy. For truly refractory cases of sight-threating uveitis, alkylating agents, such as cyclophosphamide and chlorambucil, have been employed in patients with IBD [32].

Though relatively newer to the scene, TNF-alpha inhibitors have proven remarkably successful in controlling both ocular and gastrointestinal inflammation in IBD, even in the setting of highly refractory cases [8, 50, 51]. In particular, infliximab has demonstrated efficacy in treating the extraintestinal manifestations of Crohn's disease, including acute and recurrent uveitis, as well as gastrointestinal manifestations refractory to other treatment [52–54]. Paradoxically, infliximab has been implicated as a cause of anterior uveitis in a patient with ulcerative colitis [55]. Though rare, these cases remind us that, while TNF antagonism generally has high success rates, the introduction of foreign proteins (biologic therapy) into patients with a predisposition for autoimmunity may rarely induce unanticipated and contrary results.

While the evidence is limited to small case series and case reports, adalimumab and infliximab are superior to etanercept for controlling uveitis refractory to other immunomodulatory therapy [56, 57]. Most uveitis specialists do not recommend etanercept for the treatment of uveitis; [58] hence, a patient with active uveitis while taking etanercept for underlying bowel disease may appropriately be switched to another TNF-inhibitor with the consent of the prescribing physician.

Salicylazosulfapyridine (sulfasalazine), a prodrug composed of 5-aminosalicylic acid (5-ASA) and sulfapyridine, is a common first-line therapy for IBD. As such, ophthalmologists treating IBD-associated uveitis will likely encounter patients already under therapy with sulfasalazine. It is important to note that, despite a lack of proven efficacy as a primary therapy for uveitis, sulfasalazine significantly decreases the number of annual flares of anterior uveitis, at least in patients with ankylosing spondylitis [59, 60]. The data for IBD patients with uveitis treated with sulfasalazine are limited, but similar conclusions may be extrapolated. In a prospective study of 10 patients with three or more flares annually of acute anterior uveitis, there was one IBD patient in the cohort; sulfasalazine reduced the annual flares of uveitis in this patient from four to zero [59].

Except in managing the complications of uveitis (cataract, glaucoma, epiretinal membranes, etc.), surgery has a limited role in managing IBD-associated uveitis. However, colectomy or revision of bowel anastomosis primarily for gastrointestinal inflammation has been shown to have a positive effect on control of ocular inflammation [8, 23, 61].

Conclusion

IBD comprises a spectrum of gastrointestinal disease characterized by chronic inflammation of unknown etiology, although certain environmental and genetic factors likely play a role in the pathogenesis. Uveitis is a common extraintestinal manifestation of IBD and most often presents as an acute, recurrent, bilateral anterior uveitis; however, intermediate, posterior, and panuveitides may also be encountered in these patients. While many cases may be adequately treated with topical corticosteroids, other patients will require systemic treatment with both oral steroids and immunomodulatory therapy. Several options exist for treatment, though for severe or refractory gastrointestinal and/or ocular inflammation, the TNF-alpha antagonists are increasingly employed.

References

1. Shivananda S, Lennard-Jones J, Logan R, et al. Incidence of inflammatory bowel disease across Europe: is there a difference between north and south? Results of the European collaborative study on inflammatory bowel disease (EC-IBD). Gut. 1996;39(5):690–7.
2. Ghanchi FD, Rembacken BJ. Inflammatory bowel disease and the eye. Surv Ophthalmol. 2003;48 (6):663–76.
3. Dhar A. Environmental factors associated with Crohn's disease in India-there's more to it than meets the eye. Indian J Gastroenterol Off J Indian Soc Gastroenterol. 2011;30(6):255–6.
4. Gent AE, Hellier MD, Grace RH, Swarbrick ET, Coggon D. Inflammatory bowel disease and domestic hygiene in infancy. Lancet. 1994;343(8900):766–7.
5. Greenstein AJ, Janowitz HD, Sachar DB. The extra-intestinal complications of Crohn's disease and ulcerative colitis: a study of 700 patients. Medicine. 1976;55(5):401–12.
6. Vavricka SR, Brun L, Ballabeni P, et al. Frequency and risk factors for extraintestinal manifestations in the Swiss inflammatory bowel disease cohort. Am J Gastroenterol. 2011;106(1):110–9.
7. Juillerat P, Mottet C, Froehlich F, et al. Extraintestinal manifestations of Crohn's disease. Digestion. 2005;71(1):31–6.
8. Taylor SR, McCluskey P, Lightman S. The ocular manifestations of inflammatory bowel disease. Curr Opin Ophthalmol. 2006;17(6):538–44.
9. Felekis T, Katsanos K, Kitsanou M, et al. Spectrum and frequency of ophthalmologic manifestations in patients with inflammatory bowel disease: a prospective single-center study. Inflamm Bowel Dis. 2009;15(1):29–34.
10. Cury DB, Moss AC. Ocular manifestations in a community-based cohort of patients with inflammatory bowel disease. Inflamm Bowel Dis. 2010;16 (8):1393–6.
11. Cheng S, Vu P. Recurrent orbital myositis with radiological feature mimicking thyroid eye disease in a patient with Crohn's disease. Orbit. 2009;28(6):368–70.
12. Lange AP, Bahar I, Sansanayudh W, Kaisermann I, Slomovic AR. Salzmann nodules—a possible new ocular manifestation of Crohn's disease: a case report. Cornea. 2009;28(1):85–6.
13. Soomro H, Armstrong M, Graham EM, Stanford MR. Sudden loss of vision caused by a vasculitic ophthalmic artery occlusion in a patient with ankylosing spondylitis and Crohn's disease. Br J Ophthalmol. 2006;90(11):1438.
14. Leibovitch I, Galanopoulos A, Selva D. Suppurative granulomatous myositis of an extra-ocular muscle in Crohn's disease. Am J Gastroenterol. 2005;100 (9):2136–7.
15. Foroozan R, Sambursky R. Ocular myasthenia gravis and inflammatory bowel disease: a case report and literature review. Br J Ophthalmol. 2003;87(9):1186–7.
16. Chowers I, Siganos CS, Solomon A, Frucht-Pery J. Deep stromal inflammation–a possible new ocular manifestation of Crohn's disease. Ocul Immunol Inflamm. 1998;6(1):59–62.
17. Durno CA, Ehrlich R, Taylor R, Buncic JR, Hughes P, Griffiths AM. Keeping an eye on Crohn's disease: orbital myositis as the presenting symptom. Can J Gastroenterol (Journal canadien de gastroenterologie). 1997;11(6):497–500.
18. Strauss RE. Ocular manifestations of Crohn's disease: literature review. Mt Sinai J Med N Y. 1988;55 (4):353–6.
19. Petrelli EA, McKinley M, Troncale FJ. Ocular manifestations of inflammatory bowel disease. Ann Ophthalmol. 1982;14(4):356–60.
20. Cojocaru IM, Cojocaru M, Tanasescu R, et al. Some clinico-immunological aspects in patients with ocular myasthenia gravis associated with inflammatory bowel disease. Romanian J Intern Med (Revue roumaine de medecine interne). 2008;46(2):165–68.
21. Ernst BB, Lowder CY, Meisler DM, Gutman FA. Posterior segment manifestations of inflammatory bowel disease. Ophthalmology. 1991;98(8):1272–80.
22. Hopkins DJ, Horan E, Burton IL, Clamp SE, de Dombal FT, Goligher JC. Ocular disorders in a series of 332 patients with Crohn's disease. Br J Ophthalmol. 1974;58(8):732–7.
23. Knox DL, Schachat AP, Mustonen E. Primary, secondary and coincidental ocular complications of Crohn's disease. Ophthalmology. 1984;91(2):163–73.
24. Billson FA, De Dombal FT, Watkinson G, Goligher JC. Ocular complications of ulcerative colitis. Gut. 1967;8(2):102–6.
25. Wright R, Lumsden K, Luntz MH, Sevel D, Truelove SC. Abnormalities of the Sacro-iliac joints and uveitis in ulcerative colitis. Quarter J Med. 1965;34:229–36.
26. Dotson JL, Hyams JS, Markowitz J, et al. Extraintestinal manifestations of pediatric inflammatory bowel disease and their relation to disease type and severity. J Pediatr Gastroenterol Nutr. 2010;51(2):140–5.
27. Das KM. Relationship of extraintestinal involvements in inflammatory bowel disease: new insights into autoimmune pathogenesis. Dig Dis Sci. 1999;44(1):1–13.
28. Salmon JF, Wright JP, Murray AD. Ocular inflammation in Crohn's disease. Ophthalmology. 1991;98 (4):480–4.
29. Lyons JL, Rosenbaum JT. Uveitis associated with inflammatory bowel disease compared with uveitis associated with spondyloarthropathy. Arch Ophthalmol. 1997;115(1):61–4.
30. Turkcapar N, Toruner M, Soykan I, et al. The prevalence of extraintestinal manifestations and HLA association in patients with inflammatory bowel disease. Rheumatol Int. 2006;26(7):663–8.

31. Roussomoustakaki M, Satsangi J, Welsh K, et al. Genetic markers may predict disease behavior in patients with ulcerative colitis. Gastroenterology. 1997;112(6):1845–53.
32. Soukiasian SH, Foster CS, Raizman MB. Treatment strategies for scleritis and uveitis associated with inflammatory bowel disease. Am J Ophthalmol. 1994;118(5):601–11.
33. Korelitz BI, Coles RS. Uveitis (iritis) associated with ulcerative and granulomatous colitis. Gastroenterology. 1967;52(1):78–82.
34. Zaidman GW, Coles RS. Peripheral uveitis and ulcerative colitis. Ann Ophthalmol. 1981;13(1):73–6.
35. Singleton EM, Hutson SE. Anterior uveitis, inflammatory bowel disease, and ankylosing spondylitis in a HLA-B27-positive woman. South Med J. 2006;99 (5):531–3.
36. Paroli MP, Spinucci G, Bruscolini A, La Cava M, Abicca I. Uveitis preceding Crohn's disease by 8 years. Int Ophthalmol. 2011;31(5):413–5.
37. Banares A, Jover JA, Fernandez-Gutierrez B, et al. Patterns of uveitis as a guide in making rheumatologic and immunologic diagnoses. Arthritis Rheum. 1997;40(2):358–70.
38. Salmon JF, Wright JP, Bowen RM, Murray AD. Granulomatous uveitis in Crohn's disease. A clinicopathologic case report. Arch Ophthalmol. 1989;107 (5):718–9.
39. Liu MP, Hwang FS, Dunn JP, Stark WJ, Bower KS. Hypopyon uveitis following LASIK in a patient with ulcerative colitis. J Refract Surg. 2012;28(8):589–91.
40. Tappeiner C, Dohrmann J, Spital G, Heiligenhaus A. Multifocal posterior uveitis in Crohn's disease. Graefe's Arch Clin Exp Ophthalmol (Albrecht von Graefes Archiv fur klinische und experimentelle Ophthalmologie). 2007;245(3):457–59.
41. Gass JDM. Stereoscopic atlas of macular diseases: diagnosis and treatment. 3rd ed. St. Louis: Mosby; 1987.
42. Fuentes-Paez G, Martinez-Osorio H, Herreras JM, Calonge M. Subretinal fibrosis and uveitis syndrome associated with ulcerative colitis. Int J Colorectal Dis. 2007;22(3):333–4.
43. Verbraak FD, Schreinemachers MC, Tiller A, van Deventer SJ, de Smet MD. Prevalence of subclinical anterior uveitis in adult patients with inflammatory bowel disease. Br J Ophthalmol. 2001;85(2):219–21.
44. Cloche V, Buisson A, Trechot F, et al. Ocular symptoms are not predictive of ophthalmologic inflammation in inflammatory bowel disease. Digestive Liver Dis Off J Italian Soc Gastroenterol Italian Assoc Stud Liver. 2013;45(3):195–9.
45. Hofley P, Roarty J, McGinnity G, et al. Asymptomatic uveitis in children with chronic inflammatory bowel diseases. J Pediatr Gastroenterol Nutr. 1993;17 (4):397–400.
46. Daum F, Gould HB, Gold D, et al. Asymptomatic transient uveitis in children with inflammatory bowel disease. Am J Dis Child. 1979;133(2):170–1.
47. Rychwalski PJ, Cruz OA, Alanis-Lambreton G, Foy TM, Kane RE. Asymptomatic uveitis in young people with inflammatory bowel disease. J AAPOS Off Publ Am Assoc Pediatr Ophthalmol Strabismus Am Assoc Pediatr Ophthalmol Strabismus. 1997;1(2):111–4.
48. Samson CM, Waheed N, Baltatzis S, Foster CS. Methotrexate therapy for chronic noninfectious uveitis: analysis of a case series of 160 patients. Ophthalmology. 2001;108(6):1134–9.
49. Thorne JE, Jabs DA, Qazi FA, Nguyen QD, Kempen JH, Dunn JP. Mycophenolate mofetil therapy for inflammatory eye disease. Ophthalmology. 2005;112 (8):1472–7.
50. Peyrin-Biroulet L, Deltenre P, de Suray N, Branche J, Sandborn WJ, Colombel JF. Efficacy and safety of tumor necrosis factor antagonists in Crohn's disease: meta-analysis of placebo-controlled trials. Clin Gastroenterol Hepatol Off Clin Pract J Am Gastroenterol Assoc. 2008;6(6):644–53.
51. Hanauer SB, Feagan BG, Lichtenstein GR, et al. Maintenance infliximab for Crohn's disease: the ACCENT I randomised trial. Lancet. 2002;359(9317):1541–9.
52. Hale S, Lightman S. Anti-TNF therapies in the management of acute and chronic uveitis. Cytokine. 2006;33(4):231–7.
53. Fries W, Giofre MR, Catanoso M, Lo Gullo R. Treatment of acute uveitis associated with Crohn's disease and sacroileitis with infliximab. Am J Gastroenterol. 2002;97(2):499–500.
54. Ally MR, Veerappan GR, Koff JM. Treatment of recurrent Crohn's uveitis with infliximab. Am J Gastroenterol. 2008;103(8):2150–1.
55. Singla MB, Hodge DK, Moawad FJ. Infliximab-induced anterior uveitis in a patient with ulcerative colitis. J Crohn's Colitis. 16 Feb 2015.
56. Schmeling H, Horneff G. Etanercept and uveitis in patients with juvenile idiopathic arthritis. Rheumatology (Oxford). 2005;44(8):1008–11.
57. Murray PI, Sivaraj RR. Anti-TNF-alpha therapy for uveitis: Behcet and beyond. Eye (London). 2005;19 (8):831–3.
58. Rifkin LM, Birnbaum AD, Goldstein DA. TNF inhibition for ophthalmic indications: current status and outlook. BioDrugs Clin Immunotherapeutics, Biopharmaceuticals Gene Ther. 2013;27(4):347–57.
59. Munoz-Fernandez S, Hidalgo V, Fernandez-Melon J, et al. Sulfasalazine reduces the number of flares of acute anterior uveitis over a one-year period. J Rheumatol. 2003;30(6):1277–9.
60. Benitez-Del-Castillo JM, Garcia-Sanchez J, Iradier T, Banares A. Sulfasalazine in the prevention of anterior uveitis associated with ankylosing spondylitis. Eye (London). 2000;14(Pt 3A):340–3.
61. Mintz R, Feller ER, Bahr RL, Shah SA. Ocular manifestations of inflammatory bowel disease. Inflamm Bowel Dis. 2004;10(2):135–9.

Juvenile Idiopathic Arthritis

25

Ann-Marie Lobo

Juvenile idiopathic arthritis (JIA) refers to a group of heterogeneous arthritides that has an age of onset before 16 years and is often associated with chronic uveitis.

Epidemiology

JIA associated uveitis is the most common type of pediatric uveitis associated with a systemic disease [1]. JIA uveitis has a variable prevalence worldwide, with the majority of cases reported in North America and Europe. The disease is more common in girls and patients with positive anti-nuclear antibodies (ANA).

Pathogenesis and Risk Factors

Genetic and environmental factors play a role in the development of JIA. The risk of JIA is 15–30-fold higher in siblings of JIA patients than the general population. HLA types DRB1*11 and DBR1*13 have been associated with a higher susceptibility of developing JIA uveitis [2]. T cell activation and increased levels of pro-inflammatory cytokines such as tumor necrosis factor alpha (TNF) and IL-6 have been implicated in the pathogenesis of JIA.

Risk factors associated with the development of JIA uveitis include ANA positivity, oligoarticular form of arthritis, early age of onset of disease of less than 4 years, and female gender (Table 25.1). In most patients, arthritis presents before uveitis. 90 % of patients who develop uveitis do so within 4 years of diagnosis of arthritis [3]. A younger age of onset of arthritis is associated with a higher likelihood of developing uveitis in girls but not in boys [4].

Diagnostic Criteria and Clinical Presentation

There are several different types of JIA which can be classified by the number of joints involved. Specific types of JIA have higher associations with the development of uveitis. The American College of Rheumatology divides JIA into three categories based on number of joints involved: systemic, oligoarticular (persistent or extended), or polyarticular (Table 25.2). The International League of Associations for Rheumatology (ILAR) classification also includes Rheumatoid factor (RF) positive polyarthritis, RF negative polyarthritis, psoriatic arthritis, and enthesitis-related arthritis. Uveitis is most often associated with the extended

A.-M. Lobo (✉)
Department of Ophthalmology, Harvard Medical School, Massachusetts Eye and Ear Infirmary, Boston, MA 02114, USA
e-mail: Ann-Marie_Lobo@meei.harvard.edu

G.N. Papaliodis (ed.), *Uveitis*,
DOI 10.1007/978-3-319-09126-6_25

Table 25.1 Risk factors for JIA uveitis requiring frequent screening

ANA positive
Oligoarthritis
Age <7
Duration of disease <4 years
Rheumatoid factor negative polyarthritis

oligoarthritis type of JIA in 25 % of patients followed by the persistent oligoarthritis type in 16 % [3]. Systemic JIA is rarely associated with uveitis.

Unlike most forms of uveitis, JIA uveitis is associated with an insidious onset of nongranulomatous anterior uveitis in a white, quiet eye. Children generally report no symptoms and may present to an ophthalmologist after failing a school vision screen or because of diagnosis of arthritis. Clinical signs include anterior uveitis with cells and flare. Anterior chamber cells are present when there is active inflammation, but most eyes with chronic inflammation may exhibit flare associated with leakage of proteins from the ciliary body vasculature. Inflammation is most commonly bilateral, but there can be unilateral

Table 25.2 JIA subtypes and screening guidelines

JIA subtypes by ACR*	Clinical features	Uveitis	Screening Guidelines: [23] ANA, age of onset, duration of disease(years): frequency of screens (months)
Systemic*	Fever with arthritis, skin rash, lymphadenopathy, hepatosplenomegaly	Rare	12
Oligoarticular/pauciarticular*	Arthritis of ≤4 joints in first 6 months of disease	Common	ANA+, onset ≤6 yrs, duration ≤4 yrs:3
Persistent	≤4 joints entire disease course		ANA+, duration >4 yrs:6
			ANA+, duration ≥7 yrs:12
Extended	>5 joints after first 6 months		ANA+, onset > 6 yrs, duration ≤2 yrs:6
			ANA+, duration >4 yrs:12
			ANA−, onset ≤6 yrs, duration ≤4 yrs:6
			ANA−, duration >4 yrs:12
Polyarticular*	Arthritis of >5 joints in first 6 months of disease	Common in RF negative	See guidelines for Oligoarticular
Additional JIA subtypes by ILAR			
RF positive polyarticular	Arthritis of >5 joints in first 6 months of disease	Rare	See guidelines for Oligoarticular
RF negative polyarticular		common	
Psoriatic	Arthritis and psoriasis	Common	See guidelines for Oligoarticular
	Dactylitis, nail pitting, Psoriasis in 1st degree relative		
Enthesitis	Arthritis and/or enthesitis HLA-B27	Often symptomatic acute anterior uveitis in males over age 6	Based on symptoms or 12 months if asymptomatic
Undifferentiated	Arthritis that does not fit other categories		

*Subtypes defined by American College of Rheumatology

inflammation or asymmetric involvement. Other common clinical features include band keratopathy, nongranulomatous keratic precipitates, posterior synechiae, and elevated intraocular pressure. Patients can have posterior segment involvement including vitritis, cystoid macular edema, and optic disc edema.

Patients with enthesitis-related arthritis who develop uveitis may present with symptoms of acute anterior uveitis, including pain, photophobia, redness, and blurred vision. These patients are generally male adolescent patients with positive HLA-B27.

Diagnostic Workup and Differential Diagnosis

The diagnosis of JIA uveitis is made based on careful history, physical exam, and ancillary tests. Patients and family members should be asked about a history of joint swelling or restriction of movements as well as family history of autoimmune diseases, especially inflammatory arthritis or psoriasis. Children with uveitis should have a thorough physical examination for evidence of joint disease, preferably by a pediatric rheumatologist. Serologic testing may be helpful in ruling out other entities for uveitis (Table 25.3). ANA positivity is a major risk factor for the development of uveitis in patients with oligoarticular arthritis, with up to 30 % of these patients developing uveitis. RF positivity is associated with a low risk for uveitis.

The differential diagnosis of uveitis with arthritis in children includes infectious and noninfectious entities. Lyme disease is an important infectious cause of uveitis and arthritis in children and serologic testing (both screening enzyme linked immunoassay and confirmatory Western blot) should be performed for patients who live in endemic areas. Cat scratch disease can also present with uveitis and Bartonella serologies should be obtained if the history is suggestive. Viral processes such as the herpes family of viruses can cause uveitis in children and should be considered in the differential diagnosis.

Table 25.3 Laboratory workup for pediatric uveitis and associated diagnoses

Anti-nuclear antibody (ANA)	JIA
Rheumatoid factor (RF)	RF positive polyarthritis
HLA-B27	Seronegative spondyloarthropathies (ankylosing spondylitis, psoriatic arthritis, reactive arthritis)
Angiotensin converting enzyme (ACE), Lysozyme	Sarcoidosis, Blau syndrome
Sedimentation rate (ESR)	Generalized inflammatory markers
C-reactive protein (CRP)	
BUN/creatinine	TINU
Urinalysis	TINU
Lyme screen and Western blot	Lyme disease

Other noninfectious causes of uveitis in the pediatric population include sarcoidosis, which can present with arthritis and anterior uveitis in children. Familial juvenile systemic granulomatosis, also known as Blau syndrome, can also present with arthritis and uveitis in children; however, the uveitis is most often a bilateral granulomatous panuveitis which differs from JIA uveitis. Tubulointerstitial nephritis with uveitis syndrome can present as bilateral anterior uveitis, often with fevers, malaise, and flank pain. Definitive diagnosis is made with renal biopsy demonstrating interstitial nephritis. Behcet's disease can also present with uveitis and pauciarticular arthritis; diagnostic criteria include the presence of oral and/or genital ulcers. Behcet's is rare in children and is characterized by more extensive vasculitis.

Treatment

JIA uveitis is most often associated with a chronic course with 60–80 % of patients having inflammation lasting longer than 3 months. JIA is associated with a low incidence of remission of anterior uveitis [5]. The goal of treatment in

JIA uveitis should be to eliminate active inflammation in order to prevent long-term ocular complications. While topical and systemic corticosteroids may be initial treatments for uveitis, they should be used sparingly due to significant side effects related to chronic exposure. Systemic nonsteroidal medications may be helpful for arthritis symptoms, but generally do not adequately control ocular inflammation. Patients diagnosed with JIA uveitis, particularly those with ocular complications at presentation and duration of uveitis greater than 3 months should be treated with steroid-sparing immunosuppressive therapies (Table 25.4). Methotrexate is the most commonly used first-line treatment for JIA uveitis and is effective for both joint and eye disease. Other anti-metabolite therapies such as azathioprine and mycophenolate mofetil and T cell inhibitors like cyclosporine have been used in JIA uveitis with variable results [6]. The advent of biologic response modifier therapies has had a significant impact on the treatment and control of ocular inflammation in JIA. In patients with severe disease that is recalcitrant to standard immunosuppressive therapy, TNF alpha inhibitors such as infliximab and adalimumab are safe and effective second-line treatments for JIA uveitis [7–9]. TNF inhibitors are usually used in conjunction with methotrexate for improved efficacy and to prevent the development of human anti-chimeric antibodies in patients treated with infliximab, although they can be used as monotherapy. Other biologic agents such as abatacept and rituximab have also been used in patients with severe JIA uveitis who have failed multiple immunosuppressive therapies [10, 11].

Table 25.4 Treatments for JIA uveitis

Initial Treatment	Indications
Corticosteroids	
Topical	Initial treatment of uveitis, should not be used long term
Systemic	Reserved for significant joint/eye inflammation, can have significant adverse effects with chronic use
Nonsteroidal agents	Treatment of mild joint/eye inflammation
First-line immunosuppression	
Antimetabolites	
Methotrexate (MTX)	Considered first-line immunosuppressive therapy; oral or subcutaneous dosing
Mycophenolate mofetil	Can be used instead of MTX
Azathioprine	Can be used instead of MTX
Leflunomide	Can be used as additional therapy
T cell inhibitors	
Cyclosporine	Can be used as additional therapy
Second-line immunosuppression	
TNF alpha inhibitors	
Infliximab	Chimeric monoclonal antibody, intravenous infusion
Adalimumab	Fully humanized monoclonal antibody, subcutaneous
Golimumab	Fully humanized monoclonal antibody, subcutaneous
Etanercept	Fusion protein for soluble TNF, subcutaneous, minimally effective for uveitis
Other treatments	
Abatacept	CTLA-4 fusion protein that inhibits T cell costimulation, subcutaneous
Rituximab	Chimeric monoclonal antibody to CD 20, infusion

Surgical management of ocular complications in JIA uveitis should be undertaken only after a prolonged period of quiescence of inflammation of at least 3–6 months. EDTA chelation can be performed to remove band keratopathy in the visual axis (Fig. 25.1). Cataract surgery should be performed in young patients in the amblyogenic age range. Perioperative management for JIA uveitic cataracts involves systemic immunosuppression, aggressive topical steroids, intraoperative intravenous steroids, and peri- or intraocular steroids. A posterior capsulotomy and pars plana vitrectomy can also be performed at the time of cataract surgery. Placement of an intraocular lens is still considered controversial because of the risk of posterior synechiae

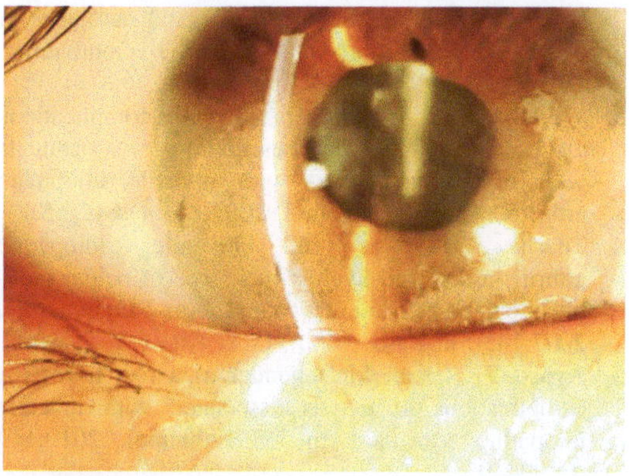

Fig. 25.1 Slit lamp photograph OD—14 year old boy with JIA-associated uveitis status post cataract removal and EDTA chelation for band keratopathy. Vision improved from 20/400 preoperatively to 20/40

formation, pupillary and cyclitic membranes, posterior capsular opacification, and hypotony. In very young patients with history of severe inflammation or hypotony, lens placement should be avoided. Improved control of inflammation and lens materials has been associated with good visual outcomes in patients who have an intraocular lens placed [10]. A surgical iridectomy is advisable at the time of lens placement to avoid potential for pupillary block.

In JIA uveitis patients who develop glaucoma recalcitrant to medical management, goniotomy surgery is an effective first-line surgery in patients without significant peripheral anterior synechiae [12]. Glaucoma drainage devices can be used in patients who have significant angle closure or who are unresponsive to goniotomy.

Complications and Prognosis

JIA uveitis has been associated with significant morbidity due to the development of ocular complications. In several studies, 45–60 % of JIA uveitis patients developed at least one ocular complication, including cataract, glaucoma, posterior synechiae formation, band keratopathy, hypotony, or macular edema [3, 13, 14]. Rates of development of each of these complications vary widely from population-based to tertiary care center studies, but regardless of the study, complication rates increase with duration of disease. Other risk factors for increased rate of ocular complications related to timing of disease presentation include diagnosis of uveitis prior to arthritis and shorter duration between diagnosis of arthritis and uveitis. Risk factors for ocular complications related to clinical features at initial presentation include presence of posterior synechiae and active inflammation (>1 + cell). Male gender has also been found to be a risk factor for more ocular complications and poorer visual prognosis in JIA uveitis [15].

Cataracts are one of the most common complications in JIA uveitis with up to 80 % prevalence in patients by the time they reach adulthood. Risk factors for the development of cataract formation include posterior synechiae at initial presentation, use of topical steroids >3 drops per day, use of systemic corticosteroids, and active ongoing inflammation [16, 17].

The development of ocular complications is significant since most complications can lead to vision loss. Historically, JIA uveitis patients have had a guarded prognosis, with up to 30 % of patients developing significant vision loss of less than 20/50 and 24 % with vision less than 20/200 [14, 18–21]. A large study of JIA patients from North America revealed that risk factors for moderate to severe vision loss included active anterior chamber inflammation (>1 + anterior chamber cell), posterior synechiae formation, and intraocular surgery [22]. However, the use of immunosuppressive treatment for JIA uveitis can result in a 60 % decrease in the risk for significant vision loss.

Conclusion

JIA is associated with chronic uveitis and can result in significant ocular morbidity. Early screening and aggressive treatment with immunosuppressive therapy are important factors in preventing ocular complications and vision loss.

References

1. Smith JA, et al. Epidemiology and course of disease in childhood uveitis. Ophthalmology 2009;116 (8):1544–51, 1551 e1.
2. Macaubas C, et al. Oligoarticular and polyarticular JIA: epidemiology and pathogenesis. Nat Rev Rheumatol. 2009;5(11):616–26.
3. Heiligenhaus A, et al. Prevalence and complications of uveitis in juvenile idiopathic arthritis in a population-based nation-wide study in Germany: suggested modification of the current screening guidelines. Rheumatology (Oxford). 2007;46 (6):1015–9.
4. Saurenmann RK, et al. Risk factors for development of uveitis differ between girls and boys with juvenile idiopathic arthritis. Arthritis Rheum. 2010;62 (6):1824–8.
5. Artornsombudh P, et al. Factors predictive of remission of new-onset anterior uveitis. Ophthalmology. 2014;121(3):778–84.
6. Heiligenhaus A, et al. Evidence-based, interdisciplinary guidelines for anti-inflammatory treatment of uveitis associated with juvenile idiopathic arthritis. Rheumatol Int. 2012;32(5):1121–33.
7. Levy-Clarke G, et al. Expert panel recommendations for the use of anti-tumor necrosis factor biologic agents in patients with ocular inflammatory disorders. Ophthalmology 2014;121(3):785–96 e3.
8. Zannin ME, et al. Safety and efficacy of infliximab and adalimumab for refractory uveitis in juvenile idiopathic arthritis: 1-year followup data from the Italian Registry. J Rheumatol. 2013;40(1):74–9.
9. Foeldvari I, et al. Tumor necrosis factor-alpha blocker in treatment of juvenile idiopathic arthritis-associated uveitis refractory to second-line agents: results of a multinational survey. J Rheumatol. 2007;34(5):1146–50.
10. Heiligenhaus A, et al. Treatment of severe uveitis associated with juvenile idiopathic arthritis with anti-CD20 monoclonal antibody (rituximab). Rheumatology (Oxford). 2011;50(8):1390–4.
11. Zulian F, et al. Abatacept for severe anti-tumor necrosis factor alpha refractory juvenile idiopathic arthritis-related uveitis. Arthritis Care Res (Hoboken). 2010;62(6):821–5.
12. Bohnsack BL, Freedman SF. Surgical outcomes in childhood uveitic glaucoma. Am J Ophthalmol. 2013;155(1):134–42.
13. Woreta F, et al. Risk factors for ocular complications and poor visual acuity at presentation among patients with uveitis associated with juvenile idiopathic arthritis. Am J Ophthalmol. 2007;143(4):647–55.
14. Thorne JE, et al. Juvenile idiopathic arthritis-associated uveitis: incidence of ocular complications and visual acuity loss. Am J Ophthalmol. 2007;143(5):840–6.
15. Ayuso VK, et al. Male gender as a risk factor for complications in uveitis associated with juvenile idiopathic arthritis. Am J Ophthalmol. 2010;149 (6):994–9.
16. Thorne JE, et al. Risk of cataract development among children with juvenile idiopathic arthritis-related uveitis treated with topical corticosteroids. Ophthalmology. 2010;117(7):1436–41.
17. Angeles-Han S, Yeh S. Prevention and management of cataracts in children with juvenile idiopathic arthritis-associated uveitis. Curr Rheumatol Rep. 2012;14(2):142–9.
18. Kump LI, et al. Visual outcomes in children with juvenile idiopathic arthritis-associated uveitis. Ophthalmology. 2006;113(10):1874–7.
19. Dana MR, et al. Visual outcomes prognosticators in juvenile rheumatoid arthritis-associated uveitis. Ophthalmology. 1997;104(2):236–44.
20. Yu EN, et al. Outcomes of treatment with immunomodulatory therapy in patients with corticosteroid-resistant juvenile idiopathic arthritis-associated chronic iridocyclitis. Ocul Immunol Inflamm. 2005;13(5):353–60.
21. Ozdal PC, Vianna RN, Deschenes J. Visual outcome of juvenile rheumatoid arthritis-associated uveitis in adults. Ocul Immunol Inflamm. 2005;13(1):33–8.
22. Gregory AC 2nd, et al. Risk factors for loss of visual acuity among patients with uveitis associated with juvenile idiopathic arthritis: the systemic immunosuppressive therapy for eye diseases study. Ophthalmology. 2013;120(1):186–92.
23. Cassidy J, et al. Ophthalmologic examinations in children with juvenile rheumatoid arthritis. Pediatrics. 2006;117(5):1843–5.

26 Lens Induced

George N. Papaliodis

Introduction

Lens induced or phacogenic uveitis is an uncommon cause of intraocular inflammation presumably due to an immune reaction against lens proteins. This entity has been described after rupture of the lens capsule (from trauma or surgery) and also in hypermature lenses with leakage of lens proteins despite an intact capsule. Recognition of this condition is imperative as prompt removal of the lens is typically curative.

Epidemiology and Pathogenesis

The exact incidence of phacogenic uveitis is unknown but typically accounts for less than 1 % of all cases of uveitis in multiple case series [1, 2]. The pathogenesis of the disorder is similarly not well characterized, but the condition is generally viewed as a localized form of autoimmune disease. It has been hypothesized that the anterior chamber can tolerate some limited quantity of lens proteins without inducing an inflammatory response. The tolerance to the lens proteins may be altered due to trauma and rupture of the capsule. Others have hypothesized that immune tolerance is compromised due to the quantity of lens proteins in the anterior chamber. The exact inciting mechanism of the disorder and the role of anterior chamber associated immune deviation are unclear.

Clinical Manifestations

Patients with lens induced intraocular inflammation typically develop anterior uveitis (granulomatous or nongranulomatous depending upon severity) with associated vitritis involving the intermediate zone of the eye [3]. Younger patients more typically have a history of recent or old trauma. The anterior uveitis can be severe and associated with hypopyon. Patients may similarly have elevated intraocular pressures due to lens proteins obstructing trabecular meshwork outflow.

Diagnosis

The diagnosis of phacogenic uveitis is typically established via supportive history and appropriate clinical features along with exclusion of other potential etiologies. In cases that remain uncertain, anterior chamber aspirate demonstrating the presence of giant macrophages engorged with lens material will confirm the diagnosis.

G.N. Papaliodis (✉)
Department of Ophthalmology, Harvard Medical School, Massachusetts Eye and Ear Infirmary, Boston, MA 02114, USA
e-mail: George_Papaliodis@meei.harvard.edu

G.N. Papaliodis (ed.), *Uveitis*,
DOI 10.1007/978-3-319-09126-6_26

Treatment

Phacogenic uveitis typically resolves completely by removal of all lens material. Adjunctive treatment (for any residual lens material) may require prolonged use of topical corticosteroids or rarely systemic corticosteroids. If the intraocular inflammation fails to respond to the surgical removal of all lens material, an alternative diagnosis should be considered.

Conclusion

Lens induced or phacogenic uveitis is an uncommon clinical entity inducing intraocular inflammation and is generally viewed as a focal autoimmune disorder triggered by intolerance to intraocular lens proteins (either via trauma and rupture of the capsule or hypermature lens). The treatment that is often curative is complete removal of all lens material.

References

1. Henderly DE, Genstler AJ, Smith RE, Rao NA. Changing patterns of uveitis. Am J Ophthalmol. 1987;103:131–6.
2. Rodriguez A, Calonge M, Pedroza-Seres M, et al. Referral patterns of uveitis in a tertiary eye care center. Arch Ophthalmol. 1996;114:593–9.
3. Khalil MK, Lorenzetti DW. Lens induced inflammations. Can J Ophthalmol. 1986;21:96–102.

Masquerade Syndromes

27

Emmett T. Cunningham Jr, Carol L. Shields
and Jerry A. Shields

Introduction

Uveitis masquerade syndromes include conditions that either mimic uveitis or cause intraocular inflammation as a secondary effect [1–12]. Most masquerade syndromes in uveitis are neoplastic, although non-neoplastic masquerade syndromes also well recognized. While population-based estimates of the prevalence of uveitis masquerade syndromes are not available, data from uveitis referral clinics suggest that such conditions constitute less than 3 % of cases in that setting [13–16], and well below 1 % of patients with uveitis seen in a general ophthalmology practice [17].

The more commonly encountered non-neoplastic and neoplastic uveitis masquerade syndromes are listed in Table 27.1 and summarized below. We have not included infections in this chapter, although undiagnosed and inappropriately treated infectious uveitis can produce paradoxical and/or transient responses to therapy similar to those seen with some noninfectious masquerade syndromes. Endogenous endophthalmitis and infectious causes of exaggerated, prolonged or delayed postoperative inflammation can be particularly difficult to diagnose [1, 18, 19].

Non-neoplastic Masquerade Syndromes

Anterior Uveitis

Corneal Epithelial Defects

Large or persistent defects in the corneal epithelium can produce moderate to severe anterior chamber inflammation—including hypopyon [20–23]. This can occur following large corneal abrasions, after chemical burns, in eyes with neurotrophic keratopathy following herpetic keratitis, in the setting of an underlying

Financial Conflicts: The authors have no relevant financial conflicts.

E.T. Cunningham Jr (✉)
California Pacific Medical Center, San Francisco, CA, USA
e-mail: emmett_cunningham@yahoo.com

E.T. Cunningham Jr
Stanford University School of Medicine, Stanford, CA, USA

E.T. Cunningham Jr
UCSF School of Medicine, San Francisco, CA, USA

E.T. Cunningham Jr
West Coast Retina Medical Group, 1445 Bush St, San Francisco, CA 94109, USA

C.L. Shields · J.A. Shields
Ocular Oncology Service, Thomas Jefferson University, Philadelphia, PA, USA

C.L. Shields · J.A. Shields
Ocular Oncology Service, Wills Eye Hospital, Philadelphia, PA, USA

G.N. Papaliodis (ed.), *Uveitis*,
DOI 10.1007/978-3-319-09126-6_27

Table 27.1 Uveitis masquerade syndromes—classified by primary location of the inflammation

Non-neoplastic
Anterior
Corneal epithelial defects
Angle closure glaucoma
Pigment dispersion syndrome
Occult intraocular foreign body
Drug- and vaccine-induced uveitis
Juvenile xanthogranuloma[a]
Intermediate
Vitreous hemorrhage
Asteroid hyalosis
Retinitis pigmentosa
Amyloidosis
synchysis scintillans (cholesterolosis bulbi)
Posterior
Ocular ischemic syndrome
Central serous chorioretinopathy
Panuveitis
Scleritis
Rhegmatogenous retinal detachment (Schwartz-Matsu syndrome)
Neoplastic
Anterior
Iris/ciliary body metastasis
Leukemia[a]
Langerhans cell histiocytosis[a]
Iris stromal cyst leakage or rupture[a]
Intermediate
Primary vitreoretinal lymphoma
Posterior
Choroidal lymphoma
Choroidal melanoma
Choroidal metastasis
Retinal metastasis
Paraneopastic syndromes (CAR, MAR, AEPPVM, BDUMP)
Panuveitis
Retinoblastoma[a]

CAR cancer-associated retinopathy; *MAR* melanoma associated retinopathy; *BDUMP* bilateral diffuse uveal melanocytic proliferation; *AEPPVM* acute exudative paraneoplastic polymorphous vitelliform maculopathy
[a]Occur more often in Children

corneal dystrophy, or following surgery. It is important to rule out an active infection in such patients.

Primary Acute Angle Closure

Primary acute closure of the anterior chamber angle can produce anterior chamber inflammation associated with elevated intraocular pressure [24, 25], which together can be confused for inflammatory ocular hypertensive syndrome (IOHS) of the sort seen in patients with herpetic anterior uveitis due to herpes simplex, varicella, or cytomegalovirus, sarcoidosis, toxoplasmic retinochoroiditis, and syphilis [26]. Careful examination of the fellow eye can reveal clues to the diagnosis, including an at-risk angle structure and evidence of prior angle closure attacks, such as glaucomflecken on the anterior lens capsule. Unlike IOHS, the anterior chamber inflammation seen in primary acute angle closure tends to resolve promptly with normalization of intraocular pressure (IOP). The prevalence of angle closure is higher in Asians and Asian Indians than in European and Western populations.

Pigment Dispersion Syndrome

Free-floating pigment in the anterior chamber can be mistaken for inflammatory cells. This occurs most commonly in patients with pigment dispersion syndrome (PDS), pigmentary glaucoma, or pigment release following anterior chamber surgery or laser treatment. Pigment dispersion syndrome, in particular, can be confused with chronic anterior uveitis [27]. While high-power slitlamp biomicroscopy can usually distinguish fine, copper-color pigment particles from slightly larger and non-pigmented leukocytes (Fig. 27.1), additional clues that support a diagnosis of PDS include backward bowing of and/or radial slit- or wedge-like transillumination defects in the iris pigment epithelium, pigment deposition on the lens capsule, iris, trabecular meshwork, and corneal endothelium (Krukenberg spindle), and failure to improve following topical corticosteroid treatment. Intraocular pressure may or may not be elevated. Patients with PDS are often relatively young and myopic.

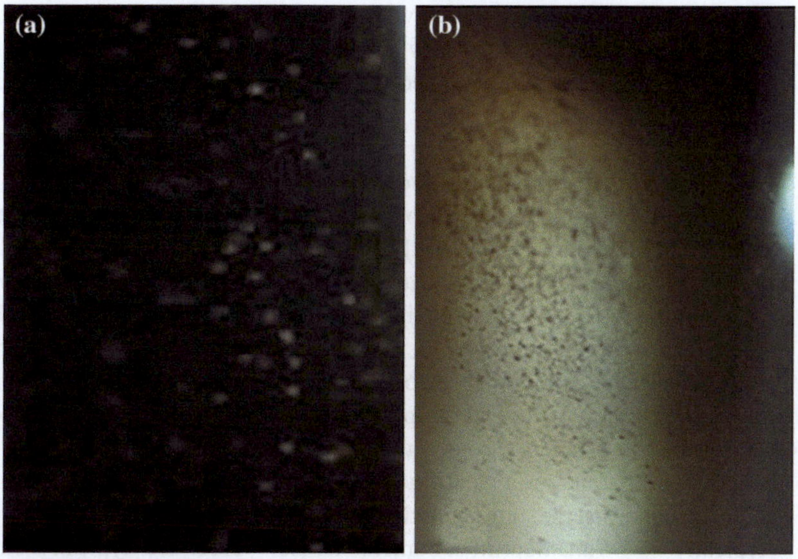

Fig. 27.1 High-power slitlamp biomicroscopic photographs of the mid-anterior chamber showing relatively larger, non-pigmented leukocytes in a patient with anterior uveitis (**a**) verses fine, copper-color pigment particles in a patient with pigment dispersion syndrome (**b**)

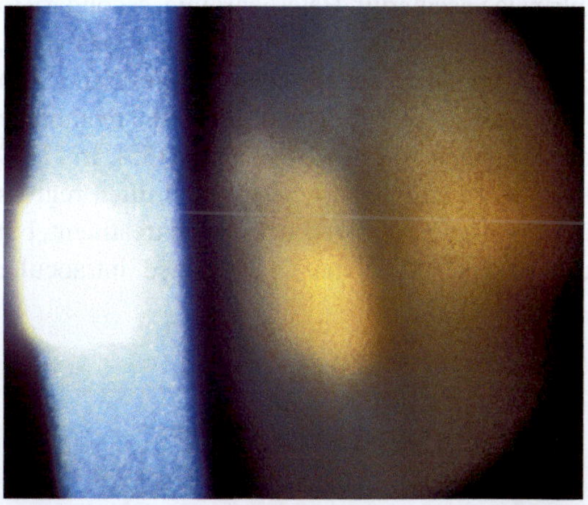

Fig. 27.2 High-power slitlamp biomicroscopic photograph showing rusty brown pigment on the anterior lens capsule in a patient with a retained piece of iron resulting in siderosis

Intraocular Foreign Body

Intraocular foreign bodies (IOFB) frequently produce some degree of intraocular inflammation. Traumatic endophthalmitis occurs in a high proportion of such patients and must be considered in the acute setting [28]. Less frequently, a retained IOFB may produce chronic uveitis, which is often only transiently or incompletely responsive to topical corticosteroids [29, 30]. A retained IOFB made of iron can produce the clinical syndrome known as ocular siderosis, which is characterized by deposition of rusty brown pigment on the lens capsule (Fig. 27.2), iris and cornea, mydriasis, pigmentary changes in the retina, attenuation of the retinal vessels, and either hyperemia, or palor of the optic disc, depending on duration. In contrast, a retained IOFB made of copper can produce ocular chalcosis, signs of which include a greenish-blue ring near the limbus (Kayser–Fleisher ring), a sunflower anterior subcapsular cataract, and metallic refractile particles in the anterior chamber and on the retina. A history or signs eye trauma can support the diagnosis. Professions and activities at greatest risk include those involving metal working and the use of motorized machines. Patients with retained IOFB tend to be young and male. Various imaging techniques have been used to locate occult IOFBs, including B-scan ultrasonography, X-rays, magnetic resonance imaging (MRI), and computed tomography (CT). Magnetic resonance imaging should be avoided in eyes suspected of a having a retained metallic IOFB because the IOFB can shift from the magnetic field and lead to ocular damage. High-resolution CT with thin cuts through the orbit is perhaps the most sensitive technique for identifying metal, stone, or glass, but can miss less radio-opaque objects. While listed here as primarily anterior uveitis, patients with retained IOFB may also have inflammatory cells in the vitreous. Some patients with retained IOFB have no active intraocular inflammation.

Drug- and Vaccine-Induced Uveitis

Although uncommon, a number of drugs and vaccines can induce uveitis [31, 32]. The mechanism(s) of drug-induced uveitis are generally unclear, although both toxic and inflammatory reactions have been suggested to play a role. Systemic agents commonly associated with ocular inflammation include the bisphosphonates—most notably pamidronate sodium, used to treat osteoporosis and to prevent fractures due to malignant bone disease; sulfonamide antibiotics—typically trimethoprim-sulfamethoxazole; tumor necrosis factor-alpha (TNF-α) inhibitors—most notably etanercept [33], and fluoroquinolone antibiotics—especially oral moxifloxacin and to a lesser extent ciprofloxacin [34]. Topical medications strongly implicated as causing uveitis in a minority of patients include the intraocular pressure lowering agents metopranolol, brimonidine, and the prostaglandin analogues. Intraocular agents associated with uveitis include cidofovir, used infrequently to treat viral retinitis, and the anti-vascular endothelial growth factor (VEGF) agents. Uveitis may also occur following vaccination, most notably with Bacille Calmette-Guerin (BCG).

Juvenile Xanthogranuloma

Juvenile xanthogranuloma (JXG) is an uncommon systemic histiocytosis associated with multiple cutaneous papules and, in 0.3–0.4 % of cases, ocular involvement. Infants and children are affected most commonly. While JXG lesions involving the orbit, eyelids and adnexa, conjunctiva, and both anterior and posterior segments have been described, the iris is the most frequently reported site (Fig. 27.3). Iris lesions in JXG are typically circumscribed, nodular, and yellow-white or orange in color—often with intrinsic vascularity. Heterochromia, secondary to recurrent hyphema, may or may not be present [1, 3–10]. Juvenile xanthogranuloma presenting as a more diffuse and transparent, epi-iridic membrane has also been described, but is rare [35]. Iris JXG lesions are intrinsically benign and often regress in response to topical corticosteroid treatment, but can produce hyphema and elevated intraocular

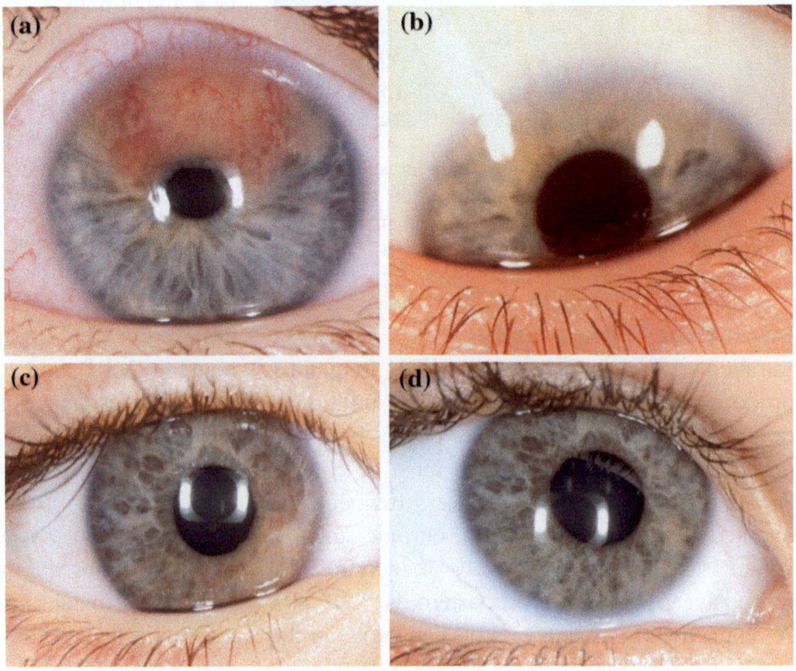

Fig. 27.3 Iris juvenile xanthogranuloma (JXG). Young child with visible iris JXG (**a**) with intense vascularity that responded to topical corticosteroids (**b**) over a 1 month period. Young child with ill-defined iris JXG (**c**) and stringy vascularity that responded to topical corticosteroids (**b**) over a 2 month period

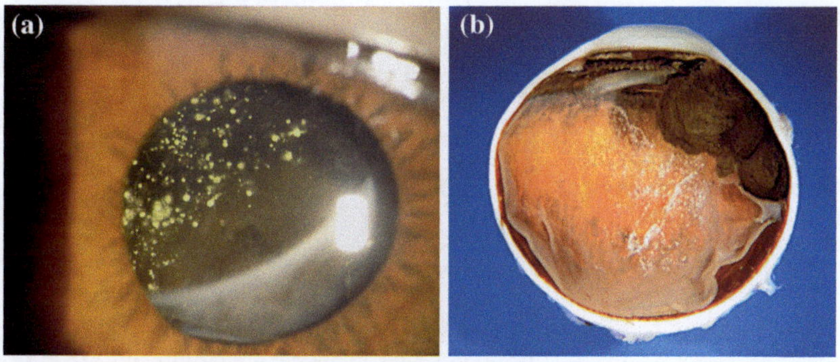

Fig. 27.4 Asteroid hyalosis (**a**) found coincidentally in an eye with uveal melanoma, shown on gross pathology (**b**) following enucleation

pressure requiring more aggressive treatment. Intra-cameral bevacizumab has been used recently with success [36, 37]. Children with JXG are at increased risk for both neurofibromatosis type 1 (NF1) and juvenile myelomonocytic leukemia (JMML) [35].

Intermediate Uveitis

Vitreous Hemorrhage

Vitreous hemorrhage occurs in a number of clinical settings, including patients with proliferative diabetic retinopathy, vitreous or retinal detachment, occlusive retinal vascular disease, intraocular tumors, and trauma [38, 39]. While the clinical recognition of red blood cells in patients with acute vitreous hemorrhage usually offers little challenge, red blood cells can, within one to three weeks, loose both their characteristic biconcave shape and hemoglobin, becoming smaller, round, tan-colored 'ghost cells' that may be mistaken for leukocytes. Elevated intraocular pressure that occurs in this setting is referred to as 'ghost cell glaucoma' or hemophthalmitis. Formation of a ghost cell pseudohypopyon has also been described [39].

Asteroid Hyalosis

Asteroid hyalosis is an age-related vitreous degeneration of unknown etiology, typically unilateral and more common in men and let common in eyes with posterior vitreous detachment [40] (Fig. 27.4). The characteristic aggregates are composed of calcium hydoxyapatite [41], and far larger than leukocytes, but when relatively few in number and distributed preferentially to the deep vitreous may be mistaken for leukocytes. Prolapse of vitreous hyalosis into the anterior chamber of either aphakic or pseudophakic eyes has been reported to mimic both endophthalmitis and an iris mass [42].

Retinitis Pigmentosa

Retinitis pigmentosa (RP) refers to a group of hereditary retinal degenerative disorders characterised by progressive loss of photoreceptors, visual field constriction, worsening night blindness, and decreased or abnormal electroretinographic findings. The condition is bilateral in most patients and is typically diagnoses in childhood or adolescence. Over time, most patients develop widespread disruption of the retinal pigment epithelium with bone spicule formation, arteriolar attenuation, and waxy pallor of the optic disc. Findings usually associated with uveitis, including anterior chamber cell, posterior subcapsular cataract, vitritis, macular edema, vasculitis, and epiretinal membrane formation are not uncommon [1, 3–10]. Geographic areas of RPE disruption, vascular narrowing, and optic atrophy can also occur following congenital infection by syphilis, toxoplasmosis, rubella, or one of the herpes viruses [43].

Amyloidosis

Amyloidosis refers to a heterogeneous group of disorders characterized by the production and tissue deposition of insoluble, fibrillar proteins known as amyloid. Over two-dozen individual proteins are

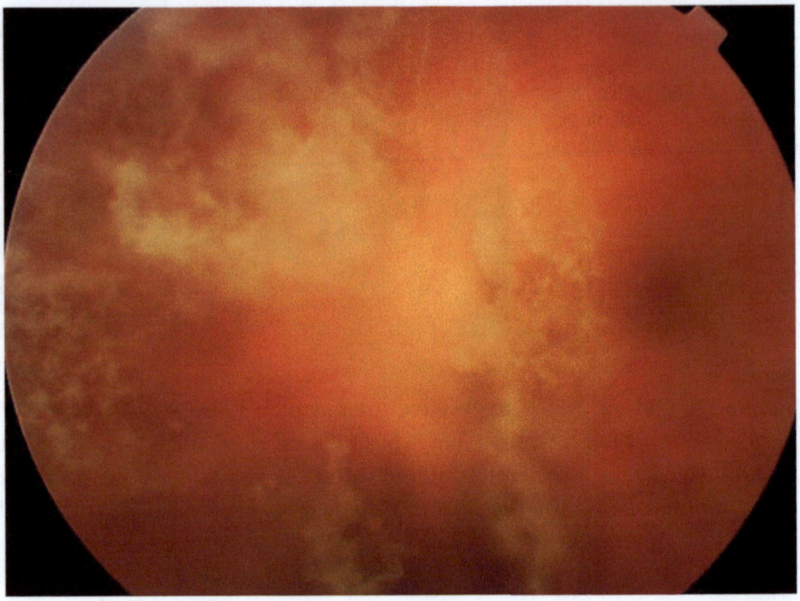

Fig. 27.5 Color fundus photograph of a patient with amyloidosis showing typical 'glass-wool' appearance. High-power slitlamp biomicroscopy of the anterior vitreous would reveal a conspicuous absence of vitreous cells

capable of producing amyloidosis in humans. While the proteins themselves are different, the protein aggregates in amyloidosis share a common beta-pleated sheet configuration. Vitreous amyloidosis, a rare condition that usually occurs in the setting of a hereditary condition known as familial amyloidotic polyneuropathy (FAP), can mimic vitreous inflammation, but can be differentiated by a complete lack of cells and a its characteristically wispy, "glass-wool" appearance (Fig. 27.5). Histological analysis of the vitreous shows positive Congo Red dye staining with "apple-green" birefringence under polarized light [44].

Synchysis Scintillans (Cholesterolosis Bulbi)

Synchysis scintillans, also known as cholesterolosis bulbi, is a degenerative process of the vitreous characterized by the deposition of cholesterol crystals in the vitreous cavity. While synchysis scintillans can resemble vitritis, the particles in synchysis scintillans have a yellow, glisening appearance, whereas inflammatory cells in the vitreous tend to be more white in appearance and non-glisening. Cholesterol crystals in eyes with synchysis scintillans are typically quite mobile due to advance syneresis.

Posterior Uveitis

Ocular Ischemic Syndrome

Ocular ischemic syndrome (OIS) is an uncommon disorder caused by chronically decreased perfusion of the ophthalmic artery, most typically as a result of ipsilateral carotid artery disease and less frequently as a result of vasculitis. Common symptoms include decreased vision and pain. Anterior segment findings include chemosis, conjunctival or episcleral injection, anterior chamber inflammation, and rubeosis. Posterior segment findings include mild vitreous inflammation, retinal venous congestion, dot-blot hemorrhages in the mid-periphery, and neovascularization. Fluorescein angiography reveals delayed retinal and choroidal perfusion. Patients suspected of having OIS should undergo imaging of their carotid arteries and aortic arch, as well as testing for giant cell arteritis [45–47]. Rarely, OIS can occur as a complication of strabismus or scleral buckle surgery [19].

Central Serous Chorioretinopathy

Central serous chorioretinopathy (CSC) is characterized by relative choroidal hyperperfusion producing both retinal pigment epithelial and serous retinal detachments. Men are affected more commonly than woman and many patients have what has been described as a "type A personality" [48]. Serous retinal detachment similar to what is seen in patients with CSC is a well-recognized feature of ocular inflammatory disease, particularly uveitis caused by Vogt–Koyanagi–Harada (VKH) disease [15] and sympathetic ophthalmia [49], leading to occasional misdiagnosis [50, 51]. Whereas the detachments in patients with VKH disease and sympathetic ophthalmia are typically bilateral and invariably associated with vitreous cell, CSC tends to be unilateral and has no vitreous inflammation. In addition, fluorescein angiography of active CSC often reveals distinctive focal RPE leakage and, when chronic, can reveal RPE tracks known as 'guttering' that are due to the gravitational effects of persistent subretinal fluid. Corticosteroid administration is an important risk factor for the development of CSC and, infrequently, CSC can occur as a therapeutic complication in uveitis patients receiving corticosteroids [52].

Scleritis

Scleritis is an uncommon disorder characterized by inflammation of the sclera. Whereas anterior scleritis typically produces pain and redness, and is often associated with an underlying systemic vasculitis, pain is less common in posterior scleritis, which is most often idiopathic. Intraocular inflammation, or uveitis, occurs secondarily in approximately 25 % of patients with both anterior and posterior scleritis [53]. The scleral source of the uveitis can be overlooked if the anterior sclera is not examined thoroughly or, in the case of posterior scleritis, B-scan ultrasonography is not performed.

Rhegmatogenous Retinal Detachment (Schwartz-Matsu Syndrome)

Common symptoms of rhegmatogenous retinal detachment (RRD) include floaters, flashes (photopsias or phosphenes) and cloudy or decreased vision –symptoms similar to those experienced by patients with intermediate and posterior uveitis. To complicate matters further, hemorrhage, pigmented cells referred to as 'tobacco dust,' (Shafer's sign) and inflammation can all occur in eyes with RRD. It is important, therefore, that RRD be considered in all eyes with uveitis [1, 3–10]. A subset of patients with chronic RRD will develop ocular hypertension—a condition known as Schwartz-Matsu syndrome shown to be due to phagocytosed photoreceptor outer segments migrating to and obstructing the trabecular outflow channels [54, 55]. Retinal breaks in patients with Schwartz-Matsu syndrome are often anterior and difficult to localize.

Neoplastic Masquerade Syndromes

Anterior Uveitis

Iris/Ciliary Body Metastasis

Metastasis to the eye is the most common cause of ocular malignancy, occurring in approximately 5–25 % of cancers as a function of both cancer type and stage. Most metastases involve the uveal tract, with the choroid comprising roughly 90 % and iris/ciliary body metastasis constituting the remaining 10 %. Breast and lung cancer are the most common primary sites, with breast cancer tending to occur later in the course of disease, once the diagnosis is established, and lung cancer tending to metastasis earlier (Fig. 27.6). Lung cancer is currently the most common source of iris and ciliary body metastases [3, 8, 10–12]. In a large analysis of 104 patients with iris metastases, the primary malignancy arose from cancer of the breast (33 %), lung (27 %), or skin (melanoma) (12 %) [56]. Systemic lymphoma, often aggressive, can also metastasis to the iris. Most lymphomatous iris lesions are B-cell in origin [57]. Anterior chamber inflammation occurs in approximately half of all patients with iris/ciliary body metastasis. Iris neovascularization, hyphema, and ocular hypertension can also occur. Gonioscopy and ultrasonography are important for identifying metastatic lesions as the source of anterior chamber inflammation or hyphema. Fine needle aspiration biopsy and cytopathology can be used to confirm the diagnosis in cases where the diagnosis is uncertain.

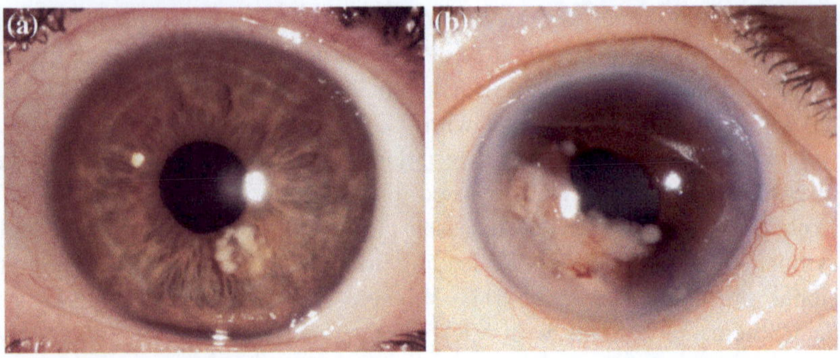

Fig. 27.6 Iris metastasis from breast cancer (**a**, **b**) in two different patients, simulating anterior uveitis

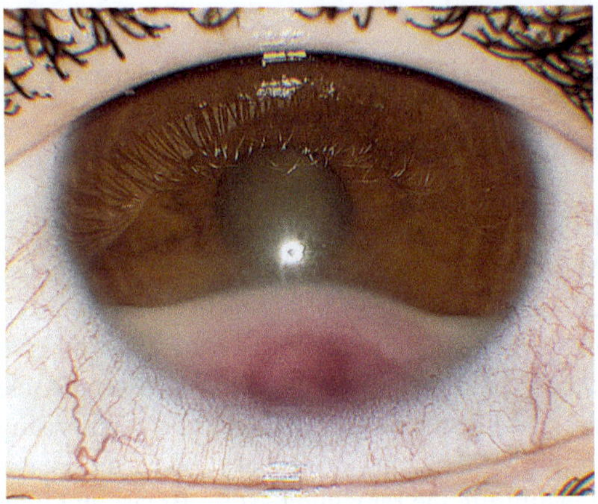

Fig. 27.7 A hemorrhagic, or 'pink' hypopyon in a patient with recurrent acute lymphocytic leukemia (ALL)

Leukemia

Hematopoietic stem cell malignancies are known as leukemias, and may be either acute or chronic, and either lymphocytic or myelocytic. The acute leukemias tend to be comprised of less mature cells and, consequently, are more often aggressive and more likely to involve the eye. While leukemic cells frequently infiltrate the retina and choroid producing leukemic retinopathy and choroidopathy, respectively, these presentations are infrequently mistaken for uveitis. Iris and anterior segment involvement, in contrast, can be confused for uveitis, as the most common signs are iritis and hypopyon, often associated with hyphema, producing a so-called 'pink hypopyon' (Fig. 27.7). While iris and anterior segment involvement can be the presenting sign of leukemia, it is more often a sign of relapse [3, 8, 10–12]. All patients with a known history of leukemia who develop anterior chamber inflammation should be considered to have a leukemic relapse until proven otherwise.

Langerhans Cell Histiocytosis

Langerhans Cell Histiocytosis (LCH) is a proliferative disorder of the bone marrow-derived histiocytic cell, the Langerhans cell. Langerhans cell histiocytosis is believed to be either an immune dysregulation or a neoplastic disorder. This condition can be unifocal or multifocal and may affect the skin, bone, other tissues, and the eye. With ocular involvement, there is generally a solid mass of Langerhans cells with overlying free-floating cells in the aqueous or vitreous [58]. While history may suggest LCH as the cause of intraocular cells, definitive diagnosis often requires fine needle aspiration biopsy. Langerhans cells display the unique feature of CD1a positivity on immunostaining. Management involves either systemic chemotherapy or local radiotherapy.

Iris Stromal Cyst

Iris stromal cyst is a translucent mass that typically arises on the iris surface, resulting from aberrant implantation of corneal or conjunctival epithelium inside the eye. Occasionally, the cyst can leak, leading to severe photophobia with anterior chamber cell and flare. In some cases, the cyst can rupture, producing severe anterior uveitis with or without hypopyon formation, an intense fibrin reaction, and high IOP [59]. Topical or subTenon's corticosteroids or anterior chamber washout can be helpful.

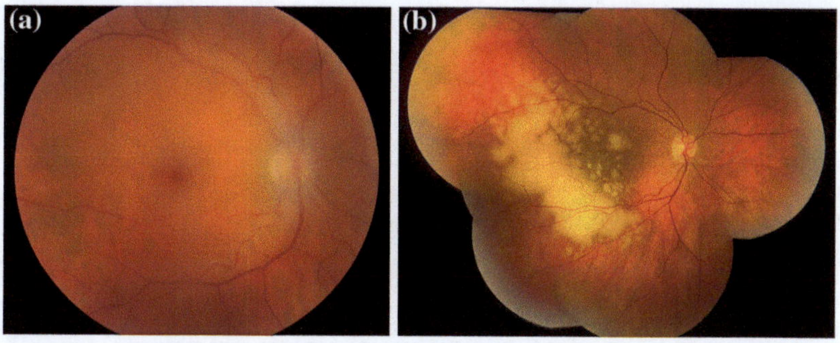

Fig. 27.8 Vitreoretinal lymphoma with primarily vitreous cells (**a**) in one patient and sub retinal pigment epithelial tumor (**b**) in another patient

Intermediate Uveitis

Primary Vitreoretinal Lymphoma

Primary vitreoretinal lymphoma (PVRL) is an uncommon non-Hodgkin's lymphoma, most often B-cell in origin that can involve the vitreous, retina, and/or optic nerve. Primary iris and ciliary involvement also occurs, but is uncommon. Findings are frequently bilateral. Approximately 80 % of patients who present with PVRL eventually develop central nervous system involvement, whereas about 20 % of central nervous system involvement also has PVRL. Fifty percent of patients with PVRL are over 60 year of age and men outnumber women. Suggestive clinical findings include abnormal sheets or clumps of vitreous cells and the presence of subretinal pigment epithelial (subRPE) infiltrates (Fig. 27.8). Some degree of anterior chamber inflammation is typically present. It should be noted, however, that most patients over 60 years of age with chronic vitritis do not have lymphoma. Infection by HIV dramatically increases the risk of PVRL. Patients suspected of having PVRL should undergo MRI of the brain with contrast and cerebrospinal fluid analysis for cytology. If these tests are negative, vitreous and/or retinal biopsy should be considered [60].

Posterior Uveitis

Uveal Lymphoma

Like PVRL, lymphomatous involvement of the uveal tract is typically non-Hodgkin's in type and B-cell in origin. Unlike PVRL, however, uveal lymphoma is often composed of extranodal marginal zone B-cells, and hence tends to be indolent, is frequently unilateral, and associated with systemic lymphoma in approximately 20–30 % of patients. The occurrence of central nervous system lymphoma in patients with uveal lymphoma is rare. More than half of all patients with uveal lymphoma are over 65, and it is uncommon for patients to be less than 40 years of age. Choroidal lymphomas occur more frequently than lymphomatous involvement of the iris and ciliary body and are characterized most typically by either multifocal choroidal infiltrates similar in size and appearance to those seen in patient with birdshot chorioretinopathy or sarcoid involvement of the choroid, or by diffuse choroidal thickening. Both anterior and posterior episcleral extension are common, occurring in up to 50 % of patients. Patients suspected of having uveal lymphoma should undergo thorough visual inspection of the anterior episcleral surface for the classic "salmon patch" infiltration of lymphoma, followed by B-scan ultrasonography of the posterior episcleral surface, to rule out episcleral extension. When identified, such episcleral lesions provide a good site for biopsy. A CBC with differential should also be performed and consideration should also be given to full body CT or CT-PET imaging to rule out systemic lymphoma [60, 61].

Uveal Melanoma

Uveal melanoma results from malignant proliferation of uveal melanocytes and is typically focal. Involvement of the choroid is much more

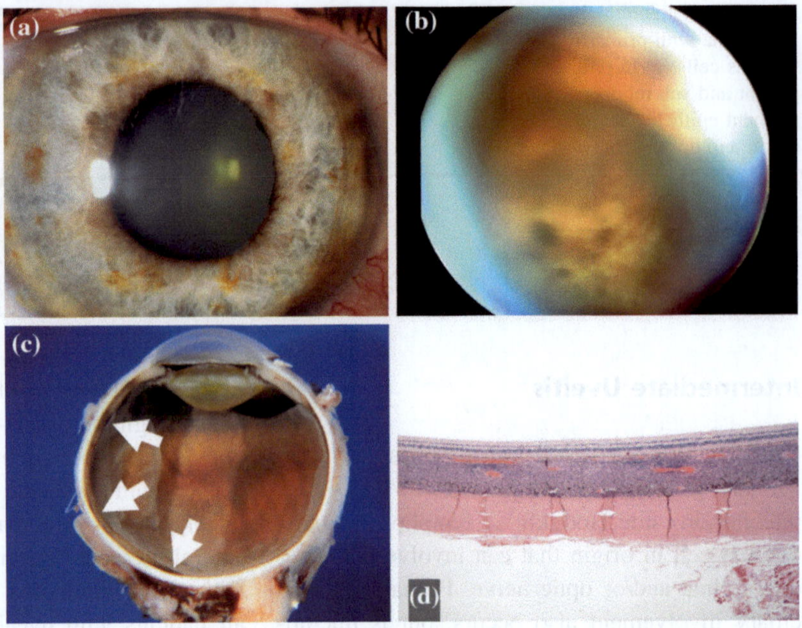

Fig. 27.9 Diffuse choroidal melanoma followed for presumed chronic uveitis for several months. Note the iris pigmentation near the angle (**a**), poor view of a pigmented choroidal mass (**b**), flat appearance on gross pathology (**c**), and thickened choroidal infiltration of melanoma on histopathology (D)

common than the ciliary body or iris Diffuse uveal melanoma also occurs, but is rare [62] (Fig. 27.9). Uveal melanomas tend to occur after age 40, and are much more common in Caucasians than either African Americans or Asians. Approximately 5 % of patients with uveal melanoma have anterior chamber or vitreous inflammation that may mimic primary uveitis. Moreover, lightly pigmented or amelanotic lesions can resemble choroidal granulomas. Patients suspected of having uveal melanoma should undergo ultrasonography and be considered for fine needle aspiration biopsy followed by melanoma treatment [63, 64].

Choroidal Metastasis

As with anterior uveal metastases, breast, and lung cancer are the most common primary sources for choroidal metastasis. At presentation, choroidal metastases are typically yellow- or gray-white in appearance, two or more disc-diameters in size, multiple, and bilateral; although solitary, unilateral lesions also occur. Serous detachment of the overlying retina is common. As with amelanotic uveal melanoma, such lesions can be mistaken for choroidal granulomas, scleritis, or other inflammatory processes, particularly when anterior chamber or vitreous cells are present (Fig. 27.10). Choroidal lesions occurring in patients with a history of cancer should be considered to be metastases until proven otherwise. Multimodal imaging and ultrasonography can aid in distinguishing choroidal metastasis from amelanotic uveal melanoma and choroiditis. The diagnosis can be confirmed by biopsy as indicated [65].

Retinal Metastasis

Metastases to the retina are rare, constituting less than 1 % of ocular involvement by systemic malignancies. Cutaneous melanoma, breast, and lung cancer are the most frequently reported primary sites. Lesions are typically unilateral, solitary, yellow- or gray-white, and flat—resembling infectious retinitis (Fig. 27.11). Vitreous seeding and serous retinal detachment can occur, further complicating the clinical presentation. A history of metastatic cancer usually suggests the diagnosis, which can be confirmed by biopsy if necessary [66].

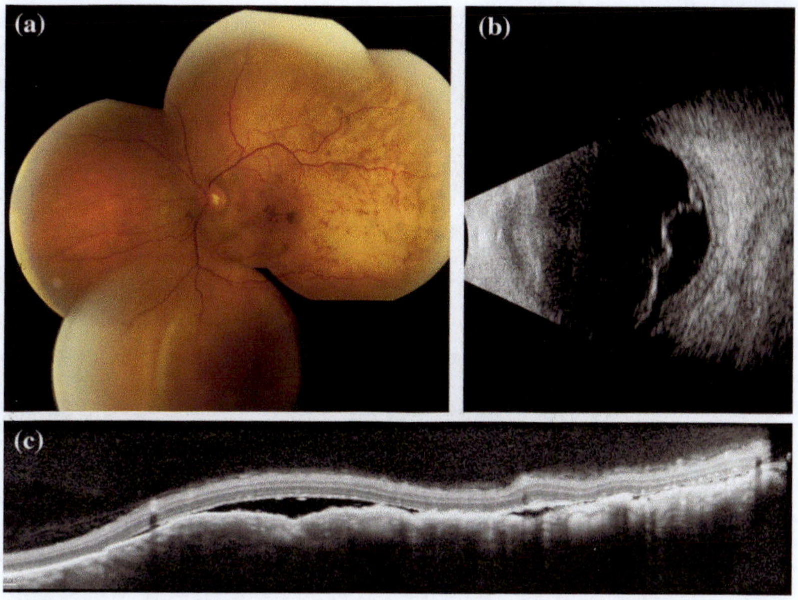

Fig. 27.10 Choroidal metastasis (**a**) follow for 8 months as atypical uveal inflammation but later found to be diffuse metastasis with serous retinal detachment on ultrasonography (**b**) and optical coherence tomography (**c**) and with the classic "lumpy bumpy" surface of choroidal metastasis (**c**)

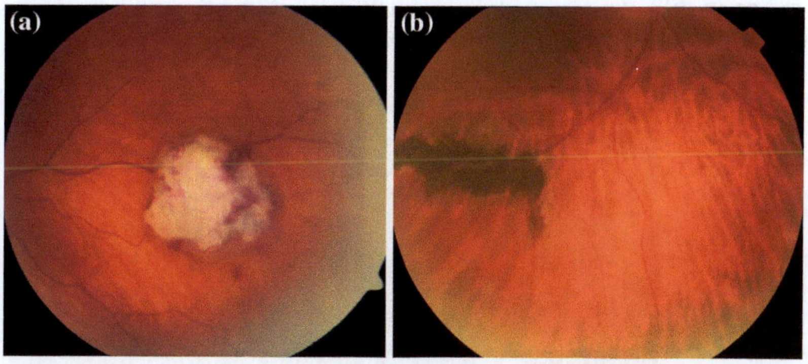

Fig. 27.11 Retinal metastasis from lung cancer (**a**) in one patient and cutaneous melanoma (**b**) in another patient simulating retinitis

Paraneopastic Syndromes (CAR, MAR, AEPPVM, BDUMP)

Symptoms and signs of outer retinal degeneration due to tumor-induced anti-retinal antibody formation can occur in the setting of systemic malignancy and has been termed cancer-associated retinopathy (CAR). Most patients with CAR have a small cell lung carcinoma as the primary site, although findings typical of CAR have been described in the setting of other cancers, including cutaneous melanoma, in which case the syndrome is referred to as melanoma associated retinopathy (MAR). Vision loss can be rapid, often pre-dates the diagnosis of cancer, and is frequently associated with nyctalopia and positive visual symptoms, such halos, shimmering, and photopsias. Examination of the anterior segment is often unremarkable. Vitreous inflammation may be present, but is typically mild. The fundus per se is often normal, but can show arteriolar narrowing and atrophy of the optic disc over time. Abnormal electroretinographic testing and identification of anti-retinal antibodies support the diagnosis, but even with these results it can sometimes be difficult to distinguish CAR from other causes of diffuse outer retinal disfunction, most notably acute zonal occult outer retinopathy (AZOOR). Of the nearly twenty retinal antigens implicated in CAR, anti-recovering and anti-α-enolase

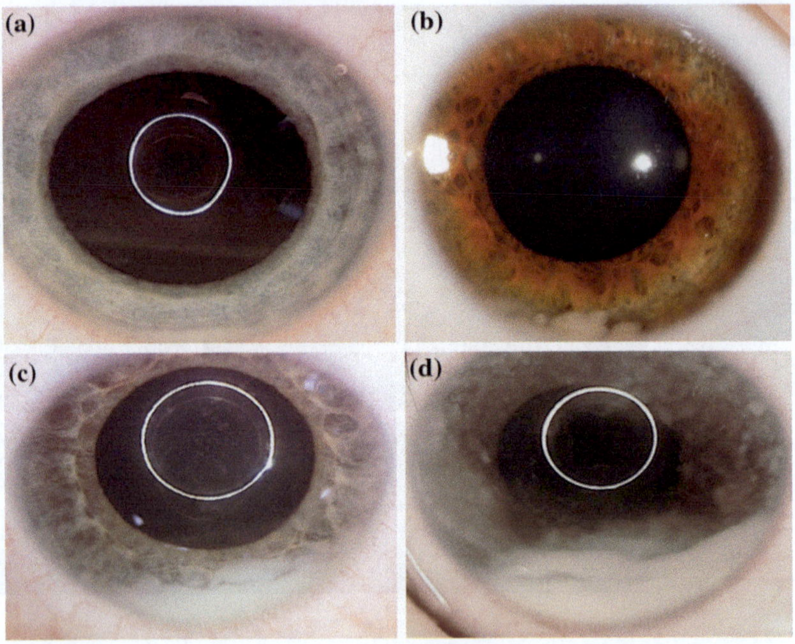

Fig. 27.12 Retinoblastoma in the anterior chamber in four different patients demonstrating mild (**a**), moderate (**b**), advanced (**c**), and severe (**d**) involvement. All eyes came to enucleation

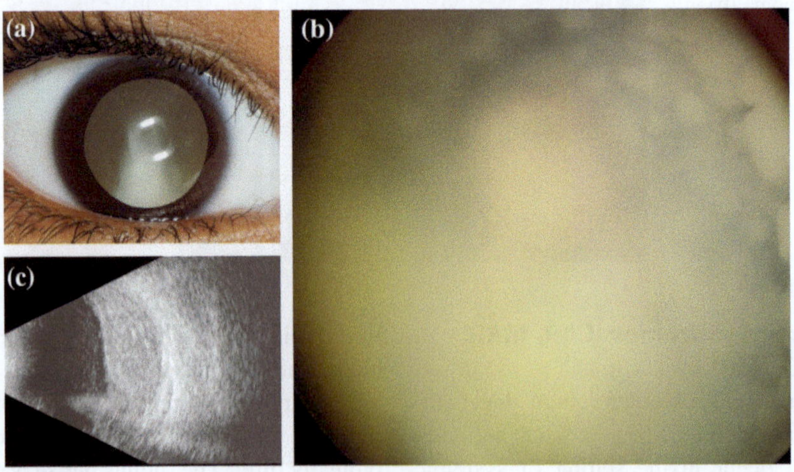

Fig. 27.13 Eight-year-old girl with retinoblastoma who was treated for chronic unrelenting uveitis for several months demonstrating white vitreous neoplastic cells on external (**a**) and posterior segment (**b**) examination with no view of the retina. Ultrasound (**c**) shows minimally calcified, extensive retinoblastoma

provide the strongest support for the diagnosis. In addition to the signs of MAR described above, melanoma has also been associated with an Acute Exudative Paraneoplastic Polymorphous Vitelliform Maculopathy (AEPPVM) that can mimic PVRL, as well as a Vogt–Koyanagi–Harada (VKH) -like syndrome. Bilateral Diffuse Uveal Melanocytic Proliferation (BDUMP) is a rare related paraneoplastic syndrome characterized by the occurrence of polygonal patches of RPE atrophy surrounded by aggregates of hypertrophied RPE cells—so-called "giraffe pattern", diffuse thickening of the uveal tract, and rapidly progressive cataracts. Heavily pigmented melanocytes are found in the choroid underlying areas of RPE atrophy. Identification of the associated malignancy in patients with BDUMP is often delayed for many months. Reproductive tract malignancies associated are common in women with BDUMP, whereas lung, pancreas and colon carcinomas have been reported in men [67].

Panuveitis

Retinoblastoma

Retinoblastoma is an ocular tumor composed of photoreceptor precursor cells. Retinoblastoma is the most common intraocular cancer in children, presenting almost always prior to five years of age. Diffuse infiltrating retinoblastoma tends to occur in older children and presents with diffuse vitreous neoplastic cells with flat retinal infiltration and often no classic solid retinoblastoma tumor, simulating uveitis or retinitis [68]. Approximately one-third of tumors are bilateral. Common reasons for referral include leukocoria and strabismus. True intraocular inflammation, while uncommon, can occur in eyes with retinoblastoma in response to tumor necrosis. Pseudo inflammation is perhaps more common and is produced by seeding of the aqueous and vitreous by tumor cells (Figs. 27.12 and 27.13). Anterior chamber seeding, in particular, can mimic granulomatous uveitis and, when dense, produce a pseudohypopyon—which is typically gray-white in appearance and characterized by irregular or lumpy layering. Conversely, both toxocariasis and toxoplasmosis can mimic retinoblastoma [69].

Summary

A number of ocular and systemic diseases can masquerade as uveitis, both in children and adults. These conditions include both non-neoplastic diseases—such as angle closure glaucoma, pigment dispersion syndrome, JXG, and others, as well as neoplastic conditions—such as vitreoretinal lymphoma, uveal metastasis, and retinoblastoma. Masquerade syndromes should be considered in all patients with uveitis, but particularly when clinical findings and/or response to therapy are suggestive.

References

1. Moorthy RS, Valluri S. Masquerade syndromes. American Academy of Ophthalmology, Focal Points 2013, vol XXXI, no 8 (Module 2 of 3).
2. Jones N. Masquerade syndromes. In: Uveitis. 2nd ed. London: Jaypee Brothers Medical Publishers; 2013 p. 337–348 (chapter 20).
3. Waheed NK, Foster CS. Masquerade syndromes: malignancies. In: Foster CS, Vitale AT, editors. Diagnosis & treatment of uveitis. 2nd ed. London: Jaypee Brothers Medical Publishers; 2013. p. 705–735 (chapter 51).
4. Palafox K, Foster CS. Nonmalignant, noninfectious, masquerade syndromes In: Foster CS and Vitale AT. Editors. Diagnosis & treatment of uveitis. 2nd ed. London: Jaypee Brothers Medical Publishers; 2013. p. 750–789 (chapter 53).
5. Whitcup SM. Masquerade syndromes. In: Nussenblatt RB, Whitcup SM, editors. Uveitis. Fundamentals and clinical practice. 4th ed. New York: Mosby Elsevier; 2010. p. 401–410 (chapter 30).
6. Shields JA, Shields CL. Intraocular tumors: an atlas and textbook. 2nd ed. Philadelphia: Lippincott, Williams & Wilkins;2008.
7. Madigan WP, Raymond WR, Wroblewski KJ, Thebpatiphat N, Birdsong RH, Jaafar MS. A review of pediatric uveitis: Part I. Infectious causes and the masquerade syndromes. J Pediatr Ophthalmol Strabismus. 2008;45(3):140–149.
8. Kubicka-Trzaska A, Romanowska-Dixon B. Malignant uveitis masquerade syndromes. Klin Oczna. 2008;110(4–6):199–202.
9. Kubicka-Trzaska A, Romanowska-Dixon B. Non-malignant uveitis masquerade syndromes. Klin Oczna. 2008;110(4–6):203–6.
10. Schüler A, Coupland SE, Krause L, Bornfeld N. Malignant and non-malignant uveitis-masquerade syndromes in childhood. Klin Monbl Augenheilkd. 2007;224(6):477–82.
11. Tsai T, O'Brien JM. Masquerade syndromes: malignancies mimicking inflammation in the eye. Int Ophthalmol Clin. 2002;42(1):115–31.
12. Read RW, Zamir E, Rao NA. Neoplastic masquerade syndromes. Surv Ophthalmol. 2002;47(2):81–124.
13. Grange LK, Kouchouk A, Dalal MD, Vitale S, Nussenblatt RB, Chan CC, Sen HN. Neoplastic masquerade syndromes in patients with uveitis. Am J Ophthalmol. 2014;157(3):526–31.

14. Ohguro N, Sonoda KH, Takeuchi M, Matsumura M, Mochizuki M. The 2009 prospective multi-center epidemiologic survey of uveitis in Japan. Jpn J Ophthalmol. 2012;56(5):432–5.
15. Rao NA, Gupta A, Dustin L, Chee SP, Okada AA, Khairallah M, Bodaghi B, Lehoang P, Accorinti M, Mochizuki M, Prabriputaloong T, Read RW. Frequency of distinguishing clinical features in Vogt-Koyanagi-Harada disease. Ophthalmology. 2010;117(3):591–9.
16. Rothova A, Ooijman F, Kerkhoff F, Van Der Lelij A, Lokhorst HM. Uveitis masquerade syndromes. Ophthalmology. 2001;108(2):386–99.
17. McCannel CA, Holland GN, Helm CJ, Cornell PJ, Winston JV, Rimmer TG. Causes of uveitis in the general practice of ophthalmology. UCLA Community-Based Uveitis Study Group. Am J Ophthalmol. 1996;121(1):35–46.
18. Diaz V, Samson CM, Foster CS. Masquerade syndromes: Endophthalmitis. In: Foster CS and Vitale AT, editors. Diagnosis & treatment of uveitis. 2nd ed. London: Jaypee Brothers Medical Publishers; 2013. p. 736–749 (chapter 52).
19. Doshi RR, Arevalo JF, Flynn HW Jr, Cunningham ET Jr. Evaluating exaggerated, prolonged, or delayed postoperative intraocular inflammation. Am J Ophthalmol. 2010;150(3):295–304.
20. Sun R, Gimbel HV. Corneal epithelial defect may affect anterior chamber flare. J Refract Surg. 1996;12(7):755.
21. Nishiwaki-Dantas, Maria Cristina; Abbott, Richard L; Dantas, Paulo Elias Correa; Hartong, Toby J. Sterile corneal epithelial defect associated with hypopyon. Arq Bras Oftalmol 1996;59(3):229–233.
22. Ionides ACW, Tuft SJ, Ferguson VMG, Matheson MM, Hykin PG. Corneal infiltration after recurrent corneal epithelial erosion. Br J Ophthalmol 1997;81:537–540.
23. Papathanassiou M, Gartry D. Sterile corneal ulcer with ring infiltrate and hypopyon after recurrent erosions. Eye. 2007;21:124–6.
24. Schwartz SD, Borchert M, Oberman A. Hypopyon keratouveitis in acute angle-closure glaucoma. Am J Ophthalmol. 1987;104(4):430–1.
25. Moorthy RS, Mermoud A, Baerveldt G, Minckler DS, Lee PP, Rao NA. Glaucoma associated with uveitis. Surv Ophthalmol. 1997;41(5):361–94.
26. Zelefsky JR, Cunningham ET Jr. Evaluation and management of elevated intraocular pressure in patients with uveitis. American Academy of Ophthalmology. Focal Points, June 2010.
27. Gonzalez-Gonzalez LA, Rodríguez-García A, Foster CS. Pigment dispersion syndrome masquerading as acute anterior uveitis. Ocul Immunol Inflamm. 2011;19(3):158–66.
28. Palioura S, Eliott D. Traumatic endophthalmitis, retinal detachment, and metallosis after intraocular foreign body injuries. Int Ophthalmol Clin. 2013;53(4):93–104.
29. Mete G, Turgut Y, Osman A, Gülşen U, Hakan A. Anterior segment intraocular metallic foreign body causing chronic hypopyon uveitis. J Ophthalmic Inflamm Infect. 2011;1(2):85–7.
30. Sychev YV, Verner-Cole EA, Suhler EB, Stout JT, Vemulakonda GA. Occult nonmetallic intraocular foreign bodies presenting as fulminant uveitis: a case series and review of the literature. Clin Ophthalmol. 2013;7:1747–51.
31. Moorthy RS, London NJ, Garg SJ, Cunningham ET Jr. Drug-induced uveitis. Curr Opin Ophthalmol. 2013;24(6):589–97.
32. London NJ, Garg SJ, Moorthy RS, Cunningham ET Jr. Drug-induced uveitis. J Ophthalmic Inflamm Infect. 2013;3(1):43.
33. Cunningham ET Jr, Pasadhika S, Suhler EB, Zierhut M. Drug-induced inflammation in patients on TNFα inhibitors. Ocul Immunol Inflamm. 2012;20(1):2–5.
34. Eadie B, Etminan M, Mikelberg FS. Risk for uveitis with oral moxifloxacin: a comparative safety study. JAMA Ophthalmol. 2014 Oct 2. doi:10.1001/jamaophthalmol.2014.3598. [Epub ahead of print].
35. Manjandavida FP, Arepalli S, Tarlan B, Shields CL. Optical coherence tomography characteristics of epi-iridic membrane in a child with recurrent hyphema and presumed juvenile xanthogranuloma. J AAPOS. 2014;18(1):93–5.
36. Shields CL, Hogarty MD, Kligman BE, Christian C, Ehya H, Shields JA. Langerhans cell histiocytosis of the uvea with neovascular glaucoma: diagnosis by fine-needle aspiration biopsy and management with intraocular bevacizumab and brachytherapy. J AAPOS. 2010;14(6):534–7.
37. Ashkenazy N, Henry CR, Abbey AM, McKeown CA, Berrocal AM, Murray TG. Successful treatment of juvenile xanthogranuloma using bevacizumab. J AAPOS. 2014;18(3):295–7.
38. Goff MJ, McDonald HR, Johnson RN, Ai E, Jumper JM, Fu AD. Causes and treatment of vitreous hemorrhage. Compr Ophthalmol Update. 2006;7(3):97–111.
39. Spraul CW, Grossniklaus HE. Vitreous Hemorrhage. Surv Ophthalmol. 1997;42(1):3–39.
40. Fawzi AA, Vo B, Kriwanek R, Ramkumar HL, Cha C, Carts A, Heckenlively JR, Foos RY, Glasgow BJ. Asteroid hyalosis in an autopsy population: The University of California at Los Angeles (UCLA) experience. Arch Ophthalmol. 2005;123(4):486–90.
41. Winkler J, Lünsdorf H. Ultrastructure and composition of asteroid bodies. Invest Ophthalmol Vis Sci. 2001;42(5):902–7.
42. Shields CL, Romanelli-Gobbi M, Lally SE, Shields JA. Vitreous asteroid hyalosis prolapse into the anterior chamber simulating iris metastasis. Middle East Afr J Ophthalmol. 2012;19(3):346–8.
43. Mets MB, Chhabra MS. Eye manifestations of intrauterine infections and their impact on childhood blindness. Surv Ophthalmol. 2008;53(2):95–111.

44. Roe RH, Fisher Y, Eagle RC Jr, Fine HF, Cunningham ET Jr. Oculoleptomeningeal amyloidosis in a patient with a TTR Val30Gly mutation in the transthyretin gene. Ophthalmology. 2007;114(11): e33–7.
45. Brown GC, Green WR. The ocular ischemic syndrome. Curr Opin Ophthalmol. 1994;5:14–20.
46. Mizener JB, Podhajsky P, Hayreh SS. Ocular ischemic syndrome. Ophthalmology. 1997;104:859–64.
47. Mendrinos E, Machinis TG, Pournaras CJ. Ocular ischemic syndrome. Surv Ophthalmol. 2010;55:2–34.
48. Nicholson B, Noble J, Forooghian F, Meyerle C. Central serous chorioretinopathy: update on pathophysiology and treatment. Surv Ophthalmol. 2013;58 (2):103–26.
49. Castiblanco CP, Adelman RA. Sympathetic ophthalmia. Graefes Arch Clin Exp Ophthalmol. 2009;247(3):289–302.
50. Arantes TE, Garcia CR, Rossi MR, Muccioli C. Spectral domain optical coherence tomography and angiographic findings in central serous chorioretinopathy complicated by bilateral nonrhegmatogenous retinal detachment associated with systemic corticosteroids. Ocul Immunol Inflamm. 2009;17(5):316–8.
51. Yang P, Ren Y, Li B, Fang W, Meng Q, Kijlstra A. Clinical characteristics of Vogt-Koyanagi-Harada syndrome in Chinese patients. Ophthalmology. 2007;114(3):606–14.
52. Khairallah M, Kahloun R, Tugal-Tutkun I. Central serous chorioretinopathy, corticosteroids, and uveitis. Ocul Immunol Inflamm. 2012;20(2):76–85.
53. Gonzalez-Gonzalez LA, Molina-Prat N, Doctor P, Tauber J, Sainz de la Maza M, Foster CS. Clinical features and presentation of posterior scleritis: a report of 31 cases. Ocul Immunol Inflamm. 2014;22 (3):203–207.
54. Schwartz A. Chronic open-angle glaucoma secondary to rhegmatogenous retinal detachment. Am J Ophthalmol. 1973;75(2):205–11.
55. Matsuo N, Takabatake M, Ueno H, Nakayama T, Matsuo T. Photoreceptor outer segments in the aqueous humor in rhegmatogenous retinal detachment. Am J Ophthalmol. 1986;101(6):673–9.
56. Shields CL, Kaliki S, Crabtree GS, Peshtani A, Morton S, Anand RA, Coco G, Shields JA. Iris metastasis from systemic cancer in 104 patients: the 2014 Jerry A Shields Lecture. Cornea. 2015;34 (1):42–8.
57. Mashayekhi A, Shields CL, Shields JA. Iris involvement by lymphoma: a review of 13 cases. Clin Exp Ophthalmol. 2013;41(1):19–26.
58. Shields CL, Hogarty MD, Kligman, et al. Langerhans cell histiocytosis of the uvea with neovascular glaucoma. Diagnosis by needle biopsy and management with intraocular bevacizumab and brachytherapy. J Am Assoc Ped Ophthalm Strab 2010;14 (6):534–537.
59. Shields CL, Arepalli S, Lally SE, Lally EB, Shields JA. Iris stromal cyst management with absolute alcohol-induced sclerosis in 16 patients. JAMA Ophthamol. 2014;132:703–8.
60. Chan C-C, Sen HN. Current concepts in diagnosing and managing primary vitreoretinal (intraocular) lymphoma. Discov Med. 2013;15(81):93–100.
61. Mashayekhi A, Shukla SY, Shields JA, Shields CL. Choroidal lymphoma: clinical features and association with systemic lymphoma. Ophthalmology. 2014;121(1):342–51.
62. Shields CL, Kaliki S, Furuta M, Shields JA. Diffuse versus non-diffuse small (<3 millimeters thickness) choroidal melanoma: comparative analysis in 1751 cases. The 2012 F. Phinizy Calhoun Lecture 2012. Retina. 2013;33:1763–76.
63. Aronow ME, Portell CA, Sweetenham JW, Singh AD. Uveal lymphoma: clinical features, diagnostic studies, treatment selection, and outcomes. Ophthalmology. 2014;121(1):334–41.
64. Shields CL, Manalac J, Das C, Ferguson K, Shields JA. Choroidal melanoma: clinical features, classification, and top 10 pseudomelanomas. Curr Opin Ophthalmol. 2014;25(3):177–85.
65. Shields CL, Shields JA, Gross NE, Schwartz GP, Lally SE. Survey of 520 eyes with uveal metastases. Ophthalmology. 1997;104(8):1265–76.
66. Shields CL, McMahon JF, Atalay HT, Hasanreisoglu M, Shields JA. Retinal metastasis from systemic cancer in 8 cases. JAMA Ophthalmol. 2014 Jul 17.
67. Rahimy E, Sarraf D. Paraneoplastic and non-paraneoplastic retinopathy and optic neuropathy: evaluation and management. Surv Ophthalmol. 2013;58(5):430–58.
68. Shields CL, Ghassemi F, Tuncer S, Thangappan A, Shields JA. Clinical spectrum of diffuse infiltrating retinoblastoma in 34 consecutive eyes. Ophthalmology. 2008;115:2253–8.
69. Shields CL, Fulco EM, Arias JD, Alarcon C, Pellegrini M, Rishi P, Kaliki S, Bianciotto CG, Shields JA. Retinoblastoma frontiers with intravenous, intra-arterial, periocular, and intravitreal chemotherapy. Eye (Lond). 2013;27(2):253–64.

Medication Induced

28

George N. Papaliodis

Introduction

Medication- or drug-induced uveitis is a relatively rare adverse effect related to drug administration. The potential offending agents can be administered systemically, intraocularly, or topically. The frequency of drug administration leading to intraocular inflammation is difficult to establish. In a series by Fraunfelder et al. [1] at a large tertiary referral uveitis clinic, medication-associated uveitis represented 0.5 % of cases. Many agents have been potentially implicated with sparse supporting data to confirm the observation. In 1981, Naranjo and colleagues published a series of criteria which should be fulfilled to ascribe causality of adverse effects to drugs [2] including:

1. The reaction is frequently described and documented
2. Recovery from symptoms occurs when the drug is tapered or discontinued
3. Other causes for symptoms have been excluded
4. Symptoms worsen when the dose of the drug is increased
5. The adverse event is documented by objective evidence
6. Similar effects occur in a patient with similar drugs
7. Symptoms recur with rechallenge of the suspected drug

Based on the number of fulfilled criteria, Naranjo stratified the adverse effect as certain, probable, possible, or unlikely.

Clinical Characteristics

With rare exception, drug-induced uveitis is generally mild to moderate in severity. The intraocular inflammation is usually non-granulomatous and may involve the anterior and posterior segments of the eye. Visual acuity typically correlates with the degree of intraocular inflammation. The treatment of choice for these events is cessation of the offending agent. The associated ocular inflammation generally responds well to the topical administration of corticosteroids for iritis and systemic corticosteroids for posterior segment inflammation. Table 28.1 represents medications that have been stratified as definite or probable by the Naranjo algorithm.

G.N. Papaliodis (✉)
Department of Ophthalmology, Harvard Medical School, Massachusetts Eye and Ear Infirmary, 243 Charles Street, Boston, MA 02114, USA
e-mail: George_Papaliodis@meei.harvard.edu

G.N. Papaliodis (ed.), *Uveitis*,
DOI 10.1007/978-3-319-09126-6_28

Table 28.1 Medications

Systemic drugs	Type of Uveitis/Severity
Bisphosphonates (alendronate [8], ibandronate, risedronate, zoledronic acid [9], pamidronate [7])	Anterior uveitis (mild to severe)
Cidofovir [5, 6]	Anterior uveitis (mild to severe)
Diethylcarbamazine [19]	Anterior to posterior uveitis (mild to severe)
Fluoroquinolones (ciprofloxacin, ofloxacin, gatifloxacin, levofloxacin, moxifloxacin [1, 11, 12], norfloxacin)	Anterior uveitis (mild to severe); may be associated with iris transillumination defects
Ibuprofen [17]	Anterior uveitis (mild)
Oral Contraceptives [17]	Anterior uveitis/retinal vasculitis
Quinidine [16]	Anterior uveitis (mild to moderate)
Rifabutin [3, 4]	Anterior uveitis (moderate to severe); hypopyon; retinal vasculitis
Sulfonamides [10]	Anterior uveitis (mild to moderate)
Topiramate [15]	Anterior uveitis (mild to severe); hypopyon
Tumor necrosis factor inhibitors (Etanercept, Infliximab, Adalimumab) [13, 14]	Anterior uveitis (mild to moderate)
Topical agents	**Type of Uveitis/Severity**
Metipranolol [18]	Anterior uveitis (mild to moderate)
Glucocorticosteroids [20]	Anterior uveitis (mild to moderate; may be related to steroid withdrawal)
Brimonidine [21]	Anterior uveitis (mild to moderate; may be granulomatous)
Prostaglandin analogs (latanoprost [22], travoprost, bimatoprost)	Anterior uveitis (mild; may be associated with cystoid macular edema)
Intraocular agents	**Type of Uveitis/Severity**
Anti-VEGF agents (ranibizumab, bevacizumab, pegaptanib, afilbercept) [23]	Panuveitis (mild to severe)
Cidofovir [5, 6]	Panuveitis (mild to severe)
Triamcinolone acetonide [24]	Panuveitis (mild to severe)
Vaccinations	**Type of Uveitis/Severity**
Bacille Calmette-Guerin (BCG) [25]	Anterior uveitis to panuveitis (mild to severe)
Measles, mumps, rubella (MMR) [26]	Anterior uveitis to panuveitis (mild to severe)
Influenza [27]	Anterior uveitis to panuveitis (mild to severe)
Hepatitis B [28]	Anterior uveitis to panuveitis (mild to severe)

Conclusion

Medication-associated uveitis is a rare adverse effect of drug administration that can typically induce mild to moderate intraocular inflammation. The prognosis is generally favorable as the uveitis responds well to cessation of the offending agent and use of topical and/or systemic corticosteroids. With the expanding armamentarium of available therapeutic agents, the list of drugs that can potentially induce uveitis continues to increase. At the time of this publication, multiple case series have reported uveitis associated with use of ipilimumab (a CTLA-4 inhibitor) in the treatment of metastatic melanoma [29]. The physician must be cognizant that certain medications may be associated with intraocular inflammation and have a high index of suspicion if established Naranjo criteria are fulfilled.

References

1. Fraunfelder FW, Rosenbaum JT. Drug-induced uveitis. Incidence, prevention and treatment. Drug Saf. 1997;17(3):197–207.
2. Naranjo CA, Busto U, Sellers EM, et al. A method for estimating the probability of adverse drug reactions. Clin Pharmacol Ther. 1981;30:224–39.
3. Tseng AL, Walmsley SL. Rifabutin-associated uveitis. Ann Pharmacother. 1995;29:1149–55.
4. Siegal FP, Eilbott D, Burger H, Gehan K, Davidson B, Kaell AT, Weiser B. Dose-limiting toxicity of rifabutin in AIDS-related complex: syndrome of arthralgia/arthritis. AIDS. 1990;4(5):433–41.
5. Akler ME, Johnson DW, Burman WJ, Johnson SC. Anterior uveitis and hypotony after intravenous cidofovir for the treatment of cytomegalovirus retinitis. Ophthalmology. 1998;105(4):651–7.
6. Ambati JK, Wynne KB, Angerame MC, Robinson MR. Anterior uveitis associated with intravenous cidofovir use in patients with cytomegalovirus retinitis. Br J Ophthal. 1999;83(10):1153–8.
7. Fraunfelder FW, Fraunfelder FT, Jensvold B. Scleritis and other ocular side effects associated with pamidronate disodium. Am J Ophthal. 2003;135 (2):219–22.
8. Fraunfelder FW. Ocular side effects associated with bisphosphonates. Drugs Today (Barc). 2003;39: 829–35.
9. Durnian JM, Olujohungbe A, Kyle G. Bilateral acute uveitis and conjunctivitis after zoledronic acid therapy. Eye. 2005;19(2):221–2.
10. Tilden ME, Rosenbaum JT, Fraunfelder FT. Systemic Sulfonamides as a cause of bilateral, anterior uveitis. Arch Ophthal. 1991;109(1):67–9.
11. Bringas CR, Iglesias CD. Acute and bilateral uveitis secondary to moxifloxacin. Arch Soc Esp Oftalmol. 2004;79(7):357–9.
12. Wefers BR, Brouwers K, et al. Uveitis-like syndrome and iris transillumination after the use of oral moxifloxacin. Eye (Lond). 2009;23(12):2260–2.
13. Ramos-Casals M, Diaz-Lagares C, Cuadrado MJ, Khamashta MA. BIOGEAS Study Group. Autoimmune diseases induced by biological agents: a double-edged sword? Autoimmun Rev. 2010;9 (3):188–93.
14. Lim LL, Fraunfelder FW, Rosenbaum JT. Do tumor necrosis factor inhibitors cause uveitis? Registry-Based Study. Arthritis Rheum. 2007;56(10): 3248–52.
15. Jabbarpoor Bonyadi MH, Soheilian R, Soheilian M. Topiramate-induced bilateral anterior uveitis associated with hypopyon formation. Ocular Immunol Inflamm. 2011;19(1):86–8.
16. Caraco Y, Arnon R, Raveh D. Quinidine-induced uveitis. Isr J Med Sci. 1992;28(10):741–3.
17. Cano PJ, Diaz-Llopis M. Drug induced uveitis. Archivos de la Sociedad Espanola de Oftalmologia. 2005;80(3):137–49.
18. Kinshuck D. Glauline (metipranolol) induced uveitis and increase in intraocular pressure. Br J Ophthalmol. 1991;75(9):575.
19. Taylor HR, Murphy RP, Newland HS, White AT, D'Anna SA, Keyvan-Larijani E, Aziz MA, Cupp EW, Greene BM. Treatment of onchocerciasis. The ocular effects of ivermectin and diethylcarbamazine. Arch Ophthalmol. 1986;104(6):863–70.
20. Martins JC, Wilensky JT, Asseff CF, Obstbaum SA. Buerk KM Corticosteroid-induced uveitis. Am J Ophthalmol. 1974;77(4):433–7.
21. Byles DB, Frith P, Salmon JF. Anterior uveitis as a side effect of topical brimonidine. Am J Ophthalmol. 2000;130(3):287–91.
22. Warwar RE, Bullock JD, Ballal D. Cystoid macular edema and anterior uveitis associated with latanoprost use. Experience and incidence in a retrospective review of 94 patients. Ophthalmology. 1998;105 (2):263–8.
23. Ladas ID, Karagiannis DA, Rouvas AA, Kotsolis AI, Liotsou A, Vergados I. Safety of repeat intravitreal injections of bevacizumab versus ranibizumab: our experience after 2,000 injections. Retina. 2009;29 (3):313–8.
24. Wang LC, Yang CM. Sterile endophthalmitis following intravitreal injection of triamcinolone acetonide. Ocul Immunol Inflamm. 2005;13(4):295–300.
25. Jacob M, Gambrelle J, Fleury J, Durieu I, Kodjikian L, Duquesne N, Grange JD. Panuveitis following intravesical bacille Calmette-Guerin therapy. J Fr Ophtalmol. 2006;29(5):552–5.
26. Islam SM, El-Sheikh HF, Tabbara KF. Anterior uveitis following combined vaccination for measles, mumps and rubella (MMR): a report of two cases. Acta Ophthalmol Scand. 2000;78(5):590–2.
27. Blanche P, Decrette C, Sicard D. Development of uveitis following vaccination for influenza. Clin Infect Dis. 1994;19(5):979.
28. Fraunfelder FW, Suhler EB, Fraunfelder FT. Hepatitis B vaccine and uveitis: an emerging hypothesis suggested by review of 32 case reports. Cutan Ocul Toxicol. 2010;29(1):26–9.
29. Papavasileiou E, Prasad S, Freitag SK, Sobrin L, Lobo AM. Ipilimumab-induced ocular and orbital inflammation-a case series and review of the literature. Ocul Immunol Inflamm. 2015;24:1–7.

Multiple Sclerosis

29

Olga Rosenvald and Dean M. Cestari

Introduction

Uveitis has been described in association with a number of disorders affecting the central nervous system (CNS), including inflammatory, infectious, neoplastic, and idiopathic. Multiple sclerosis (MS) is a demyelinating disease that frequently presents with visual signs and symptoms resulting from involvement of both afferent and efferent pathways. Most commonly MS is associated with optic neuritis, internuclear ophthalmoplegia (resulting from lesions at the medial longitudinal fasciculus), and varying other eye movement manifestations including nystagmus. The clinical presentation of uveitis varies greatly in patients with multiple sclerosis and has a prevalence ranging from 0.4 to 28.5 % [1]. Among patients with intermediate uveitis approximately 8–20 % have MS [1]. The association of uveitis and CNS diseases may result from the common embryogenesis of the posterior segment of the eye and the CNS. Similarities between the blood–brain barrier and the blood–retinal barrier also reflect this common development and may help explain the frequency of ocular manifestations in CNS diseases [2].

Multiple Sclerosis: Pathology

Multiple sclerosis is a chronic and degenerative disease of the CNS in which destruction of myelin, or demyelination, is the most prominent feature. Clinically, the disease is characterized by episodes of focal neurological manifestations which remit to a varying extent and recur over a period of time and are often progressive (Fig. 29.1).

The pathologic examination of the CNS usually reveals sharply delineated plaques that represent lesions with loss of myelin mainly affecting the white matter. These plaques have a very typical topography because they extend through periventricular white matter, optic nerves and chiasm, bilateral brainstem, and spinal cord. The histologic appearance varies by age and more recent lesions show destruction of myelin and variable astrocytic reaction with perivascular infiltration of mononuclear cells and lymphocytes [3].

O. Rosenvald
Department of Neurology, Massachusetts General Hospital and Brigham and Women's Hospital, Boston 6 Whittier Place, MA 02114, USA
e-mail: olga.rosenvald@gmail.com

D.M. Cestari (✉)
Department of Neuro-Opthalmology, Massachusetts Eye and Ear Infirmary, 243 Charles Street, Boston, MA 02114, USA
e-mail: dean_cestari@meei.harvard.edu

G.N. Papaliodis (ed.), *Uveitis*,
DOI 10.1007/978-3-319-09126-6_29

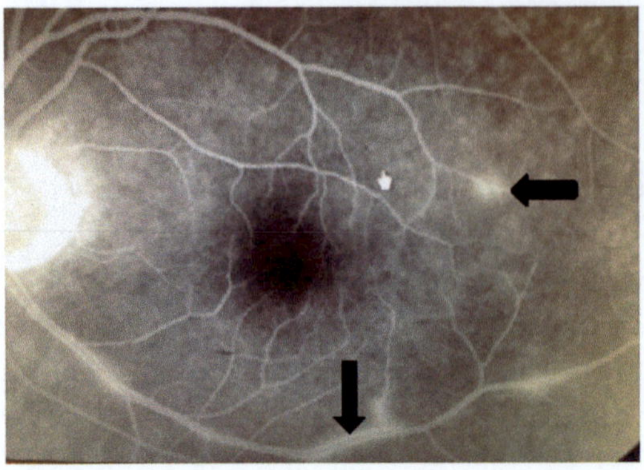

Fig. 29.1 Fluorescein angiogram demonstrating focal areas of retinal vasculitis in a patient with multiple sclerosis

Multiple Sclerosis: Epidemiology

For unclear reasons, the incidence of MS is two to three times higher in women than in men, but it is largely thought to be due to the higher susceptibility of women to autoimmune and inflammatory diseases. Although the etiology of MS remains unclear, there have been a number of established epidemiological associations. While its prevalence is reported as 1 per 100,000 in equatorial areas of the world, it increases to 6 to 14 per 100,000 in the southern US and Europe; 30 to 80 per 100,000 in Canada; northern US and northern Europe and as high as 177 per 100,000 in Minnesota; suggesting a gradient in the Northern hemisphere [4]. Recent research suggests that MS might be associated with the lack of sun exposure and reduced levels of vitamin D [5] which could partially explain the latitudinal gradient. Analysis of groups that had migrated from high to low prevalence zones suggests that at least part of the risk for developing MS depends on when the migration occurs. It has been observed that people who immigrate before the age of 15 have the same risk as people born in that area, whereas people who immigrate at a later age retain the risk associated with the region of their birthplace [6]. Although it has been suggested that possible exposure to various infections including specific viral agents is a risk factor for the development of MS, no studies have shown relevant evidence of a possible culprit [7].

Familial aggregation and heritability have also been implicated in multiple studies, with observed higher prevalence of MS in full siblings when compared to half siblings [8], as well as in monozygotic versus dizygotic twins. A genetic component is further supported by the presence of increased frequency of certain histocompatibility locus antigen (HLA) subtypes within patients with MS, namely HLA-DR6 and HLA-DR2, which are thought to be markers for “MS susceptibility” [7]. Although the presence of these HLA types is not specific for MS, those who have these genetic markers have an increased risk of developing MS by three- to fivefold [7].

Given the higher predisposition observed in patients with pars planitis to develop MS, Raja et al. evaluated a group of 53 patients with pars planitis looking for MS prevalence as well as possible genomic associations. Of 37 patients with pars planitis who underwent neurologic evaluations, 6 (16.2 %) developed multiple sclerosis. The HLA-DR15 allele, coding for one of the two HLA-DR2 subtypes, was associated with pars planitis (odds ratio = 2.86, $P = 0.004$). In addition, there was a suggestion that the association with HLA-DR15 was greater in patients with both pars planitis and multiple sclerosis, with three of the five patients with multiple sclerosis, pars planitis, and HLA typing expressing the HLA-DR15 allele [9].

Diagnosis

Traditionally, MS was diagnosed after a patient experienced two separate clinical attacks in two distinct areas of the CNS separated by at least 6 months. Today, the diagnosis is based on the widely accepted McDonald criteria in which MRI brain imaging and/or spinal fluid analysis can serve as objective clinical evidence of the disease [10]. A recent revision of this criterion by Polman et al. [11] includes the advent of refined neurological imaging, in which the presence of older lesions identified by MRI is adequate to satisfy this criterion, and the physician does not necessarily need to wait for new clinical events to establish the diagnosis of MS.

History of Ocular Inflammatory Disease and MS

Retinal venous sheathing in association with multiple sclerosis (Fig. 29.2) was first reported by Rucker in 1944 and subsequently followed by case reports describing similar findings [12]. Archambeau et al. [13] in 1965 reported the presence of vitreous cells in 10 patients with multiple sclerosis. One year later Breger et al. [14] evaluated patients with uveitis and MS and described retinal vein exudation associated with retinal ischemia and neovascularization.

Nearly two decades later Arnold et al. [15] described autopsy findings in 47 MS patients, including granulomatous retinal periphlebitis in four cases (7 eyes) and focal lymphocytic or granulomatous retinitis in three cases (5 eyes). Chester et al. [16] evaluated a cohort of 51 patients with pars planitis and found eight (16 %) cases of demyelinating disease (MS or optic neuritis), although the timing of the diagnosis in relation to the uveitis is unclear. Additional larger case series have continued to demonstrate the relationship between MS and ocular inflammation, particularly chronic anterior uveitis, intermediate uveitis, and retinal vasculitis [17].

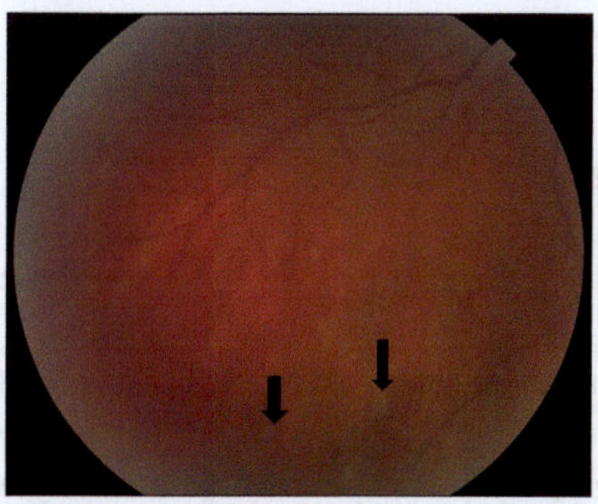

Fig. 29.2 Color fundus photograph demonstrating vitreous "snow balls" extending to the periphery in a patient with MS

Epidemiology of Uveitis and MS

Multiple population studies have investigated the prevalence of uveitis and other ocular disorders in patients with MS with varying results.

One large retrospective study of 4300 patients using the Lyon MS database found 28 patients with uveitis, with a prevalence of uveitis of 0.65 % (28/4300). Uveitis preceded the onset of MS in 46 % of the patients, occurred simultaneously in 18 % and presented following the diagnosis of MS in 36 % of cases. The area of ocular involvement and timing of uveitis were not associated with any significant difference in MS course and prognosis. There was also no difference in the course and prognosis of the CNS disease in patients with or without uveitis. The prevalence of uveitis (from all causes) in that local area was reported as 38 cases per 100,000; uveitis was 17 times more common in MS patients when compared to the general population [18].

A smaller prospective study performed in Croatia followed 42 patients with multiple sclerosis and identified intermediate uveitis in 28.5 % of these patients. This is a much higher prevalence of uveitis than previously reported in other published reports. This population also included a high number of patients with optic neuritis as a manifestation of MS. It was unclear why this cohort of patients had significantly greater ocular manifestations [19].

The neuro-ophthalmology group from Emory University evaluated patients in two large clinics, one with MS patients and the other with uveitis patients, and identified 28 patients with concomitant disease (20 women and 8 men; mean age, 47 years; range, 28 to 67 years) out of a total of 2628 patients (1 %). The mean age at onset of neurologic symptoms was 34.2 years (range, 15–55 years). MS was relapsing remitting in 19 of 28 patients (67.8 %), secondary progressive in 8 of 28 patients (28.6 %), and primary progressive in one patient [20].

A German uveitis center performed a similar retrospective evaluation of 1916 uveitis patients and found 3.1 % to also have MS. Of those, 74.6 % were female, highlighting the gender disparity of the underlying autoimmune disease [21].

Zein et al. evaluated 1254 patients with uveitis at a large tertiary care center in Boston and reported 16 cases of MS (0.013 %). Most of the patients with MS-associated uveitis were white females (88 %) between 20 and 50 years of age. The onset of uveitis fell within 5 years of the diagnosis of MS in 63 % of the patients; nine had MS diagnosed prior to the onset of uveitis by an interval of 1–19 years. Uveitis and MS were diagnosed concurrently in three patients. Interestingly, they have also observed that optic neuritis was one of the most common neurological manifestations, present in 44 % of those patients [1].

Uveitis Subtypes and MS

Patients with MS can develop intraocular inflammation involving multiple anatomic regions of the eye including optic neuritis, intermediate uveitis (image 2), iritis, panuveitis, and retina vasculitis (image 1). A large series of 2619 patients with uveitis followed at the University of Vienna identified 0.9 % (25 patients) had the concomitant diagnosis of MS. The majority of those patients (19) had intermediate uveitis, four had anterior, and two had posterior uveitis. No patients were described in this series to have panuveitis [22].

In the group of 16 patients with concomitant MS and uveitis evaluated by Zein et. al, the majority of the patients (15 of 16, 94 %) had posterior or intermediate uveitis. Anterior uveitis was present in 81 % of patients. Retinal vascular exudates were noted in 56 %. Thirteen patients (81 %) had inflammatory exudates or collagen bands at the pars plana. Cystoid macular edema was present in 31 % of the patients and optic atrophy in 19 %. They also noted that the uveitis was bilateral in 15 of the 16 patients [1].

The German uveitis group described that anterior uveitis accounted for 10 % of patients with MS, whereas intermediate uveitis comprised 78 % of the uveitis seen in patients with MS. There was a higher prevalence of MS within the subgroup of patients with intermediate uveitis (10.3 % of 438 patients) [21].

In a small prospective study of 21 patients with intermediate uveitis by Prieto et al, 47.6 % demonstrated demyelinating lesions on MRI and 33.3 % were diagnosed with definitive MS. This series was one of the highest reported associations with MS in patients with intermediate uveitis [23].

The large population study from Emory demonstrated that uveitis was bilateral in most patients (22 of 28; 78.5 %). One of the most common types of uveitis was intermediate uveitis (in 10 of 28 patients; 35.7 %) and panuveitis (in 11 of 28 patients; 39.3 %). Isolated anterior uveitis was observed in 4 of 28 patients (14.3 %) and posterior uveitis was observed in 3 of 28 patients (10.7 %). Retinal periphlebitis (venous sheathing) was noted in 11 of 28 patients (39.3 %) [20].

The results from the Lyon MS database revealed a predominance of posterior uveitis (10 patients, 35.7 %). Isolated anterior uveitis was observed in eight patients (28.6 %), panuveitis in eight patients (28.6 %), and intermediate uveitis in two patients (7.1 %). Retinal periphlebitis was noted in five patients (17.8 %) [18].

Birnbaum et al. [24] performed a large retrospective study evaluating over 1800 patients with chronic anterior uveitis. They identified 30 patients with MS (1.6 %) and noted an increase in the incidence of MS-associated uveitis diagnosed in the last decade. They have attributed this increase to refinements in the neuroimaging facilitating the diagnosis.

Therapy

There have been many recent therapeutic trials for MS, and most use antiinflammatory and immunosuppressive regimens. Glucocorticoids (such as oral Prednisone or IV methylprednisolone) temporarily ameliorate the symptoms of the disorder but do not alter the course of the disease [25]. The typical relapsing remitting pattern of MS is most responsive to immunomodulatory therapy which is not as effective for chronic progressive patterns. In patients with uveitis, a neurologic diagnosis may have important implications for management as certain medications may induce further disease. Tumor necrosis factor (TNF) blockers can exacerbate or precipitate demyelination; thus, these drugs are specifically contraindicated for patients with MS-associated uveitis.

While it was not the focus of their study, Zein et al. reported that 69 % of their MS-associated uveitis patients were treated with topical steroids, 63 % with trans-septal steroids, 38 % with oral steroids, as well as 1 patient with Azathioprine, 1 with cyclosporine, and 1 with methotrexate. They have not described different outcomes based on treatment option [1].

It remains unclear whether the various therapeutic options used in the management of disease manifestation in the CNS are effective for MS-associated uveitis. Uveitis specialists have often approached the ocular manifestations of disease in similar manner to idiopathic intermediate uveitis with regional/ intraocular corticosteroids. For progressive or more severe ocular disease, systemic immunomodulatory therapy with methotrexate, azathioprine, mycophenolate mofetil, and cyclosporine has been used (often in collaboration with neurology).

Conclusion

The clinical association of uveitis with multiple sclerosis has been reported with varying prevalence ranging from 0.4 to 28.5 %. Intermediate uveitis is the most commonly observed subtype of uveitis found in MS patients. MS-associated uveitis is typically bilateral and can have anterior and posterior manifestations.

References

1. Zein G, Berta A, Foster CS. Multiple sclerosis-associated uveitis. Ocul Immunol Inflamm. 2004;12:137–42.
2. Allegri P, Rissotto R, Herbort CP, Murialdo U. CNS diseases and uveitis. J Ophthalmic Vis Res. 2011;6 (4):284–308.
3. Lucchinetti C, Bruck W, Parisi J, Scheithauer B, Rodriguez M, Lassmann H. Heterogeneity of multiple sclerosis lesions: implications for the pathogenesis of demyelination. Ann Neurol. 2000;47:707–17.
4. Mayr WT, Pittock SJ, McClelland RL, Jorgensen NW, Noseworthy JH, Rodriguez M. Incidence and prevalence of multiple sclerosis in Olmsted County, Minnesota, 1985–2000. Neurology. 2003;61(10):1373–7.
5. Munger KL, Levin LI, Hollis BW, et al. Serum 25-hydroxyvitamin D levels and risk of multiple sclerosis. JAMA. 2006;296:2832.
6. Dean G, Kurtzke JF. On the risk of multiple sclerosis according to age at immigration to South Africa. Br Med J. 1971;3(5777):725–9.
7. Ropper AH, Samuels MA, Klein JP. Adams and Victor's principles of neurology, 10th ed.
8. Sadovnick AD, Yee IM, Ebers GC; Canadian collaborative study group. Multiple sclerosis and birth order: a longitudinal cohort study. Lancet Neurol. 2005;4(10):611–7.
9. Raja SC, Jabs DA, Dunn JP, Fekrat S, Machan CH, Marsh MJ, Bressler NM. Pars planitis: clinical features and class II HLA associations. Ophthalmology. 1999;106(3):594–9.
10. McDonald WI, Halliday AM. Diagnosis and classification of multiple sclerosis. Br Med Bull. 1977;33 (1):4–9.
11. Polman CH, Reingold SC, Banwell B, Clanet M, Cohen JA, Filippi M, Fujihara K, Havrdova E, Hutchinson M, Kappos L, Lublin FD, Montalban X, O'Connor P, Sandberg-Wollheim M, Thompson AJ, Waubant E, Weinshenker B, Wolinsky JS. Diagnostic criteria for multiple sclerosis: 2010 revisions to the McDonald criteria. Ann Neurol. 2011;69(2):292–302. doi:10.1002/ana.22366.
12. Rucker CW. Sheathing of the retinal veins in multiple sclerosis. JAMA. 1945;127:970–3.
13. Archambeau PL, Hollenhorst RW. Posterior uveitis as a manifestation of multiple sclerosis. Mayo Clin Proc. 1965;40:544–51.
14. Breger BC, Leopold IH. The incidence of uveitis in multiple sclerosis. Am J Ophthalmol I966;62:540–545.
15. Arnold AC, Pepose JS, Hepler RS, Foos RY. Retinal periphlebitis and retinitis in multiple sclerosis. I. Pathologic characteristics. Ophthalmology. 1984;91(3):255–62.
16. Chester GH, Blach RK, Cleary PE. Inflammation in the region of the vitreous base: pars planitis. Trans Ophthamol Soc UK. I976;96:151–157.
17. Gordon LK, Goldstein DA. Gender and uveitis in patients with multiple sclerosis. J Ophthalmol. 2014;2014:565262.
18. Le Scanff J, Sève P, Renoux C, Broussolle C, Confavreux C, Vukusic S. Uveitis associated with multiple sclerosis. Mult Scler. 2008;14(3):415–7.

19. T. Vidovi´c, B. Cerovski, T. Juki´c. The appearance of pars planitis in multiple sclerosis. Collegium Antropologicum. 2005;29(1):203–206.
20. Biousse V, Trichet C, Bloch-Michel E, Roullet E. Multiple sclerosis associated with uveitis in two large clinic-based series. Neurology. 1999;52(1):179–81.
21. Jakob E, Reuland MS, Mackensen F, Harsch N, Fleckenstein M, Lorenz HM, Max R, Becker MD. Uveitis subtypes in a german interdisciplinary uveitis center-analysis of 1916 patients. J Rheumatol. 2009;36(1):127–36.
22. Barisani-Asenbauer T, Maca SM, Mejdoubi L, Emminger W, Machold K, Auer H. Uveitis- a rare disease often associated with systemic diseases and infections- a systematic review of 2619 patients. Orphanet J Rare Dis. 2012;29(7):57. doi:10.1186/1750-1172-7-57. Review.
23. Prieto JF, Dios E, Gutierrez JM, Mayo A, Calonge M, Herreras JM. Pars planitis: epidemiology, treatment, and association with multiple sclerosis. Ocul Immunol Inflamm. 2001;9(2):93–102.
24. Birnbaum AD, Little DM, Tessler HH, Goldstein DA. Etiologies of chronic anterior uveitis at a tertiary referral center over 35 years. Ocul Immunol Inflamm. 2011;19(1):19–25.
25. Becker CC, Gidal BE, Fleming JO. Immunotherapy in multiple sclerosis. Part I. Am J Health Syst Pharm. 1995;52:1985–2000.
26. Smith JR, Rosenbaum JT. Neurological concomitants of uveitis. Br J Ophthalmol. 2004;88:1498–9.

30 Multiple Evanescent White Dot Syndrome

George N. Papaliodis

Introduction

Multiple evanescent white dot syndrome (MEWDS) is a rare idiopathic ocular inflammatory disorder that typically ensues after a viral prodrome. Jampol et al. [1] described the condition in 1984 in a series of 11 adults who transiently had decreased vision and the presence of white dots in the fundus. The disease is more common in young, white, healthy females and is usually unilateral although bilateral cases have been reported. The disorder is characterized by the presence of white to yellow-white lesions at the level of the retinal pigment epithelium distributed over the posterior fundus. The lesions resolve spontaneously and visual prognosis is excellent.

Epidemiology

From 1984–1994, there were approximately 80 cases of MEWDS reported in the literature (via Pubmed search). This condition typically affects younger patients (range of 17–47 years) and is more common in females (1:3 male to female ratio).

Etiology

The etiology of MEWDS is unknown although there are multiple plausible theories that have been proposed including a possible infectious etiology (given the prodromal flu-like symptoms) and autoimmune disorder. No specific infectious agent has been identified. The autoimmune basis of the disease is supported by the finding that 44.4 % of these patients are HLA-B51 positive [2].

Clinical Manifestations

Patients with MEWDS complain about blurry vision, photopsias, floaters, and visual field deficits. The most prominent characteristic of the disease is the presence of multiple, small (100–200 microns) white to yellow-white spots distributed over the posterior fundus. The lesions tend to concentrate around the optic nerve and vascular arcades and extend to the mid-periphery of the retina. Other features that have been reported include anterior chamber and vitreous cells, macular granularity, and optic nerve swelling [1, 3]. The lesions are present during the acute phase of the disorder and then spontaneously resolve without treatment.

G.N. Papaliodis (✉)
Department of Ophthalmology, Harvard Medical School, Massachusetts Eye and Ear Infirmary, 243 Charles Street, Boston, MA 02114, USA
e-mail: George_Papaliodis@meei.harvard.edu

G.N. Papaliodis (ed.), *Uveitis*,
DOI 10.1007/978-3-319-09126-6_30

Diagnosis

The diagnosis of MEWDS is primarily established clinically based on the typical fundus findings, transient nature of these lesions, and excellent visual outcome without therapy. Serologic studies may be obtained to exclude other potential entities that can mimic the findings of this disorder (e.g., syphilis, tuberculosis, toxoplasmosis, sarcoidosis). Fluorescein angiography demonstrates early punctate hyperfluorescence and late staining in areas corresponding to the white dots.

Treatment

There is no specific treatment required for this condition. The white dots resolve spontaneously (thus the term "evanescent") and the visual prognosis is excellent.

Conclusion

MEWDS is a rare idiopathic ocular inflammatory disorder manifesting as white to yellow-white lesions in the posterior fundus that ensues after a "flu-like" prodromal syndrome. The disorder is characterized by spontaneous resolution of the lesions and excellent visual prognosis.

References

1. Jampol LM, Sieving PA, Pugh D, et al. Multiple evanescent white dot syndrome. Clin Find Arch Ophthalmol. 1984;102(5):671–4.
3. Desarnaulds AB, Borruat FX, Herbort CP, Spertini F. Le Multiple Evanescent White Dot Syndrome: une prédisposition génétique? Klinische Monatsblätter für Augenheilkunde. 1996;208(05):301–2.
2. Quillen D, Davis J, et al. Perspective: the White Dot Syndromes. Am J Ophthalmol. 2004;137:538–50.

Punctate Inner Choroidopathy

31

George N. Papaliodis

Introduction

Punctate inner choroidopathy (PIC) is an idiopathic inflammatory disorder of the eye, which is more commonly affecting young myopic females. The etiology of this condition remains unknown. Patients usually develop yellow-white chorioretinal lesions at the level of the inner choroid and retinal pigment epithelium in the absence of intraocular inflammation. The condition is typically bilateral but asymmetric.

Epidemiology

The exact incidence and prevalence of PIC is unknown as this a relatively uncommon ocular inflammatory disorder. In a case series from Moorfields Hospital in London with 136 patients diagnosed with PIC over a 16 year period, 93 % of the patients were female with a mean age at initial presentation of 32 and 84 % were myopes [1].

Etiology

The etiology of the condition remains unknown although there are multiple postulated theories. Some researchers have suggested that PIC is a limited variant of myopic degeneration, as it occurs more commonly in myopic females. In the original series by Watzke et al. [2] myopia ranged from −3.25 to −10 diopters. Others have proposed that PIC represents a mild form of multifocal choroiditis. Tiedman et al. [3] theorized that there may be an association with *Epstein–Barr* virus infection and the development of the disorder. An autoimmune etiology has similarly been considered given an association with the development of PIC and the serotype HLA-DR2 [4], and there have been familial case reports involving mother–daughter who are affected [5].

Clinical Manifestations

The most common symptoms reported from patients with PIC are blurry vision, floaters, and photopsias. Slit lamp exam demonstrates absence of intraocular inflammation. Fundoscopy is characterized by multiple, small (50–300 microns in diameter), yellow or white, opaque, and round lesions scattered throughout the posterior pole. The condition is typically bilateral

G.N. Papaliodis (✉)
Department of Ophthalmology, Harvard Medical School, Massachusetts Eye and Ear Infirmary, 243 Charles Street, Boston, MA 02114, USA
e-mail: George_Papaliodis@meei.harvard.edu

G.N. Papaliodis (ed.), *Uveitis*,
DOI 10.1007/978-3-319-09126-6_31

but asymmetric. The clinical appearance is similar to presumed ocular histoplasmosis syndrome (POHS). These entities are differentiated based on lack of exposure to the causative fungal species in the latter and different demographics in the former (PIC affects young, myopic females). The most significant complication of PIC is the development of choroidal neovascular membranes (CNVM) (estimated to occur in 17–40 % of patients with PIC lesions) [2, 6] and are the leading cause of poor visual outcome from this disorder [6].

Diagnosis

The diagnosis of PIC is based on history and clinical examination (absence of intraocular inflammation and characteristic lesions in the posterior pole). Fluorescein angiography demonstrates early hyperfluorescence of the lesions with variable late staining. Electroretinogram (ERG) is typically normal.

Treatment

PIC is generally viewed as a benign disease with favorable prognosis and resolution of acute lesions within weeks after the initial presentation. Therefore, no treatment is typically recommended. Systemic corticosteroids have been used successfully in those with compromised visual acuity on presentation. Multiple treatments have been used for the CNVMs secondary to PIC including systemic and intraocular steroids, surgical excision of the membranes, photodynamic therapy (PDT), and intraocular injection of anti-VEGF agents (bevacizumab and ranibizumab).

Conclusion

Punctate inner choroidopathy (PIC) is an idiopathic inflammatory disorder of the eye, which is more commonly affecting young, myopic females. The etiology is unknown and the prognosis is generally favorable in the absence of macular CNVMs.

References

1. Essex RW, Wong J, Fraser-Bell S, Sandbach J, Tufail A, Bird AC, Dowler J. Punctate inner choroidopathy: clinical features and outcomes. Arch Ophthalmol. 2010;128(8):982–7.
2. Watzke RC, Packer AJ, Folk JC, Benson WE, Burgess D, Ober RR. Punctate inner choroidopathy. Am J Ophthalmol. 1984;98(5):572–84.
3. Tiedman JS. Epstein-Barr viral antibodies in multifocal choroiditis and panuveitis. Am J Ophthalmol. 1987;103:659–63.
4. Spaide RF, Skerry JE, Yannuzzi LA, DeRosa JT. Lack of the HLA-DR2 specificity in multifocal choroiditis and panuveitis. Br J Ophthalmol. 1990;74:536–7.
5. Sugawara E, Machida S, Fujiwara T, Kurosaka D, Hayakawa M. Punctate inner choroidopathy in mother and daughter. Jpn J Ophthalmol. 2010;54(5):505–7.
6. Brown J Jr, Folk JC, Reddy CV, Kimura AE, et al. Visual prognosis of multifocal choroiditis, punctate inner choroidopathy, and the diffuse subretinal fibrosis syndrome. Ophthalmology. 1996;103:1100–5.

Psoriasis Associated

32

Rebecca Hunter

Psoriasis

Psoriasis is a common inflammatory skin disease with a prevalence of 1–2 % in Caucasians. Skin manifestations of psoriasis vulgaris, the most common variant of psoriasis, typically involve sharply demarcated areas of erythematous plaques that are covered with silver or white scales (Fig. 32.1). These lesions usually involve the elbows, knees, scalp and lumbar area. Another variant is pustular psoriasis that is characterized by red erythematous areas and pustules as the name suggests. These pustules can combine and form large areas of pus [1].

Psoriatic Arthritis

There are various extracutaneous manifestations of psoriasis. Of these, psoriatic arthritis (PsA), a seronegative spondyloarthropathy (SpA), is one. This entity was first recognized more than 100 years ago, but its clinical manifestations and pathogenesis are still being delineated to this date [2]. The prevalence of arthritis in patients with psoriasis varies. Studies have shown that PsA affects from 5 to 25 % of patients with psoriasis and can vary not just by degree of skin involvement but also by geographic area [1, 3, 4]. The clinical spectrum of the disease can be influenced by diet, climate, and microorganisms which differ by geographic locations [5].

PsA is defined as a SpA with characteristic skin and nail findings. There are a variety of articular features that can occur in patients with PsA. The most common is polyarthritis, a symmetric arthritis involving more than 5 joints. Other clinical subsets are spondylitis with or without peripheral arthritis, distal interphalangeal arthritis (see Fig. 32.2), asymmetric mono-oligoarthritis, and arthritis mutilans [2]. It may also be grouped into patients that show peripheral articular disease or axial disease with radiologic sacroiliitis. The peripheral pattern occurs more commonly than the axial pattern. Of patients with axial disease, nearly half of the patients are HLA-B27 positive [2]. Patients who are HLA-B27 positive have earlier disease and have been noted to have a shorter interval between onset of skin manifestations and joint disease [6, 7]. Given these distinct subsets, the clinical course of PsA may vary. Some studies, however, have shown that men show less disease progression than women [8]. In addition, the relationship between skin manifestations and severity of joint disease is still unclear. Most

R. Hunter (✉)
Department of Ophthalmology, Harvard Vanguard Medical Associates, 133 Brookline Avenue, Boston, MA 02115, USA
e-mail: rebecca.s.hunter@gmail.com

G.N. Papaliodis (ed.), *Uveitis*,
DOI 10.1007/978-3-319-09126-6_32

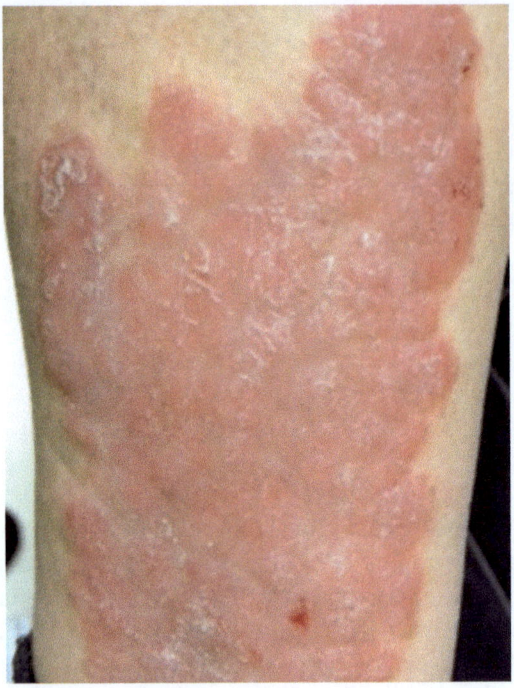

Fig. 32.1 Skin lesion in psoriasis vulgaris

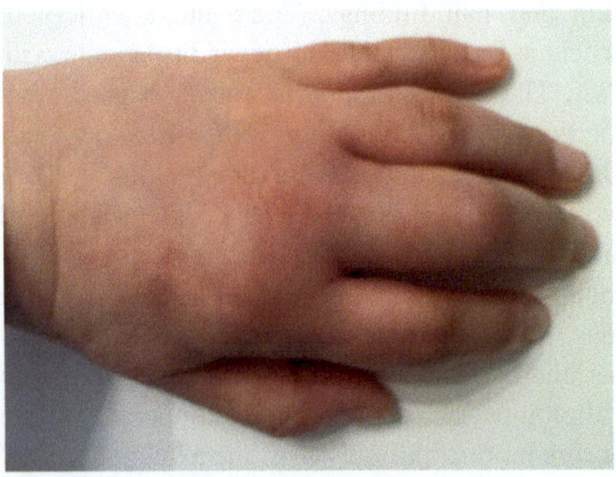

Fig. 32.2 Marked swelling of the metacarpophalangeal joints and "sausage" like swelling of the digits in a patient with psoriatic arthritis

patients develop skin lesions prior to joint disease. Some studies have found that patients with active arthritis tend to have milder skin disease but others have found an inverse relationship [9, 10]. Other studies have found no relationship between skin disease and severity of joint disease [11].

Non-ophthalmic Extra-Articular Manifestations of PsA

The correlation between severity of extra-articular manifestations and joint inflammation has been evaluated. Nail involvement can be seen in all forms of psoriasis but is more common in patients with psoriatic arthritis occurring in 50–90 % of patients with the disease [10, 12, 13]. The nail findings most commonly consist of pitting and yellow discoloration of the fingernails. In more severe cases there may be onycholysis. As opposed to skin disease, it has been noted that the severity of a patients' nail findings correlates with their joint disease [14].

Psoriatic Arthritis Associated Uveitis

Uveitis is reported to be the most common extra-articular manifestation of the SpAs [15]. The association between PsA and uveitis has been well documented. The likelihood of a patient with acute anterior uveitis to have PsA is reported to be less than 1 %, however the occurrence of uveitis is up to 25 % in patients with PsA (Table 32.1 and 32.2) [16, 17]. The prevalence of uveitis has been reported to be higher in women however this is variable [20–22]. Joint disease generally precedes eye manifestations but some reports have shown ocular inflammation as the initial presentation of PsA [18].

The first report of the association between eye manifestations and PsA was in the 1970s [19]. Lambert and Wright described the eye manifestations of 112 patients with PsA. The authors noted 31 % of patients had some form of ocular inflammation. Conjunctivitis was the most common followed by iritis, episcleritis, and keratoconjunctivitis sicca (Table 32.3). Of the patients found to have iritis, 43 % had sacroiliitis and 28.5 % had spondylitis. There was a higher prevalence of iritis in patients with axial disease when compared to other patients. The authors were the first to conclude that eye inflammation was a frequent complication of psoriatic arthritis, and this was the first study to address the concept of PsA as a seronegative SpA.

Table 32.1 Reported frequency series

Author/year	% patients with ocular inflammation	Types of inflammation
Lambert and Wright [19]	8.9	Episcleritis, AU
Leonard et al. [9]	3.3	AU
Gladman et al. [13]	7	AU
Torre-Alonso et al. [12]	2.8	AU
Jones et al. [11]	5	AU
Quiero et al. [21]	18	AU, PU
Taylor et al. [38]	10.5	AU
Collantes et al. [39]	1	AU
Zeboulon et al. [17]	25.1	AU,PU
Niccoli et al. [22]	9	AU
Canoui-Poitrine et al. [40]	11.1	AU
De Lima et al. [41]	5	AU

AU: Anterior uveitis designates iritis, iridocyclitis
PU: Posterior uveitis designates choroiditis, retinitis, vasculitis

Table 32.2 Uveitis in the SpA from clinical series [18, 21, 22, 35, 37, 39, 40, 42, 43]

	PsA	AS	ReA	IBD
Prevalence (%)	1–25	20–40	12–26	2–37
Onset	Acute/Insiduous	Acute	Acute	Insiduous
Location	AU/PU	AU	AU	AU/PU
Laterality	Bilateral	Unilateral	Unilateral	Bilateral
HLA-B27	+/−	+	+	+/−
Joints	Before	Before	After	After
Age	39–48	33	30's	37
M:F	Varies	2:1	2:1	Varies
Likelihood of uveitis (%)	7–16	20–50	12–37	3–11

Table 32.3 Types of ocular inflammation associated with PsA [12, 19, 35]

Conjunctivitis (6.7–19.6 %)
Anterior uveitis (Variable, See Table 32.2)
Keratoconjunctivitis sicca (2.7 %)
Episcleritis (1.8)
Posterior uveitis[a] (44%)

[a]Not specific as to type of posterior uveitis

Most of the literature since has evaluated PsA associated uveitis in comparison to the uveitis found in other seronegative SpAs which includes ankylosing spondylitis (AS), reactive arthritis (formerly known as Reiters syndrome), arthritis associated with inflammatory bowel disease (IBD), PsA and undifferentiated SpA [17, 20]. These studies have shown that the prevalence and clinical characteristics of uveitis associated with each type of SpA can vary significantly (Table 32.2).

Patients with PsA predominantly have uveitis that is insidious in onset, continuous and bilateral with a high rate of recurrence (Table 32.2). [20, 21] In addition, this patient population is more likely to have posterior involvement than seen in other types of SpAs. Uveitis is equally represented among patients with axial and peripheral joint disease with half of patient cohorts having peripheral joint disease alone and the other half having a combination of axial disease alone or both [22]. However, other authors have found variable risk factors such as extensive axial involvement, specifically sacroiliitis, and dactylitis [21, 22]. It has been noted that patients with axial disease and uveitis tend to have a distinct clinical picture from the more common presentation and is clinically more similar to the uveitis seen in patients with AS. [21] This presentation is more often of acute onset with predominantly anterior chamber inflammation.

Juvenile Psoriatic Arthritis and Uveitis

Given the unique features that are associated with pediatric uveitis, special attention should be given to PsA associated uveitis in children. Juvenile psoriatic arthritis (JPsA) is a distinct clinical entity, defined as a chronic inflammatory arthritis associated with psoriasis. It is considered a distinct subtype of juvenile idiopathic arthritis (JIA) based on observations that patients with JPsA have a form of juvenile idiopathic arthritis that differs both in its clinical manifestations and in its outcome than that noted in adults [23]. JPsA represents up to 10 % of all JIA subtypes and has a predilection for females. Anti-nuclear antibodies (ANAs) are positive in more than 50 % of affected patients [24]. Uveitis has been reported to occur in 10–15 % of JPsA patients. Other series have reported a much higher prevalence (Table 32.4). In addition, it has been reported that up to 13 % of children with chronic uveitis will have JPsA [28].

Table 32.4 Reported frequency of uveitis in juvenile psoriatic arthritis series

Author/year	% patients with ocular inflammation	Types of inflammation
Stoll et al. [46]	7.9	CAU
Heiligenhaus et al. [25]	10	CAU
Butbal et al. [26]	18.8–23.8	CAU, AAU

Heiligenhaus et al. [35] looked at the prevalence and complication rates of uveitis in the different subtypes of JIA. The authors noted 75 % of patients with early-onset JPsA had asymptomatic uveitis and inflammation present on routine screening. This was the same in both oligoarticular and polyarticular arthritis patients. This was in contrast to JIA patients with HLAB27 associated eye inflammation and late onset JPsA (>6 years) that was typically symptomatic. The authors also noted a low rate of complications compared to the other subtypes of JIA patients with only 25 % developing ocular complications [25].

Butbal et al. [26] compared the clinical features of patients with JPsA and JIA. The authors divided each group into patients with oligoarticular disease and polyarticular disease. They found that in patients with oligoarticular disease there was no difference in the rate of uveitis between the two groups, at 19 %. However in patients with polyarticular disease, the prevalence of uveitis in patients with JPsA was 23.8 % compared to 0 % of the JIA patients. However, the authors noted that this low prevalence of uveitis in their polyarticular JIA cohort had not been previously reported and was likely due to small sample size. Otherwise there was no statistical difference between ANA positivity, type of uveitis (acute versus chronic), or rates of complications between the two groups.

In summary, the uveitis in JPsA patients tends to be more similar to that seen in JIA patients and different than adult PsA associated uveitis. Additionally, pediatric patients should be monitored closely for asymptomatic ocular inflammation as they may have a worse visual prognosis.

Psoriasis and Uveitis

The association between psoriasis without arthritis and uveitis is not as well established but will be briefly discussed. The first report that associated psoriasis with uveitis was in 1979. Knox reported 10 patients with uveitis diagnosed with psoriasis [27]. They concluded that there was a rare but important correlation between eye inflammation and skin disease. Following this, more comprehensive studies found that most patients with uveitis and psoriasis also have arthritis at presentation [28, 29]. Given this correlation, some feel the prevalence of uveitis in patients with psoriasis without arthritis is not significant. However, more recent studies have shown evidence that an entity of psoriatic uveitis without arthritis does exist.

Durrani et al. [30] set out to establish the relationship between psoriasis without arthritis and uveitis. Prior to this there had been scattered case reports documenting patients with skin psoriasis and uveitis (Table 32.5). They compared patients with AAU and psoriasis against patients with idiopathic AAU and HLA-B27 associated uveitis. Thirty-six patients with a diagnosis of psoriasis and uveitis were found. Almost half of patients were HLAB27 positive. The authors noted that the age of presentation of ocular inflammation in patients with psoriasis was significantly higher than the other AAU groups. They commonly had recurrent uveitis that was acute in onset and non-granulomatous which was similar to the other subtypes of AAU. However, patients with psoriasis were more likely to have bilateral and persistent inflammatory episodes and respond to NSAIDs more so than with other types of AAU.

Table 32.5 Reported frequency of uveitis in psoriasis series

Author/year	% patients with ocular inflammation	% Joint involvement
Casarou-Catsari et al. [28]	3	100
Chandran et al. [31]	2	50

Chandran et al. [31] evaluated 105 Singaporean patients with psoriasis and attempted to identify all ocular abnormalities (not limited to uveitis). They noted a varied range of eye pathology in their patient population. Only 2 had uveitis and 1 of these had an associated arthritis. Interestingly both patients had extensive skin disease and the authors concluded that the severity of skin disease may be an important risk factor for the development of uveitis. This has yet to be assessed in a large population study.

In summary, there is currently minimal data to show an association between psoriasis and uveitis without arthritis although some authors, as noted, support its existence [30, 32]. Most studies do support an entity of ocular psoriasis that includes other ophthalmic disease but does not show an increased risk of uveitis [31, 33]. Other ocular manifestations of psoriasis include blepharitis, conjunctivitis, keratitis sicca, and peripheral keratitis [33].

Pathogenesis

The pathogenesis of PsA associated uveitis is unknown but likely multifactorial with genetic, environmental and immunologic factors.

The HLA-B27 haplotype has been associated with arthritis and uveitis. This was described for the first time in 1973 by Brewerton et al. [34]. HLA-B27 is implicated in a large portion of patients with PsA. This relation is particularly seen in patients with axial-type disease [35]. Some literature has reported an increased risk of developing uveitis in patients with HLA-B27 and SpA [17]. Some have found that 40 % of patients with HLAB27 have uveitis compared to 14 % in HLA-B27 negative patients, with an odds ratio of 4.2. That said, the link between autoimmune inflammatory diseases and HLA-B27 remains speculative. Interestingly, animal studies of

Table 32.6 HLA haplotypes associated with Ps/PsA uveitis

HLA type	Joint disease
HLAB27 [17, 35]	Axial
HLAB51 [44, 45]	None
HLADR13 [21]	Axial and Peripheral

HLA-B27 transgenic rats and mice that develop spontaneous inflammatory disease affecting the gastrointestinal tract, peripheral and vertebral joints, male genital tract, skin, and nails, rarely develop anterior uveitis [36].

Other haplotypes have also been associated with PsA associated uveitis (Table 32.6). Queiro found a genetic association between the HLA-DR13 haplotype and PsA and uveitis. They found that HLA-DR13 was the best predictor of developing uveitis in patients with PsA rather than HLA-B27 [21]. The authors found an increased incidence of HLAB27 in their patient population with uveitis, however, in multivariate analysis concluded that the gene predisposes to arthritis, specifically SI and spondylitis, but not uveitis and is not a true genetic risk factor for uveitis in SpA.

Treatment

The treatment strategies of PsA associated uveitis are similar to those directed at any type of immune-mediated ocular inflammatory disease. The location of inflammation (anterior or posterior), duration of inflammation, and comorbidities affect the clinician's therapeutic alternatives. As discussed, patients with PsA associated uveitis have a variety of ocular manifestations and therefore the treatment can vary. For patients with anterior segment inflammation, topical steroids and cycloplegia may be sufficient. However, if indolent inflammation is the case, requiring chronic steroid use, ocular complications such as cataract formation and elevated intraocular pressure become more concerning. For posterior inflammation, topical steroids are usually inadequate to suppress inflammation. Other alternatives include local steroid injections given either tran-septally sub-tenons, or intraocularly. These options, however, do not obviate the aforementioned complications. Systemic steroids are also an initial alternative for patients who have posterior segment inflammation or vision threatening inflammation. However if patients have recurrent disease on tapering systemic steroids or require high doses of steroids for prolonged periods to maintain disease quiescence, they should be transitioned to steroid-sparing immunosuppressive therapy.

Although the treatment of PsA and all SpA has significantly changed over the past decade, first line therapy after failure of systemic and local steroids are conventional disease-modifying antirheumatic drugs (DMARDs) which are steroid-sparing agents that include antimetabolites such as methotrexate, mycophenolate mofetil, and azathioprine; T-cell inhibitors such as cyclosporine; and alkylating agents such as cyclophosphamide and chlorambucil. This is also true for ocular manifestations of PsA.

If the patient fails conventional DMARDs or develop associated toxicity, tumor necrosis factor inhibitors (TNF-i) are usually initiated. This class of drug has revolutionized the treatment of PsA [47]. TNF-i have been associated with significant reduction in the signs and symptoms of inflammation in PsA. Four TNF-i have been in use for more than 5 years: etanercept, infliximab, adalimumab, and golimumab. These medications have been shown to be superior to placebo in the treatment of inflammatory arthritis and cutaneous manifestations of PsA. Case reports have demonstrated the use of these medications in ocular inflammatory disease. Although most of the literature focuses on the use of these medications on all SpA-associated uveitis, one study specifically addressed the use of infliximab and adalimumab in PsA associated uveitis [48]. The authors noted that 7 of 8 patients with PsA uveitis achieved remission of their ocular inflammation on TNF-i with an average time of therapy of 6 months. Six of these patients were concurrently treated with methotrexate.

More recent studies have interestingly found a lower rate of recurrence of uveitis likely related

Table 32.7 Complications in patients with PsA uveitis [35]

Complication	Rate	Rate in other SpA
Cataracts	25	28
Glaucoma	19	13
CME	31	25
Posterior synechiae	28	48

to the increased use of newer therapeutic drugs such as TNF inhibitors over the last 10 years with improved control of systemic inflammation in patients with PsA that would also significantly reduce the incidence of ocular inflammation [22].

There are also newer therapeutic agents on the horizon that have been studied in the treatment of PsA [47]. These include a TNF-i, certolizumab pegol, and the fully human monoclonal antibody against IL-12 and IL-23, ustekinumab. Studies have yet to show their efficacy in PsA associated uveitis.

Ocular Complications of Psoriatic Arthritis Associated Uveitis

The types of complications associated with PsA-associated uveitis are the same as those associated with intraocular inflammation from any cause. The complications rates have been found to be similar to those associated with other SpAs and include cataracts, glaucoma, CME, and posterior synechiae formation (Table 32.7) [35]. Children with JPsA have shown to have a worsened visual prognosis in comparison to JIA associated uveitis. [28]

Conclusion

Psoriasis is a common inflammatory skin disease that can affect various extracutaneous manifestations (most notably joints and eyes). The treatment of the associated uveitis should be guided by the location of the intraocular inflammation, duration of active disease, and concern about steroid associated ocular toxicity. For those with frequent disease exacerbations or chronic uveitis, some consideration should be given to the use of steroid sparing immunomodulatory therapy. Conventional DMARDs (Methotrexate, Azathioprine, etc) are effective treatment options as are the newer TNF alpha inhibitors.

References

1. Schon MP, Boehncke WH. Psoriasis. N Engl J Med. 2005;352(18):1899–912.
2. Scarpa R, Mathieu A. Psoriatic arthritis: evolving concepts. Curr Opin Rheumatol. 2000;12(4):274–80.
3. Zachariae H. Prevalence of joint disease in patients with psoriasis: implications for therapy. Am J Clin Dermatol. 2003;4(7):441–7.
4. Espinoza LR, Cuellar ML, Silveira LH. Psoriatic arthritis. Curr Opin Rheumatol. 1992;4(4):470–8.
5. Marchesoni A, Helliwell P, Gallazzi M, Gibertini P, Rossetti A, Galli L. Psoriatic arthritis in British and Italian patients: a comparative clinical, radiologic, and scintigraphic study. J Rheumatol. 1999;26 (12):2619–21.
6. Queiro R, Alperi M, Alonso-Castro S, et al. Patients with psoriatic arthritis may show differences in their clinical and genetic profiles depending on their age at psoriasis onset. Clin Exp Rheumatol. 2012;30 (4):476–80.
7. Queiro R, Torre JC, Gonzalez S, Lopez-Larrea C, Tinture T, Lopez-Lagunas I. HLA antigens may influence the age of onset of psoriasis and psoriatic arthritis. J Rheumatol. 2003;30(3):505–7.
8. Queiro R, Tejon P, Coto P, et al. Clinical differences between men and women with psoriatic arthritis: relevance of the analysis of genes and polymorphisms in the major histocompatibility complex region and of the age at onset of psoriasis. Clin Dev Immunol. 2013;2013:482691.
9. Leonard DG, O'Duffy JD, Rogers RS. Prospective analysis of psoriatic arthritis in patients hospitalized for psoriasis. Mayo Clin Proc. 1978;53(8):511–8.
10. Fitzgerald O, Dougados M. Psoriatic arthritis: one or more diseases? Best Pract Res Clin Rheumatol. 2006;20(3):435–50.
11. Jones SM, Armas JB, Cohen MG, Lovell CR, Evison G, McHugh NJ. Psoriatic arthritis: outcome of disease subsets and relationship of joint disease to nail and skin disease. Br J Rheumatol. 1994;33 (9):834–9.
12. Torre Alonso JC, Rodriguez Perez A, Arribas Castrillo JM, Ballina Garcia J, Riestra Noriega JL, Lopez Larrea C. Psoriatic arthritis (PA): a clinical,

immunological and radiological study of 180 patients. Br J Rheumatol. 1991;30(4):245–250.
13. Gladman DD, Shuckett R, Russell ML, Thorne JC, Schachter RK. Psoriatic arthritis (PSA)–an analysis of 220 patients. Q J Med. 1987;62(238):127–41.
14. Cohen MR, Reda DJ, Clegg DO. Baseline relationships between psoriasis and psoriatic arthritis: analysis of 221 patients with active psoriatic arthritis. Department of veterans affairs cooperative study group on seronegative spondyloarthropathies. J Rheumatol. 1999;26(8):1752–6.
15. Keck KM, Choi D, Savage LM, Rosenbaum JT. Insights into uveitis in association with spondyloarthritis from a large patient survey. J Clin Rheumatol Pract Rep Rheum Musculoskelet Dis. 2014;20(3):141–5.
16. Kammer GM, Soter NA, Gibson DJ, Schur PH. Psoriatic arthritis: a clinical, immunologic and HLA study of 100 patients. Semin Arthritis Rheum. 1979;9 (2):75–97.
17. Zeboulon N, Dougados M, Gossec L. Prevalence and characteristics of uveitis in the spondyloarthropathies: a systematic literature review. Ann Rheum Dis. 2008;67(7):955–9.
18. Monnet D, Breban M, Hudry C, Dougados M, Brezin AP. Ophthalmic findings and frequency of extraocular manifestations in patients with HLA-B27 uveitis: a study of 175 cases. Ophthalmology. 2004;111(4):802–9.
19. Lambert JR, Wright V. Eye inflammation in psoriatic arthritis. Ann Rheum Dis. 1976;35(4):354–6.
20. Sampaio-Barros PD, Conde RA, Bonfiglioli R, Bertolo MB, Samara AM. Characterization and outcome of uveitis in 350 patients with spondyloarthropathies. Rheumatol Int. 2006;26(12):1143–6.
21. Queiro R, Torre JC, Belzunegui J, et al. Clinical features and predictive factors in psoriatic arthritis-related uveitis. Semin Arthritis Rheum. 2002;31(4):264–70.
22. Niccoli L, Nannini C, Cassara E, et al. Frequency of iridocyclitis in patients with early psoriatic arthritis: a prospective, follow up study. Int J Rheum Dis. 2012;15(4):414–8.
23. Shore A, Ansell BM. Juvenile psoriatic arthritis–an analysis of 60 cases. J pediatr. 1982;100(4):529–35.
24. Petty RE, Southwood TR, Manners P, et al. International league of associations for rheumatology classification of juvenile idiopathic arthritis: second revision, Edmonton, 2001. J Rheumatol. 2004;31 (2):390–2.
25. Heiligenhaus A, Niewerth M, Ganser G, Heinz C, Minden K. German Uveitis in Childhood Study G. Prevalence and complications of uveitis in juvenile idiopathic arthritis in a population-based nation-wide study in Germany: suggested modification of the current screening guidelines. Rheumatology. 2007;46 (6):1015–9.
26. Butbul YA, Tyrrell PN, Schneider R, et al. Comparison of patients with juvenile psoriatic arthritis and nonpsoriatic juvenile idiopathic arthritis: how different are they? J Rheumatol. 2009;36(9):2033–41.
27. Knox DL. Psoriasis and intraocular inflammation. Trans Am Ophthalmol Soc. 1979;77:210–24.
28. Catsarou-Catsari A, Katsambas A, Theodoropoulos P, Stratigos J. Ophthalmological manifestations in patients with psoriasis. Acta dermato-venereologica. 1984;64(6):557–9.
29. Iijima S, Iwata M, Otsuka F. Psoriatic arthritis and hypopyon-iridocyclitis. Possible mechanism of the association of psoriasis and anterior uveitis. Dermatology. 1996;193(4):295–9.
30. Durrani K, Foster CS. Psoriatic uveitis: a distinct clinical entity? Am J Ophthalmol. 2005;139(1):106–11.
31. Chandran NS, Greaves M, Gao F, Lim L, Cheng BC. Psoriasis and the eye: prevalence of eye disease in Singaporean Asian patients with psoriasis. J Dermatol. 2007;34(12):805–10.
32. Burden-Teh E, Murphy R. Psoriasis and uveitis–should we be asking about eye symptoms? Br J Dermatol. 2014;170(3):756–7.
33. Rehal B, Modjtahedi BS, Morse LS, Schwab IR, Maibach HI. Ocular psoriasis. J Am Acad Dermatol. 2011;65(6):1202–12.
34. Brewerton DA, Caffrey M, Nicholls A, Walters D, James DC. Acute anterior uveitis and HL-A 27. Lancet. 1973;302(7836):994–6.
35. Paiva ES, Macaluso DC, Edwards A, Rosenbaum JT. Characterisation of uveitis in patients with psoriatic arthritis. Ann Rheum Dis. 2000;59(1):67–70.
36. Hammer RE, Maika SD, Richardson JA, Tang JP, Taurog JD. Spontaneous inflammatory disease in transgenic rats expressing HLA-B27 and human beta 2 m: an animal model of HLA-B27-associated human disorders. Cell. 1990;63(5):1099–112.
37. Rosenbaum JT. Acute anterior uveitis and spondyloarthropathies. Rheum Dis Clin North Am. 1992;18 (1):143–51.
38. Taylor W, Gladman D, Helliwell P, et al. Classification criteria for psoriatic arthritis: development of new criteria from a large international study. Arthritis Rheum. 2006;54(8):2665–73.
39. Collantes E, Zarco P, Munoz E, et al. Disease pattern of spondyloarthropathies in Spain: description of the first national registry (REGISPONSER) extended report. Rheumatology. 2007;46(8):1309–15.
40. Canoui-Poitrine F, Lekpa FK, Farrenq V, et al. Prevalence and factors associated with uveitis in spondylarthritis patients in France: results from an observational survey. Arthritis Care Res. 2012;64 (6):919–24.
41. Lima FB, Abalem MF, Ruiz DG, et al. Prevalence of eye disease in Brazilian patients with psoriatic arthritis. Clinics. 2012;67(3):249–53.
42. Banares A, Hernandez-Garcia C, Fernandez-Gutierrez B, Jover JA. Eye involvement in the spondyloarthropathies. Rheum Dis Clin North Am. 1998;24(4):771–784, ix.

43. Lyons JL, Rosenbaum JT. Uveitis associated with inflammatory bowel disease compared with uveitis associated with spondyloarthropathy. Arch Ophthalmol. 1997;115(1):61–4.
44. Hatchome N, Tagami H. Hypopyon-iridocyclitis as a complication of pustular psoriasis. J Am Acad Dermatol. 1985;13(5 Pt 1):828–9.
45. Morita E, Sato S, Yamamoto S. Uveitis in psoriasis associated with HLA-B51; a link to Behcet's disease? Br J Dermatol. 1997;136(6):979–80.
46. Stoll ML, Zurakowski D, Nigrovic LE, Nichols DP, Sundel RP, Nigrovic PA. Patients with juvenile psoriatic arthritis comprise two distinct populations. Arthritis Rheum. 2006;54(11):3564–72.
47. Ash Z, Gauioux-Viala C, Gossec L, Hensor EM, Fitzgerald O, Winthrop K, van der Heijde D, Emery P, Smolen JS, Marzo-Ortega H. A systematic literature review of drug therapies for the treatment of psoriatic arthritis: current evidence and meta-analysis informing the EULAR recommendations for the management of psoriatic arthritis. Ann Rheum Dis. 2012;71(3):319–26.
48. Huynh N, Cervantes-Castaneda RA, Bhat P, Gallagher MJ, Foster CS. Biologica response modifier therapy for psoriatic ocular inflammatory disease. Ocular Immunol Inflamm. 2008;16(3):89–93.

Reactive Arthritis/Uveitis Syndrome

33

George N. Papaliodis

Introduction

Reactive arthritis/uveitis syndrome (also described as Reiter's syndrome) is an autoimmune condition that develops in response to an infection in other regions of the body (following diarrheal illnesses, cervicitis, urethritis). The original description in the literature included a triad of associated inflammatory events including: (1) arthritis; (2) conjunctivitis; (3) urethritis. Anterior uveitis has been described in 3–12 % of affected patients [1].

In 1916, Hans Conrad Julius Reiter reported a German lieutenant who developed non-gonococcal urethritis, arthritis, and conjunctivitis [2]. Reiter was not the first to describe this syndrome, but his name became affiliated with the condition. In 1977, a campaign to rename the syndrome "reactive arthritis" was initiated as others had described the constellation of findings in the literature prior to Reiter, and Reiter had been convicted at the Nuremberg trials for war crimes as a member of the Nazi party (enthusiastic support of enforced racial sterilization and euthanasia).

The exact incidence and prevalence of the disorder is difficult to establish as the classic triad is only found in approximately 33 % of the patients, and there is often a lag between the development of the infectious illness and the resultant inflammatory events (typically 1–4 weeks later). Additionally, some of the predisposing infectious agents (eg Chlamydia urethritis) may be relatively silent with few if any clinical symptoms. In a US population-based study in Oregon and Minnesota, the incidence of reactive arthritis following documented enteric bacterial infections ranged from 0.6 to 3.1 cases per 100,000 (and varied depending upon the organism) [3].

Clinical Manifestations

The syndrome can affect many organ systems in the body including

1. joints—patients develop a painful, inflammatory, asymmetric oligoarthritis which can involve the phalanges, ankles, hips, sacroiliac joint, and knees
2. ligaments and tendons—inflammation at the site of insertion into the bone (aka enthesitis)
3. eyes—conjunctivitis, iritis, keratitis, scleritis; Conjunctivitis is found in 58 % of patients with reactive arthritis syndrome and is typically bilateral and mild

G.N. Papaliodis (✉)
Department of Opthalmology, Harvard Medical School, Massachusetts Eye and Ear Infirmary, 243 Charles Street, Boston, MA 02114, USA
e-mail: George_Papaliodis@meei.harvard.edu

G.N. Papaliodis (ed.), *Uveitis*,
DOI 10.1007/978-3-319-09126-6_33

4. skin—keratoderma blennorrhagica (patches of scaly skin on the palms, soles, trunk, or scalp)
5. genitourinary system—urethritis, cervicitis, prostatitis, cystitis
6. mouth—oral ulcerations
7. cardiac—valvular incompetence (aortic insufficiency) has been very rarely described [4]

Causes

Multiple infectious agents have been implicated as potential inciting etiologies of the syndrome. Antecedent urinary tract infection with Chlamydia *trachomatis* or *Ureaplasma urealyticum* has been associated as a trigger for reactive arthritis. In other cases, patients have developed the symptoms following a diarrheal illness due to intestinal infection with *Shigella*, *Salmonella*, *Yersinia*, *Campylobacter*, *E. coli*, and *C. difficile*. The inability to identify the exact pathogen does not exclude the condition. Even in well controlled case series, the success in isolating the microbe is approximately 50 %.

Interestingly, approximately 30–50 % of those who develop reactive arthritis/uveitis syndrome are HLA-B27 positive (although values vary widely). The development of the syndrome has been theorized to require the correct genetic predisposition and appropriate environmental exposure (infectious process) to initiate the inflammatory autoimmune condition. The clinical manifestations and severity depend upon the triggering infection and epidemiologic setting [5].

Testing

Confirmation of the antecedent infectious process by laboratory testing is often difficult to establish as there is commonly a delay between the infectious agent that initiated the process and the development of the inflammatory sequelae. In patients who have localizing symptoms (diarrhea, dysuria, cervical discharge, etc.), stool cultures, urine culture, and/or vaginal swabs are obtained. Erythrocyte sedimentation rate (ESR) and c-reactive protein (CRP) may be elevated, although in one large study, elevations in ESR and CRP were found in less than 50 % of the patients [6]. HLA-B27 testing (as noted above) may also be of some clinical utility. Synovial fluid findings are typically nonspecific and characteristic of inflammatory arthritis with elevated leukocyte counts.

Treatment

There are multiple considerations in the treatment of this condition as numerous organ systems are often involved. Treatment of the inciting infectious process (urologic or gastrointestinal) has not demonstrated efficacy in reducing or controlling the inflammatory events in other areas of the body [7].

Patients with acute arthritis are treated with oral nonsteroidal anti-inflammatory drugs (NSAIDs). This category of agents is the most common form of therapy (Naproxen 500 mg BID to TID; Indocin 50 mg TID to QID; Diclofenac 50 mg TID). Those with refractory disease can be treated with intra-articular or systemic corticosteroids.

Those resistant to oral NSAIDs and subsequently fail systemic steroids or patients who develop chronic arthritis (defined as greater than 6 months duration) should be considered for non-biologic disease modifying antirheumatic drugs (DMARDs). The most commonly used agent in this category is methotrexate. Patients who do not respond to methotrexate at maximal dosing are typically treated with TNF alpha inhibitors. Meyer et al. [8] published a series of patients with refractory reactive arthritis (having failed NSAIDs and non-biologic DMARDs) and demonstrated that anti TNF alpha therapy was rapidly effective in 90 % of the patients.

The conjunctivitis associated with this syndrome is bilateral and mild and often requires no treatment. Acute anterior uveitis can be treated with topical corticosteroids and cycloplegic agents. In patients with frequently recurring or chronic intraocular inflammation, systemic immunomodulatory therapy should be considered with the agents previously described in this section. Patients are initiated on treatment with oral NSAIDs and then converted to Methotrexate for treatment failures. Those with recalcitrant disease may warrant therapy with TNF alpha inhibitors.

Conclusion

Reactive arthritis/Reiter's syndrome is classically defined as a clinical triad of inflammatory events manifesting as arthritis, urethritis, and conjunctivitis. The aforementioned findings ensue after a predisposing infectious illness typically involving the urethra, urinary tract, or bowel. HLA-B27 is present in approximately 30–50 % of patients who develop reactive arthritis. Some studies have demonstrated a higher association in those who are HLA-B27 positive (75–90 %) [9]. The conjunctivitis is often bilateral and mild requiring no treatment. Anterior uveitis is treated with topical steroids along with cycloplegics. In those with frequently recurring or chronic inflammation, therapy with daily oral NSAIDs or more aggressive pharmacologic options like Methotrexate or a TNF alpha inhibitor may be indicated.

References

1. Lee DA, Barker SM, Su WD, Allen GL, Liesegang TJ, Ilstrup DM. The clinical diagnosis of Reiter's syndrome: ophthalmic and nonophthalmic aspects. Ophthalmology. 1986;93(3):350–6.
2. Reiter H. Ueber eine bisher unerkannte Spirochaeten-infection. Dtsch Med Wochenschr. 1916;42:1435.
3. Leirisalo-Repo M, Sieper J. Reactive arthritis: epidemiology, clinical features, and treatment. In: Weisman MH, van der Heijde D, Reveille JD, editors. Ankylosing spondylitis and the spondyloarthropathies. Elsevier: Philadelphia; 2006;53.
4. Brown LE, Forfia P, Flynn JA. Aortic insufficiency in a patient with reactive arthritis: case report and review of the literature. HSS J. 2011;7:187.
5. Leirisalo-Repo M, Hannu T, Mattila L. Microbial factors in spondyloarthropathies: insights from population studies. Curr Opin Rheumatol. 2003;15(4):408–12.
6. Townes JM, Deodhar AA, Laine ES, Smith K, Krug HE, Barkhuizen A, Thompson ME, Cieslak PR, Sobel J. Reactive arthritis following culture-confirmed infections with bacterial enteric pathogens in Minnesota and Oregon: a population-based study. Ann Rheum Dis. 2008;67(12):1689.
7. Barber CE, Kim J, Inman RD, Esdaile JM, James MT. Antibiotics for treatment of reactive arthritis: a systematic review and metaanalysis. J Rheumatol. 2013;40(6):916–28 Epub 2013 Apr 15.
8. Meyer A1, Chatelus E, Wendling D, Berthelot JM, Dernis E, Houvenagel E, Morel J, Richer O, Schaeverbeke T, Gottenberg JE, Sibilia J. Club Rhumatisme et Inflammation. Safety and efficacy of anti-tumor necrosis factor α therapy in ten patients with recent-onset refractory reactive arthritis. Arthritis Rheum. 2011;63(5):1274–80.
9. Keat A. Reiter's syndrome and reactive arthritis in perspective. New Eng J of Med. 1983;309:1606.

Relapsing Polychondritis

34

Jose Daniel Diaz

Introduction

Relapsing polychondritis (RP) is a rare, recurrent, and often progressive multisystem autoimmune disorder characterized by destructive inflammation of cartilaginous and connective tissues in many organs. Initially described in 1923 as a polychrondropathy, [1] the episodic nature of the inflammatory events ultimately lead to its characterization as relapsing polychondritis in 1960 by Pearson et al. [2] The pathogenesis remains largely unknown, and the diagnosis is usually made based on the presence of chondritis in two of three anatomic sites (auricular, nasal, laryngotracheal). Alternatively, patients may meet criteria by one of the aforementioned and two additional features such as ocular inflammation, audiovestibular damage, or seronegative arthritis [3]. As the manifestations are unusual and there is no confirmatory blood study, early diagnosis can be difficult but crucial to avoid severe life-threatening complications such as renal failure or laryngotracheal collapse [4]. In 1986, the 5 and 10 year survival rates after diagnosis was 74 and 55 %, respectively [5]. Advances in awareness, treatment options, and improved management of complications since that initial study have increased survival to a reported 94 % at 8 years in 1998 [6].

Epidemiology and Ocular Manifestations

RP is a very rare condition, with a reported incidence of 3.5 cases per million worldwide [3]. It is most commonly diagnosed in middle age, usually between 40–50 years of age; however, it can appear in childhood and as late as during the eighth decade [5, 7]. There is a male to female ratio of approximately 1:3, and it affects all ethnic groups, however there have been reports of predominance in Caucasian populations [8, 9].

As ocular manifestations are common in patients with RP, ophthalmologists can play a significant role in diagnosis. Ocular involvement has been reported in 60–70 % of cases, with episcleritis (39 %) and scleritis (14 %) representing the most common manifestations [10]. Other ocular manifestations include uveitis, exudative retinal detachment, chorioretinitis, ocular muscle paresis, optic neuritis, and peripheral ulcerative keratitis [10, 11]. Importantly, up to a third of patients with RP present with ocular symptoms, which may be a marker of

J.D. Diaz (✉)
Department of Ophthalmology, Massachusetts Eye and Ear Infirmary, Boston, MA 02114, USA
e-mail: Jose_Diaz@MEEI.harvard.edu

G.N. Papaliodis (ed.), *Uveitis*,
DOI 10.1007/978-3-319-09126-6_34

disease severity as patients with ocular involvement tend to develop multisystem manifestations [6, 10–12].

In those who develop uveitis, nongranulomatous iritis is the most common manifestation, reported in up to 22 % of RP patients [5, 10]. This may occur independently or concomitantly with scleritis (as a sclerouveitis) [13, 14]. Dense cyclitic membranes and hypopyon have also been reported as sequelae of severe intraocular inflammation [15–17]. Several case reports have described posterior uveitis and panuveitis although these are exceedingly rare [18, 19].

Laboratory Investigation

There are no specific laboratory tests for the diagnosis of RP. Antibodies to type II collagen are elevated in the acute phase of RP and have been shown to correlate with disease activity [20–23]. Antibodies to type IX and XI collagen have also been described, however they generally lack sensitivity and specificity. Serologic testing for the presence of antinuclear antibodies (ANA), anti-neutrophil cytoplasmic antibodies (ANCA), rheumatoid factor, or complement levels can suggest the presence of concomitant autoimmune or inflammatory disorders, but are generally unhelpful in the diagnosis of RP [24, 25].

Laboratory investigation can be used to assist in following the course of the disease, most notably during an acute flare. Anemia, leukocytosis, thrombocytosis, and elevated ESR are often seen during the active phase [10, 26].

Treatment

Given the rarity of RP, there is a general lack of randomized clinical trials to confirm the efficacy and optimal dosing of treatment regimens used in patients with RP. Most data is anecdotal with treatment generally being empiric and titrated according to disease activity. Furthermore, it must be noted that treatment for the ocular manifestations of RP often overlaps with treatment of other systemic involvement.

Patients with mild ocular disease including episcleritis, mild scleritis, and iritis can respond well to topical corticosteroids which may also be combined with systemic nonsteroidal anti-inflammatory drugs (NSAIDs). Patients with more severe evidence of ophthalmic involvement such as peripheral ulcerative keratitis, nodular and necrotizing scleritis typically require systemic corticosteroids (prednisone 1 mg/kg daily) and/or more potent cytotoxic agents such as methotrexate, azathioprine, mycophenolate mofetil, cyclophosphamide, and TNF-alpha inhibitors (adalimumab and infliximab) [27–29].

Immunomodulatory agents are often needed in patients with signs of systemic vasculitis or those who develop resistance to or chronic dependence on systemic steroids to remain clinically stable. Methotrexate, although contraindicated in patients with hepatic impairment, is considered effective at treating those with RP associated ocular inflammation. A starting dose of Methotrexate typically 7.5–10 mg/week is used, which can be titrated up to 25 mg/week as dictated by disease activity [30]. Infliximab, an anti-TNF-alpha agent has been reported to be effective in patients with refractory RP, especially in those with necrotizing scleritis refractory to treatment with methotrexate.

Conclusion

RP continues to be an elusive autoimmune disease characterized by recurrent inflammatory episodes of cartilaginous tissue. Given the numerous typical and atypical presentations, combined with the rarity of the disorder, the correct diagnosis is often delayed. Ocular manifestations of disease such as episcleritis and scleritis are common while uveitis is more uncommon. Although extensive case reports and case series of RP are available in the literature, there is still limited data regarding its pathogenesis and optimal treatment in patients with uveitis. Topical and systemic corticosteroids continue to be the mainstay of treatment, with steroid-sparing agents available for patients requiring long-term management. Continued multicenter studies are warranted in order to establish a logical treatment approach and guidelines.

References

1. Jaksch-Wartenhorst R. Polychrondropatha. Wien Arch Med. 1923;6:93–100.
2. Pearson C, Kline HM, Newcomer VD. Relapsing polychondritis. N Engl J Med. 1960;263:51–8. doi:10.1056/NEJM196007142630201.
3. Kent PD, Michet CJJ, Luthra HS. Relapsing polychondritis. Curr Opin Rheumatol. 2004;16(1):56–61.
4. Vitale A, Sota J, Rigante D, et al. Relapsing polychondritis: an update on pathogenesis, clinical features, diagnostic tools, and therapeutic perspectives. Curr Rheumatol Rep. 2016;18(1):3. doi:10.1007/s11926-015-0549-5.
5. Michet CJJ, McKenna CH, Luthra HS, O'Fallon WM. Relapsing polychondritis. Survival and predictive role of early disease manifestations. Ann Intern Med. 1986;104(1):74–8.
6. Letko E, Zafirakis P, Baltatzis S, Voudouri A, Livir-Rallatos C, Foster CS. Relapsing polychondritis: a clinical review. Semin Arthritis Rheum. 2002;31(6):384–95.
7. Belot A, Duquesne A, Job-Deslandre C, et al. Pediatric-onset relapsing polychondritis: case series and systematic review. J Pediatr. 2010;156(3):484–9. doi:10.1016/j.jpeds.2009.09.045.
8. Ananthakrishna R, Goel R, Padhan P, Mathew J, Danda D. Relapsing polychondritis–case series from South India. Clin Rheumatol. 2009;28(1):S7–10. doi:10.1007/s10067-008-1016-8.
9. Trentham DE, Le CH. Relapsing polychondritis. Ann Intern Med. 1998;129(2):114–22.
10. Isaak BL, Liesegang TJ, Michet CJJ. Ocular and systemic findings in relapsing polychondritis. Ophthalmology. 1986;93(5):681–9.
11. Magargal LE, Donoso LA, Goldberg RE, Gonder J, Brodsky I. Ocular manifestations of relapsing polychondritis. Retina. 1981;1(2):96–9.
12. Zeuner M, Straub RH, Rauh G, Albert ED, Scholmerich J, Lang B. Relapsing polychondritis: clinical and immunogenetic analysis of 62 patients. J Rheumatol. 1997;24(1):96–101.
13. Matas BR. Iridocyclitis associated with relapsing polychondritis. Arch Ophthalmol. 1970;84(4):474–6.
14. Zion VM, Brackup AH, Weingeist S. Relapsing polychondritis, erythema nodosum and sclerouveitis. A case report with anterior segment angiography. Surv Ophthalmol. 1974;19(2):107–14.
15. Anderson NG, Garcia-Valenzuela E, Martin DF. Hypopyon uveitis and relapsing polychondritis: a report of 2 patients and review of autoimmune hypopyon uveitis. Ophthalmology. 2004;111(6):1251–4. doi:10.1016/j.ophtha.2003.09.026.
16. Hilding A. Syndrome of cartilage pathology, destructive iridocyclitis, multiple joint dislocations; comparison with concurrent eye and joint diseases described in literature. AMA Arch Ophthalmol. 1952;48(4):420–7.
17. Ben Salah R, Frikha F, Hentati Y, Kallel S, Ghorbel A, Mnif Z, Bahloul Z. Recurrent anterior uveitis with hypopyon revealing relapsing polychondritis. Intern Med. 2012;51(22):3173–3176.
18. Guignier B, Messer L, Subilia A, Michel G. Inaugural bilateral panuveitis in relapsing polychondritis. J Fr Ophtalmol. 2010;33(10):741–51. doi:10.1016/j.jfo.2010.07.018.
19. Paroli MP, Priori R, Spinucci G, Abicca I, Valesini G. Uveitis with retinal occlusive vasculitis and sensorineural hypoacusia as first symptoms of relapsing polychondritis. Clin Exp Rheumatol. 2012;30(1–70):S101–3.
20. Ebringer R, Rook G, Swana GT, Bottazzo GF, Doniach D. Autoantibodies to cartilage and type II collagen in relapsing polychondritis and other rheumatic diseases. Ann Rheum Dis. 1981;40(5):473–9.
21. Foidart JM, Abe S, Martin GR, et al. Antibodies to type II collagen in relapsing polychondritis. N Engl J Med. 1978;299(22):1203–7. doi:10.1056/NEJM197811302992202.
22. Rodriguez ML, Caeiro F, Romero-Piffiguer MD, Juarez CP, Luna JD. Bilateral vitreous hemorrhages in a patient with relapsing polychondritis and high levels of type II collagen antibodies. Retina. 2000;20(3):299–301.
23. Tani N, Ogoshi M, Kawakubo C, et al. Case of relapsing polychondritis showing elevation of anti-type II collagen antibody titer. J Dermatol. 2013;40(9):767–8. doi:10.1111/1346-8138.12244.
24. Papo T, Piette JC. Antineutrophil cytoplasmic antibodies in polychondritis. Ann Rheum Dis. 1993;52(5):384.
25. Piette JC, El-Rassi R, Amoura Z. Antinuclear antibodies in relapsing polychondritis. Ann Rheum Dis. 1999;58(10):656–7.
26. Chow MT, Anderson SF. Relapsing polychondritis. Optom Vis Sci. 2000;77(6):286–92.
27. Hoang-Xaun T, Foster CS, Rice BA. Scleritis in relapsing polychondritis. Response Ther Ophthalmol. 1990;97(7):892–8.
28. Jabbarvand M, Fard MA. Infliximab in a patient with refractory necrotizing scleritis associated with relapsing polychondritis. Ocul Immunol Inflamm. 2010;18(3):216–7. doi:10.3109/09273941003624914.
29. Messmer EM, Foster CS. Vasculitic peripheral ulcerative keratitis. Surv Ophthalmol. 1999;43(5):379–96.
30. Lahmer T, Treiber M, von Werder A, et al. Relapsing polychondritis: an autoimmune disease with many faces. Autoimmun Rev. 2010;9(8):540–6. doi:10.1016/j.autrev.2010.02.016.

Adult Rheumatoid Arthritis

35

Evangelia Papavasileiou, Katarzyna Brodowska and George N. Papaliodis

Introduction

Rheumatoid arthritis (RA) is a common, chronic systemic inflammatory disease of unknown etiology that primarily involves the joints. Extra-articular manifestations are also observed including ophthalmologic involvement in approximately 25 % of RA patients. The clinical course of the ocular disease may be quite variable. The importance of early diagnosis of ophthalmic disease in the patient with RA cannot be overemphasized since it permits the timely management of potentially serious, sight-threatening complications. The presence of ocular disease may also be an indication of ongoing systemic disease activity [1, 2]. However, ocular involvement and severity of ocular disease may exist independently from articular inflammation and should be evaluated in all RA patients regardless of extra-ophthalmic manifestations [3].

E. Papavasileiou (✉) · K. Brodowska · G.N. Papaliodis
Department of Ophthalmology, Harvard Medical School, Massachusetts Eye and Ear Infirmary, 12th Floor, 243 Charles Street, Boston, MA 02114, USA
e-mail: Evangelia_Papavasileiou@meei.harvard.edu

K. Brodowska
e-mail: Katarzyna_Brodowska@meei.harvard.edu

G.N. Papaliodis
e-mail: George_Papaliodis@meei.harvard.edu

G.N. Papaliodis (ed.), *Uveitis*,
DOI 10.1007/978-3-319-09126-6_35

Epidemiology

RA is found worldwide and has no racial predilection; the prevalence is 0.8–1 % of the general population [4] affecting women approximately three times more often than men. Worldwide the annual incidence of RA is approximately three cases per 10,000. The disease is more commonly diagnosed after age 40 [4] but patients of any age can be afflicted. The onset of RA is most frequent during the fourth and fifth decades of life (peak between ages 35–50) [5]. The disease prevalence increases with age, and the threefold difference between the sexes diminishes in older age groups [6].

Diagnosis

The revised criteria for the diagnosis of rheumatoid arthritis (RA) are as follows: (1) morning stiffness in and around joints lasting at least 1 h before maximal improvement; (2) soft tissue swelling (arthritis) of three or more joint areas observed by a physician; (3) swelling (arthritis) of the proximal interphalangeal, metacarpophalangeal, or wrist joints; (4) symmetric swelling (arthritis); (5) rheumatoid nodules; (6) the presence of rheumatoid factor; and (7) radiographic erosions and/or peri-articular osteopenia in hand and/or wrist joints. The diagnosis of rheumatoid arthritis is established by the presence of four or more of the aforementioned criteria (Criteria 1 through 4 must have been present for at least 6 weeks to merit significance). The presence of rheumatoid factor (RF) is found in approximately 75 % of patients with RA and is not independently diagnostic of the disease. Anti-cyclic citrullinated peptide (anti CCP) antibodies are as sensitive as RF and more specific in early and established disease. Anti CCP may be detected in patients prior to the onset of clinical manifestations of RA [7–13].

Ocular Manifestations

The most common ocular manifestation of adult RA is keratoconjunctivitis sicca occurring in 9–31 % of patients. Other ocular manifestations include: episcleritis (0.17–5.7 % of RA patients); scleritis (0.15–6.3 % of RA patients) [5]; scleromalacia perforans, peripheral and central corneal ulceration have also been reported but are less common.

Uveitis is rare in adult RA in the absence of concomitant inflammatory disease involving the cornea or sclera (this is theorized via progression of inflammatory disease in contiguous ocular structures). In a series of 32 patients with rheumatoid scleritis, 14 (44 %) had at least one episode of anterior uveitis; of those, 7 patients (50 %) had necrotizing anterior scleritis, 5 patients had diffuse anterior scleritis, and 2 patients had nodular anterior scleritis [14]. None of the patients had isolated iritis in the absence of scleritis. Other case series have reported correlation with the degree of scleral inflammation and presence of uveitis.

Rheumatoid arthritis associated vasculitis was described in the 1960s in patients who developed severe clinical manifestations (skin rash, cutaneous ulcerations, gangrene, peripheral neuropathy, and visceral infarction) [15]. In one case series by Giordano and colleagues, 18.3 % of patients with RA had fluorescein angiographic evidence of retinal vasculitis [16] without clinical signs on fundoscopy.

Etiology

The etiology of rheumatoid arthritis (RA) is unknown but suspected to have both genetic and environmental factors (as with most autoimmune diseases). Severe RA is 4 fold more common than the general population in those with first-degree relatives who have rheumatoid factor positive RA. Approximately 10 % of patients with RA will have an affected first-degree relative [4].

In a study reported by Lawrence, there was a 32 % concordance rate of rheumatoid arthritis in monozygotic twins [17]. There have also been HLA types identified more commonly in patients with rheumatoid arthritis. The HLA-DRB1×0401/0404 genotype is particularly associated with severe, erosive, seropositive RA [18–21].

Treatment

The treatment of adult rheumatoid arthritis associated uveitis is dictated by the location of the intraocular inflammation (anterior versus posterior), severity of disease, and associated scleral involvement. The treatment of the concomitant scleritis is often the key determinant in selection of an anti-inflammatory agent.

Anterior uveitis is typically treated with topical steroid drops and cycloplegics. Posterior uveitis is treated with local steroid injections (trans-septal), systemic corticosteroids, or DMARDS (disease modifying anti-rheumatic drugs). If the associated scleritis is mild, an oral NSAID in combination with topical steroids may be a reasonable initial therapy (Naprosyn 375–500 mg BID to TID; Indocin 75 mg BID). For moderate to severe associated scleritis (e.g., severe diffuse or nodular scleritis), systemic corticosteroids are preferred given rapidity of action and control of inflammation (Prednisone one mg/kg/day). For those with severe/necrotizing scleritis, initiation of treatment with a DMARD in addition to systemic corticosteroids is recommended to achieve disease remission. The response to therapy is monitored closely and altered as necessary. The DMARDs currently used include:

- Leflunomide (Arava)
- Cyclosporine (Neoral)
- Methotrexate (Rheumatrex, Trexall)
- Azathioprine (Imuran)
- Cyclophosphamide (Cytoxan)

Biologics (Actemra, Cimzia, Enbrel, Humira, Kineret, Orencia, Remicade, Rituxan, Simponi) have also been used in this disorder with efficacy.

A detailed discussion of each medication is beyond the scope of this section but more thoroughly covered in the chapter on Medical Treatment for Uveitis.

Due to the destructive nature of the joint disease, potential involvement of multiple organ systems, and possible complications that may ensue from systemic immune suppression, patients are often managed by a rheumatologist and collaborating ophthalmologist [20–25].

Conclusion

RA is a common, chronic, destructive, and generally progressive systemic inflammatory disease with a long-term outcome that is characterized by significant morbidity and associated premature mortality. The most common ocular manifestation of RA is dry eye and associated sequelae. Uveitis in adult RA is usually due to associated scleritis and/or keratitis. The treatment of choice is often dictated by the severity of the associated scleral inflammation.

References

1. McGavin DD, Williamson J, Forrester JV, et al. Episcleritis and scleritis. A study of their clinical manifestations and association with rheumatoid arthritis. Br J Ophthalmol. 1976;60:192.
2. Foster CS, Forstot SL, Wilson LA. Mortality rate in rheumatoid arthritis patients developing necrotizing scleritis or peripheral ulcerative keratitis. Effects of systemic immunosuppression. Ophthalmology. 1984;91:1253.
3. Franklin Jr AN, William WB, Bruce SB, Stephen TH, Estelle F, Simons R, Robert F, Lemanske Jr. Albert & Jakobiec's Principles & Practice of Ophthalmology, 3rd Edition Book Chapter 323. Adult Rheumatoid Arthritis: Saunders Publishing; 2008.
4. Lipsky PE. Rheumatoid Arthritis. In: Fauci AS, Kasper DL, Longo DL, editors. Harrison's principles of internal medicine. 17th ed. New York: McGraw-Hill; 2008.
5. Matsuo T, Kono R, Matsuo N, et al. Incidence of ocular complications in rheumatoid arthritis and the relation of keratoconjuntivitis sicca with its systemic activity. Scand J Rheumatol. 1997;26:113–6.
6. Anitha B. Ocular manifestations of rheumatoid arthritis: Correlation with disease activity and management protocols.Masters Thesis. Rajiv Gandhi University of Health Sciences: Bangalore; 2011.
7. Gregerson PK, Silver J, Winchester RJ. The share epitope hypothesis: an approach to understanding the molecular genetics of susceptibility to rheumatoid arthritis. Arthritis Rheum. 1987;30:1205–13.
8. Ollier WE, MacGregor A. Genetic epidemiology of rheumatic disease. Br Med Bull. 1995;51:267–85.
9. Fuerst DJ, Tanzer DJ, Smith RE. Rheumatoid diseases. Int Ophthalmol Clin. 1998;38(4):47–80.
10. Bloch KJ, Buchanan WW, Wohl MJ, et al. Sjögren's syndrome: A clinical, pathological, and serological study of sixty-two cases. Med (Baltimore). 1965;44 (5):187–231.
11. Sjögren's Syndrome Foundation. About Sjogren's. http://www.sjogrens.org/home/about-sjogrens-syndrome. Accessed 6 Jan 2013.
12. Harper SL, Foster CS. The ocular manifestations of rheumatoid disease. Int Ophthalmol Clin. 1998;38 (1):1–19.
13. Hughes GRV, Whaley K. Sjögren's syndrome. Br Med J. 1972;4(5839):533–6.
14. de la Maza MS, Foster CS, Jabbur NS. Sderitis associated with rheumatoid arthritis and with other systemic immunemediated diseases. Ophthalmology. 1994;101(7):1281–8.
15. Wikinson M, Torrance WN. Clinical background of rheumatoid vascular disease. Ann Rheum Dis. 1967;26:475.
16. Dana R, Chong E, Foster CS. Adult rheumatoid arthritis. In Albert DM, Miller JW, editors. Albert & Jakobiec's Principles and Practice of Ophthalmology, 3rd edn. Saunders: Philadelphia; 2008.
17. Olier WE, MacGregor A. Genetic epidemiology of rheumatoid disease. Br Med Bull. 1995;51(2):267–85.
18. Scott DG, Bacon PA, Tribe CR. Systemic rheumatoid vasculitis: a clinical and laboratory study of 50 cases. Med (Balitmore). 1981;60:288–97.
19. Giordano N, D'Ettorre M, Biasi G, Fioravanti A, Moretti L, Marcolongo R. Retinal vasculitis in rheumatoid arthritis: an angiographic study. Clin Exp Rheumatol. 1990;8(2):121–5.

20. de la Maza MS, Foster CS, Jabbur NS. Sderitis associated with rheumatoid arthritis and with other systemic immunemediated diseases. Ophthalmology. 1994;101(7):1281–8.
21. Patel SJ, Lundy DC. Ocular manifestations of autoimmune disease. Am Fam Physician. 2002;66 (6):991–8.
22. McCluskey PJ, Wakefield D. Scleritis and episcleritis. In: Pepose JS, Holland GN, Wilhelmus KR editors. Ocular Infection and Immunity, Mosby: St. Louis; 1996. p. 642.
23. Pinckers A, Broekhuyse RM. The EOG in rheumatoid arthritis. Acta Ophthalmol (Copenh). 1983; 61:831.
24. McCormick SA, DiBartolomeo AG, Raju VK, Schwab IR. Ocular chrysiasis. Ophthalmology. 1985; 92:1432.
25. Sigal LH. The neurologic presentation of vasculitic and rheumatologic syndromes. Rev Med (Baltimore). 1987;66:157.

Sarcoidosis

36

Kathryn L. Pepple and Russell N. Van Gelder

Introduction

Sarcoidosis is a multisystem inflammatory disease of unclear etiology characterized by the presence of noncaseating granulomas. Any system can be involved, although the lungs, lymph nodes, skin, and the eye are most commonly involved [1]. 25–60 % of patients with systemic sarcoidosis will present with ophthalmic involvement at some point in the course of their disease [2], and any part of the eye and orbit can be involved (see Table 36.1). In some patients ophthalmic manifestations can be the initial manifestation of systemic disease [3, 4]. Uveitis is the most common ocular presentation. Sarcoidosis is responsible for 3–10 % of uveitis cases in referral practices [4–8].

Systemic Manifestations of Sarcoidosis

The primary organ affected by sarcoidosis is the lung, with up to 95 % of patients demonstrating involvement by chest X-ray [1]. X-ray findings have been classified into five categories by the modified Scadding system [9]. Stage zero patients have no evidence of hilar adenopathy or pulmonary infiltrate. Stage 1 disease shows bilateral hilar lymphadenopathy without pulmonary infiltration. Stage 2 shows bilateral hilar lymphadenopathy with pulmonary infiltration. Stage 3 patients demonstrate just pulmonary infiltration without hilar lymphadenopathy, and Stage 4 patients demonstrate evidence of pulmonary fibrosis. Prognostic information can be gained by scoring pulmonary involvement, with 90 % of Stage 1 patients entering disease remission within 2 years of diagnosis, while 30 % or less of patients with stage III disease will enter remission. Overall half of patients with systemic sarcoidosis will experience remission within 3 years of diagnosis with two-thirds experiencing remission by 10 years [10]. However, one-third of patients will have persistent, progressive disease that can lead to significant organ damage and functional impairment. Fortunately, the disease is only rarely fatal with <5 % mortality, usually as a result of pulmonary fibrosis, cardiac, or neurologic involvement [10].

Skin involvement is also common, occurring in 25–35 % of patients [10]. Erythema nodosum only occurs in about 10 % of patients, but is a classic rash that can present as part of Lofgren's syndrome (Erythema nodosum, fever, arthralgias, and bilateral hilar lymphadenopathy).

K.L. Pepple (✉) · R.N. Van Gelder
Department of Ophthalmology, University of Washington, 908 Jefferson St., 7th Floor, Seattle, WA 98104, USA
e-mail: kpepple@uw.edu

G.N. Papaliodis (ed.), *Uveitis*,
DOI 10.1007/978-3-319-09126-6_36

Table 36.1 Ophthalmic manifestations of sarcoidosis

Orbital granuloma
Lacrimal gland enlargement and keratoconjunctivits sicca
Conjunctival granuloma
Interstitial keratitis
Episcleritis
Scleritis
Anterior uveitis –Acute and chronic –Granulomatous and nongranulomatous
Intermediate uveitis
Posterior uveitis –Retinal vasculitis –Choroiditis –Retinitis –Optic neuritis

Lupus pernio is another distinctive sarcoid-associated rash that appears as indurated violaceous lesions on the nose, cheeks, lips, and ears. Other less specific skin findings include macules, papules, and plaques on the trunk and extremities. When present, skin findings provide good tissue to biopsy for diagnostic histology.

Almost any tissue can be affected in sarcoidosis, and many patients will present with clinical involvement of the liver (11 %), central nervous system (5 %), the parotid gland (4 %), the bone marrow (4 %), or within the heart (2 %) [1]. On autopsy, more widespread organ involvement can be documented. Some organ systems will manifest simultaneous involvement as part of well-described acute clinical syndromes. The eye is involved in the acute presentation known as Heerfordt's syndrome with uveitis, fever, parotid gland enlargement, and cranial nerve palsies. The potential for widespread and variable organ involvement in sarcoidosis emphasizes the importance of a good review of systems and complete exam in patients with this disease.

Epidemiology

Sarcoidosis is found throughout the world, but prevalence and typical presentation can vary by region and ethnicity [11]. The highest incidence is reported in Finland at 28 cases for 100,000 people. In comparison, Japan has the lowest reported incidence of 3.7 cases per 100,000 people [12]. In the United States, African Americans are affected three times more often than Caucasians, and are more likely to develop chronic disease [13].

Most patients will present in their third or fourth decade, and most are diagnosed before the age of 50 [10]. Peak incidence is around age 30, but sarcoidosis can present at any age. While older children and adolescents typically present with a similar array of organ involvement as seen in adults, pediatric patients with the early onset form of the disease present more commonly with joint involvement [14]. Blau–Jabs syndrome, which presents with granulomatous arthritis, uveitis, and dermatitis, is a familial form of early onset sarcoidosis due to mutations in the CARD15/NOD2 gene [15].

Differences in ocular disease prevalence have also been identified in association with gender, race, and geographic location [4, 11, 16, 17]. Reports of ocular involvement in systemic sarcoidosis range widely from <10 % in Finland [18], to 12–80 % in the United States [1, 2, 7, 19], 27–50 % in England [20, 21], 41 % in the Netherlands [4], and to 50–80 % in Japan [18, 22]. Ocular involvement has different definitions in these studies, and prevalence rates exceeding 50 % usually reflects the inclusion of kerato-conjuctivitis sicca as a manifestation of ocular sarcoidosis. Ocular involvement can also be influenced by race and gender, with multiple studies identifying an increased risk for eye involvement in women and black patients [1, 4]. A further racial predisposition toward anterior uveitis in black patients and posterior uveitis in white patients has also been described [4, 23].

Etiology

The etiology of sarcoidosis remains unknown, but there is increasing evidence for an infectious or environmental trigger that in susceptible populations leads to the characteristic chronic granulomatous inflammatory response [24]. Possible infectious agents vary by population with nontuberculosis mycobacterial exposure linked to patients in North American and Europe, while *Propionibacterium* has been linked with Japanese cases [25]. An infectious agent is also implicated by the transmission of sarcoidosis from affected donors to previously unaffected patients undergoing bone marrow [26, 27] and cardiac [28] transplantation. The case for mycobacterial exposure is strongly support by the results of biochemical exploration of the Kveim reagent. This reagent was used in the Kveim-Siltzbach test, a historical clinical test for sarcoidosis. The test utilized a protease resistant extract of spleen or lymph node tissue from patients with known sarcoidosis. This extract was injected subcutaneously into patients with suspected sarcoidosis. A positive test consisted of a granulomatous reaction occurring at the injection site [29]. Within the insoluble and protease resistant fraction of the Kveim reagent, mycobacterial catalase was identified [30]. Subsequent studies found that a significant number of sarcoidosis patients demonstrate a specific immune response to catalase peptides, supporting a role for mycobacterial exposure in the development of sarcoidosis [31]. Other environmental factors have also been suggested by studies identifying sarcoidosis in association with exposure to inorganic particles [32, 33], increased incidence in the spring [34], and in association with certain occupations such as metal working, firefighting, nursing, and first responders to the World Trade Center attack in 2001 [35–38].

In addition to an environmental trigger, genetic susceptibility influences disease development and pathogenesis. Case-controlled epidemiology studies, candidate gene studies, and genome wide association studies (GWAS) have identified an increased prevalence of sarcoidosis among family members as well as susceptibility and phenotype modifying gene associations [39–42]. Many susceptibility genes have a known role in immune function and regulation, most notably two HLA class II antigens HLA-DRB1 and HLA-DQB1 which have been repeatedly associated with disease [43, 44].

Genetic factors have also been implicated in influencing the ocular manifestations of sarcoidosis. Association studies have identified an increased likelihood of ocular involvement developing in the siblings of patients with known ocular disease (OR 3.0, 95 % CI 1.7–5.4) [45]. And a recent study suggests the complement factor H (CFH) polymorphism Tyrosine 402 histidine genotype may predispose to more severe posterior segment disease [40].

Pathogenesis

The immunopathologic hallmarks of sarcoidosis includes epitheliod noncaseating granulomas with activated CD4+ T cells and macrophages, a Th1 polarized cytokine response, and local tissue production of immunoregulatory cytokines such as TNF-α, IL-10, IL-12, and IL-18 [46, 47]. The stimulus for granuloma formation and maintenance in sarcoidosis is still not completely understood. However, a growing body of evidence supports a two-step model of disease [48]. The first step entails exposure to an environmental agent such as infection with a *Mycobacterium* or *Propionibacterium* species. The infection is rendered inactive by the host immune response, but clearance of certain protease resistant or other insoluble antigens is delayed and activates the characteristic sterile granulomatous response. The course of this second stage of the disease (i.e., acute vs. chronic) would then be modified by genetically encoded immune systems variations leading to the protean phenotypic manifestations.

Ocular Manifestations

Ocular sarcoidosis most commonly presents as uveitis. However, any part of the orbit or adnexa can be affected, and sarcoidosis should be considered in the differential diagnosis of any patient with inflammatory disease. Classic findings that suggest sarcoidosis include granulomatous or "mutton fat" keratic precipitates (Fig. 36.1), iris nodules (Fig. 36.2), vitreous snowballs, nodular segmental periphlebitis (Fig. 36.3), atrophic peripheral chorioretinal lesions (Fig. 36.4), and active granulomas of the retina (Fig. 36.5), optic nerve (Fig. 36.6), or choroid [49]. Bilateral involvement is typical (86–98 %), but involvement can be asymmetric [32, 50]. Keratoconjunctivitis sicca is an another common manifestation of ocular sarcoidosis, second only

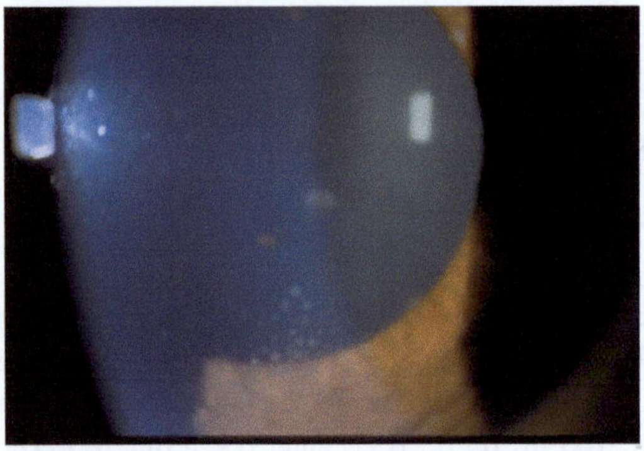

Fig. 36.1 Granulomatous keratic precipitates in sarcoid anterior uveitis

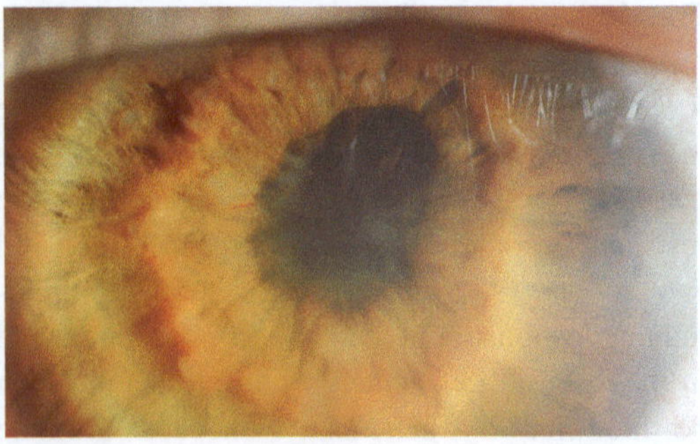

Fig. 36.2 Bussaca nodules of the iris in a pediatric patient with sarcoid panuveitis (photo courtesy of Debra Goldstein)

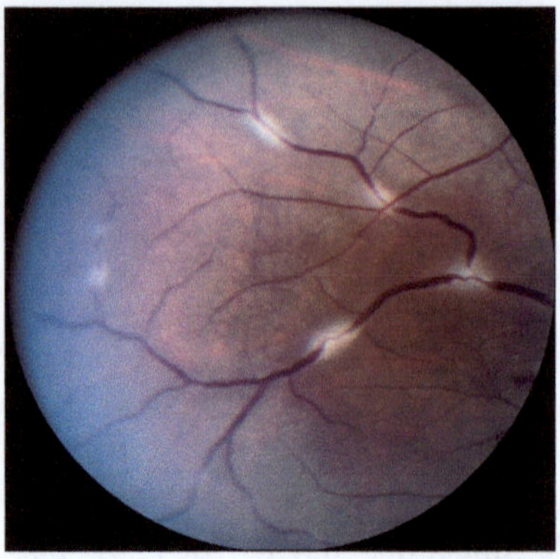

Fig. 36.3 Segmental periphlebitis without vascular occlusion is a common posterior segment manifestation of sarcoid uveitis (photo courtesy of Debra Goldstein)

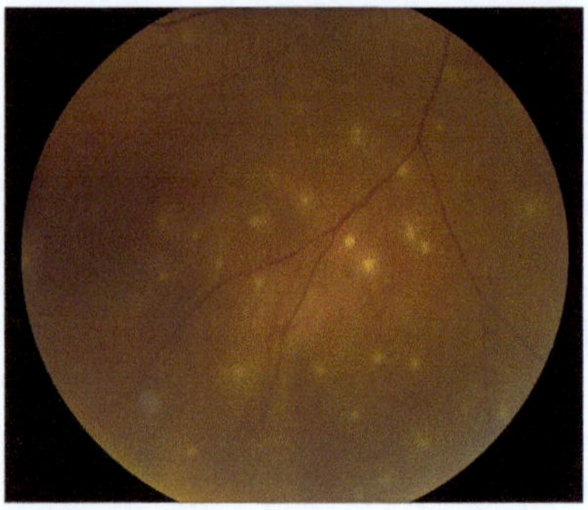

Fig. 36.4 Inactive, punched out chorioretinal scars in the inferior periphery in an older Caucasian female with primarily posterior segment involvement

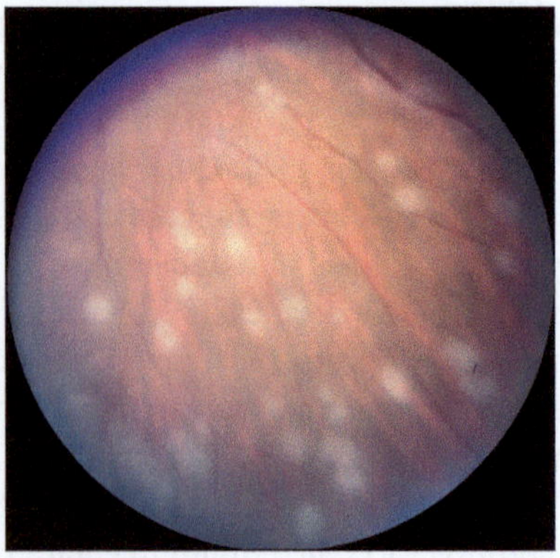

Fig. 36.5 Active retinal granulomas (photo courtesy of Debra Goldstein)

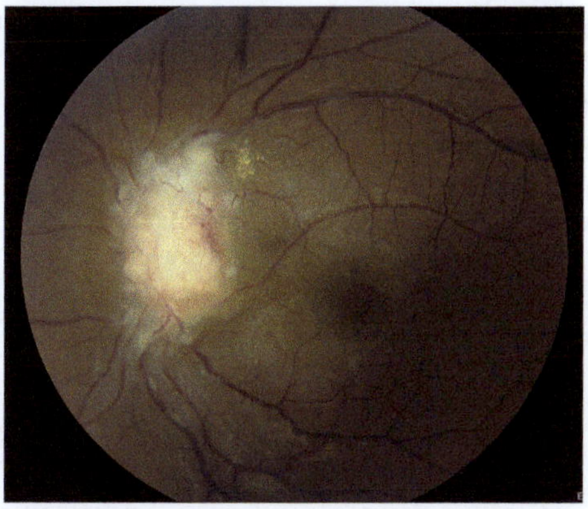

Fig. 36.6 Sarcoid granuloma of the optic nerve head

to uveitis in one case series [7], with lacrimal gland involvement described in almost one-third of patients with chronic disease [2]. A full discussion of all ophthalmic manifestations of sarcoidosis is beyond the scope of this chapter. We will focus on the intraocular and uveitic manifestations of sarcoidosis except to note that when the eyelids or conjunctiva are involved, biopsy of these structures can be an excellent and minimally invasive source of tissue for pathological diagnosis, with yields of 36–75 % [51, 52]. Nondirected biopsy, on the other hand, is of very low yield and not advised. In cases where suspicion is high, but initial biopsy results are negative, additional analysis of biopsy samples with multiplane sectioning may increase yield [53].

Most patients with sarcoid uveitis will present with symptoms such as redness, sensitivity to light, and decreased vision. However some patients with will be asymptomatic, or have minimal complaints such as floaters and ocular disease will only be identified on screening evaluation [4]. The International Workshop on Ocular Sarcoidosis (IWOS) identified seven clinical signs that are suggestive of ocular sarcoidosis (Table 36.3). These are considered characteristic, but not pathognomonic for sarcoid uveitis since they can also be found in other forms of uveitis, particularly infection with TB.

Anterior Uveitis

Anterior uveitis is the most common form of uveitis presenting in around two-thirds of patients. Most patients will have a single occurrence that corresponds to the initial diagnosis of systemic disease, but some patients will develop chronic anterior uveitis [2]. Granulomatous features such as mutton fat keratic precipitates (KP) or iris nodules are classic. Nodules at the papillary margin (Koeppe), on the iris surface (Busacca), and in the angle (Berlin nodules) are present during disease activity. As the peripheral granulomas resolve spontaneously or with treatment, they can form synechia to the anterior lens capsule, or tent-shaped peripheral anterior synechia (PAS) [54]. Extensive PAS and posterior synechia can lead to chronic or acute angle closure glaucoma which portends a poor visual prognosis [55]. Documentation of the new synechia and PAS can help detect episodes of disease activity between office visits, and prompt reevaluation of the treatment strategy before permanent damage has occurred.

Intermediate Uveitis

Intermediate uveitis is a less frequent manifestation of ocular sarcoidosis (4–21 %) [7, 56], however it is important to identify and treat effectively as it can be significantly associated with decreased vision [55]. Symptomatic patients will report blurred vision or floaters with minimal pain and redness. Vitreous signs classic for sarcoid include snowballs and "strings of pearls" vitreous opacities. Intermediate uveitis can also present with segmental periphlebitis that may take on the classic appearance of "candle wax drippings" also known as "taches de bougie". Complications of intermediate uveitis such as cystoid macular edema can occur, and can lead to permanent vision loss if untreated.

Posterior Uveitis

Posterior involvement is second to anterior uveitis in prevalence occurring in around a third of patients, but is associated with a higher risk for poor visual prognosis [55]. Vitritis and vasculitis are frequent findings. Involvement of the retinal venules with segmental periphlebitis is typical, but less commonly vascular involvement can be significant and include arteriolitis, aneurysm formation, and branch retinal vein occlusion with neovascularization [57, 58]. Round punched out choroidal lesions, most often in the inferior peripheral retina are common, particularly in elderly Caucasian women [59]. Posterior segment granulomas, appearing as solitary or multiple elevated whitish masses, are uncommon (~6 % of patients), but can involve the retina, choroid, and optic nerve [50].

Diagnosis

The gold standard for diagnosis of ocular sarcoidosis requires identification of noncaseating granulomas in ocular tissue samples. However, due to the low diagnostic yield from nondirected conjunctival biopsy and the risk of morbidity associated with in intraocular biopsy, this gold standard is rarely achieved. Therefore a validated criteria based on a combination of seven clinical and five laboratory or imaging findings has been established in order provide a standardized level of diagnostic certainty for ocular sarcoidosis [49, 50]. Using the International Workshop on Ocular Sarcoidosis (IOWS) criteria for the diagnosis ocular sarcoidosis (Table 36.2), four levels of diagnostic certainty were established. The highest level of certainty "definitive ocular sarcoidosis" requires the combination of a compatible clinical presentation (Table 36.3) with a positive biopsy of any involved tissue (eye biopsy not required). Other laboratory and imaging studies have varying positive and negative predictive values for establishing the diagnosis of ocular sarcoidosis (Table 36.4), but can be used to support the lower levels of certainty in the absence of biopsy confirmation [50]. Due to the presence of lung involvement in 90 % of patients with systemic sarcoidosis, demonstration of bilateral hilar lymphadenopathy by chest X-ray or CT is considered strong support for the

Table 36.2 IOWS criteria for the diagnosis of ocular sarcoidosis

Definite ocular sarcoidosis	Biopsy proven with compatible uveitis
Presumed ocular sarcoidosis	Biopsy not performed Bilateral hilar lymphadenopathy with compatible uveitis
Probable ocular sarcoidosis	Biopsy not performed Normal chest X-ray three suggestive eye findings (Table 36.3) two positive lab tests (Table 36.4)
Possible ocular sarcoidosis	Biopsy negative four suggestive eye findings two positive lab tests

Table 36.3 Clinical signs suggestive of ocular sarcoidosis

1. Mutton fat keratic precipitates OR Iris nodules at the papillary margin (Koeppe) or in the stroma (Bussacca)
2. Nodules in the trabecular meshwork OR tent-shaped peripheral anterior synechia
3. Vitreous snowballs OR string of pearls vitreous opacities
4. Multifocal peripheral chorioretinal lesions
5. Periphlebitis with a nodular or segmental appearance OR macroaneurysm in an inflamed eye
6. Granuloma of the optic nerve OR choroid
7. Bilateral ocular inflammation

Table 36.4 Laboratory investigations for ocular sarcoidosis

1. Chest X-ray with bilateral hilar lymphadenopathy
2. Chest CT in a patient with a negative chest X-ray
3. Elevated serum angiotensin converting enzyme OR elevated serum lysozyme
4. Two abnormal liver enzymes test (ALP, AST, ALT, GGT, or LDH)
5. Negative tuberculin test

ALP alkaline phosphatase, *AST* aspartate aminotransferase, *ALT* alanine aminotransferase, *GGT* gamma-glutamyl transferase, or *LDH* lactate dehydrogenase diagnosis of ocular sarcoidosis, and confers the diagnosis of "presumed ocular sarcoidosis." Any evidence of pulmonary involvement should prompt further evaluation with a pulmonary specialist for pulmonary function testing and consideration of bronchoalveolar lavage and transbronchial lymph node biopsy. In the absence of hilar lymphadenopathy and without biopsy confirmation, a patient can still be diagnosed with "probable" sarcoidosis or "possible" sarcoidosis in the presence of a compatible uveitis and the specified combination of supportive ocular findings and laboratory studies.

Additional investigational tests that have been used to suggest the diagnosis of sarcoidosis including elevated angiotensin converting enzyme (ACE), elevated serum lysozyme, abnormal liver enzymes, and anergy to PPD testing [60]. None have sufficient positive or negative predictive values to definitively diagnose or rule out disease in isolation. However, in the correct clinical context two or more positive tests can support the diagnosis of "probable or possible ocular sarcoidosis." Among these tests, serum ACE and lysozyme levels are commonly ordered despite the low sensitivity or specificity. Angiotensin converting enzyme is generated by the macrophages involved in granuloma formation, and serum ACE levels can reflect the total granuloma burden present in a systemic granulomatous disease like sarcoidosis. An elevated serum ACE can be identified in 60 % of patients with sarcoidosis [50, 60], but a normal or low ACE level does no rule out disease. ACE levels will also be lowered in patients taking ACE inhibitor medications for hypertension. Particular care needs to exercised in the interpretation of ACE levels in the pediatric population as ACE activity can be markedly increased through puberty in normal healthy children [61]. Although not included in the IWOS criteria, gallium scintigraphy in combination with serum ACE levels has been reported to have a high specificity for the diagnosis of sarcoidosis in patients with a negative chest X-ray [62]. However gallium scanning can be difficult to interpret, and a negative test does not rule out disease so it is not routinely recommended. Like ACE, lysozyme is also produced by granulomata, and can be elevated in patients with sarcoidosis. Typically elevations in lysozyme and ACE will occur together, but occasionally, patients with sarcoidosis will only demonstrate an elevation in serum lysozyme. However, once again this result is not specific for sarcoidosis, and lysozyme can also be elevated in other conditions such as leprosy, tuberculosis, acute leukemia, pernicious anemia, and osteoarthritis [60].

In addition to the above tests and considerations, two critical components in the evaluation of any patient with ocular sarcoidosis include the exclusion of other granulomatous diseases, particularly tuberculosis, and a complete examination to determine the presence and extent of any systemic involvement with appropriate subspecialty referral.

Treatment

Patients with ocular sarcoidosis are at risk for vision loss from complications such as cataract, glaucoma, macular edema, retinal ischemia, and optic nerve involvement [2, 55, 56, 63]. The first goal of treatment is to control inflammation using corticosteroids. The route of delivery should be tailored to best target the anatomic location or locations of inflammation. In addition, medical management of complications including elevated pressure and cystoid macular edema (CME) should be initiated as indicated. Surgical management for complications such as cataract, vitreous opacity, CME, and advanced glaucoma requiring surgical intervention should ideally be planned after 3 months of quiescence has been achieved [64–67].

Topical therapy is generally effective for anterior segment involvement, with periocular steroids reserved for refractory cases or for treatment of any associated cystoid macular edema. For acute anterior uveitis, frequent administration, of a topical steroid is recommended until improvement in the inflammation is noted. Once improvement has been achieved (by SUN criteria [68]), topical steroids should be tapered to the minimal required to maintain quiescence. During periods of active inflammation, a cycloplegic may also be administered to reduce the development of posterior synechia and minimize photosensivity. For many patients, topical therapy will provide sufficient control for anterior disease. However, in patients with persistent inflammation and frequent (more than 4 per year) or vision threatening recurrences, systemic therapy may be needed.

Intermediate and posterior segment involvement generally requires the use of oral corticosteroids. However, in cases of unilateral or asymmetric involvement periocular or intraocular steroids can be effective. Before institution of oral therapy or local depot steroid therapy, infectious etiologies must be excluded. Consensus guidelines for the use of systemic corticosteroids in patients with ocular inflammatory disease suggests the initial dose for treatment of active disease with Prednisone at 1 mg per kg per day for adult patients [69, 70]. For most patients this equals a dose of 60–80 mg of oral prednisone a day followed by tapering to low dose therapy (<10 mg per day) with disease activity monitoring. Some patients may require low dose corticosteroid therapy to maintain disease quiescence.

In some cases, steroid sparing immunomodulatory agents may be required for the management of patients with ocular sarcoidosis. Indications for corticosteroid sparing agents include a chronic requirement for greater than 10 mg of prednisone daily to maintain disease control, the development of corticosteroid intolerance, or the desire to avoid steroid-related side effects [69]. There are few studies that have evaluated the use of the various immunomodulatory agents in the specific treatment of patients with ocular sarcoidosis [71–76], but there are two pivotal studies that outline the summation of available data from retrospective and prospective case series, and provide expert panel recommendations on the use of immunomodulatory agents in patients with uveitis [69, 77]. These recommendations form the basis of the following treatment algorithm, but adjustments should be made for individual patient circumstances.

Methotrexate (MTX) has demonstrated efficacy in both systemic and ocular sarcoidosis [73, 74], and in the absence of contraindications it is generally the first line agent used. Prescribing practices vary, but in general patients are treated with 15–25 mg dosed on a weekly basis. Liver function tests should be monitored monthly over the first 3 months of therapy, and every 3 months subsequently. In addition to MTX, other oral agents including mycofenolate mofetil and azathioprine are considered efficacious in treating ocular inflammatory disease, and may offer a more compatible side effect profile for individual patients [78–81]. Although systemic cyclosporine is used in the management of refractory/steroid dependent uveitis, there is evidence in pulmonary medicine to suggest that this drug may not be effective in sarcoidosis. A randomized controlled trial compared the efficacy of Cyclosporine in progressive pulmonary sarcoid to standard medical therapy (Prednisone). The investigators could show no benefit in the group treated with Cyclosporine and Prednisone compared to those treated with Prednisone alone, and more adverse events were observed in the patients treated with Cyclosporine [93]. Tacrolimus is another promising steroid sparing agent, however as a newer agent in the uveitis literature there is less information about this agent in patients with sarcoid uveitis [82, 83]. Alkylating agents such as cyclophosphamide and chlorambucil have significant systemic toxicities that make them less desirable options for patients that fail other immunomodulatory agents, and they are not used as first line agents for the treatment of sarcoid uveitis.

When conventional first line immunomodulation fail, blockade of tumor necrosis alpha (TNFα) appears efficacious for patients with sarcoid related uveitis. There are five anti-TNFα agents available at this time in the United States; infliximab (Remicade), adalimumab (Humira), etanercept (Enbrel), golimumab (Simponi), and certolizumab (Cimzia). All the anti-TNF agents have been used in the treatment of noninfectious uveitis, but the evidence for use of golimumab and certolizumab is still limited at this time [84]. Good evidence exists for efficacy of infliximab [85–88] and adalimumab in the treatment of ocular sarcoidosis, and current guidelines recommend these two agents as second line agents in patients failing or intolerant to other immunomodulators [77]. Etanercept has not demonstrated efficacy for treatment of eye disease [76], and may lead to worsening of ocular inflammation in sarcoid patients [89]. Therefore current recommendations state that etanercept should not be used in the treatment of ocular sarcoidosis. A paradoxical sarcoid like reaction has been reported in association with use of each of the anti-TNFα agents [90]. Thus it is theoretically possible that worsening inflammation in the face of treatment could be misinterpreted as treatment failure rather than a drug effect in patients with sarcoid uvietis.

Prognosis

Visual prognosis in patients with sarcoid uveitis is most impacted by the development of chronic inflammation, posterior segment involvement, and the presence of complications such as glaucoma, cataract, and cystoid macular edema [55, 91, 92]. However, most cases will respond well to a combination of topical, local or low-dose systemic corticosteroids.

Summary

Sarcoidosis is a multisystem granulomatous disease that affects the eye in one-third of patients. Bilateral involvement and granulomatous features are classic features to suggest the diagnosis. Screening for pulmonary involvement with a chest X-ray or CT, and ruling out other infectious etiologies are required as part of the diagnostic evaluation. Treatment begins with corticosteroids, which are typically very effective for patients with sarcoid uveitis. Immunomodulation may be required for patients that develop chronic disease.

References

1. Baughman RP, Teirstein AS, Judson MA, et al. Clinical characteristics of patients in a case control study of sarcoidosis. Am J Respir Crit Care Med. 2001;164(10 Pt 1):1885–9.
2. Jabs DA, Johns CJ. Ocular involvement in chronic sarcoidosis. Am J Ophthalmol. 1986;102(3):297–301.
3. Sivakumar M, Chee SP. A case series of ocular disease as the primary manifestation in sarcoidosis. Ann Acad Med Singapore. 1998;27(4):560–6.
4. Rothova A, Alberts C, Glasius E, Kijlstra A, Buitenhuis HJ, Breebaart AC. Risk factors for ocular sarcoidosis. Doc Ophthalmol. 1989;72(3–4):287–96.
5. Blaise P, Fardeau C, Chapelon C, Bodaghi B, Le Hoang P. Minor salivary gland biopsy in diagnosing ocular sarcoidosis. Br J Ophthalmol. 2011;95(12):1731–4.
6. Jones NP. Sarcoidosis and uveitis. Ophthalmol Clin North Am. 2002;15(3):319–326.
7. Evans M, Sharma O, LaBree L, Smith RE, Rao NA. Differences in clinical findings between Caucasians and African Americans with biopsy-proven sarcoidosis. Ophthalmology. 2007;114(2):325–33.
8. Jones NP. The manchester uveitis clinic: the first 3000 patients-epidemiology and casemix. Ocul Immunol Inflamm. 2013.
9. Scadding JG. Prognosis of intrathoracic sarcoidosis in England. A review of 136 cases after five years' observation. Br Med J. 1961;2(5261):1165–72.
10. Iannuzzi MC, Rybicki BA, Teirstein AS. Sarcoidosis. N Engl J Med. 2007;357(21):2153–65.
11. Jones N, Mochizuki M. Sarcoidosis: epidemiology and clinical features. Ocul Immunol Inflamm. 2010;18(2):72–9.
12. Pietinalho A, Hiraga Y, Hosoda Y, Lofroos AB, Yamaguchi M, Selroos O. The frequency of sarcoidosis in Finland and Hokkaido Japan. A comparative epidemiological study. Sarcoidosis. 1995;12(1):61–7.
13. Rybicki BA, Major M, Popovich J Jr, Maliarik MJ, Iannuzzi MC. Racial differences in sarcoidosis incidence: a 5-year study in a health maintenance organization. Am J Epidemiol. 1997;145(3):234–41.
14. Cimaz R, Ansell BM. Sarcoidosis in the pediatric age. Clin Exp Rheumatol. 2002;20(2):231–7.
15. Miceli-Richard C, Lesage S, Rybojad M, et al. CARD15 mutations in Blau syndrome. Nat Genet. 2001;29(1):19–20.
16. Siltzbach LE, James DG, Neville E, et al. Course and prognosis of sarcoidosis around the world. Am J Med. 1974;57(6):847–52.
17. Baughman RP, Lower EE, Kaufman AH. Ocular sarcoidosis. Semin Respir Crit Care Med. 2010;31(4):452–62.
18. Pietinalho A, Ohmichi M, Hiraga Y, Lofroos AB, Selroos O. The mode of presentation of sarcoidosis in

Finland and Hokkaido, Japan. A comparative analysis of 571 Finnish and 686 Japanese patients. Sarcoidosis Vasc Diffuse Lung Dis. 1996;13(2):159–66.
19. Obenauf CD, Shaw HE, Sydnor CF, Klintworth GK. Sarcoidosis and its ophthalmic manifestations. Am J Ophthalmol. 1978;86(5):648–55.
20. Crick RP, Hoyle C, Smellie H. The eyes in sarcoidosis. Br J Ophthalmol. 1961;45(7):461–81.
21. James DG, Anderson R, Langley D, Ainslie D. Ocular sarcoidosis. Br J Ophthalmol. 1964;48:461–470.
22. Ohara K, Okubo A, Sasaki H, Kamata K. Intraocular manifestations of systemic sarcoidosis. Jpn J Ophthalmol. 1992;36(4):452–7.
23. Khalatbari D, Stinnett S, McCallum RM, Jaffe GJ. Demographic-related variations in posterior segment ocular sarcoidosis. Ophthalmology. 2004;111(2):357–62.
24. Brownell I, Ramirez-Valle F, Sanchez M, Prystowsky S. Evidence for mycobacteria in sarcoidosis. Am J Respir Cell Mol Biol. 2011;45(5):899–905.
25. Eishi Y, Suga M, Ishige I, et al. Quantitative analysis of mycobacterial and propionibacterial DNA in lymph nodes of Japanese and European patients with sarcoidosis. J Clin Microbiol. 2002;40(1):198–204.
26. Heyll A, Meckenstock G, Aul C, et al. Possible transmission of sarcoidosis via allogeneic bone marrow transplantation. Bone Marrow Transplant. 1994;14(1):161–4.
27. Tauro S, Mahendra P. Resolution of sarcoidosis after allogeneic bone marrow transplantation with donor lymphocyte infusions. Bone Marrow Transplant. 2001;27(7):757–9.
28. Burke WM, Keogh A, Maloney PJ, Delprado W, Bryant DH, Spratt P. Transmission of sarcoidosis via cardiac transplantation. Lancet. 1990;336(8730):1579.
29. Siltzbach LE. The Kveim test in sarcoidosis. A study of 750 patients. JAMA. 1961;178:476–82.
30. Song Z, Marzilli L, Greenlee BM, et al. Mycobacterial catalase-peroxidase is a tissue antigen and target of the adaptive immune response in systemic sarcoidosis. J Exp Med. 2005;201(5):755–67.
31. Drake WP, Dhason MS, Nadaf M, et al. Cellular recognition of Mycobacterium tuberculosis ESAT-6 and KatG peptides in systemic sarcoidosis. Infect Immun. 2007;75(1):527–30.
32. Newman LS, Rose CS, Bresnitz EA, et al. A case control etiologic study of sarcoidosis: environmental and occupational risk factors. Am J Respir Crit Care Med. 2004;170(12):1324–30.
33. Rybicki BA, Amend KL, Maliarik MJ, Iannuzzi MC. Photocopier exposure and risk of sarcoidosis in African-American sibs. Sarcoidosis Vasc Diffuse Lung Dis. 2004;21(1):49–55.
34. Demirkok SS, Basaranoglu M, Coker E, Karayel T. Seasonality of the onset of symptoms, tuberculin test anergy and Kveim positive reaction in a large cohort of patients with sarcoidosis. Respirology. 2007;12(4):591–3.
35. Kucera GP, Rybicki BA, Kirkey KL, et al. Occupational risk factors for sarcoidosis in African-American siblings. Chest. 2003;123(5):1527–35.
36. Prezant DJ, Dhala A, Goldstein A, et al. The incidence, prevalence, and severity of sarcoidosis in New York City firefighters. Chest. 1999;116(5):1183–93.
37. Parkes SA, Baker SB, Bourdillon RE, et al. Incidence of sarcoidosis in the Isle of Man. Thorax. 1985;40(4):284–7.
38. Izbicki G, Chavko R, Banauch GI, et al. World Trade Center "sarcoid-like" granulomatous pulmonary disease in New York City Fire Department rescue workers. Chest. 2007;131(5):1414–23.
39. Kawagoe T, Mizuki N. Sarcoidosis. Curr Opin Ophthalmol. 2011;22(6):502–7.
40. Thompson IA, Liu B, Sen HN, et al. Association of complement factor H tyrosine 402 histidine genotype with posterior involvement in sarcoid-related uveitis. Am J Ophthalmol. 2013;155(6):1068–1074 e1061.
41. Rybicki BA, Iannuzzi MC, Frederick MM, et al. Familial aggregation of sarcoidosis. a case-control etiologic study of sarcoidosis (ACCESS). Am J Respir Crit Care Med. 2001;164(11):2085–91.
42. Spagnolo P, Grunewald J. Recent advances in the genetics of sarcoidosis. J Med Genet. 2013;50(5):290–7.
43. Rossman MD, Thompson B, Frederick M, et al. HLA-DRB1*1101: a significant risk factor for sarcoidosis in blacks and whites. Am J Hum Genet. 2003;73(4):720–35.
44. Iannuzzi MC, Maliarik MJ, Poisson LM, Rybicki BA. Sarcoidosis susceptibility and resistance HLA-DQB1 alleles in African Americans. Am J Respir Crit Care Med. 2003;167(9):1225–31.
45. Judson MA, Hirst K, Iyengar SK, et al. Comparison of sarcoidosis phenotypes among affected African-American siblings. Chest. 2006;130(3):855–62.
46. Mitchell DN, Scadding JG, Heard BE, Hinson KF. Sarcoidosis: histopathological definition and clinical diagnosis. J Clin Pathol. 1977;30(5):395–408.
47. Chan CC, Wetzig RP, Palestine AG, Kuwabara T, Nusenblatt RB. Immunohistopathology of ocular sarcoidosis. Report of a case and discussion of immunopathogenesis. Arch Ophthalmol. 1987;105(10):1398–402.
48. Chen ES, Song Z, Willett MH, et al. Serum amyloid A regulates granulomatous inflammation in sarcoidosis through Toll-like receptor-2. Am J Respir Crit Care Med. 2010;181(4):360–73.
49. Herbort CP, Rao NA, Mochizuki M. International criteria for the diagnosis of ocular sarcoidosis: results of the first International Workshop On Ocular Sarcoidosis (IWOS). Ocul Immunol Inflamm. 2009;17(3):160–9.

50. Takase H, Shimizu K, Yamada Y, Hanada A, Takahashi H, Mochizuki M. Validation of international criteria for the diagnosis of ocular sarcoidosis proposed by the first international workshop on ocular sarcoidosis. Jpn J Ophthalmol. 2010;54(6):529–36.
51. Crick R, Hoyle C, Mather G. Conjunctival biopsy in sarcoidosis. Br Med J. 1955;2(4949):1180–1.
52. Merritt JC, Lipper SL, Peiffer RL, Hale LM. Conjunctival biopsy in sarcoidosis. J Natl Med Assoc. 1980;72(4):347–9.
53. Bui KM, Garcia-Gonzalez JM, Patel SS, Lin AY, Edward DP, Goldstein DA. Directed conjunctival biopsy and impact of histologic sectioning methodology on the diagnosis of ocular sarcoidosis. J Ophthalmic Inflamm Infect. 2014;4(1):8.
54. Kawaguchi T, Hanada A, Horie S, Sugamoto Y, Sugita S, Mochizuki M. Evaluation of characteristic ocular signs and systemic investigations in ocular sarcoidosis patients. Jpn J Ophthalmol. 2007;51 (2):121–6.
55. Dana MR, Merayo-Lloves J, Schaumberg DA, Foster CS. Prognosticators for visual outcome in sarcoid uveitis. Ophthalmology. 1996;103(11): 1846–53.
56. Lobo A, Barton K, Minassian D, du Bois RM, Lightman S. Visual loss in sarcoid-related uveitis. Clin Experiment Ophthalmol. 2003;31(4):310–6.
57. Rothova A, Lardenoye C. Arterial macroaneurysms in peripheral multifocal chorioretinitis associated with sarcoidosis. Ophthalmology. 1998;105 (8):1393–7.
58. Verougstraete C, Snyers B, Leys A, Caspers-Velu LE. Multiple arterial ectasias in patients with sarcoidosis and uveitis. Am J Ophthalmol. 2001; 131(2):223–31.
59. Lardenoye CW, Van der Lelij A, de Loos WS, Treffers WF, Rothova A. Peripheral multifocal chorioretinitis: a distinct clinical entity? Ophthalmology. 1997;104(11):1820–6.
60. Weinreb RN, Tessler H. Laboratory diagnosis of ophthalmic sarcoidosis. Surv Ophthalmol. 1984;28 (6):653–64.
61. Rodriguez GE, Shin BC, Abernathy RS, Kendig EL Jr. Serum angiotensin-converting enzyme activity in normal children and in those with sarcoidosis. J Pediatr. 1981;99(1):68–72.
62. Power WJ, Neves RA, Rodriguez A, Pedroza-Seres M, Foster CS. The value of combined serum angiotensin-converting enzyme and gallium scan in diagnosing ocular sarcoidosis. Ophthalmology. 1995;102(12):2007–11.
63. Rothova A. Suttorp-van Schulten MS, Frits Treffers W, Kijlstra A. Causes and frequency of blindness in patients with intraocular inflammatory disease. Br J Ophthalmol. 1996;80(4):332–6.
64. Kiryu J, Kita M, Tanabe T, Yamashiro K, Miyamoto N, Ieki Y. Pars plana vitrectomy for cystoid macular edema secondary to sarcoid uveitis. Ophthalmology. 2001;108(6):1140–4.
65. Ieki Y, Kiryu J, Kita M, et al. Pars plana vitrectomy for vitreous opacity associated with ocular sarcoidosis resistant to medical treatment. Ocul Immunol Inflamm. 2004;12(1):35–43.
66. Akova YA, Foster CS. Cataract surgery in patients with sarcoidosis-associated uveitis. Ophthalmology. 1994;101(3):473–9.
67. Van Gelder RN, Leveque TK. Cataract surgery in the setting of uveitis. Curr Opin Ophthalmol. 2009;20 (1):42–5.
68. Jabs DA, Nussenblatt RB, Rosenbaum JT. Standardization of uveitis nomenclature for reporting clinical data. Results of the First International Workshop. Am J Ophthalmol. 2005;140(3):509–16.
69. Jabs DA, Rosenbaum JT, Foster CS, et al. Guidelines for the use of immunosuppressive drugs in patients with ocular inflammatory disorders: recommendations of an expert panel. Am J Ophthalmol. 2000;130 (4):492–513.
70. Hunninghake GW, Costabel U, Ando M, et al. ATS/ERS/WASOG statement on sarcoidosis. American Thoracic Society/European Respiratory Society/World Association of Sarcoidosis and other Granulomatous Disorders. Sarcoidosis Vasc Diffuse Lung Dis. 1999;16(2):149–73.
71. Murray PI, Bodaghi B, Sharma OP. Systemic treatment of sarcoidosis. Ocul Immunol Inflamm. 2011;19(2):145–50.
72. Bhat P, Cervantes-Castaneda RA, Doctor PP, Anzaar F, Foster CS. Mycophenolate mofetil therapy for sarcoidosis-associated uveitis. Ocul Immunol Inflamm. 2009;17(3):185–90.
73. Baughman RP, Lower EE, Ingledue R, Kaufman AH. Management of ocular sarcoidosis. Sarcoidosis Vasc Diffuse Lung Dis. 2012;29(1):26–33.
74. Dev S, McCallum RM, Jaffe GJ. Methotrexate treatment for sarcoid-associated panuveitis. Ophthalmology. 1999;106(1):111–8.
75. Erckens RJ, Mostard RL, Wijnen PA, Schouten JS, Drent M. Adalimumab successful in sarcoidosis patients with refractory chronic non-infectious uveitis. Graefes Arch Clin Exp Ophthalmol. 2012;250 (5):713–20.
76. Baughman RP, Lower EE, Bradley DA, Raymond LA, Kaufman A. Etanercept for refractory ocular sarcoidosis: results of a double-blind randomized trial. Chest. 2005;128(2):1047–62.
77. Levy-Clarke G, Jabs DA, Read RW, Rosenbaum JT, Vitale A, Van Gelder RN. Expert panel recommendations for the use of anti-tumor necrosis factor biologic agents in patients with ocular inflammatory disorders. Ophthalmology. 2014;121(3):785–796 e783.
78. Daniel E, Thorne JE, Newcomb CW, et al. Mycophenolate mofetil for ocular inflammation. Am J Ophthalmol. 2010;149(3):423–432 e421–422.
79. Gangaputra S, Newcomb CW, Liesegang TL, et al. Methotrexate for ocular inflammatory diseases. Ophthalmology. 2009;116(11):2188–2198 e2181.

80. Pasadhika S, Kempen JH, Newcomb CW, et al. Azathioprine for ocular inflammatory diseases. Am J Ophthalmol. 2009;148(4):500–509 e502.
81. Kacmaz RO, Kempen JH, Newcomb C, et al. Cyclosporine for ocular inflammatory diseases. Ophthalmology. 2010;117(3):576–84.
82. Lee RW, Greenwood R, Taylor H, et al. A randomized trial of tacrolimus versus tacrolimus and prednisone for the maintenance of disease remission in noninfectious uveitis. Ophthalmology. 2012;119(6):1223–30.
83. Zhai J, Gu J, Yuan J, Chen J. Tacrolimus in the treatment of ocular diseases. BioDrugs. 2011;25(2):89–103.
84. Sanchez-Cano D, Callejas-Rubio JL, Ruiz-Villaverde R, Rios-Fernandez R, Ortego-Centeno N. Off-label uses of anti-TNF therapy in three frequent disorders: Behcet's disease, sarcoidosis, and noninfectious uveitis. Mediators Inflamm. 2013;2013:286857.
85. Lindstedt EW, Baarsma GS, Kuijpers RW, van Hagen PM. Anti-TNF-alpha therapy for sight threatening uveitis. Br J Ophthalmol. 2005;89(5):533–6.
86. Cruz BA, Reis DD, Araujo CA. Refractory retinal vasculitis due to sarcoidosis successfully treated with infliximab. Rheumatol Int. 2007;27(12):1181–3.
87. Baughman RP, Bradley DA, Lower EE. Infliximab in chronic ocular inflammation. Int J Clin Pharmacol Ther. 2005;43(1):7–11.
88. Doty JD, Mazur JE, Judson MA. Treatment of sarcoidosis with infliximab. Chest. 2005;127(3):1064–71.
89. Hashkes PJ, Shajrawi I. Sarcoid-related uveitis occurring during etanercept therapy. Clin Exp Rheumatol. 2003;21(5):645–6.
90. Cunningham ET Jr, Pasadhika S, Suhler EB, Zierhut M. Drug-induced inflammation in patients on TNFalpha inhibitors. Ocul Immunol Inflamm. 2012;20(1):2–5.
91. Edelsten C, Pearson A, Joynes E, Stanford MR, Graham EM. The ocular and systemic prognosis of patients presenting with sarcoid uveitis. Eye (Lond). 1999;13(Pt 6):748–53.
92. Miserocchi E, Modorati G, Di Matteo F, Galli L, Rama P, Bandello F. Visual outcome in ocular sarcoidosis: retrospective evaluation of risk factors. Eur J Ophthalmol. 2011;21(6):802–10.
93. Wyser CP, van Schalkwyk EM, Alheit B, Bardin Pg, Joubert Jr. Treatment of progressive pulmonary sarcoidosis with cyclosporin A. A randomized controlled trial. Am J Respir Crit Care Med. 1997 Nov;156(5):1371–6.

Sympathetic Ophthalmia

37

Anna Marmalidou and Chukwuemeka Nwanze

Introduction

In 1813 the 3-year-old son of a harness maker stabbed himself in the right eye while playing with one of his father's awls resulting in loss of vision in the traumatized eye. Shortly thereafter, the boy's left eye became inflamed, and 2 years later he had lost vision in the non-traumatized eye leaving him completely blind. Approximately 10 years later, this boy, Louis Braille, invented the most commonly used tactile writing system for the blind [1]. This alphabet was named braille after the inventor.

The clinical scenario depicted above is the typical presentation of patients afflicted with sympathetic ophthalmia (SO). SO is a rare, bilateral, and diffuse granulomatous intraocular inflammation that occurs in most cases within days or months after either surgery or penetrating trauma to one eye. The clinical features of SO have been known since antiquity. The earliest known description of SO in literature is a paper by Agathias in an anthology compiled from Constantius Cephalis dating from 1000 AD [2]. SO was initially named sympathetic ophthalmitis in 1840 by Sir William Mackenzie, a Scottish ophthalmologist, who presented a series of six cases in which a penetrating injury to one eye led to bilateral blindness [3].

A. Marmalidou (✉)
Department of Ophthalmology, Massachusetts Eye and Ear Infirmary, Harvard Medical School, 243 Charles Street, Boston, MA 02114, USA
e-mail: anna_marmalidou@meei.harvard.edu

C. Nwanze
Department of Ophthalmology, Boston Medical Center, 85 East Concord St., Boston, MA 02118, USA

G.N. Papaliodis (ed.), *Uveitis*,
DOI 10.1007/978-3-319-09126-6_37

Epidemiology

Most of the literature about the incidence of SO dates from the 1960s to 1980s [4–8]. These studies suggest an incidence with a range of 0.2–0.5 % following penetrating ocular injuries and 0.01 % after intraocular surgery. There are two more recent studies from the United Kingdom (2000) [9] and China (2009) [10]. The UK study estimated the minimum rate of SO to be 0.03 per 100,000. The Chinese study estimated that SO occurred at a rate of 0.37 % after open globe injury. The results of both of these studies are within the range of previously published articles. There are approximately 3.1 penetrating eye injuries per 100,000 person/year in the United States [11]. This implies approximately 9,800 penetrating eye injuries in the United States during 2013 [12]. These estimates suggest that during 2013 there were approximately 98 new cases of SO in the US.

Males are at increased risk for eye trauma compared to females [13–15], thus SO resulting from ocular trauma tends to affect males more commonly [2, 5, 8, 16]. Similarly, given the higher rates of ocular trauma in younger patients, the age distribution of trauma-related SO cases is skewed lower [8, 17]. However, contemporary trends such as increased child safety monitoring and prophylactic medical/surgical measures may be reversing these trends in SO [16]. Surgery-induced SO does not show any gender predilection. Since older patients undergo more ocular surgery, surgical-induced SO tends to affect older patients [9, 17].

Clinical Presentation

SO has been reported to occur as early as 10 days [18] or as late as 66 years [19] after the penetrating trauma/surgical procedure. The peak incidence of SO occurs between 1 and 2 months after the inciting injury [20]. Most cases of SO (70–80 %) occur between 2 weeks and 3 months of the causative event [21]. 90 % of SO occurs within 1 year of the injury [20].

Patients who have SO typically present with ocular injection, pain, photophobia, epiphora, and insidious loss of vision in the non-injured eye [8, 22, 23]. These patients may also present with diminished near vision, a result of changes in accommodative amplitude [23, 24]. These symptoms are often accompanied by worsened inflammation in the injured eye [25]. Non-ocular symptoms are rare and include hearing disturbances, high-frequency deafness, vitiligo, poliosis, alopecia, and meningismus [23, 26, 27]. Clinical symptoms and signs are variable and can range from mild to severe [25, 28].

The slit lamp exam of patients with SO can reveal conjunctival injection and ciliary flush (limbal injection) [8, 22, 23]. The cornea may have granulomatous (mutton fat) precipitates or small white keratic precipitates [23, 28]. The anterior chamber has cell and flare in approximately 67 % of cases [8]. The iris may be thickened from lymphocytic infiltration and posterior synechiae may form. Intraocular pressure may be elevated as a result of synechiae and clogging of the trabecular meshwork with inflammatory debris. Alternatively, the eye pressure may be low secondary to ciliary body shutdown from the inflammation [22].

The posterior segment exam reveals moderate-to-severe vitritis (see Fig. 37.2). Papillitis, choroiditis, macular edema, migration of pigment into inner retinal layers, retinal vasculitis, and serous retinal detachments may also occur [21, 24]. Yellow-white choroidal lesions occur in the posterior pole and mid-equatorial region. These lesions may become confluent over time. These lesions correspond pathologically to Dalen-Fuchs nodules (see Fig. 37.1) [22, 25]. Dalen-Fuchs nodules appear in approximately one-third of eyes enucleated for SO [21, 29]. The Dalen-Fuchs nodules are not pathognomonic of sympathetic ophthalmia as they may be seen in other granulomatous inflammatory diseases such as Vogt–Koyanagi–Harada syndrome and sarcoidosis [25, 30]. Dalen-Fuchs nodules may represent the more severe spectrum of SO [25, 31].

Findings in chronic SO include cataract, glaucoma, choroidal neovascularization, subretinal fibrosis, atrophy of the optic nerve/retina/choroid, and finally phthisis bulbi [22, 24].

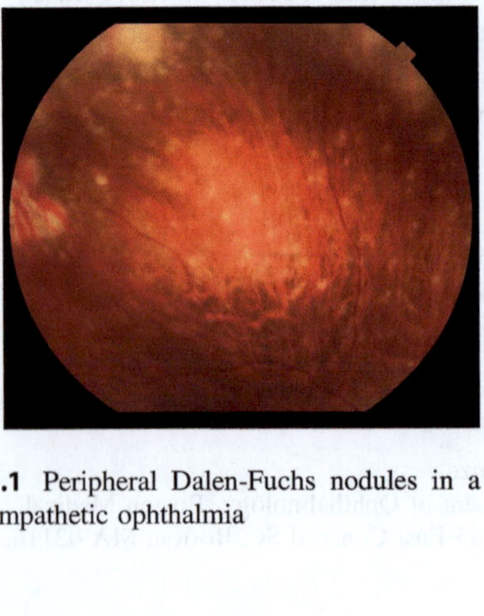

Fig. 37.1 Peripheral Dalen-Fuchs nodules in a patient with sympathetic ophthalmia

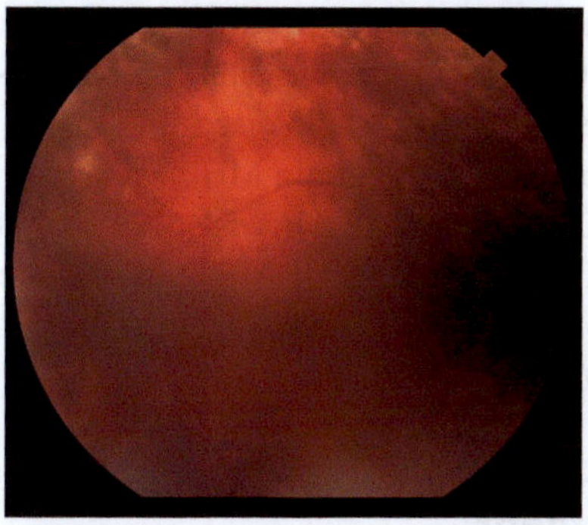

Fig. 37.2 Retinal vasculitis, vitritis, and inferior serous retinal detachment in a patient with sympathetic ophthalmia

Testing

There are no blood studies to confirm the diagnosis of sympathetic ophthalmia. Clinical investigations in SO include fluorescein angiography (FA), indocyanine green angiography (ICG), B-scan ultrasonography (US), optical coherence tomography (OCT), and pathological sections of enucleated eyes.

FA in the early venous phase demonstrates multiple hyperfluorescent areas that then demonstrate late leakage at the level of the RPE [22, 29]. Leakage occurs in Dalen-Fuchs nodules and areas of retinal vasculitis [24]. Early blocking is seen in areas occupied by Dalen-Fuchs nodules. The optic nerve head often stains in SO even in cases without optic nerve head edema [24]. Late pooling can be seen in the posterior pole representing multiple, lobular, serous retinal detachments [32].

ICG shows multiple hypofluorescent spots without a hyperfluorescent collar in the intermediate phase. Some of these areas become isofluorescent in the late stage [33–35]. These hypofluorescent areas are thought to correspond to choroidal edema and choroidal inflammatory infiltration [24]. Large areas of hypofluorescence can be detected in the late phase of ICG [35].

US in SO is used to detect gross anatomic changes in the retina and choroid. US can demonstrate diffuse thickening of the choroid as well as serous retinal detachments [36–38].

OCT in SO can be used to detect micro-anatomic changes within the retina. Observable OCT findings in SO include serous retinal detachments, intra-retinal edema, disintegration of RPE, tears in the RPE, elongation of photoreceptors, and disorganization of the retinal layers [29, 38–40]. Dalen-Fuchs nodules on OCT appear as hyper-reflective lesions at the level of the RPE with disruption of the inner segment/outer segment (IS/OS) junction [38, 41].

Pathological sections of eyes with SO (both the injured and the secondarily involved eye) demonstrate marked swelling of the choroid that corresponds to lymphocytic infiltration of the choroid. The inflammatory response is characterized as a diffuse, non-necrotizing, granulomatous inflammation of the entire uvea [22, 29, 42, 43]. Major cell types include epithelioid cells and some giant cells [2]. However, the cellular response is variable from case to case which may explain the wide spectrum of clinical presentations [44]. In severe cases, eosinophils and plasma cells can be observed, especially around the inner choroid [45]. Severe cases are also associated with the presence of pigment in the epithelioid cells [46]. The inflammation, typically but not always, spares the choriocapillaris [21, 45, 47].

Dalen-Fuchs nodules appear in approximately one-third of SO cases [21, 22]. Dalen-Fuchs nodules on pathological sections appear as yellow-white lesions of the mid-periphery, located in the choroid, typically between the RPE and Bruch's membrane [22, 25]. The RPE overlying the nodules is usually intact, but can vary from atrophic to hypertrophic [42, 44]. Histologically, the Dalen-Fuchs nodules are composed of lymphocytes, histiocytes, and epithelioid cells covered by an intact dome of RPE [22, 42, 44].

Pathogenesis

SO has been reported after trauma to the eye including non-penetrating trauma with hyphema, perforated corneal ulcers, penetrating foreign bodies, perforating foreign bodies, and malignant melanoma [21, 48–50]. SO has similarly been described as a sequelae from surgical procedures such as trans-scleral cyclo-destructive laser, cataract surgery, paracentesis incisions, iridectomy, irradiation of choroidal melanomas, evisceration, retinal surgeries such as pars plana vitrectomy, and scleral buckling. SO has also resulted from accidental surgical perforation of the eye and from post-surgical endophthalmitis [29, 51–60]. Regardless of the nature of the instigating injury, the ultimate initiating factor is the disruption of the immune privilege of the eye. The immune privilege of the eye is a result of blood–ocular barriers in the retinal vascular endothelium, epithelium of the RPE, retinal and ciliary blood vessels; the absence of lymphatics in the eye, except for the conjunctiva; and a host of tightly regulated molecular expression profiles and atypical immunologic cascades [25, 61–68]. Once these barriers are breached, intraocular proteins are exposed to the immune system and an immunologic reaction against these antigens is initiated. Animal studies have shown that an SO-like syndrome can be induced in mammals with the peripheral (non-ocular) injection of proteins such as rhodopsin, interphotoreceptor retinoid-binding protein, recoverin, and soluble retinal antigen (S antigen) [69–73].

The initial presentation of the intraocular antigens to immune cells is via major histocompatibility molecules (MHC) and the process is regulated via several cytokines. It is hypothesized that certain MHC molecules, as a result of differential inter-molecular interactions, present intraocular proteins more successfully to immune cells. Similarly, certain cytokine variants are more or less able to induce a successful immune reaction. Thus, individuals with certain MHC and/or cytokine types are more likely to develop SO. It follows that the severity of the manifestations of SO might also be affected by the specific types of cytokines or MHC molecules that the individual possesses. Several variants of cytokines and their associated proteins, for example tumor necrosis factor (TNF)-α, TNF-β, TNF receptor 2, and cytotoxic T-lymphocyte-associated protein (CTLA) 4 and interleukin 10 (IL-10), have been shown to be either promote or protect against SO. Patients with these cytokine variants differ both in the severity of their clinical presentation and the amount of steroids they required to control their disease [74, 75]. Similarly, patients with certain MHC variants, such as HLA-DR4, HLA-DRw54, HLA-Bw54, HLA-DRB1*04, and HLA-DQA1*03, are more susceptible to SO and develop more severe variants of SO [76, 77].

Treatment

There are essentially two broad approaches to the management of SO: preventative by removal of the inciting ocular tissues and/or therapeutic with immunosuppressive/anti-inflammatory treatment.

Enucleation of the injured eye as a treatment for SO was first advocated for by Pritchard in 1851 who suggested that enucleation be performed once the uninjured eye showed signs of serious inflammation [78]. This recommendation was controversial because in some cases enucleation did not impact the course of the disease [2]. A study by Reynard et al. [79] demonstrated that early enucleation, which was defined as enucleation within 2 weeks of the inciting injury, resulted in better visual acuity in the uninjured eye, irrespective of treatment with corticosteroids. A subsequent multivariate logistic regression analysis of these data reaffirmed the conclusion that enucleation prior to 2 weeks after the injury resulted in reduced rates of SO. However, it was noted that eyes with good visual potential should not be enucleated [80]. Generally, enucleation of injured eyes with poor visual potential within 2 weeks of injury reduces but does not eliminate the risk of SO. Evisceration of the eye has also been used as a method to prevent SO [81]. There is a healthy ongoing controversy about the relative benefits of evisceration (improved cosmesis, surgical ease, and surgical risk) vs. enucleation (reduced risk of SO) [82–88].

Immunosuppression is used to treat sympathetic ophthalmia after it becomes manifest. Prior to the use of corticosteroids, approximately 50–60 % of eyes affected by SO became permanently blind [7, 23, 47]. By the last 1970 (well after the introduction of corticosteroids), as many as 64 % of patients who had been treated with corticosteroids had vision 20/60 or better. The cost of visual preservation in these patients was the steroid-associated side effects, with most patients developing Cushing's syndrome [7]. More modern corticosteroid treatment involves high-dose oral corticosteroids (e.g., 1.0–2.0 mg/kg/day prednisone) continued for a period of 3 months. This is administered with adjunctive topical steroids and cycloplegics as dictated by anterior chamber inflammation. Steroids are subsequently tapered off and the response to treatment is evaluated. Pulsed intravenous steroids (methylprednisolone 1 g/day for 3 days), followed by oral steroids, may be beneficial in severe cases [22, 89].

In an effort to reduce the systemic side effects of corticosteroids, the use of intravitreal steroids may enable reduction of the quantity of systemic steroids that may be required [22].

Some cases of SO are refractory to steroids or require high doses of steroids for prolonged duration that can cause systemic side effects. These cases have been managed with steroid sparing immunomodulatory therapy including cyclosporine, tacrolimus, chlorambucil, cyclophosphamide, methotrexate, mycophenolate mofetil, and azathioprine [22, 25, 90–95]. The preceding drugs can be toxic and can have severe long-term sequelae including infertility and secondary malignancies [28]. Moreover, these agents require the physician to have competence in prescribing these agents and managing complications that may ensue. Current therapy has shifted toward less toxic and more directed immunomodulatory molecules. There have been several reports of SO patients that have responded to treatment with anti-TNF-α monoclonal antibodies including adalimumab and infliximab [96–98].

In the future, with the advent of "personalized medicine," patients may be genotyped to risk stratify those who are more likely to develop severe variants of SO and treated more aggressively to prevent ocular damage.

Conclusion

Sympathetic ophthalmia is a relatively rare, bilateral granulomatous panuveitis that occurs more commonly after penetrating trauma but also described after intraocular surgical procedures. The initiating event compromises the immune privilege of the eye and induces intraocular inflammation. Systemic corticosteroids are the initial treatment implemented, but these patients often require steroid sparing immunomodulatory therapy to control the uveitis and avoid steroid-associated toxicity.

References

1. Bullock JD, Galst JM. The story of Louis Braille. Arch Ophthalmol. 2009;127:1532–3.
2. Albert DM, Diaz-Rohena R. A historical review of sympathetic ophthalmia and its epidemiology. Surv Ophthalmol. 1989;34:1–14.
3. MacKenzie W. A practical treatise on diseases of the eye. 3rd ed. London: Longmans; 1840.
4. Allen JC. Sympathetic ophthalmia, a disappearing disease. JAMA. 1969;209:1090.
5. Liddy L, Stuart J. Sympathetic ophthalmia in Canada. Can J Ophthalmol J Can Ophtalmol. 1972;7:157–9.
6. Gass JD. Sympathetic ophthalmia following vitrectomy. Am J Ophthalmol. 1982;93:552–8.
7. Makley TA Jr, Azar A. Sympathetic ophthalmia. A long-term follow-up. Arch Ophthalmol. 1978;96:257–62.
8. Marak GE Jr. Recent advances in sympathetic ophthalmia. Surv Ophthalmol. 1979;24:141–56.
9. Kilmartin DJ, Dick AD, Forrester JV. Prospective surveillance of sympathetic ophthalmia in the UK and Republic of Ireland. Br J Ophthalmol. 2000;84:259–63.
10. Zhang Y, Zhang MN, Jiang CH, Yao Y. Development of sympathetic ophthalmia following globe injury. Chin Med J. 2009;122:2961–6.
11. Smith D, Wrenn K, Stack LB. The epidemiology and diagnosis of penetrating eye injuries. Acad Emerg Med Official J Soc Acad Emerg Med. 2002;9: 209–13.
12. Annual Estimates of the Resident Population for Selected Age Groups by Sex for the United States, States, Counties, and Puerto Rico Commonwealth and Municipios: April 1, 2010 to July 1, 2013 In: U. S. Census Bureau PD, editor. June 2014.

13. Wong TY, Klein BE, Klein R. The prevalence and 5-year incidence of ocular trauma. The Beaver Dam eye study. Ophthalmology. 2000;107:2196–202.
14. May DR, Kuhn FP, Morris RE, et al. The epidemiology of serious eye injuries from the United States Eye Injury Registry. Graefe's Arch Clin Exp Ophthalmol (Albrecht von Graefes Archiv fur klinische und experimentelle Ophthalmologie). 2000;238:153–7.
15. Wong TY, Lincoln A, Tielsch JM, Baker SP. The epidemiology of ocular injury in a major US automobile corporation. Eye (London, England) 1998;12(Pt 5):870–4.
16. Sen HN, Nussenblatt RB. Sympathetic ophthalmia: what have we learned? Am J Ophthalmol. 2009;148:632–3.
17. Chan CC, Mochizuki M. Sympathetic ophthalmia: an autoimmune ocular inflammatory disease. Springer Semin Immunopathol. 1999;21:125–34.
18. Stafford WR. Sympathetic ophthalmia. Report of a case occurring ten and one-half days after injury. Arch Ophthalmol. 1965;74:521–4.
19. Zaharia MA, Lamarche J, Laurin M. Sympathetic uveitis 66 years after injury. Can J Ophthalmol J Can Ophtalmol. 1984;19:240–3.
20. Goto H, Rao NA. Sympathetic ophthalmia and Vogt-Koyanagi-Harada syndrome. Int Ophthalmol Clin. 1990;30:279–85.
21. Lubin JR, Albert DM, Weinstein M. Sixty-five years of sympathetic ophthalmia. A clinicopathologic review of 105 cases (1913–1978). Ophthalmology. 1980;87:109–21.
22. Damico FM, Kiss S, Young LH. Sympathetic ophthalmia. Semin Ophthalmol. 2005;20:191–7.
23. Chaithanyaa N, Devireddy SK, Kishore Kumar RV, Gali RS, Aneja V. Sympathetic ophthalmia: a review of literature. Oral Surg Oral Med Oral Pathol Oral Radiol. 2012;113:172–6.
24. Chu DS, Foster CS. Sympathetic ophthalmia. Int Ophthalmol Clin. 2002;42:179–85.
25. Albert DM, Miller JW, Azar DT. Albert & Jakobiec's principles and practice of ophthalmology. Philadelphia: Saunders/Elsevier; 2008.
26. Nirankari MS, Khanna KK, Chawla GD, Mathur RP. Sympathetic ophthalmitis with total deafness (a case report). J All India Ophthalmol Soc. 1970;18:29–32.
27. Comer M, Taylor C, Chen S, Martin K, Jordan K, Meyer P. Sympathetic ophthalmia associated with high frequent deafness. Br J Ophthalmol. 2001;85:496.
28. Nussenblatt RB. Sympathetic Ophthalmia. In: Uveitis Fundamental and Clinical Practice. St. Louis: Mosby; 2004. pp. 311–23.
29. Chu XK, Chan CC. Sympathetic ophthalmia: to the twenty-first century and beyond. J Ophthalmic Inflammation Infect. 2013;3:49.
30. Moorthy RS, Inomata H, Rao NA. Vogt-Koyanagi-Harada syndrome. Surv Ophthalmol. 1995;39:265–92.
31. Jennings T, Tessler HH. Twenty cases of sympathetic ophthalmia. Br J Ophthalmol. 1989;73:140–5.
32. Burkholder BM, Dunn JP. Multiple serous retinal detachments seen on wide-field imaging in a patient with sympathetic ophthalmia. JAMA Ophthalmol. 2014;132:1220.
33. Bernasconi O, Auer C, Zografos L, Herbort CP. Indocyanine green angiographic findings in sympathetic ophthalmia. Graefe's Arch Clin Exp Ophthalmol (Albrecht von Graefes Archiv fur klinische und experimentelle Ophthalmologie). 1998;236:635–8.
34. Moshfeghi AA, Harrison SA, Ferrone PJ. Indocyanine green angiography findings in sympathetic ophthalmia. Ophthalmic Surg Lasers Imaging Official J Int Soc Imaging Eye. 2005;36:163–6.
35. Saatci AO, Pasa E, Soylev MF, Kocak N, Durak I, Kaynak S. Sympathetic ophthalmia and indocyanine green angiography. Arch Ophthalmol. 2004;122: 1568–9.
36. Castiblanco C, Adelman RA. Imaging for sympathetic ophthalmia: impact on the diagnosis and management. Int Ophthalmol Clin. 2012;52: 173–81.
37. Arevalo JF, Garcia RA, Al-Dhibi HA, Sanchez JG, Suarez-Tata L. Update on sympathetic ophthalmia. Middle East Afr J Ophthalmol. 2012;19:13–21.
38. Varghese M, Raghavendra R. Dalen Fuch's nodules and serous retinal detachment on optical coherence tomography in sympathetic ophthalmitis. Indian J Ophthalmol. 2013;61:245–6.
39. Mahendradas P, Avadhani K, Madhavarao B, et al. High definition spectral domain optical coherence tomography of retinal pigment epithelial rip in a case of sympathetic ophthalmia. J Ophthalmic Inflamm Infect. 2013;3:19.
40. Gupta V, Gupta A, Dogra MR, Singh I. Reversible retinal changes in the acute stage of sympathetic ophthalmia seen on spectral domain optical coherence tomography. Int Ophthalmol. 2011;31:105–10.
41. Muakkassa NW, Witkin AJ. Spectral-Domain optical coherence tomography of sympathetic ophthalmia with Dalen-Fuchs nodules. Ophthalmic Surg Lasers Imaging Retina. 2014:1–3.
42. Jakobiec FA, Marboe CC, Knowles DM 2nd, et al. Human sympathetic ophthalmia. An analysis of the inflammatory infiltrate by hybridoma-monoclonal antibodies, immunochemistry, and correlative electron microscopy. Ophthalmology. 1983;90:76–95.
43. Chan CC, Nussenblatt RB, Fujikawa LS, et al. Sympathetic ophthalmia. Immunopathological findings. Ophthalmology. 1986;93:690–5.
44. Reynard M, Riffenburgh RS, Minckler DS. Morphological variation of Dalen-Fuchs nodules in sympathetic ophthalmia. Br J Ophthalmol. 1985;69:197–201.
45. Croxatto JO, Rao NA, McLean IW, Marak GE. Atypical histopathologic features in sympathetic ophthalmia. A study of a hundred cases. Int Ophthalmol. 1982;4:129–35.
46. Marak GE Jr, Font RL, Zimmerman LE. Histologic variations related to race in sympathetic ophthalmia. Am J Ophthalmol. 1974;78:935–8.

47. Winter FC. Sympathetic uveitis; a clinical and pathologic study of the visual result. Am J Ophthalmol. 1955;39:340–7.
48. Dada T, Kumar A, Sharma N. Sympathetic ophthalmia associated with antecedent adherent leucoma–a rare association. Acta Ophthalmol Scand. 1998;76:380–1.
49. Easom HA. Sympathetic Ophthalmia Associated with Malignant Melanoma. Arch Ophthalmol. 1963;70:786–90.
50. Bakri SJ, Peters GB 3rd. Sympathetic ophthalmia after a hyphema due to nonpenetrating trauma. Ocular Immunol Inflamm. 2005;13:85–6.
51. Fankhauser F, Kwasniewska S, Van der Zypen E. Cyclodestructive procedures. I. Clinical and morphological aspects: a review. Ophthalmol J Int Ophthalmol Int J Ophthalmol Zeitschrift fur Augenheilkunde 2004;218:77–95.
52. Wang WJ. Clinical and histopathological report of sympathetic ophthalmia after retinal detachment surgery. Br J Ophthalmol. 1983;67:150–2.
53. Chan CC, Roberge RG, Whitcup SM, Nussenblatt RB. 32 cases of sympathetic ophthalmia. A retrospective study at the National Eye Institute, Bethesda, Md., from 1982 to 1992. Arch Ophthalmol. 1995;113:597–600.
54. Abu El-Asrar AM, Al Kuraya H, Al-Ghamdi A. Sympathetic ophthalmia after successful retinal reattachment surgery with vitrectomy. Eur J Ophthalmol. 2006;16:891–4.
55. Lyons C, Tuft S, Lightman S. Sympathetic ophthalmia from inadvertent ocular perforation during conventional retinal detachment surgery. Br J Ophthalmol. 1997;81:612.
56. Bechrakis NE, Muller-Stolzenburg NW, Helbig H, Foerster MH. Sympathetic ophthalmia following laser cyclocoagulation. Arch Ophthalmol. 1994;112:80–4.
57. Edward DP, Brown SV, Higginbotham E, Jennings T, Tessler HH, Tso MO. Sympathetic ophthalmia following neodymium:YAG cyclotherapy. Ophthalmic Surg. 1989;20:544–6.
58. Fries PD, Char DH, Crawford JB, Waterhouse W. Sympathetic ophthalmia complicating helium ion irradiation of a choroidal melanoma. Arch Ophthalmol. 1987;105:1561–4.
59. Brour J, Desjardins L, Lehoang P, et al. Sympathetic ophthalmia after proton beam irradiation for choroidal melanoma. Ocular Immunol Inflamm. 2012;20:273–6.
60. Rathinam SR, Rao NA. Sympathetic ophthalmia following postoperative bacterial endophthalmitis: a clinicopathologic study. Am J Ophthalmol. 2006;141:498–507.
61. Zhou R, Caspi RR. Ocular immune privilege. F1000 biology reports 2010;2.
62. Yamada J, Streilein JW. Induction of anterior chamber-associated immune deviation by corneal allografts placed in the anterior chamber. Invest Ophthalmol Vis Sci. 1997;38:2833–43.
63. Streilein JW. Molecular basis of ACAID. Ocular Immunol Inflamm. 1997;5:217–8.
64. Streilein JW. Regulation of ocular immune responses. Eye (London, England) 1997;11(Pt 2):171–5.
65. Streilein JW, Dana MR, Ksander BR. Immunity causing blindness: five different paths to herpes stromal keratitis. Immunol Today. 1997;18:443–9.
66. Streilein JW, Ksander BR, Taylor AW. Immune deviation in relation to ocular immune privilege. J Immunol. 1997;158:3557–60.
67. Streilein JW, Takeuchi M, Taylor AW. Immune privilege, T-cell tolerance, and tissue-restricted autoimmunity. Hum Immunol. 1997;52:138–43.
68. Taylor AW, Alard P, Yee DG, Streilein JW. Aqueous humor induces transforming growth factor-beta (TGF-beta)-producing regulatory T-cells. Curr Eye Res. 1997;16:900–8.
69. Schalken JJ, Winkens HJ, Van Vugt AH, De Grip WJ, Broekhuyse RM. Rhodopsin-induced experimental autoimmune uveoretinitis in monkeys. Br J Ophthalmol. 1989;73:168–72.
70. de Kozak Y, Sakai J, Thillaye B, Faure JP. S antigen-induced experimental autoimmune uveo-retinitis in rats. Curr Eye Res. 1981;1:327–37.
71. Gery I, Chanaud NP 3rd, Anglade E. Recoverin is highly uveitogenic in Lewis rats. Invest Ophthalmol Vis Sci. 1994;35:3342–5.
72. Gery I, Wiggert B, Redmond TM, et al. Uveoretinitis and pinealitis induced by immunization with interphotoreceptor retinoid-binding protein. Invest Ophthalmol Vis Sci. 1986;27:1296–300.
73. Hirose S, Kuwabara T, Nussenblatt RB, Wiggert B, Redmond TM, Gery I. Uveitis induced in primates by interphotoreceptor retinoid-binding protein. Arch Ophthalmol. 1986;104:1698–702.
74. Atan D, Turner SJ, Kilmartin DJ, et al. Cytokine gene polymorphism in sympathetic ophthalmia. Invest Ophthalmol Vis Sci. 2005;46:4245–50.
75. Glover N, Ah-Chan JJ, Frith P, Downes S, Atan D. Unremitting sympathetic ophthalmia associated with homozygous interleukin-10-1082A single nucleotide polymorphism. Br J Ophthalmol. 2008;92:155–6.
76. Kilmartin DJ, Wilson D, Liversidge J, et al. Immunogenetics and clinical phenotype of sympathetic ophthalmia in British and Irish patients. Br J Ophthalmol. 2001;85:281–6.
77. Davis JL, Mittal KK, Freidlin V, et al. HLA associations and ancestry in Vogt-Koyanagi-Harada disease and sympathetic ophthalmia. Ophthalmology. 1990;97:1137–42.
78. Pritchard A. Srugical cases admitted under Augustine Pritchard, Esq, Surgeon to the Infirmary. Bristol R Infirmary Provincial Med Surg J. 1851;18:66–7.
79. Reynard M, Riffenburgh RS, Maes EF. Effect of corticosteroid treatment and enucleation on the visual prognosis of sympathetic ophthalmia. Am J Ophthalmol. 1983;96:290–4.
80. lubin JR, Albert, D.M. Sympathetic Ophthalmia (letter). Ophthalmology 1982;89:1291–2.

81. Levine MR, Pou CR, Lash RH. The 1998 Wendell Hughes Lecture. Evisceration: is sympathetic ophthalmia a concern in the new millennium? Ophthalmic Plast Reconstr Surg. 1999;15:4–8.
82. Migliori ME. Enucleation versus evisceration. Curr Opin Ophthalmol. 2002;13:298–302.
83. Zheng C, Wu AY. Enucleation versus evisceration in ocular trauma: a retrospective review and study of current literature. Orbit. 2013;32:356–61.
84. Yousuf SJ, Jones LS, Kidwell ED Jr. Enucleation and evisceration: 20 years of experience. Orbit. 2012;31:211–5.
85. Manandhar A. Sympathetic ophthalmia: enucleation or evisceration? Nepalese J Ophthalmol Biannual Peer-Rev Acad J Nepal Ophthalmic Soc NEPJOPH. 2011;3:181–7.
86. du Toit N, Motala MI, Richards J, Murray AD, Maitra S. The risk of sympathetic ophthalmia following evisceration for penetrating eye injuries at Groote Schuur Hospital. Br J Ophthalmol. 2008;92:61–3.
87. O'Donnell BA, Kersten R, McNab A, Rose G, Rosser P. Enucleation versus evisceration. Clin Exp Ophthalmol. 2005;33:5–9.
88. Gurdal C, Erdener U, Irkec M, Orhan M. Incidence of sympathetic ophthalmia after penetrating eye injury and choice of treatment. Ocular Immunol Inflamm. 2002;10:223–7.
89. Hebestreit H, Huppertz HI, Sold JE, Dammrich J. Steroid-pulse therapy may suppress inflammation in severe sympathetic ophthalmia. J Pediatr Ophthalmol Strabismus. 1997;34:124–6.
90. Kilmartin DJ, Forrester JV, Dick AD. Cyclosporin A therapy in refractory non-infectious childhood uveitis. Br J Ophthalmol. 1998;82:737–42.
91. Kilmartin DJ, Forrester JV, Dick AD. Cyclosporine-induced resolution of choroidal neovascularization associated with sympathetic ophthalmia. Arch Ophthalmol. 1998;116:249–50.
92. Yang CS, Liu JH. Chlorambucil therapy in sympathetic ophthalmia. Am J Ophthalmol. 1995; 119:482–8.
93. Tessler HH, Jennings T. High-dose short-term chlorambucil for intractable sympathetic ophthalmia and Behcet's disease. Br J Ophthalmol. 1990;74:353–7.
94. Goldstein DA, Fontanilla FA, Kaul S, Sahin O, Tessler HH. Long-term follow-up of patients treated with short-term high-dose chlorambucil for sight-threatening ocular inflammation. Ophthalmology. 2002;109:370–7.
95. Moore CE. Sympathetic ophthalmitis treated with azathioprine. Br J Ophthalmol. 1968;52:688–90.
96. Kim JB, Jeroudi A, Angeles-Han ST, Grossniklaus HE, Yeh S. Adalimumab for pediatric sympathetic ophthalmia. JAMA Ophthalmol. 2014; 132:1022–4.
97. Menghini M, Frimmel SA, Windisch R, Meier FM. Efficacy of infliximab therapy in two patients with sympathetic ophthalmia. Klin Monatsbl Augenheilkd. 2011;228:362–3.
98. Gupta SR, Phan IT, Suhler EB. Successful treatment of refractory sympathetic ophthalmia in a child with infliximab. Arch Ophthalmol. 2011;129:250–2.

Systemic Lupus Erythematosus 38

Khayyam Durrani

Introduction

Systemic lupus erythematosus (SLE) is a chronic, multisystem autoimmune disorder characterized by the production of antibodies directed against components of the cell nucleus, termed antinuclear antibodies [1, 2]. The condition can be life-threatening, and in some patients with ocular involvement, may result in irreversible vision loss [3, 4].

Epidemiology

The prevalence of SLE is estimated to be 40 cases per 100,000 persons in individuals of northern European descent, and more than 200 cases per 100,000 in individuals of African descent [5]. The vast majority of patients are females, with a female-to-male ratio of 9:1, and a peak age of onset between the second and fourth decades of life [6]. In addition to individuals of African descent, Hispanics, and Asians are also at higher risk of developing SLE [5].

K. Durrani (✉)
Division of Ophthalmology, Cornea & External Disease, and Ocular Immunology & Uveitis Services, University of Connecticut Health Center, 263 Farmington Avenue, Farmington, CT 06030, USA
e-mail: kdurrani@uchc.edu

G.N. Papaliodis (ed.), *Uveitis*,
DOI 10.1007/978-3-319-09126-6_38

Clinical Features

Systemic Manifestations

The American College of Rheumatology (ACR) developed revised consensus criteria for the diagnosis of SLE in 1997, which were further modified by the Systemic Lupus International Collaborating Clinics (SLICC) group in 2012 [7–9]. According the SLICC criteria, a diagnosis of SLE can be confirmed on the basis of biopsy-proven lupus nephritis in the presence of ANA or anti-dsDNA antibodies, or if 4 of 17 diagnostic criteria, including at least 1 clinical and 1 immunologic criteria, are met (Table 38.1). Although almost any organ system may be involved, the most common systemic manifestations of SLE are arthralgia, skin rash, including the characteristic butterfly rash involving the nose and cheeks, as well as the raised, erythematous, scaly lesions of discoid lupus, and constitutional symptoms, such as fatigue, feverishness, and anorexia [10, 11]. These are followed in frequency by renal involvement, resulting in either lupus nephritis, nephrotic syndrome, or renal failure, and central nervous system involvement, resulting from cerebral vasculitis or CNS autoantibodies, which may manifest as headache, psychosis, seizures, and focal neurologic deficits [12, 13]. Other systemic manifestations of SLE include serositis, pleurisy, and cardiac

Table 38.1 Systemic Lupus International Collaborating Clinics (SLICC) classification criteria for the diagnosis of systemic lupus erythematosus

Clinical criteria
Acute cutaneous lupus
Chronic cutaneous lupus
Nonscarring alopecia
Oral or nasal ulcers
Joint disease
Serositis
Renal manifestation
Neurologic manifestation
Hemolytic anemia
Leukopenia or Lymphopenia
Thrombocytopenia
Immunologic criteria
ANA
Anti-dsDNA
Anti-Sm
Antiphospholipid
Low complement
Direct Coombs' test

ANA Antinuclear antibodies; *anti-dsDNA* anti-double-stranded DNA; *anti-Sm* anti-Smith antibody. A diagnosis of SLE is made if 4 of the above criteria, including 1 clinical criterion and 1 immunologic criterion are met, OR in patients with biopsy-proven nephritis compatible with SLE, in the presence of ANAs or anti-dsDNA antibodies

involvement including pericarditis, Libman–Sacks endocarditis, and myocarditis [14].

Ocular Manifestations

SLE may affect any structure of the eye and its adnexae, and ocular involvement has been reported to occur in up to one-third of patients [15].

Lupus may result in periorbital skin involvement occurring as an extension of the characteristic malar rash seen in the condition. In addition, discoid lupus may primarily affect the lids, presenting as a chronic, intractable blepharitis, or as raised scaly lesions typically affecting the lateral third of the lower lids [16, 17].

Keratoconjunctivitis sicca (KCS) is the most common ocular manifestation of SLE, occurring in up to one-third of patients [15]. KCS is associated with the HLA-DRW52 antigen and anti-Ro (SSA) and anti-La (SSB) antibodies [18]. Affected patients demonstrate typical stippling of the corneal and conjunctival epithelia with fluorescein and Rose Bengal stains, as well as abnormal Schirmer testing. Filamentary keratitis and fibrosis of the corneal stroma and conjunctiva may occur in severe cases [19, 20]. Scleritis and episcleritis are less common manifestations of SLE, with lupus being responsible for 4 % of cases of scleritis, and 11 % of cases episcleritis in some studies [21, 22]. The presence of scleritis may also be an indicator of systemic disease activity [23]. Peripheral ulcerative keratitis, interstitial keratitis, and anterior uveitis are less common manifestations of SLE, but should always be considered in the differential diagnosis of these conditions [24, 25].

Retinal involvement is the second most common ophthalmic manifestation of lupus, occurring in some studies in 3–29 % of patients [26]. Retinal vascular changes have been shown to correlate with systemic disease activity, and the waxing and waning of retinal lesions parallels the course of the systemic disease [27]. In one prospective study of patients with lupus retinopathy, 88 % of patients had active systemic disease, 73 % had active CNS involvement, and patients with retinal involvement had a higher mortality rate compared to patients without retinal involvement [28]. The most common retinal manifestations of SLE are cotton wool spots and intraretinal hemorrhages [29]. In patients with retinal vascular involvement, lupus typically results in an arteriolitis, and although venular inflammation may occur, the latter is a less common manifestation of the disease. Vasculitis will manifest as vascular tortuosity and sheathing. Other findings may include microaneurysms, retinal edema, and exudates [19, 26, 30]. A less common but more destructive complication is severe vaso-occlusive retinopathy, a syndrome which occurs as a consequence of severe, widespread arteriolitis and venulitis resulting in multiple branch retinal artery occlusions, extensive capillary non-perfusion, and if untreated, may culminate in retinal neovascularization and vitreous hemorrhage, with associated poor visual prognosis [31, 32]. Patients with antiphospholipid antibodies such as lupus anticoagulant and anti-cardiolipin antibodies are at a higher risk of developing severe vascular occlusive disease [33, 34].

Choroidal involvement is also highly correlated with systemic disease activity, and may result in fluid accumulation beneath the neurosensory retina and retinal pigment epithelium, and progress to large exudative retinal and RPE detachments [35–37]. Uveal effusions have also been reported in SLE, and may lead to secondary angle closure glaucoma [38].

Central nervous system involvement in SLE may result in cranial nerve palsies, as well as optic neuritis, the latter of which may occur with transverse myelitis [39, 40]. Anterior ischemic optic neuropathy, as well as chiasmal and retrochiasmal inflammation are other neuro-ophthalmic manifestations of the disease [41].

Lupus may, in addition, result in orbital inflammation, which may manifest as periorbital edema, panniculitis, trochleitis, orbital myositis and orbital infarction [42–47].

Pathophysiology

The pathogenesis of SLE is incompletely understood, and the disease is thought to occur as a consequence of environmental factors in genetically predisposed individuals. A genetic susceptibility to lupus is evidenced by the increased risk in siblings of patients with SLE of developing the disease, the concordance rate of 24 % for identical twins, and the association with the major histocompatibility genes HLA-DR2, DR3, B7, and B8 [48]. In addition to genetic factors, both patient and external environmental factors, such as sunlight exposure, endogenous estrogen production, hormone replacement therapy, Epstein–Barr virus infection, and defective clearance of apoptotic cells resulting in the release of autoantigens, are thought to play a role in the pathogenesis of the disease [6, 49–52]. Other factors, including deficiency in components of the classical complement pathway, mannan-binding protein deficiencies, and genetic polymorphisms in cytokines, such as TNF-α and IL-6 have also been implicated in the underlying immune dysregulation that occurs in SLE, resulting in suppressor T-cell dysfunction, B-cell hyperreactivity, polyclonal B-cell activation, and autoantibody production [53–55].

Such autoantibody production includes, among others, those directed against nuclear antigens, such as the anti-single-stranded and double-stranded DNA antibodies, as well as those against annexins, Ro, La, CD45 cell surface glycoprotein, and histones [6, 48, 56, 57]. These antibodies result in tissue damage by the Coombs and Gell Type II hypersensitivity reaction, with direct toxic effects on targeted cells, resulting in thrombocytopenia, hemolytic anemia, and CNS disease from antiplatelet, anti-red blood cell and antineuronal antibodies, respectively [48]. Type III hypersensitivity reactions, with antigen-antibody deposition, are thought to be responsible for renal dysfunction as well as the ocular manifestations of lupus, and such immune complexes have been identified in retinal and cerebral endothelium, ciliary body, choroid, and conjunctival basement membrane [58]. Such immune complex deposition activates the complement cascade by the classical pathway, resulting the C3a and C5a mediated chemotaxis, and the release of hydrolytic enzymes and proinflammatory cytokines by neutrophils, resulting in tissue damage [48, 59].

Diagnosis

The diagnosis of lupus is based on a combination of clinical features and immunologic tests. It should be kept in mind, however, that ocular involvement may be the first manifestation of SLE in some patients [23]. In addition, ocular manifestations are not included in the ACR or SLICC diagnostic criteria, and although such criteria are useful in identifying patients in a clinical research setting, a diagnosis of SLE can be made and treatment initiated even if not all criteria are met [23]. More than 95 % of patients demonstrate antinuclear antibody (ANA) production, and the test is an effective screening tool for SLE. However, it is nonspecific, and additional testing for anti-double-stranded DNA, Smith antigen, and anti-Ku, and anti-PCNA/cyclin are more specific for the disease [60]. Low levels of C3 and C4 occur in patients with active SLE.

In patients with suspected keratoconjunctivitis sicca, fluorescein and Rose Bengal staining, and Schirmer testing are useful in determining the underlying mechanism of dry eye. Keratoconjunctivitis sicca associated with SLE is typically associated with aqueous deficiency rather than evaporative dry eye syndrome [1].

Fluorescein angiography is a valuable tool in detecting subtle retinal vasculitis, as well as retinal ischemia, edema and neovascularization, and is useful in gauging retinal vasculitic disease activity [26]. Magnetic resonance imaging with contrast in patients with optic nerve involvement may help differentiate lupus optic neuritis from anterior ischemic optic neuropathy, as most patients with neuritis demonstrate enhancement of the optic nerve [61].

Treatment

Patients with lupus and ocular involvement require systemic therapy to control disease activity. In individuals with arthritis, serositis, and dermatologic manifestations without additional systemic involvement, oral nonsteroidal anti-inflammatory drugs (NSAIDs) or aminoquinolines, such as chloroquine or hydroxychloroquine, with careful monitoring for associated retinopathy, may be adequate to control disease activity [62, 63]. However, barring patients with mild keratoconjunctivitis sicca, individuals with ocular involvement typically require initial therapy with systemic corticosteroids, either oral, or intravenous, followed by systemic steroid-sparing immunomodulatory therapy. This typically includes the use of cyclophosphamide, mycophenolate mofetil, azathioprine, or methotrexate [62, 64].

Cyclophosphamide, an alkylating agent that causes cross-linking of DNA bases, inhibits the rapid proliferation of lymphocytes, and has a long track record of safety and efficacy in patients with SLE, particularly lupus nephritis, as well as in patients with severe ocular involvement [65, 66]. Mycophenolate mofetil is an inhibitor of inosine monophosphate dehydrogenase, an enzyme involved in purine synthesis, and has also been shown to be effective, with one meta-analysis suggesting superiority to cyclophosphamide in patients with lupus nephritis [67]. Azathioprine, a prodrug that is converted to 6-mercaptopurine, is also an inhibitor of purine synthesis with proven efficacy in systemic SLE, including patients with ocular involvement [68]. Rituximab is a monoclonal anti-B lymphocyte antibody that may be effective in controlling inflammation patients with recalcitrant SLE, and case reports suggest it may be useful in selected patients with associated retinal vasculitis and optic neuritis [69, 70]. Belimumab, another recently developed biologic response modifier, is a monoclonal antibody to B-cell activating factor (BAFF). It was the first biologic response modifier approved for SLE, receiving FDA approval in 2011 [71, 72]. Although Phase III trials demonstrated modest efficacy in patients with active lupus, its role in patients with ocular involvement remains to be seen [71, 73]. In patients with severe, recalcitrant uveitis, plasmapheresis has been shown to decrease inflammation and improve vision in selected cases [74].

Prognosis

The 5-and 10-year survival rates in patients with lupus have improved significantly with the advent of steroid-sparing immunomodulatory therapy, and currently exceed 85 % [75]. With appropriate therapy, the majority of patients with ocular involvement have a good visual prognosis, including most patients with retinal manifestations [26, 28]. However, patients with widespread retinal occlusive disease have a much poorer prognosis, with over half of patients in one study having a final visual acuity of worse than 20/200 [31].

Conclusion

SLE is a chronic, multisystem autoimmune disorder that can affect almost any ocular and adnexal structure. End-organ damage occurs as a result of autoantibody production resulting in direct cytotoxicity as well as immune complex deposition. Systemic disease activity has been shown to correlate with the activity of retinal vascular manifestations. With appropriate therapy, most patients with ocular involvement have a good visual prognosis. However, patients with severe occlusive retinopathy are at higher risk systemic morbidity and severe vision loss.

References

1. Davies JB, Rao PK. Ocular manifestations of systemic lupus erythematosus. Curr Opin Ophthalmol. 2008;19(6):512–8.
2. Sivaraj RR, Durrani OM, Denniston AK, Murray PI, Gordon C. Ocular manifestations of systemic lupus erythematosus. Rheumatology (Oxford). 2007;46 (12):1757–62.
3. Read RW. Clinical mini-review: systemic lupus erythematosus and the eye. Ocul Immunol Inflamm. 2004;12(2):87–99.
4. Arevalo JF, Lowder CY, Muci-Mendoza R. Ocular manifestations of systemic lupus erythematosus. Curr Opin Ophthalmol. 2002;13(6):404–10.
5. Johnson AE, Gordon C, Palmer RG, Bacon PA. The prevalence and incidence of systemic lupus erythematosus in Birmingham, England. Relationship to ethnicity and country of birth. Arthritis Rheum. 1995;38(4):551–8.
6. D'Cruz DP, Khamashta MA, Hughes GR. Systemic lupus erythematosus. Lancet. 2007;369(9561):587–96.
7. Tan EM, Cohen AS, Fries JF, et al. The 1982 revised criteria for the classification of systemic lupus erythematosus. Arthritis Rheum. 1982;25(11):1271–7.
8. Hochberg MC. Updating the American College of Rheumatology revised criteria for the classification of systemic lupus erythematosus. Arthritis Rheum. 1997;40(9):1725.
9. Petri M, Orbai AM, Alarcon GS, et al. Derivation and validation of the Systemic Lupus International Collaborating Clinics classification criteria for systemic lupus erythematosus. Arthritis Rheum. 2012;64 (8):2677–86.
10. Cervera R, Khamashta MA, Font J, et al. Systemic lupus erythematosus: clinical and immunologic patterns of disease expression in a cohort of 1,000 patients. The European Working Party on Systemic Lupus Erythematosus. Medicine (Baltimore). 1993;72(2):113–24.
11. Gurevitz SL, Snyder JA, Wessel EK, Frey J, Williamson BA. Systemic lupus erythematosus: a review of the disease and treatment options. Consult Pharm. 2013;28(2):110–21.
12. Bluestein HG, Pischel KD, Woods VL Jr. Immunopathogenesis of the neuropsychiatric manifestations of systemic lupus erythematosus. Springer Semin Immunopathol. 1986;9(2–3):237–49.
13. McCune WJ, Golbus J. Neuropsychiatric lupus. Rheum Dis Clin North Am. 1988;14(1):149–67.
14. Gladman D. Systemic lupus erythematosus: clinical features. In: Klippel JWC, Wortman R, editors. Primer on the rheumatic diseases. 11th ed. Atlanta: Arthritis Foundation; 1997. p. 267–72.
15. Jensen JL, Bergem HO, Gilboe IM, Husby G, Axell T. Oral and ocular sicca symptoms and findings are prevalent in systemic lupus erythematosus. J Oral Pathol Med. 1999;28(7):317–22.
16. Huey C, Jakobiec FA, Iwamoto T, Kennedy R, Farmer ER, Green WR. Discoid lupus erythematosus of the eyelids. Ophthalmology. 1983;90(12):1389–98.
17. Kopsachilis N, Tsaousis KT, Tourtas T, Tsinopoulos IT. Severe chronic blepharitis and scarring ectropion associated with discoid lupus erythematosus. Clin Exp Optom. 2013;96(1):124–5.
18. Hochberg MC, Boyd RE, Ahearn JM, et al. Systemic lupus erythematosus: a review of clinico-laboratory features and immunogenetic markers in 150 patients with emphasis on demographic subsets. Medicine (Baltimore). 1985;64(5):285–95.
19. Gold DH, Morris DA, Henkind P. Ocular findings in systemic lupus erythematosus. Br J Ophthalmol. 1972;56(11):800–4.
20. Grennan DM, Forrester J. Involvement of the eye in SLE and scleroderma. A study using fluorescein angiography in addition to clinical ophthalmic assessment. Ann Rheum Dis. 1977;36(2):152–6.
21. Sainz de la Maza M, Foster CS, Jabbur NS. Scleritis associated with systemic vasculitic diseases. Ophthalmology. 1995;102(4):687–92.
22. Akpek EK, Uy HS, Christen W, Gurdal C, Foster CS. Severity of episcleritis and systemic disease association. Ophthalmology. 1999;106(4):729–31.
23. Nguyen QD, Foster CS. Systemic lupus erythematosus and the eye. Int Ophthalmol Clin. 1998;38(1):33–60.
24. Varga JH, Wolf TC. Bilateral transient keratoendotheliitis associated with systemic lupus erythematosus. Ann Ophthalmol. 1993;25(6):222–3.
25. Adan CB, Trevisani VF, Vasconcellos M, de Freitas D, de Souza LB, Mannis M. Bilateral deep keratitis caused by systemic lupus erythematosus. Cornea. 2004;23(2):207–9.
26. Lanham JG, Barrie T, Kohner EM, Hughes GR. SLE retinopathy: evaluation by fluorescein angiography. Ann Rheum Dis. 1982;41(5):473–8.

27. Klinkhoff AV, Beattie CW, Chalmers A. Retinopathy in systemic lupus erythematosus: relationship to disease activity. Arthritis Rheum. 1986;29(9):1152–6.
28. Stafford-Brady FJ, Urowitz MB, Gladman DD, Easterbrook M. Lupus retinopathy. Patterns, associations, and prognosis. Arthritis Rheum. 1988;31(9):1105–10.
29. Ushiyama O, Ushiyama K, Koarada S, et al. Retinal disease in patients with systemic lupus erythematosus. Ann Rheum Dis. 2000;59(9):705–8.
30. Noma H, Shimizu H, Mimura T. Unilateral macular edema with central retinal vein occlusion in systemic lupus erythematosus: a case report. Clin Ophthalmol. 2013;7:865–7.
31. Jabs DA, Fine SL, Hochberg MC, Newman SA, Heiner GG, Stevens MB. Severe retinal vaso-occlusive disease in systemic lupus erythematous. Arch Ophthalmol. 1986;104(4):558–63.
32. Ho TY, Chung YM, Lee AF, Tsai CY. Severe vaso-occlusive retinopathy as the primary manifestation in a patient with systemic lupus erythematosus. J Chin Med Assoc. 2008;71(7):377–80.
33. Au A, O'Day J. Review of severe vaso-occlusive retinopathy in systemic lupus erythematosus and the antiphospholipid syndrome: associations, visual outcomes, complications and treatment. Clin Experiment Ophthalmol. 2004;32(1):87–100.
34. Read RW, Chong LP, Rao NA. Occlusive retinal vasculitis associated with systemic lupus erythematosus. Arch Ophthalmol. 2000;118(4):588–9.
35. Nguyen QD, Uy HS, Akpek EK, Harper SL, Zacks DN, Foster CS. Choroidopathy of systemic lupus erythematosus. Lupus. 2000;9(4):288–98.
36. Khng CG, Yap EY, Au-Eong KG, Lim TH, Leong KH. Central serous retinopathy complicating systemic lupus erythematosus: a case series. Clin Exp Ophthalmol. 2000;28(4):309–13.
37. Baglio V, Gharbiya M, Balacco-Gabrieli C, et al. Choroidopathy in patients with systemic lupus erythematosus with or without nephropathy. J Nephrol. 2011;24(4):522–9.
38. Wisotsky BJ, Magat-Gordon CB, Puklin JE. Angle-closure glaucoma as an initial presentation of systemic lupus erythematosus. Ophthalmology. 1998;105(7):1170–2.
39. Jabs DA, Miller NR, Newman SA, Johnson MA, Stevens MB. Optic neuropathy in systemic lupus erythematosus. Arch Ophthalmol. 1986;104(4):564–8.
40. Saleh Z, Menassa J, Abbas O, Atweh S, Arayssi T. Cranial nerve VI palsy as a rare initial presentation of systemic lupus erythematosus: case report and review of the literature. Lupus. 2010;19(2):201–5.
41. Lessell S. The neuro-ophthalmology of systemic lupus erythematosus. Doc Ophthalmol. 1979;47(1):13–42.
42. Gomez-Puerta JA, Levy S, Khamashta MA, Hughes GR. Periorbital oedema in systemic lupus erythematosus. Lupus. 2003;12(11):866–9.
43. Amirlak I, Narchi H. Isolated orbital pseudotumor as the presenting sign of systemic lupus erythematosus. J Pediatr Ophthalmol Strabismus. 2008;45(1):51–4.
44. Jordan DR, McDonald H, Olberg B, McKim D, McKendry R. Orbital panniculitis as the initial manifestation of systemic lupus erythematosus. Ophthal Plast Reconstr Surg. 1993;9(1):71–5.
45. Arthurs BP, Khalil MK, Chagnon F, Lindley SK, Anderson DP, Burnier M Jr. Orbital infarction and melting in a patient with systemic lupus erythematosus. Ophthalmology. 1999;106(12):2387–90.
46. Grimson BS, Simons KB. Orbital inflammation, myositis, and systemic lupus erythematosus. Arch Ophthalmol. 1983;101(5):736–8.
47. Fonseca P, Manno RL, Miller NR. Bilateral sequential trochleitis as the presenting feature of systemic lupus erythematosus. J Neuroophthalmol. 2013;33(1):74–6.
48. Rahman A, Isenberg DA. Systemic lupus erythematosus. N Engl J Med. 2008;358(9):929–39.
49. Kanda N, Tsuchida T, Tamaki K. Estrogen enhancement of anti-double-stranded DNA antibody and immunoglobulin G production in peripheral blood mononuclear cells from patients with systemic lupus erythematosus. Arthritis Rheum. 1999;42(2):328–37.
50. Gross AJ, Hochberg D, Rand WM, Thorley-Lawson DA. EBV and systemic lupus erythematosus: a new perspective. J Immunol. 2005;174(11):6599–607.
51. Munoz LE, Gaipl US, Franz S, et al. SLE–a disease of clearance deficiency? Rheumatology (Oxford). 2005;44(9):1101–7.
52. Somers E, Richardson B. Environmental exposures, epigenetic changes and the risk of lupus. Lupus. 2014;23(6):568–76.
53. Rekvig OP, Van der Vlag J. The pathogenesis and diagnosis of systemic lupus erythematosus: still not resolved. Semin Immunopathol. 2014;36(3):301–11.
54. Lorenz G, Desai J, Anders HJ. Lupus nephritis: update on mechanisms of systemic autoimmunity and kidney immunopathology. Curr Opin Nephrol Hypertens. 2014;23(3):211–7.
55. Liu A, La Cava A. Epigenetic dysregulation in systemic lupus erythematosus. Autoimmunity. 2014;47(4):215–9.
56. Bastian BC. Annexins in cancer and autoimmune diseases. Cell Mol Life Sci. 1997;53(6):554–6.
57. Mamoune A, Saraux A, Delaunay JL, Le Goff P, Youinou P, Le Corre R. Autoantibodies to CD45 in systemic lupus erythematosus. J Autoimmun. 1998;11(5):485–8.
58. Aronson AJ, Ordonez NG, Diddie KR, Ernest JT. Immune-complex deposition in the eye in systemic lupus erythematosus. Arch Intern Med. 1979;139(11):1312–3.
59. Nataf S, Davoust N, Ames RS, Barnum SR. Human T cells express the C5a receptor and are chemoattracted to C5a. J Immunol. 1999;162(7):4018–23.
60. Mills JA. Systemic lupus erythematosus. N Engl J Med. 1994;330(26):1871–9.

61. Rizzo JF 3rd, Andreoli CM, Rabinov JD. Use of magnetic resonance imaging to differentiate optic neuritis and nonarteritic anterior ischemic optic neuropathy. Ophthalmology. 2002;109(9):1679–84.
62. Merrill JT. Treatment of systemic lupus erythematosus: a 2012 update. Bull NYU Hosp Jt Dis. 2012;70 (3):172–6.
63. Marmor MF, Kellner U, Lai TY, Lyons JS, Mieler WF. Revised recommendations on screening for chloroquine and hydroxychloroquine retinopathy. Ophthalmology. 2012;118(2):415–22.
64. Bertsias G, Ioannidis JP, Boletis J, et al. EULAR recommendations for the management of systemic lupus erythematosus. Report of a Task Force of the EULAR Standing Committee for International Clinical Studies Including Therapeutics. Ann Rheum Dis. 2008;67(2):195–205.
65. Durrani K, Papaliodis GN, Foster CS. Pulse IV cyclophosphamide in ocular inflammatory disease: efficacy and short-term safety. Ophthalmology. 2004;111(5):960–5.
66. Suelves AM, Arcinue CA, Gonzalez-Martin JM, Kruh JN, Foster CS. Analysis of a novel protocol of pulsed intravenous cyclophosphamide for recalcitrant or severe ocular inflammatory disease. Ophthalmology. 2013;120(6):1201–9.
67. Liu LL, Jiang Y, Wang LN, Yao L, Li ZL. Efficacy and safety of mycophenolate mofetil versus cyclophosphamide for induction therapy of lupus nephritis: a meta-analysis of randomized controlled trials. Drugs. 2012;72(11):1521–33.
68. Pasadhika S, Kempen JH, Newcomb CW, et al. Azathioprine for ocular inflammatory diseases. Am J Ophthalmol. 2009;148(4):500–09 e502.
69. Damato E, Chilov M, Lee R, Singh A, Harper S, Dick A. Plasma exchange and rituximab in the management of acute occlusive retinal vasculopathy secondary to systemic lupus erythematosus. Ocul Immunol Inflamm. 2011;19(5):379–81.
70. Wei W, Zerfoss E, Ashker L, Cantore WA. Bilateral optic neuritis in pediatric systemic lupus erythematosus associated with antiphospholipid antibodies and neuromyelitis optica immunoglobulin. J Pediatr Ophthalmol Strabismus. 2010;e1–4 (47 Online).
71. Hahn BH. Belimumab for systemic lupus erythematosus. N Engl J Med. 2013;368(16):1528–35.
72. Kandala NB, Connock M, Grove A, et al. Belimumab: a technological advance for systemic lupus erythematosus patients? Report of a systematic review and meta-analysis. BMJ Open. 2013;3(7).
73. Merrill JT, Ginzler EM, Wallace DJ, et al. Long-term safety profile of belimumab plus standard therapy in patients with systemic lupus erythematosus. Arthritis Rheum. 2012;64(10):3364–73.
74. Papadaki TG, Zacharopoulos IP, Papaliodis G, Iaccheri B, Fiore T, Foster CS. Plasmapheresis for lupus retinal vasculitis. Arch Ophthalmol. 2006;124 (11):1654–6.
75. Urowitz MB, Gladman DD, Tom BD, Ibanez D, Farewell VT. Changing patterns in mortality and disease outcomes for patients with systemic lupus erythematosus. J Rheumatol. 2008;35(11):2152–8.

39 Giant Cell Arteritis

Jing Zhang

Introduction

Giant cell arteritis (GCA), also known as temporal arteritis, is one of the most common systemic granulomatous vasculitides of the elderly [1, 2]. GCA affects large- and medium-sized arteries, especially the superficial temporal, occipital, vertebral, ophthalmic, posterior ciliary, internal and external carotid arteries [3]. The involved arteries develop intimal hyperplasia and luminal obstruction, thereby leading to ischemic manifestations and associated symptoms such as headache, scalp tenderness, jaw claudication, malaise, fever, and vision loss [4]. Elevated systemic inflammatory markers such as erythrocyte sedimentation rate (ESR), C-reactive protein (CRP), and interleukin-6 can be seen in the acute phase. Despite the associated suggestive symptoms and abnormal laboratory tests, temporal artery biopsy is widely accepted as the gold standard for the diagnosis of GCA [2].

J. Zhang (✉)
Department of Ophthalmology, Massachusetts Eye and Ear Infirmary, 243 Charles Street, Boston, MA 02114, USA
e-mail: Jing_Zhang@meei.harvard.edu

G.N. Papaliodis (ed.), *Uveitis*,
DOI 10.1007/978-3-319-09126-6_39

Epidemiology

GCA is the most frequent primary vasculitis affecting people aged over 50 years [5]. The overall incidence of GCA in people over age 50 varies from 1.1 per 100,000/year to 32.4 per 100,000/year, while European countries have the highest incidence [6]. The incidence of GCA increases with age, from 2.3 per 100,000/year among people in their sixth decade to 44.7 per 100,000/year in their ninth decade and older [7, 8]. The incidence in women is nearly twice that of men [5].

The exact etiology of GCA is unclear with a variety of infectious agents such as herpes and parainfluenza viruses as possible disease triggers [9, 10]. A genetic predisposition has also been recognized as an important component as GCA is associated with carriage of HLA-DRB1*04 alleles [11].

Ocular Manifestations

The most common ocular manifestation of GCA is anterior ischemic optic neuropathy (AION) caused by interruption of blood flow in the posterior ciliary arteries. AION caused by GCA is responsible for 78–99 % of vision loss [12, 13]. Amaurosis fugax, due to the ischemia of outer retinal segment, has an incidence of 2–30 % in patients with GCA. GCA can also induce ischemia of the oculomotor nerves or the extraocular muscles resulting in diplopia.

Uveitis is an uncommon manifestation of GCA. At the time of this publication, there are only a few case reports in the last 20 years [1, 14–17]. Ischemia of the posterior ciliary arteries and their branches can cause posterior uveitis. Choroidal ischemic lesions, which appear as peripheral chorioretinal degenerative patches, can be seen after the onset of posterior uveitis [18]. The degenerative patches have a triangular pattern with base toward the periphery and apex toward the posterior pole [18]. Vitritis and exudative retinal detachment have also been reported in posterior uveitis associated with GCA [1]. In addition, disc edema, multiple raised creamy subretinal peripapillary lesions, narrowed arterial vessels of the posterior pole, sheathing and cotton wool spots have been observed in the fundus examination [14]. The fluorescein angiography (FA) can also reveal segmental disc hyperfluorescence and signs of arterial vasculitis in the posterior pole [14].

Anterior uveitis can be caused by ischemia of anterior segment. Corneal edema, keratic precipitates, anterior chamber and vitreous cells have also been reported as associated manifestations of anterior uveitis [15, 18]. Pan uveitis can also occur due to the ischemia of both anterior and posterior segments and usually associated with optic nerve ischemia [18].

Laboratory Investigation

Elevation of ESR is commonly seen in GCA but is neither a sensitive nor specific indicator. The false negative rate can be as high 17 % in diagnostic cases, thus normal ESR cannot exclude GCA [19]. C reactive protein (CRP) is an indicator of acute inflammation with high specificity of 97.5 %. CRP is more sensitive than ESR and can be elevated even when ESR level is normal. Combining CRP and ESR together, the test sensitivity can be increased to 99 % [20].

Elevated platelet count, greater than 400×10^3/L, is a specific marker in the diagnosis of GCA [21]. Thrombocytosis has been positively correlated with biopsy proven GCA [22, 23]. In addition, serum interleukin-6 (IL-6) has been elevated in patients with GCA [24].

Temporal artery biopsy is generally recommended as the gold standard for the diagnosis of GCA. Biopsy should be performed once the diagnosis of GCA is suspected. The overall sensitivity of temporal artery biopsy is 87 %. Contralateral biopsy should be performed if the initial biopsy is negative in highly suspected cases [25]. The recommended timing of the biopsy is within the first two weeks after presentation as patients are treated with steroids which could reduce the inflammation in the artery and thus make the diagnosis of GCA more difficult [26].

Diagnostic Criteria

The diagnosis of GCA depends on at least three of the following five criteria: (1) age at onset of 50 years or older, (2) onset of new headache, (3) temporal artery tenderness or decreased pulse, (4) elevated ESR (≥50 mm/h) by the Westergren method, and (5) histologic findings, according to the American College of Rheumatology (ACR) classification in 1990 [27].

However, the ACR criteria have limitations in that 28.3 % of patients met ACR criteria but had a negative biopsy [28]. One possible explanation is that the predictive values of ACR criteria could decrease when disease prevalence is low, especially in ophthalmology or general medical clinics [29].

Treatment

The goal of treatment in GCA is to stop the vascular inflammation and prevent the progression of ischemia. There are multiple medications that have demonstrated efficacy:

1. Corticosteroids

Systemic corticosteroids are the first choice for treatment in GCA due to the rapid onset of anti-inflammatory effects. There is no generally accepted dose of corticosteroids. Some physicians recommend starting oral prednisolone 1 mg/kg up to a maximum of 80 mg daily, while others initiate treatment with intravenous methylprednisolone 1 g/daily for the first three days followed by PO Prednisone. Both treatment strategies include oral prednisone 1 mg/kg for at least one month and then subsequently tapering based on symptoms and inflammatory markers [30]. Generally, systemic symptoms improve within the first 24–72 h of steroid treatment, while ESR normalizes several weeks later [30]. It has been reported that progressive visual loss may occur despite the early administration of high-dose corticosteroids [30, 31]. Topical and/or local corticosteroids can also be used in those who develop uveitis from GCA.

2. Methotrexate

Methotrexate has been used as adjunct to systemic corticosteroids in several studies. Methotrexate may reduce the relapse rate and the dose of steroids as a steroid-sparing comedication in a meta-analysis of three randomized controlled studies [32]. Treatment with methotrexate is recommended by European League Against Rheumatism (EULAR) [33]. However, a four year clinical trial showed no beneficial effect when standard therapy with prednisone was combined with methotrexate [34].

3. Biological agents

Infliximab, a tumor necrosis factor-alpha antibody, has demonstrated no beneficial effect in GCA and may potentially be detrimental in a randomized controlled trial [35]. Conversely, tocilizumab, a humanized antihuman IL-6 receptor antibody, has demonstrated the ability to reduce the dose of corticosteroids, thus reducing the incidence of corticosteroids-associated adverse events [24].

4. Aspirin

In a retrospective study of GCA patients, Aspirin reduced the risk of ischemic events due to its anti-platelet effect [36].

Other corticosteroid sparing agents, such as acetylsalicylic acid (ASA), HMG-CoA reductase inhibitors, and mycophenolate mofetil (MMF) have been used in several cases [36–38]. However, there is no clear consensus on treatment given the limited case reports.

Conclusion

GCA can cause the pathologic obstruction of large- and medium-sized arteries and result in organ ischemia. Ocular manifestations are common while permanent vision loss can be induced by AION. GCA associated uveitis is a rare manifestation of the disorder and most likely the result of ocular ischemia. Biopsy is the gold standard in the diagnosis of GCA. High dose systemic corticosteroid treatment is the therapy of choice.

References

1. Slemp SN, Martin SE, Burgett RA, Hattab EM. Giant cell arteritis presenting with uveitis. Ocul Immunol Inflamm. 2014;22(5):391–3.
2. Lee AG. Ocular manifestations of giant cell arteritis. Am J Ophthalmol. 1998;126(5):742–4.
3. Weyand CM, Bartley GB. Giant cell arteritis: new concepts in pathogenesis and implications for management. Am J Ophthalmol. 1997;123(3):392–5.
4. Ly KH, Regent A, Tamby MC, Mouthon L. Pathogenesis of giant cell arteritis: More than just an inflammatory condition? Autoimmun Rev. 2010;9(10):635–45.
5. Borchers AT, Gershwin ME. Giant cell arteritis: a review of classification, pathophysiology, geoepidemiology and treatment. Autoimmun Rev. 2012;11(6–7):A544–54.
6. De Smit E, Palmer AJ, Hewitt AW. Projected worldwide disease burden from giant cell arteritis by 2050. J Rheumatol. 2015;42(1):119–25.
7. Bengtsson BA, Malmvall BE. The epidemiology of giant cell arteritis including temporal arteritis and polymyalgia rheumatica. Incidences of different

clinical presentations and eye complications. Arthritis Rheum. 1981;24(7):899–904.
8. Machado EB, Michet CJ, Ballard DJ, et al. Trends in incidence and clinical presentation of temporal arteritis in Olmsted County, Minnesota, 1950–1985. Arthritis Rheum. 1988;31(6):745–9.
9. Kennedy PG, Lipton HL. Varicella-zoster virus claims yet another painful scalp–Giant cell arteritis. Neurology. 2015;84(19):1918–9.
10. Duhaut P, Bosshard S, Ducroix JP. Is giant cell arteritis an infectious disease? Biological and epidemiological evidence. Presse medicale (Paris, France: 1983). 2004;33(19 Pt 2):1403–8.
11. Carmona FD, Mackie SL, Martin JE, et al. A large-scale genetic analysis reveals a strong contribution of the HLA class II region to giant cell arteritis susceptibility. Am J Hum Genet. 2015;96 (4):565–80.
12. Liu GT, Glaser JS, Schatz NJ, Smith JL. Visual morbidity in giant cell arteritis. Clinical characteristics and prognosis for vision. Ophthalmology. 1994;101(11):1779–85.
13. Foroozan R, Deramo VA, Buono LM, et al. Recovery of visual function in patients with biopsy-proven giant cell arteritis. Ophthalmology. 2003;110(3):539–42.
14. Moschos MM, Guex-Crosier Y. Giant cell arteritis: A rare cause of posterior vasculitis. Clinical ophthalmology (Auckland, N.Z.). 2009;3:111–5.
15. Rajesh CV, Cole M. Panuveitis as a presenting feature of giant cell arteritis. Br J Ophthalmol. 2000;84(3):340.
16. Bandini F, Benedetti L, Ceppa P, Corallo G. Uveitis as a presenting sign of giant cell arteritis. J Neuroophthalmol Official J North Am Neuroophthalmol Soc. 2005;25(3):247–8.
17. Dasgupta B, Pitzalis C, Panayi GS. Inflammation of the uveal tract as a presenting feature of temporal arteritis. Ann Rheum Dis. 1989;48(11):964–5.
18. Vedrine L, Algayres JP, Coutant G. Giant-cell arteritis. N Engl J Med. 2003;348(15):1497–8; author reply 1497–1498.
19. Love DC, Berler DK, O'Dowd GJ, Brooks JZ, Love RA. Erythrocyte sedimentation rate and its relationship to hematocrit giant cell arteritis. Arch Ophthalmol (Chicago, Ill.: 1960). 1988;106(3):309–310.
20. Parikh M, Miller NR, Lee AG, et al. Prevalence of a normal C-reactive protein with an elevated erythrocyte sedimentation rate in biopsy-proven giant cell arteritis. Ophthalmology. 2006;113(10):1842–5.
21. Foroozan R, Danesh-Meyer H, Savino PJ, Gamble G, Mekari-Sabbagh ON, Sergott RC. Thrombocytosis in patients with biopsy-proven giant cell arteritis. Ophthalmology. 2002;109(7):1267–71.
22. Krishna R, Kosmorsky GS. Implications of thrombocytosis in giant cell arteritis. Am J Ophthalmol. 1997;124(1):103.
23. Price N, Clearkin LG. Thrombocytosis and giant cell arteritis. Lancet (London, England). 1994;343 (8898):672.
24. Evans J, Steel L, Borg F, Dasgupta B. Long-term efficacy and safety of tocilizumab in giant cell arteritis and large vessel vasculitis. RMD open. 2016;2(1):e000137.
25. Niederkohr RD, Levin LA. Management of the patient with suspected temporal arteritis a decision-analytic approach. Ophthalmology. 2005;112(5):744–56.
26. Deacon BS, Chacko JG. Case of the missed opportunity for temporal artery biopsy. J Ark Med Soc. 2009;106(4):86–7.
27. Hunder GG, Bloch DA, Michel BA, et al. The American College of Rheumatology 1990 criteria for the classification of giant cell arteritis. Arthritis Rheum. 1990;33(8):1122–8.
28. Nesher G, Sonnenblick M, Friedlander Y. Analysis of steroid related complications and mortality in temporal arteritis: a 15-year survey of 43 patients. J Rheumatol. 1994;21(7):1283–6.
29. Rao JK, Allen NB, Pincus T. Limitations of the 1990 American College of Rheumatology classification criteria in the diagnosis of vasculitis. Ann Intern Med. 1998;129(5):345–52.
30. Proven A, Gabriel SE, Orces C, O'Fallon WM, Hunder GG. Glucocorticoid therapy in giant cell arteritis: duration and adverse outcomes. Arthritis Rheum. 2003;49(5):703–8.
31. Hayreh SS, Zimmerman B. Visual deterioration in giant cell arteritis patients while on high doses of corticosteroid therapy. Ophthalmology. 2003;110 (6):1204–15.
32. Mahr AD, Jover JA, Spiera RF, et al. Adjunctive methotrexate for treatment of giant cell arteritis: an individual patient data meta-analysis. Arthritis Rheum. 2007;56(8):2789–97.
33. Mukhtyar C, Guillevin L, Cid MC, et al. EULAR recommendations for the management of large vessel vasculitis. Ann Rheum Dis. 2009;68(3):318–23.
34. Hoffman GS, Cid MC, Hellmann DB, et al. A multicenter, randomized, double-blind, placebo-controlled trial of adjuvant methotrexate treatment for giant cell arteritis. Arthritis Rheum. 2002;46 (5):1309–18.
35. Hoffman GS, Cid MC, Rendt-Zagar KE, et al. Infliximab for maintenance of glucocorticosteroid-induced remission of giant cell arteritis: a randomized trial. Ann Intern Med. 2007;146(9):621–30.
36. Lee MS, Smith SD, Galor A, Hoffman GS. Antiplatelet and anticoagulant therapy in patients with giant cell arteritis. Arthritis Rheum. 2006;54 (10):3306–9.
37. Maron DJ, Fazio S, Linton MF. Current perspectives on statins. Circulation. 2000;101(2):207–13.
38. Sciascia S, Piras D, Baldovino S, et al. Mycophenolate mofetil as steroid-sparing treatment for elderly patients with giant cell arteritis: report of three cases. Aging Clin Exp Res. 2012;24(3):273–7.

Post-traumatic Uveitis and Post-operative Inflammation

40

Scott M. Barb

Traumatic Uveitis

Etiology

Trauma to the globe and its contents can occur in many forms including chemical, radiation, electrical, blunt force, and penetrating or perforating injury with and without intraocular foreign body. The mechanism for which ocular trauma leads to uveitis in most cases is thought to be related to disruption of the microvasculature within the uveal tissue leading to infiltration of leukocytes and other pro-inflammatory mediators into the tissue or chamber [1, 2]. There is growing belief that those with autoimmune disease and other inflammatory disorders may be predisposed to an increased risk or degree of inflammation than the normal population after ocular trauma [3, 4].

Epidemiology

The overall incidence of uveitis as a whole is reported to be 52.4/100,000 person/years with a prevalence of 115.3/100,000 persons [5]. In most epidemiological studies of uveitis, traumatic uveitis is excluded from analysis with other exogenous causes. However, in evaluations of large groups of patients with uveitis, nonsurgical traumatic uveitis appeared to represent around 0.5–4.8 % of the population with most cases presenting as anterior uveitis [2, 6, 7].

Over 2.4 million eye injuries are reported to occur annually in the United States alone and the overwhelming majority are in male patients [8]. Large studies evaluating eye injuries due to all mechanisms show that isolated traumatic uveitis is seen in around 0.5 % of cases [9]. However, uveitis often presents in the context of multiple other concomitant injuries and has been much more prevalent in studies looking specifically at severe injuries and those conducted in other parts of the world. It is possible that many cases of traumatic uveitis are overlooked due to concurrent hyphema or other more significant visually threatening injury.

In a study of electrical-burn patients, 9 % of patients were shown to have unilateral iritis [10]. Studies evaluating blunt traumatic injury to the eye demonstrate the rate of uveitis to be as high as 10 % [11]. The incidence of uveitis is not well defined in penetrating or perforating eye injury. However, there is certainly an increased likelihood of ocular inflammation and infection with the presence of an intraocular foreign body [12–14]. Perhaps, more concerning is this increased risk of infection in open globe injury. The risk of

S.M. Barb (✉)
Department of Ophthalmology, Massachusetts Eye and Ear Infirmary, 243 Charles Street, Boston, MA 02114, USA
e-mail: scott_barb@meei.harvard.edu

G.N. Papaliodis (ed.), *Uveitis*,
DOI 10.1007/978-3-319-09126-6_40

endophthalmitis in open globe injury is estimated to range from 3.3 to 30 % and increase to 1.3–61 % in those with intraocular foreign bodies [15, 16]. Epidemiological information regarding the other mechanisms of injury discussed above remains limited.

Clinical Presentation

History and physical examination of the face and eye often give clues to the type of trauma a patient has sustained. The patient will often give a history of work (metal, construction, house), assault, sports/motor vehicle injury, or fall that help the examiner understand the mechanism and force of injury.

Clinical Signs

Lacerations, ecchymoses, and edema of the surrounding face and eyelids often coincide with blunt or penetrating trauma. Orbital fractures are often commonly seen in blunt force injury involving the eye [17]. Burns of the surrounding adnexal structures often give clues to the type of burn a patient has endured.

However, slit lamp examination of the eye is always necessary to know the extent of ocular damage sustained by injury. Burns of the conjunctiva and cornea may be seen with or without fluorescein staining in chemical and electrical burns. Corneal and conjunctival abrasions may occur in the setting of both blunt and penetrating trauma. Corneal and conjunctival lacerations often occur in the setting of penetrating or sharp injury. Hyperemia of the conjunctiva and increased tearing/discharge are commonly seen in all types of injury involving the conjunctiva and cornea. Microhyphema or hyphema are often seen with blunt ocular trauma but may also be seen in penetrating trauma. Anterior chamber inflammation (flare, cell, or cell and flare) may often be seen with or without accompanying pigmented cell. Damage to the angle structures (angle recession or cyclodialysis) occurs more commonly with blunt trauma [18, 19]. Zonular damage and lens dislocation can be seen in both blunt and penetrating trauma. Vitreous hemorrhage and traumatic posterior vitreous detachment may occur in the setting of blunt and penetrating trauma. Retinal commotio or tears as well as choroidal rupture may also be seen in the setting of significant blunt trauma [20].

Open globe injury may occur with direct blunt rupture or penetrating/perforating trauma to the eye. Inspection should always be paid for intraocular foreign body especially in the setting of penetrating ocular injury. The severity of inflammation and toxicity seen with foreign bodies depends on the substance with severe toxicity typically seen in iron, copper, and vegetable matter, mild inflammation in nickel, aluminum, and zinc, and minimal to no inflammation with inert substances such as gold, glass, plastic, and stone [21, 22].

Clinical Symptoms

Patients often experience a number of clinical symptoms in the setting of traumatic uveitis. Most common among these symptoms is general discomfort, which can be seen with any type of trauma. Photophobia is also quite common especially in the setting of corneal disruption or anterior chamber reaction (pigmented or non-pigmented cell). Flashes and floaters may be experienced in the setting of vitreous hemorrhage, posterior vitreous detachment, and acute retinal break. And of course, blurred vision may occur in the setting of all traumas involving the eye.

Diagnosis

The diagnosis of ocular inflammation after trauma is often determined by history and physical examination along with the presence of inflammatory non-pigmented cells in the anterior chamber or vitreous cavity. Ancillary testing is often not necessary unless view to the fundus is limited by cataract or vitreous hemorrhage or there is concern for ruptured globe, intraocular foreign body, or orbital fracture. In these cases, B scan ultrasonography or CT scan may be indicated to determine the extent or cause of inflammation and ocular damage [23, 24].

Treatment

Treatment is directed at removing the cause of inflammation, treating the inflammation itself, and preventing any side effects related to prolonged inflammation. In the cases of radiation, electrical, and most blunt injuries, the inflammatory stimuli are typically removed at time of presentation and thus anti-inflammatory topical medication such as prednisolone may be started and titrated to the degree of inflammation present. In addition, topical cycloplegics such as cyclopentolate are often used to prevent long-term side effects of prolonged inflammation such as formation of synechiae and to reduce photophobia.

For those cases involving chemical injury, the eye must be irrigated to achieve a physiologic pH with careful examination to remove any chemical particulate matter. In these cases there are often significant corneal or conjunctival epithelial defects and the balance of treating inflammation and allowing appropriate healing of the defects must be weighed when deciding to start topical steroids [25, 26].

Finally, the main goal of treatment in cases of penetrating or perforating intraocular injury with and without intraocular foreign body is to close the eye and remove any intraocular foreign body [27]. Post-operatively, these patients are often started on topical steroid and cycloplegic medication to help control the acute inflammatory reaction and eventually tapered off while under close observation for rebound inflammation. These patients must be followed regularly given the increased risk for endophthalmitis and sympathetic ophthalmia [28].

Prognosis

The long-term outcomes of patients with isolated traumatic anterior uveitis or iritis are often excellent. However, visual outcomes may be limited by concurrent injury to other parts of the eye. In the case of blunt injury, there is a possibility of retinal and optic nerve injury or eventual cataract formation, which may limit vision [20, 29]. In addition, significant blunt injury can also result in open globe injury. Chemical injury may result in corneal scarring obstructing the visual axis [26]. Electrical and radiation injury may result in the development of cataract [30]. Finally, penetrating or perforating open globe injury limits vision in a number of ways depending on the extent of ocular injury, the presence of an intraocular foreign body, time to primary closure, presenting visual acuity, and risk of infection [31–33].

Surgical Trauma and Post-operative Inflammation

Etiology

Inflammation in the setting of surgery is a common phenomenon and a normal/expected response to the tissue trauma induced by the surgical intervention. All ophthalmic procedures including even the most standard such as cataract surgery, vitreoretinal surgery, lasers, and injections often result in post-operative inflammation.

Cataract Surgery

There have been major advances in the field of cataract surgery over the last few decades with a continued shift to small clear corneal incisions and phacoemulsification. The goal of this shift is to improve surgical times and outcomes, which includes minimizing energy usage and tissue damage to lessen post-operative inflammation and resultant side effects [34–36].

Anterior chamber inflammation, as demonstrated by the presence of cell and flare, is common after cataract surgery. Other than the surgery itself, there are a number of etiologies that may cause more severe or prolonged ocular inflammation. These include surgical complications, malpositioned intraocular lens implants, retained nuclear material, reactivated uveitis, endophthalmitis, uveitis–glaucoma–hyphema (UGH) syndrome, and retained foreign body or toxic solution in the anterior chamber [37–41].

Patients who developed more significant post-operative inflammation are at greater risk of cystoid macular edema, glaucoma, and compromising a technically successful surgical procedure. Patients who develop post-operative macular edema are often asymptomatic aside from blurry vision. The diagnosis is often established by imaging studies such as optical coherence tomography and fluorescein angiography [42].

Studies suggest that clinical CME related to post-operative inflammation can be seen in as many as 1–2 % of all uncomplicated cataract surgeries [43]. However, the rate of CME is higher in complicated surgical cases and those with pre-existing diabetic retinopathy and uveitis [44]. A ruptured posterior capsule increases the risk of CME to 10–20 % and retained nuclear fragment increases the risk to as much as 29 % [45, 46].

The pathophysiological mechanism for post-operative inflammation resulting in CME is related to the production of prostaglandin analogs and other pro-inflammatory molecules leading to the increased permeability of retinal vessels [47].

Although most cases of post-operative inflammation respond very well to topical therapy, there are resistant cases that require periocular, systemic, or intravitreal (injection or implant) steroids. In fact, infrequently, vitrectomy may aid in relieving vitreous adhesions and reduce vitreomacular traction leading to macular edema [48–51]. Additional treatment goals of post-operative inflammation due to a specific source other than the surgery itself include fragment removal in cases of retained nuclear material, treatment of infection in endophthalmitis, improved or more intense perioperative control of previously existing uveitis, and repositioning or lens exchange of the intraocular lens in cases of UGH syndrome [39, 40, 52–54].

Vitreoretinal Surgery

Similar to cataract surgery, cystoid macular edema (CME) can occur in the post-operative setting of vitreoretinal surgery. The mechanism for CME related to post-operative inflammation in vitreoretinal surgery is similar to that of cataract surgery described above [55].

However, the incidence of CME related to post-operative inflammation alone is difficult to discern since many of these patients have existing CME or cause for CME at the time of surgery including diabetic retinopathy, vein occlusion, and retinal traction. Perhaps, the most effective way to evaluate the incidence of CME due to post-operative inflammation alone is in a subset of patients undergoing vitrectomy for a benign condition such as floaters with a low likelihood of pre-operative CME. Studies evaluating these patients have shown CME in as many as 5.5 % of cases but many reports show no patients developing CME [56–58]. The incidence of CME is higher in patients undergoing vitreoretinal surgery of longer duration with more instrumentation including laser or tamponade agent [59, 60]. In addition, patients undergoing cataract surgery after vitrectomy are at an increased risk of post-operative CME as high as 26 % [61]. However, it is difficult to attribute the degree of CME due to post-operative inflammation alone since many of these patients undergoing more significant surgery often have pre-existing CME.

The diagnosis of CME after vitreoretinal surgery is mostly reliant on clinical exam and OCT. Treatment paradigms are similar to cataract surgery with evidence suggesting the combined use of topical steroid and NSAID achieves the best visual outcomes and resolution of CME [43]. In addition, it is common for patients to receive periocular or intravitreal steroids at the time of surgery especially in patients with pre-existing uveitis [62, 63].

Similar to cataract surgery, there are other causes for more extensive and prolonged post-operative inflammation after vitrectomy including retained tamponade agent, endophthalmitis, pre-existing uveitis, and sympathetic ophthalmia [64, 65]. The incidence of endophthalmitis and sympathetic ophthalmia after vitrectomy is quite low and estimated to be 0.07 % and 0.015–0.125 %, respectively [66–68]. Despite this increased risk for sympathetic ophthalmia, the number of reported cases of sympathetic ophthalmia after vitrectomy is quite small especially with sutureless 23- and 25-gage technique.

However, the role of vitrectomy in the setting of uveitis and post-operative inflammation must not be forgotten. In cases of retained dropped nuclear fragments, endophthalmitis, or uveitic diagnostic dilemmas, vitrectomy is often crucial for diagnosis and treatment [69–71].

Lasers

Mild inflammation after anterior and posterior segment laser is quite common [72, 73]. The mechanism of inflammation is similar to other surgical interventions as a result of alterations in the blood–eye barrier and production of pro-inflammatory cytokines from the laser-induced tissue damage [74, 75].

These patients typically present with anterior chamber or vitreous cell and have minimal to no discomfort. The diagnosis is often made from slit lamp exam alone. The inflammation typically peaks within the first few days post procedure. The treatment for post-operative inflammation is typically observation versus topical steroid depending on the extent of inflammation. Patients often have a quick response to these medications with minimal need for long-term use [73].

Clinically evident anterior chamber inflammation is present in 23 % of patients with primary open angle glaucoma after undergoing argon laser trabeculoplasty (ALT). This incidence is much higher in patients with pseudoexfoliation and pigmentary glaucoma [73]. As the use of selective laser trabeculoplasty (SLT) has become more common, the incidence and degree of inflammation after laser trabeculoplasty has decreased dramatically. This is likely due to the reduced tissue damage and overall energy use in SLT [76]. In fact, some studies have shown little to no clinical inflammation in eyes treated with SLT [77].

The use of cyclophotocoagulation is becoming more common for advanced or refractory glaucoma. Mild inflammation is expected given the targeted destruction of uveal tissue that occurs during this procedure. However, clinically significant inflammation is rare even in patients with inflammatory glaucoma especially with the targeted use of endocyclophotocoagulation [78, 79]. However, sympathetic ophthalmia has been rarely reported after cyclophotocoagulation [80].

Laser peripheral iridotomy (LPI) is one of the most common anterior segment laser procedures. Mild anterior chamber inflammation is often inevitable. Those with pre-existing uveitis or darkly pigmented irides are more prone to this inflammation and this has a direct impact on the rate of maintained patency of the iridotomy [81]. Iridotomies are commonly created using YAG laser or a combination of argon and YAG laser. YAG laser typically results in less inflammation due to the overall reduction in total energy used. Periprocedural topical steroids are often used but are of questionable proven benefit. LPI has been rarely shown to lead to recurrence of herpetic keratouveitis in several patients [82].

Posterior capsular opacification (PCO) occurs in nearly 33 % of pseudophakic patients after 5 years. Prolonged post-operative inflammation after cataract surgery appears to be a possible risk factor for PCO [83]. Studies have shown an increased risk of PCO in uveitic patients undergoing cataract surgery but this finding is confounded by the younger age of most of these patients [84]. Minimal inflammation is expected after YAG capsulotomy, but CME related to inflammation has been shown to occur in as many as 1 % [85]. Persistent inflammation (>6 months) in the anterior chamber and vitreous has been shown to occur in 0.4 and 0.7 % of patients after YAG capsulotomy, respectively [86]. This is often responsive to topical steroids. However, the more significant impact of mild inflammation is IOP rise after capsulotomy. This is often treated or prevented with use of a periprocedural IOP-lowering medication such as apraclonidine [87]. Interestingly, a noted but rare complication of YAG capsulotomy is the release of sequestered capsular bacterial organisms leading to severe inflammation and endophthalmitis [88].

Focal laser and panretinal photocoagulation (PRP) remain the most commonly used posterior segment lasers despite the increasing use of intravitreal anti-VEGF therapy. Retinal laser burns are known to incite inflammatory activity by disrupting the immune privilege of the eye and increasing the permeability of the blood–aqueous barrier [89]. In fact, PRP has been shown to increase pro-inflammatory cytokines in proliferative diabetic patients and actually temporarily worsen macular edema as a result [90, 91]. Aqueous flare has been reported to persist as long as 90 days after routine PRP in patients with diabetes [92]. Despite this fact, topical anti-inflammatory medications are not routinely used after focal laser or PRP.

Intravitreal Injections

The use of intravitreal injections has increased dramatically in the last decade due to the proven efficacy of anti-VEGF (vascular endothelial growth factor) medications in diabetic retinopathy and macular edema related to neovascular age-related macular degeneration (AMD) and retinal vein occlusion (RVO) [93, 94].

Inflammation in the setting of intravitreal injection can occur in the form of a sterile reaction or infectious endophthalmitis. Sterile endophthalmitis is defined as any acute intraocular inflammation without infection that resolves without antibiotic treatment. The incidence of sterile endophthalmitis after injection is reported to be between 0.033 and 2.9 % [95–97]. However, the incidence of infectious endophthalmitis appeared to also vary slightly by technique and was reported to be between 0.0075 and 0.2 % [98, 99].

The etiology of a sterile inflammatory reaction due to intravitreal injection of anti-VEGF agents remains unclear. Several theories have been proposed such as improper storage protocol, increased immune response after repeated injections, and endotoxin contamination during production. Despite clusters of these sterile reactions being explained by improper storage or production, the sporadic incidence cannot be fully accounted for by these mechanisms [100]. The increased immune response theory provides an intriguing explanation since repeated injections are often necessary for many patients. However, studies have shown that history of prior injections or inflammation does not increase the risk of future sterile reaction or worsening of current inflammation [96, 97].

It may be difficult to differentiate between sterile and infectious endophthalmitis but diagnostic clues are often available in the clinical presentation. Sterile endophthalmitis usually presents slightly earlier after injection (<1 day to 1 week) [101, 102]. The sterile group often presents with complaints of blurred vision and floaters. Also there is usually less severe anterior chamber and vitreous reaction as well as less pain [103, 104]. Typically, the duration of inflammation is also shorter in sterile endophthalmitis (2–10 weeks) but this difference is unreliable given that duration of infectious endophthalmitis is highly variable with treatment [96, 102].

Management varies quite markedly and includes topical medications, intravitreal antibiotics, and even vitrectomy. Comparisons between patients believed to have sterile endophthalmitis show similar results between each of these modalities of treatment in respect to duration of inflammation [100, 105]. However, this data is of uncertain value as those with more significant inflammation typically receive more aggressive treatment confounding outcomes. Therefore, many studies suggest that it is reasonable to maintain a low threshold for vitreous tap and inject of antibiotics especially with significant pain and inflammation [102]. Perhaps, the greatest difference between these two groups is prognosis with the sterile group often returning to baseline visual acuity regardless of treatment and the infectious group often having significantly reduced visual acuity.

Despite the relatively small risk of inflammation related to intravitreal injection, it must not be forgotten that intravitreal injections are used to treat ocular inflammatory conditions or the consequences of inflammation. This includes the use of steroid implants to treat uveitis and refractory macular edema [106, 107].

Conclusion

Multiple mechanisms of injury can lead to intraocular inflammation. The greater the associated tissue trauma is usually correlated with a more robust ocular inflammatory response. The most commonly employed treatment for the majority of these cases is topical corticosteroids.

References

1. Martin TM, Smith JR, Rosenbaum JT. Anterior uveitis: current concepts of pathogenesis and interactions with the spondyloarthropathies. Curr Opin Rheumatol. 2002;14:337–41.
2. Rosenbaum JT, Tammaro J, Robertson JE. Uveitis precipitated by nonpenetrating ocular trauma. Am J Ophthalmology. 1991;112(4):392–5.
3. Seymour R, Ramsey MS. Unusually severe traumatic uveitis associated with occult ankylosing spondylitis. Can J Ophthalmol. 1991;26(3):156–8.
4. Petrou P, Reddy MA. Unusually resistant post-traumatic uveitis with high serum ACE—an occult ocular sarcoidosis. Ocul Immunol Inflamm. 2008;16(3):117–8.
5. Read RW. Uveitis: advances in understanding of pathogenesis and treatment. Curr Rheumatol Rep. 2006;8(4):260–6.
6. Llorenc V, Mesquida M, Sainz de la Maza M, Keller J, Molins B, Espinosa G, Hernandez MV, Gonzalez-Martin J, Adan A. Epidemiology of uveitis in a Western urban multiethnic population. The challenge of globalization. Acta Ophthalmol. 2015; Epub ahead of print.
7. Cakar Ozdal MP, Yazici A, Tufek M, Ozturk F. Epidemiology of uveitis in a referral hospital in Turkey. Turk J Med Sci. 2014;44(2):337–42.
8. Feist RM, Farber MD. Ocular trauma epidemiology. Arch Ophthalmol. 1989;107(4):503–4.
9. Macewen CJ. Eye injuries: a prospective survey of 5671 cases. Br J Ophthalmol. 1989;73(11):888–94.
10. Krasny J, Broz L, Kripner J. Anterior uveitis caused by electrical discharge in whole body injuries. Cesk Slov Oftalmol. 2013;69(4):158–63.
11. Eagling EM. Ocular damage after blunt trauma to the eye. Its relationship to the nature of the injury. Br J Ophthalmol. 1974;58(2):126–40.
12. Sychev YV, Verner-Cole EA, Suhler EB, Stout JT, Vemulakonda GA. Occult nonmetallic intraocular foreign bodies presenting as fulminant uveitis: a case series and review of the literature. 2013;7:1747–51.
13. Archer DB, Davies MS, Kanski JJ. Non-metallic foreign bodies in the anterior chamber. Br J Ophthalmol. 1969;53(7):453–6.
14. Verbraeken H, Rysselaere M. Post-traumatic endophthalmitis. Eur J Ophthalmol. 1994;4(1):1–5.
15. Essex RW, Yi Q, Charles PG, Allen PJ. Posttraumatic endophthalmitis. Ophthalmology. 2004;111 (11):2015–22.
16. Brinton GS, Topping TM, Hyndiuk RA, Aaberg TM, Reeser FH, Abrams GW. Posttraumatic endophthalmitis. Arch Ophthalmol. 1984;102 (4):547–50.
17. He D, Blomquist PH, Ellis E. Association between ocular injuries and internal orbital fractures. J Oral Maxillofac Surg. 2007;65(4):713–20.
18. Malandrini A, Balesterazzi A, Martone G, Tosi GM. Caporossi. Diagnosis and management of traumatic cyclodialysis cleft. J Cataract Refract Surg. 2008;34 (7):1213–6.
19. Canavan YM, Archer DB. Anterior segment consequences of blunt ocular injury. Br J Ophthalmol. 1982;66(9):549–55.
20. Williams DF, Mieler WF, Williams GA. Posterior segment manifestations of ocular trauma. Retina. 1990;1:S35–44.
21. Billi B, Lesnoni G, Scassa C, Giuliano MA, Coppe AM, Rossi T. Copper intraocular foreign body: diagnosis and treatment. Eur J Ophthalmol. 1996;5(4):235–9.
22. Weiss MJ, Hofeldt AJ, Behrens M, Fisher K. Ocular siderosis. Diagnosis and management. Retina. 1997;105–8.
23. Mete G, Turgut Y, Osman A, Gulsen U, Hakan A. Anterior segment intraocular metallic foreign body causing chronic hypopyon uveitis. J Ophthalmic Inflamm Infect. 2011;1(2):85–7.
24. Lee HJ, Jilani M, Frohman L, Baker S. CT of orbital trauma. Emerg Radiol. 2004;10(4):168–72.
25. Brodovsky SC, McCarty CA, Snibson G, Loughnan M, Sullivan L, Daniell M, Taylor HR. Management of alkali burns: an 11-year retrospective review. Ophthalmology. 107(10):1829–35.
26. Hamill CE, Bozorg S, Chang P, Lee H, Sayegh RR, Shukla AN, Chodosh J. Corneal alkali burns: a review of the literature and proposed protocol for evaluation and treatment. Int Ophthalmol Clin. 2013;53(4):185–94.
27. Rahman I, Maino A, Devadason D, Leaterbarrow B. Open globe injuries: factors predictive of poor outcome. Eye (Lond). 2006;20(12):1336–41.
28. Gurdal C, Erdener U, Irkec M, Orhan M. Incidence of sympathetic ophthalmia after penetrating eye injury and choice of treatment. Ocul Immunol Inflamm. 2002;10(3):223–7.
29. Matthews GP, Das A, Brown S. Visual outcome and ocular survival in patients with retinal detachments secondary to open or closed globe injuries. Ophthalmic Surg Lasers. 1998;29(1):48–54.
30. Seth RK, Abedi G, Daccache AJ, Tsai JC. Cataract secondary to electrical shock from a Taser gun. J Cataract Refract Surg. 2007;33(9):1664–5.
31. Thompson WS, Rubsamen PE, Flynn HW, Schiffman J, Cousins SW. Endophthalmitis after penetrating traums. Risk factors and visual acuity outcomes. Ophthalmology. 1995;102(11):1696–701.
32. Esmaeli B, Elner SG, Schork MA, Elner VM. Visual outcome and ocular survival after penetrating trauma. A clinicopathologic study. Ophthalmology. 1995;102(3):393–400.

33. Andreoli CM, Andreoli MT, Kloek CE, Ahuero AE, Vavvas D, Durand ML. Low rate of endophthalmitis in a large series of open globe injuries. Am J Ophthalmol. 2009;147(4):601–8.
34. Pande MV, Spalton DJ, Kerr-Muir MG, Marshall J. Postoperative inflammatory response to phacoemulsification and extracapsular cataract surgery: aqueous flare and cells. J Cataract Refract Surg. 1996;22(Suppl 1):770–4.
35. Ferrari TM, Cavallo M, Durante G, et al. Macular edema induced by phacoemulsification. Doc Ophthalmol. 1999;97:325–7.
36. Chee SP, Ti SE, Sivakumar M, Tan DT. Postoperative inflammation: extracapsular cataract extraction versus phacoemulsification. J Cataract Refract Surg. 1999;25(9):1280–5.
37. Blodi BA, Flynn HW Jr, Blodi CF, et al. Retained nuclei after cataract surgery. Ophthalmology. 1992;99:41–4.
38. Cao H, Zhang L, Li L, Lo S. Risk factors for acute endophthalmitis following cataract surgery: a systematic review and meta-analysis. PLoS ONE. 2013;8(8):1–18.
39. Mehta S, Linton MM, Kempen JH. Outcomes of cataract surgery in patients with uveitis: a systematic review and meta-analysis. Am J Ophthalmol. 2014;158(4):676–92.
40. Aonuma H, Matsushita H, Nakajima K, Watase M, Tsushima K, Watanabe I. Uveitis-glaucoma-hyphema syndrome after posterior chamber intraocular lens implantation. Jpn J Ophthalmol. 1997;41(2):98–100.
41. Galloway GD, Ang GS, Shenoy R, Beigi B. Retained anterior chamber cilium causing endophthalmitis after phacoemulsification. J Cataract Refract Surg. 2004;30(2):521–2.
42. Roberts CW. Pretreatment with topical diclofenac sodium to decrease postoperative inflammation. Ophthalmology. 1996;103:636–9.
43. Ray S, D'Amico DJ. Pseudophakic macular edema. Semin Ophthalmol. 2002;17:167–80.
44. Johnson MW. Etiology and treatment of macular edema. Am J Ophthalmol. 2009;147(1):11–21.
45. Collins JF, Krol WF, Kirk GF, Gaster RN, VA Cooperative Cataract Study Group. The effect of vitreous presentation during extracapsular cataract surgery on the postoperative visual acuity at one year. Am J Ophthalmol. 2004;138:536–42.
46. Scott IU, Flynn HW Jr, Smiddy WE, et al. Clinical features and outcomes of pars plana vitrectomy in patients with retained lens fragments. Ophthalmology. 2003;110:1567–72.
47. McColgin AZ, Heier JS. Control of intraocular inflammation associated with cataract surgery. Curr Opin Ophthalmol. 2000;11:3–6.
48. Johnson MW. Etiology and treatment of macular edema. Am J Ophthalmol. 2009;147(1):11–21.
49. Conti SM, Kertes PJ. The use of intravitreal corticosteroids, evidence-based and otherwise. Curr Opin Ophthalmol. 2006;17:235–44.
50. Jaffe GJ, Martin D, Callanan D, et al. Fluocinolone acetonide implant (Retisert) for noninfectious posterior uveitis: thirty-four-week results of a multicenter randomized clinical stud. Ophthalmology. 2006;113:1020–7.
51. Harbour JW, Smiddy WE, Rubsamen PE, Murray TG, Davis JL, Flynn HW Jr. Pars plana vitrectomy for chronic pseudophakic cystoid macular edema. Am J Ophthalmol. 1995;120:302–7.
52. Bohigian GM, Wexler SA. Complications of retained nuclear fragments in the anterior chamber after phacoemulsification with posterior chamber lens implant. Am J Ophthalmol. 1997;123:546–7.
53. Kernt M, Kampik A. Endophthalmitis: pathogenesis, clinical presentation, management, and perspectives. Clinical Ophthalmol. 2010;4:121–35.
54. Lobo AM, Papaliodis GN. Perioperative evaluation and management of cataract surgery in uveitis patients. Int Ophthalmol Clin. 2010;50(1):129–37.
55. Loewenstein A, Zur D. Postsurgical cystoid macular edema. Dev Ophthalmol. 2010;47:148–59.
56. de Nie KF, Crama N, Tilanus MA, Klevering BJ, Boon CJ. Pars plana vitrectomy for disturbing primary vitreous floaters: clinical outcome and patient satisfaction. Graefes Arch Clin Exp Ophthalmol. 2013;251(5):1373–82.
57. Schiff WM, Chang S, Mandava N, Barile GR. Pars plana vitrectomy for persistent, visually significant vitreous opacities. Retina. 2000;20(6):591–6.
58. Tan HS, Mura M, Lesnik Oberstein SY, Bijl HM. Safety of vitrectomy for floaters. Am J Ophthalmol. 2011;151(6):995–8.
59. Nakamura K, Refojo MF, Crabtree DV, Pastor J, Leong F-L. Ocular toxicity of low-molecular-weight components of silicone and fluorosilicone oils. Invest Ophthalmol Vis Sci. 1991;32(12):3007–20.
60. Romano MR, Baddon C, Heimann H, Wong D, His-cott P. Histopathological findings in an epimacular membrane after intraoperative use of perfluorocarbon liquid. Eye. 2010;24(4):740–42.
61. Mylonas G, Sacu S, Deák G, et al. Macular edema following cataract surgery in eyes with previous 23-gauge vitrectomy and peeling of the internal limiting membrane. Am J Ophthalmol. 2013;155 (2):253.e2–59.e2.
62. Sonoda K-H, Enaida H, Uenoetal A. Parsplanavitrectomy assisted by triamcinolone acetonide for refractory uveitis: a case series study. Br J Ophthalmol. 2003;87(8):1010–4.
63. Leder HA, Jabs DA, Galor A, Dunn JP, Thorne JE. Periocular triamcinolone acetonide injections for cystoid macular edema complicating noninfectious uveitis. Am J Ophthalmol. 2011;152(3):441.e2–48. e2.
64. Pradeep S, Chhablani JK, Patel B, Rani P. Delayed inflammation associated with retained perfluorocarbon liquid. Indian K Ophthalmol. 2011;59(5):396–8.
65. Soheilian M, Ramezani A, Soheilian R. 25-guage vitrectomy for complicated chronic endogenous/

autoimmune uveitis: predictors of outcome. Ocul Immunol Inflamm. 2013;21(2):93–101.
66. Cohen SM, Flynn HW Jr, Murray TG, Smiddy WE. Endophthalmitis after pars plana vitrectomy. The Postvitrectomy Endophthalmitis Study Group. Ophthalmology. 1995;102(5):705–12.
67. Kilmartin D, Dick A, Forrester J. Sympathetic ophthalmia risk following vitrectomy: should we counsel patients? Br J Ophthalmol. 2000;84(5):448–9.
68. Gass JD. Sympathetic ophthalmia following vitrectomy. Am J Ophthalmol. 1982;93:552.
69. Scott IU, Flynn HW Jr, Smiddy WE, et al. Clinicalfeatures and outcomes of pars plana vitrectomy in patients with retained lens fragments. Ophthalmology. 2003;110(8):1567–72.
70. Svozilkova P, Heissigerova J, Brichova M, Kalvodova B, Dvorak J, Rihova E. The role of pars plana vitrectomy in the diagnosis and treatment of uveitis. Eur J Ophthalmol. 2011;21(1):89–97.
71. Maguire JI. Postoperative endophthalmitis: optimal management and the role and timing of vitrectomy surgery. Eye (Lond). 2008;22(10):1290–300.
72. Moster MR, Schwartz LW, Spaeth GL, Wilson RP, McAllister JA, Poryzees EM. Laser Iridectomy. A controlled study comparing argo and neodymium: YAG. Ophthalmology. 1986;93(1):20–4.
73. Mermoud A, Pittet N, Herbort CP. Inflammation patterns after laser trabeculoplasty measured with the laser flare meter. Arch Ophthalmol. 1992;110(3):368–70.
74. Mitchell PG, Blair NP, Deutsch TA, Hershey JM. The effect of neodymium: YAG laser shocks on the blood-aqueous barrier. Ophthalmology. 1987;94(5):488–90.
75. Er Doganay S, Evereklioglu C, Turkoz Y, Gunduz A, Borazan M, Ozyalin F. Comparison of the effects of argon and neurodymium:YAG laser iridotomy on cytokines in the rabbit aqueous humor. Eur J Ophthalmol. 2002;12(3):183–7.
76. Martinez-de-la-Casa JM, Garcia-Feijoo J, Castillo A, Matilla M, Macias JM, Benitez-del-Castillo JM, Garcia-Sanchez J. Selective vs. argon laser trabeculoplasty: hypotensive efficacy, anterior chamber inflammation, and postoperative pain. Eye (Lond). 2004;18(5):498–502.
77. Ayala M, Landau Hogbeck I, Chen E. Inflammation assessment after selective laser trabeculoplasty (SLT) treatment. Acta Ophthalmol. 2011;89(4):306–9.
78. Schlote T, Derse M, Zierhut M. Transscleral diode laser cyclophotocoagulation for the treatment of refractory glaucoma secondary to inflammatory eye disease. Br J Ophthalmol. 2000;84(9):999–1003.
79. McKelvie PA, Walland MJ. Pathology of cyclodiode laser: a series of nine enucleated eyes. Br J Ophthalmol. 2002;86(4):381–6.
80. Bechrakis NE, Muller-Stolzenburg NW, Helbig H, Foerster MH. Sympathetic ophthalmia following laser cyclocoagulation. Arch Ophthalmol. 1994;112(1):80–4.
81. Spencer NA, Hall AJ, Stalwell RJ. Nd:YAG laser iridotomy in uveitic glaucoma. Clin Exp Ophthalmol. 2001;29(4):217–9.
82. Hou YC, Chen CC, Wang IJ, Hu FR. Recurrent herpetic keratouveitis following YAG laser peripheral iridotomy. Cornea. 2004;23(6):641–2.
83. Elgohary MA, Dowler JG. Incidence and risk factors of Nd:YAG capsulotomy after phacoemulsification in non-diabetic and diabetic patients. Clin Exp Ophthalmol. 2006;34(6):526–34.
84. Dana MR, Chatzistefanou K, Schaumberg DA, Foster CS. Posterior capsule opacification after cataract surgery in patients with uveitis. Ophthalmology. 1997;104(9):1387–93.
85. Steinert RF, Puliafito CA, Kumar SR, Dudak SD, Patel S. Cystoid macular edema, retinal detachment, and glaucoma after Nd:YAG laser posterior capsulotomy. Am J Ophthalmol. 1991;112(4):373–80.
86. Keates RH, Steinert RF, Puliafito CA, Maxwell SK. Long-term follow-up of Nd:YAG laser posterior capsulotomy. J Am Intraocul Implant Soc. 1984;10:164–8.
87. Pollack IP, Brown RH, Crandall AS. Prevention of the rise in intraocular pressure following neodymium-YAG posterior capsulotomy using topical 1 % apraclonidine. Arch Ophthal mol. 1988;106:754–7.
88. Hollander DA, Stewart JM, Seiff SR, Poothullil AM, Jeng BH. Late-onset Corynebacterium endophthalmitis following laser posterior capsulotomy. Ophthalmic Surg Lasers Imaging. 2004;35(2):159–61.
89. Qiao H, Lucas K, Stein-Streilein J. Retinal laser burn disrupts immune privilege in the eye. Am J Pathol. 2009;174(2):414–22.
90. Shimura M, Yasuda K, Nakazawa T, Abe T, Shiono T, Iida T, Sakamoto T, Nishida K. Panretinal photocoagulation induces pro-inflammatory cytokines and macular thickening in high-risk proliferative diabetic retinopathy. Graefes Arch Clin Exp Ophthalmol. 2009;247(12):1617–24.
91. McDonald HR, Schatz H. Macular edema following panretinal photocoagulation. Retina. 1985;5(1):5–10.
92. Larsson LI, Nuija E. Increased permeability of the blood-aqueous barrier after panretinal photocoagulation for proliferative diabetic retinopathy. Acta Ophthalmol Scand. 2001;79(4):414–6.
93. Avery RL, Pieramici DJ, Rabena MD, Castellarin AA, Nasir MA, Giust MJ. Intravitral bevacizumab (Avastin) for neovascular age-related macular degeneration. Ophthalmology. 2006;113(3):363–72.
94. Avery RL, Pearlman J, Pieramici DJ, Rabena MD, Castellarin AA, Nasir MA, Giust MJ, Wendel R, Patel A. Intravitreal bevacizumab (Avastin) in the

treatment of proliferative diabetic retinopathy. Ophthalmology. 2006;113(10):1695.
95. Lima LH, Zweifel SA, Engelbert M, et al. Evaluation of safety for bilateral same-day intravitreal injections of antivascular endothelial growth factor therapy. Retina. 2009;29(9):1213–7.
96. Chong DY, Anand R, Williams PD, Qureshi JA, Callanan DG. Characterization of sterile intraocular inflammatory responses after intravitreal bevacizumab injection. Retina. 2010;30(9):1432–40.
97. Rosenfeld PJ, Brown DM, Heier JS, et al. Ranibizumab for neovascular age-related macular degeneration. N Engl J Med. 2006;355(14):1419–31.
98. Jager RD, Aiello LP, Patel SC, Cunningham ET. Risks of intravitreous injection: a comprehensive review. Retina. 2004;24:676–98.
99. Casparis H, Wolfensberger TH, Becker M, Eich G, Ambresin A, Mantel I, Michels S. Incidence of presumed endophthalmitis after intravitreal injection performed in the operating room: a retrospective multicenter study. Retina. 2014;34(1):12–7.
100. Wang F, Yu S, Liu K, et al. Acute intraocular inflammation caused by endotoxin after intravitreal injection of counterfeit bevacizumab in Shanghai, China. Ophthalmology. 2013;120:355–61.
101. Wickremasinghe SS, Michalova K, Gilhotra J, et al. Acute intraocular inflammation after intravitreous injections of bevacizumab for treatment of neovascular age-related macular degeneration. Ophthalmology. 2008;115(11):1911.e1–5.e1.
102. Shah CP, Garg SJ, Vander JF, Brown GC, Kaiser RS, Haller JA. Outcomes and risk factors associated with endophthalmitis after intravitreal injection of anti-vascular endothelial growth factor agents. Ophthalmology. 2011;118(10):2028–34.
103. Tolentino M. Systemic and Ocular Safety of Intravitreal Anti-VEGF Therapies for Ocular Neovascular Disease. Surv Ophthalmol. 2011;56(2):95–113.
104. Rosenfeld PJ, Heier JS, Hantsbarger G, Shams N. Tolerability and efficacy of multiple escalating doses of ranibizumab (lucentis) for neovascular age-related macular degeneration. Ophthalmology. 2006;113(4):623.e1–32.e1.
105. Kay CN, Tarantola RM, Gehrsetal KM. Uveitis following intravitreal bevacizumab: a non-infectious cluster. Ophthalmic Surg Lasers Imaging. 2011;42(4):292–96.
106. Arcinue CA, Ceron OM, Foster CS. A comparison between the fluocinolone acetonide (Retisert) and dexamethasone (Ozurdex) intravitreal implants in uveitis. J Ocul Pharmacol Ther. 2013;29(5):501–7.
107. Taney LS, Baumal CR, Duker JS. Sustained-release dexamethasone intravitreal implants for persistent macular edema after vitrecomy for epiretinal membrane. Ophthalmic Surg Lasers Imaging Retina. 2015;46(2):224–8.

41 Vogt-Koyanagi-Harada Syndrome

John B. Miller

History

Vogt-Koyanagi-Harada (VKH) syndrome is defined by both ophthalmic and systemic findings [1]. Vogt [2] and others [3–5] first reported a systemic association of ocular inflammation with poliosis. Harada later described cerebrospinal fluid pleocytosis associated with exudative retinal detachments and posterior uveitis [6]. Koyanagi [7] identified an even wider spectrum of uveitis-associated systemic findings; including hair loss and patchy depigmentation of the hair and skin.

It was later recognized that this constellation of findings most likely represented a broader spectrum of the same condition, termed Vogt-Koyanagi-Harada syndrome to honor those early reports [8, 9]. While both the American Uveitis Society (AUS) in 1978 [10] and the international workshop on VKH in 2001 [11] have revised the diagnostic criteria, the primary features remain as described in the early literature.

Epidemiology

VKH most often presents in the second to fifth decade of life [1]. It appears to affect women more than men, particularly in North America. It is most common in Asians, Hispanics, and both American and Asian Indians [12]. There does appear to be some variation in racial distribution within the US [12, 13], but this may be due to specific regional population demographics.

Clinical Manifestations

Bilateral panuveitis with exudative retinal detachments (Fig. 41.1) represents the classic ophthalmic findings of VKH. Associated extraocular signs include vitiligo, poliosis, alopecia, tinnitus, hearing loss, meningism (neck stiffness with photophobia) with headache, and pleocytosis of cerebrospinal fluid [14]. These systemic manifestations typically present later in the disease course and help define the classification of VKH. The complete form of VKH requires both ocular and two or more extraocular features [11]. The incomplete form is characterized by bilateral ocular involvement with just one extraocular finding. Probable VKH is defined by ophthalmic findings only. Due to the variation in the timing of the onset of systemic symptoms,

J.B. Miller (✉)
Retina Service, Massachusetts Eye and Ear Infirmary, 243 Charles Street, Boston, MA 02114, USA
e-mail: John_Miller@meei.harvard.edu

G.N. Papaliodis (ed.), *Uveitis*,
DOI 10.1007/978-3-319-09126-6_41

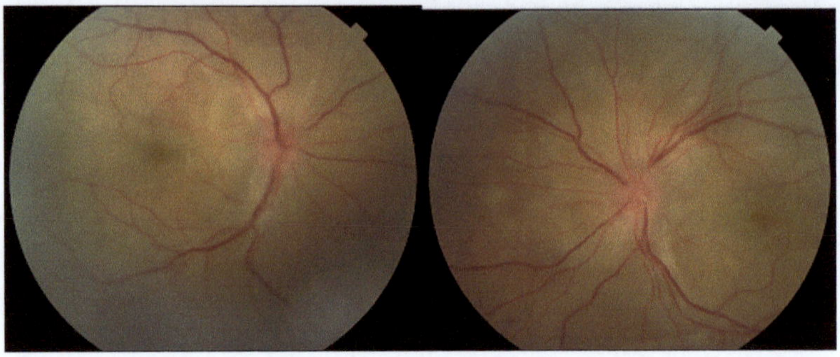

Fig. 41.1 Panuveitis with diffuse exudative retinal detachments OU in a patient with VKH

the disease classification may change over the course of the disease.

Differential Diagnosis

The entity with the most similar ophthalmic findings to VKH is sympathetic ophthalmia. Like VKH, sympathetic ophthalmia can present with bilateral panuveitis and exudative retinal detachments. While the associated extraocular findings of VKH can occur in sympathetic ophthalmia, they are incredibly rare [15]. Furthermore, a preceding sympathizing event should be identifiable in review of the patient's history when entertaining the diagnosis of sympathetic ophthalmia. This is classically thought to occur after penetrating ocular trauma, but the clinician should remember that ophthalmic surgery can also lead to sympathetic ophthalmia.

Uveal effusion syndrome and posterior scleritis are two other conditions in the differential of VKH. Uveal effusion syndrome, unlike VKH, has no intraocular inflammation. Posterior scleritis can be differentiated from VKH by the classic "T sign," posterior flattening of the globe, on ultrasonography seen with posterior scleritis.

Clinical Stages of VKH

VKH can be divided into four clinical stages: prodromal, acute uveitic, chronic uveitic, and chronic recurrent stages. Patients can present at any of these stages with a variety of signs and symptoms so it is important to understand the characteristics of each stage.

The prodromal stage of VKH is defined by a nonspecific viral-like illness. Symptoms can include fever, nausea, dizziness, headache, retrobulbar pain, and meningism. There may also be cranial nerve palsies or optic neuritis, and a lumbar puncture may reveal a lymphocytic pleocytosis even at this early time point. The prodromal stage usually lasts only a few days before progressing to more severe disease manifestations.

The acute uveitic stage follows the prodromal stage with bilateral blurry vision. While some patients may present with sequential involvement of one eye and then the other, it is most common to have bilateral posterior uveitis in the acute uveitic stage. The intraocular inflammation is defined by multiple serious retinal detachments (Fig. 41.2), optic nerve head hyperemia and edema, and thickening of the choroid.

Fluorescein angiography highlights these findings showing early hypofluorescent spots followed by hyperfluorescent spots, along with leakage and pooling in the areas of exudative

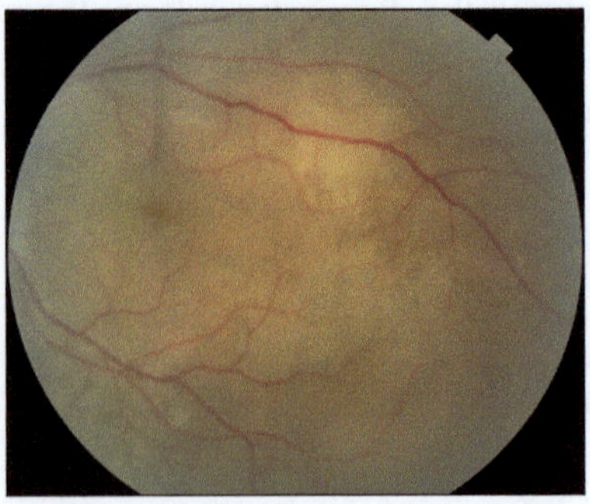

Fig. 41.2 Marked subretinal exudate and associated retinal detachment

retinal detachment in late frames. Ultrasonography can demonstrate the associated choroidal thickening. Similarly, OCT can identify this same choroidal thickening while also confirming the presence and extent of serous retinal detachments.

Typically, months after the acute uveitic stage, the chronic uveitic, or convalescent, stage begins. This stage is defined by choroidal depigmentation, vitiligo, and poliosis. Choroidal depigmentation to a red-orange choroid in conjunction with a pale disc leads to the classic sunset glow fundus, a hallmark of this stage. There can also be additional foci of hypopigmentation in the mid-periphery, particularly inferiorly. In addition to vitiligo of the skin, patients may also develop perilimbal vitiligo, or Sugiura's sign. This chronic uveitis/convalescent stage may last for months.

The chronic recurrent stage of VKH is defined by a low-grade panuveitis and intermittent recurrent episodes of granulomatous anterior uveitis. While anterior uveitis can occur in the acute stage, it is more common in the chronic recurrent phase of VKH. It is during this phase that iris nodules can arise. The most visually significant complication of this phase is choroidal neovascular membranes [16]. Additional complications secondary to recurrent bouts of inflammation can include posterior subcapsular cataract and glaucoma [17, 18].

Pathophysiology

VKH is defined by nonnecrotizing granulomatous inflammation of the uveal tract on histopathology. Uveal thickening arises from the infiltration of inflammatory cells, including lymphocytes, macrophages, and melanin filled multinucleated giant cells. Dalen-Fuchs nodules (Fig. 41.3) consist of epithelioid histiocytes that can accumulate in focal deposits between Bruch's membrane and the RPE [19].

The characteristic uveal inflammation of VKH is thought to arise from an autoimmune T-cell response to antigens within the melanocytes [20, 21]. There are strong HLA associations across specific ethnic and regional demographics. The HLA-DR4 antigen shows the greatest association in Japanese patients. Meanwhile, the HLA-DR1 and HLA-DR4 antigens are associated with VKH in 84 % of Southern California Hispanics [22] and 89 % of Mexicans [23].

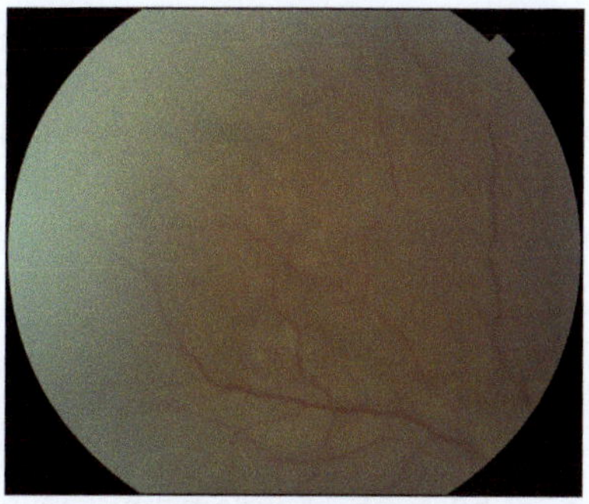

Fig. 41.3 Peripheral Dalen-Fuchs nodules in a patient with VKH

Treatment

The mainstay of treatment and accepted first line agent in the acute phase is systemic corticosteroids. The severity of the intraocular inflammation along with the extraocular findings requires systemic immunosuppression. Early intervention with aggressive steroid regimens can limit the ocular complications. The steroids are typically dosed at 1.0–2.0 mg/kg/day of oral prednisone or pulsed intravenous methylprednisolone (1000 mg daily for 3 consecutive days) followed by high-dose oral corticosteroids [14]. A multicenter study on VKH treatment found intravenous corticosteroids and high-dose oral corticosteroids equally effective as the initial treatment [24]. Tapering of the steroids typically occurs over three to six months after initiation of treatment. A slow taper of the corticosteroids has been shown to improve outcomes [14].

While steroids are quite effective in the acute phase of VKH, relapsing and recurrent inflammation has proven more steroid resistant, often requiring immunomodulatory therapy [12]. These steroid-sparing agents are also employed in cases where the steroid-related side effects are not tolerable. Cyclosporine, dosed at 5 mg/kg/day, is generally the most preferred of these options [25]. Alternatives to cyclosporine can also include the antimetabolites (Methotrexate, Mycophenolate mofetil, and Azathioprine).

Conclusions

VKH is a bilateral granulomatous panuveitis characterized by serous retinal detachments and a spectrum of extraocular findings. The disease is thought to arise from a T-cell driven autoimmune response to melanocytes. The fundus features may vary at the time of ophthalmic examination due to the multiple clinical stages of VKH, thus it is important to be aware of these different presentations. The initial treatment in the acute uveitic stage is corticosteroids with a slow taper over three to six months. Relapsing or recurrent stages may require immunomodulatory therapy. The visually significant complications of the disease include cataract, glaucoma, choroidal neovascularization, and subretinal fibrosis.

References

1. Rao NA, Moorthy RS, Inomata H. Vogt-Koyanagi-Harada syndrome. Int Ophthalmol Clin. 1995;35 (2):69–86.
2. Vogt A. Frühzeitiges Ergrauen Der Zilien Und Bemerkungen Über Den Sogenannten Plötzlichen Eintritt Dieser Veränderung. Klin Monatsbl Augenheilkd. 1906.
3. Schenkl DA. Ein Fall von plötzlich aufgetretener Poliosis circumscripta der Wimpern. Arch f Dermat. 1873;5(1):137–9. doi:10.1007/BF02430420.
4. Hutchinson J. A Case of Blanched Eyelashes. Arch Surg. 1892.
5. Pattison EM. Uveomeningoencephalitic syndrome (Vogt-Koyanagi-Harada). Arch Neurol. 1965;12 (2):197–205. doi:10.1001/archneur.1965.00460260087010.
6. Harada E. Acute Diffuse Choroiditis. Acta Soc Ophthalmol Jpn. 1926.
7. Koyanagi Y. Dysakusis, Alopecia Und Poliosis Bei Schwerer Uveitis Nicht Traumatischen Ursprungs. Klin Monatsbl Augenheilkd. 1929.
8. Babel J. Syndrome De Vogt-Koyanagi (Uveite Bilaterale, Poliosis, Alopecie, Vitiligo Et Dysacousie). Schweiz Med Wochenschr. 1932.
9. Bruno MG, McPherson SD. Harada's disease. Am J Ophthalmol. 1949;32(4):513–22.
10. Snyder DA, Tessler HH. Vogt-Koyanagi-Harada syndrome. Am J Ophthalmol. 1980;90(1):69–75.
11. Read RW, Holland GN, Rao NA, et al. Revised diagnostic criteria for Vogt-Koyanagi-Harada disease: report of an international committee on nomenclature 11. The authors constitute the International Committee on Vogt-Koyanagi-Harada Disease Nomenclature, representing the participants of the First International Workshop on Vogt-Koyanagi-Harada Disease. A full list of participants appears at the end of the article. Am J Ophthalmol. 2001;131 (5):647–52. doi:10.1016/S0002-9394(01)00925-4.
12. Moorthy RS, Inomata H, Rao NA. Vogt-Koyanagi-Harada syndrome. Surv Ophthalmol. 1995;39(4):265–92. doi:10.1016/S0039-6257(05)80105-5.
13. Ohno S, Char DH, Kimura SJ, O'Connor GR. Vogt-Koyanagi-Harada syndrome. Am J Ophthalmol. 1977;83(5):735–40.
14. Damico FM, Kiss S, Young LH. Vogt-Koyanagi-Harada Disease. Semin Ophthalmol. 2005;20 (3):183–90. doi:10.1080/08820530500232126.
15. Rao NA, Marak GE. Sympathetic ophthalmia simulating vogt-Koyanagi-Harada's disease: a clinico-pathologic study of four cases. Jpn J Ophthalmol. 1983;27(3):506–11.
16. Moorthy RS, Chong LP, Smith RE, Rao NA. Subretinal neovascular membranes in Vogt-Koyanagi-Harada syndrome. Am J Ophthalmol. 1993;116(2):164–70.
17. Moorthy RS, Rajeev B, Smith RE. Incidence and management of cataracts in Vogt-Koyanagi-Harada syndrome. Am J Ophthalmol. 1994.
18. Forster DJ, Rao NA, Hill RA, Nguyen QH, Baerveldt G. Incidence and management of glaucoma in Vogt-Koyanagi-Harada syndrome. Ophthalmology. 1993;100(5):613–8. doi:10.1016/S0161-6420(93)31604-0.
19. Inomata H, Rao NA. Depigmented atrophic lesions in sunset glow fundi of Vogt-Koyanagi-Harada disease. Am J Ophthalmol. 2001;131(5):607–14.
20. Norose K, Yano A. Melanoma specific Th1 cytotoxic T lymphocyte lines in Vogt-Koyanagi-Harada disease. Br J Ophthalmol. 1996;80(11):1002–8. doi:10.1136/bjo.80.11.1002.
21. Sugita S, Sagawa K, Mochizuki M, Shichijo S, Itoh K. Melanocyte lysis by cytotoxic T lymphocytes recognizing the MART-1 melanoma antigen in HLA-A2 patients with Vogt–Koyanagi–Harada disease. Int Immunol. 1996;8(5):799–803. doi:10.1093/intimm/8.5.799.
22. Weisz JM, Holland GN, Roer LN, et al. Association between Vogt-Koyanagi-Harada Syndrome and HLA-DR1 and -DR4 in Hispanic Patients Living in Southern California. Ophthalmology. 1995;102 (7):1012–5. doi:10.1016/S0161-6420(95)30920-7.
23. Arellanes-Garcia L, Bautista N, Mora P, Ortega-Larrocea G, Burguet A, Gorodezky C. HLA-DR is

strongly associated with Vogt-Koyanagi-Harada disease in Mexican Mestizo patients. Ocul Immunol Inflamm. 1998;6(2):93–100. doi:10.1076/ocii.6.2.93.4049.

24. Read RW, Yu F, Accorinti M, et al. Evaluation of the effect on outcomes of the route of administration of corticosteroids in acute Vogt-Koyanagi-Harada disease. Am J Ophthalmol. 2006;142(1):119–24. doi:10.1016/j.ajo.2006.02.049.
25. Wakatsuki Y, Kogure M, Takahashi Y. Combination therapy with cyclosporin a and steroid in severe case of Vogt-Koyanagi-Harada's Disease. Jpn J Ophthalmol. 1988.

Uveitis in Granulomatosis with Polyangiitis (GPA)

42

Safa Rahmani

Introduction

Granulomatosis with polyangiitis (GPA) (previously Wegener's granulomatosis) is part of the spectrum of systemic necrotizing vasculiites. It is a rare systemic inflammatory disease with necrotizing granulomatous vasculitis of the small-to-medium sized vessels. The disease usually manifests in adults but rare cases have been reported in the pediatric population [1]. GPA can affect any organ, but most commonly affects the sinuses and lungs (respiratory tract), kidneys, and the eye [2]. The granulomatosis is characterized by necrosis and thrombosis of the vessels.

Ocular Manifestations

Ophthalmologic disease is the manifesting feature of GPA in 8–16 % of patients but develops in an estimated 50–60 % of patients [4]. Orbital disease (30 %), episcleritis, scleritis, and conjunctivitis are the most common ophthalmological manifestations of GPA. Uveal involvement and granulomatous sclerouveitis are less common presentations. Uveitis (including anterior and posterior involvement) accounts for less than 10 %, and retinal involvement accounts for less than 5 % of ocular manifestations of GPA [5].

Anterior, posterior, and panuveitis have all been described in isolation or is associated with scleritis in GPA. The majority of uveitis in GPA is an anterior uveitis (70 % of uveitis cases) and more commonly occurs synchronously with anterior scleritis [6]. Anterior uveitis can be acute, granulomatous, or chronic with relapsing phases and may induce cystoid macular edema [7]. Clinical examination may range from mild ocular injection to significant inflammation with mutton fat keratic precipitates and substantial synechiae.

Posterior uveitis, including retinal vasculitis is a rare manifestation of GPA, accounting for less than 5 % of uveitis cases [6]. It can occur in conjunction with posterior scleritis and clinical presentation can range from cotton wool spots to severe vaso-occlusive disease with vasculitis, thrombosis, exudates and hemorrhages, and optic neuropathy, all with potentially significant visual morbidity [5].

Isolated choroiditis has also been reported in GPA patients that can clinically manifest as uveitis, choroidal folds, RPE changes, and occlusion of choroidal vessels. On

S. Rahmani (✉)
Department of Ophthalmology, Massachusetts Eye and Ear Infirmary, 243 Charles Street, 12th Floor Retina Service, Boston, MA 02114, USA
e-mail: Safa_Rahmani@meei.harvard.edu

G.N. Papaliodis (ed.), *Uveitis*,
DOI 10.1007/978-3-319-09126-6_42

histopathology, there is infiltration of the choroidal vessels with granulomatous inflammation [8].

Laboratory Testing

Laboratory tests that suggest GPA can be nonspecific but more indicative of inflammation such as anemia, leukocytosis, thrombocytosis, and elevated ESR and CRP. ANCA (Anti-neutrophil cytoplasmic antibody) is present in 80–90 % of patients with GPA, although positive ANCA can also be seen with other small-to-medium vessel disease such as MPA (microscopic polyangiitis) [2]. It is the clinical manifestations of end organ disease that separates these disease entities. The c-ANCA measures antibody to neutrophil serine proteinase; p-ANCA corresponds to antibody directed against lysosomal enzymes, lactoferrin, or myeloperoxidase. The ANCA titers do not necessarily correlate with disease severity and should not be used for clinical response monitoring to therapeutic interventions [3].

Treatment

Treatment of GPA requires a multidisciplinary effort as disease activity may involve multiple organ systems. Ocular GPA requires in-depth evaluation of other potential organ involvement as the eye disease may be a harbinger of more widespread systemic disease even if the patient has minimal symptoms. Treatment of ocular disease must involve control of systemic inflammation in addition to periocular or topical agents. First line therapy usually includes the use of systemic corticosteroids and cytotoxic medications. Combination of steroids and cytotoxic agents are the usual mainstay of ocular GPA, especially with use of cyclophosphamide for induction. Rituximab has similarly been shown to induce remission effectively. After initial control, many patients are able to be kept in remission with use of low dose corticosteroids with either Methotrexate, mycophenolate mofetil, or azathioprine. With aggressive management, GPA has a mean survival rates of >95 % with the current immunomodulatory therapies available [3].

Conclusion

Granulomatosis with polyangiitis (previously Wegener's granulomatosis) is a rare systemic inflammatory disease that can affect any organ but more commonly the sinuses, lungs, kidneys, and eyes. Ophthalmological disease is the manifesting feature of GPA in 8–16 % of patients but develops in an estimated 50–60 % of patients [4]. Orbital disease, episcleritis, scleritis, and conjunctivitis are the most common ophthalmological manifestations of GPA but uveitis has also been reported (less than 10 % of GPA cases). The diagnosis is established by serologic testing for ANCA (Anti-neutrophil cytoplasmic antibody) which is present in 80–90 % of patients with GPA. The mainstay of treatment is high dose corticosteroids along with cytotoxic agents (cyclophosphamide, methotrexate) and more recently biologic therapies (Rituximab).

References

1. Levi M, Kodsi SR, Rubin SE, Lyons C, Golden R, Olitsky SE, Christiansen S. Alcorn DM Ocular involvement as the initial manifestation of Wegener's granulomatosis in children. J AAPOS. 2008;12(1): 94–6.
2. Ahmed M, Niffenegger JH, Jakobiec FA, Ben-Arie-Weintrob Y, Gion N, Androudi S, Folberg R, Raizman MB, Margo CE, Smith ME, McLean IW, Caya JG, Foster CS. Diagnosis of limited ophthalmic Wegener granulomatosis: distinctive pathologic features with ANCA test confirmation. Int Ophthalmol. 2008;28(1):35–46.
3. Tarabishy AB, Schulte M, Papaliodis GN, Hoffman GS. Wegener's granulomatosis: clinical manifestations, differential diagnosis, and management of ocular and systemic disease. Surv Ophthalmol. 2010;55(5):429–44.
4. Pakrou N, Selva D, Leibovitch I. Wegener's granulomatosis: ophthalmic manifestations and management. Semin Arthritis Rheum. 2006;35(5):284–92.
5. Rothschild PR, Pagnoux C, Seror R, Brézin AP, Delair E, Guillevin L. Ophthalmologic manifestations of systemic necrotizing vasculitides at diagnosis: a

retrospective study of 1286 patients and review of the literature. Semin Arthritis Rheum. 2013;42(5):507–14.
6. Watkins AS, Kempen JH, Choi D, Liesegang TL, Pujari SS, Newcomb C, Nussenblatt RB, Rosenbaum JT, Thorne JE, Foster CS, Jabs DA. Ocular disease in patients with ANCA-positive vasculitis. J Ocul Biol Dis Infor. 2010; 3(1):12–9.
7. du Huong LT, Tran TH, Piette JC. Granulomatous uveitis revealing Wegener's granulomatosis. J Rheumatol. 2006;33(6):1209–10.
8. Proia AD. Granulomatous choroiditis in Wegener granulomatosis. Arch Ophthalmol. 2011;129(4):520–1.

Part IV
Treatment

Topical Therapies

43

George N. Papaliodis

Topical Steroids

Steroids are the most commonly prescribed anti-inflammatory drugs in all of ophthalmology and an integral component in the therapeutic armamentarium in patients with uveitis. Steroids inhibit edema, cellular infiltration, fibrin deposition, capillary dilation, leukocyte migration, capillary and fibroblast proliferation, collagen deposition, and scar formation associated with inflammation [1, 2]. There are multiple topical corticosteroid agents available in the market which vary based on anti-inflammatory potency. The high potency steroids include dexamethasone, difluprednate, and prednisolone. The lower potency steroids include fluorometholone, loteprednol, and rimexolone (Table 43.1).

Cycloplegics and Mydriatics

These agents provide notable benefits in the treatment of uveitis as adjuncts to prevent significant ocular sequelae including: anterior and posterior synechiae, pupillary block, secondary angle closure, iris bombe, and pain/photophobia associated with ciliary spasm. The most significant difference among the commercially available medications is the onset and duration of action (Table 43.2).

Nonsteroidal Anti-inflammatory Drugs (NSAIDs)

Topical ophthalmic NSAIDs have both analgesic and anti-inflammatory properties with multiple FDA approved indications including: treatment of pain and inflammation associated with cataract and refractive surgery, inhibition of intraoperative miosis, and temporary relief of ocular pruritus related to seasonal allergic conjunctivitis (Table 43.3). The role of topical NSAIDs for the treatment of macular edema is discussed in the cystoid macular edema chapter of this textbook.

G.N. Papaliodis (✉)
Department of Ophthalmology, Harvard Medical School, Massachusetts Eye and Ear Infirmary, 243 Charles Street, Boston, MA 02114, USA
e-mail: George_Papaliodis@meei.harvard.edu

G.N. Papaliodis (ed.), *Uveitis*,
DOI 10.1007/978-3-319-09126-6_43

Table 43.1 Topical steroids

Generic name	Commercial names	Concentration
Dexamethasone	Maxidex, decadron	0.1 %
Difluprednate emulsion	Durezol	0.05 %
Fluorometholone	Flarex	0.1 %
	FML forte	0.25 %
	FML	0.1 %
Loteprednol	Lotemax	0.5 % gel ointment
	Alrex	0.2 %
Prednisolone acetate	Pred forte	1 %
	Omnipred	1 %
	Pred mild	0.12 %
Prednisolone sodium phosphate	Inflamase forte	1 %
Rimexolone	Vexol	1 %

Table 43.2 Topical cycloplegics and mydriatics

Generic name	Commercial names	Concentration	Onset/Duration of action
Atropine sulfate	Isopto Atropine	1 % ointment 1 % solution	30–45 min/7–12 days
Cyclopentolate hydrochloride	Cyclogyl, AK-Pentolate	Solution 0.5, 1, 2 %	25–75 min/6–24 h
Cyclopentolate/Phenylephrine	Cyclomydril	Solution 0.2/1 %	20–60 min/3–24 h
Homatropine hydrobromide	Isopto Homatropine AK-Homatropine	Solution 5 %	30–90 min/1–4 days
Hydroxyamphetamine/Tropicamide	Paremyd	Solution 1/0.25 %	<15 min/6–8 h
Phenylephrine hydrochloride	AK-Dilate, Neo-Synephrine	Solution 2.5, 10 %	30–60 min/3–5 h
Scopolamine hydrobromide	Isopto Hyoscine	Solution 0.25 %	30–60 min/4–7 days
Tropicamide	Mydriacyl, Tropicacyl	Solution 0.5, 1 %	20–40 min/4–6 h

Table 43.3 Topical NSAIDs

Generic name	Commercial names	Concentration (%)
Bromfenac	Bromday	0.09
	Prolensa	0.07
Diclofenac sodium	Voltaren	0.1
Flurbiprofen sodium	Ocufen	0.03
Ketorolac	Acular	0.5
	Acular LS	0.4
	Acuvail	0.45
Nepafenac ophthalmic	Ilevro	0.3
	Nevanac	0.1

References

1. Drug Facts and Comparisons 4.0 (database on the Internet). St. Louis: Wolters Kluwer Health, Inc.; 2013 (cited 10 Jan 2013). Available at: http://online.factsandcomparisons.com.

2. Micromedex® Healthcare Series (database on the Internet). Greenwood Village (CO): Thomson Micromedex; 2013 (cited 10 Jan 2013). Available from: http://www.thomsonhc.com.

Medical Therapy

44

Sergio Schwartzman

Introduction

Uveitis is not a disease; rather, it is the ultimate phenotypic expression of an immunologic abnormality that may be idiopathic or associated with a recognized systemic illness. The exact genetic, cellular, and cytokine/chemokine spectrum of specific forms of uveitis is currently being delineated. Therapeutic studies and data are frequently flawed based on patient populations studied, trial design, and outcome measures. In the absence of absolute data, treatment is to some extent empiric. The therapeutic approach to uveitis requires consideration of etiology, anatomic site involved, chronicity, prior medication failure and potential ophthalmic and systemic risks of the underlying disease and proposed therapy.

As primary systemic illnesses can be identified in a significant number of patients with uveitis, it is rational, in this population, to optimally treat the underlying systemic disease first. It is important to employ a team approach in treating patients with recalcitrant uveitis as particularly in patients with systemic diseases there are medical subspecialists (Rheumatologists, Immunologists, Dermatologists, Gastroenterologists, Pulmonologists, Hematologists, Neurologists, and Internists) that can contribute greatly to the outcomes of these patients. It is critical that the autoimmune ophthalmologist lead this team. This review will focus on the medical therapy of patients with recalcitrant uveitis. Therapies for specific underlying diseases will be covered independently in individual chapters.

S. Schwartzman (✉)
Rheumatology, Hospital for Special Surgery, New York Presbyterian Hospital, Weill Medical College of Cornell University, 535 East 70th Street, New York, NY 10021, USA
e-mail: SchwartzmanS@HSS.EDU

G.N. Papaliodis (ed.), *Uveitis*,
DOI 10.1007/978-3-319-09126-6_44

Corticosteroids

Patients with a single or infrequent episode of anterior uveitis generally respond well to topical corticosteroids, cycloplegic, and/or mydriatic agents. It is the patient with chronic disease, intermediate, posterior, or panuveitis that requires aggressive therapy. Systemic steroids are generally the first therapeutic intervention. The recommended initial therapy is usually prednisone at doses of 40–80 mg per day. It is interesting that in rheumatic diseases the concept of a "window of opportunity" for treating patients with Rheumatoid Arthritis (RA) has been accepted as standard of care therapy [1]. This strategy employs the use of potent immunomodulators such as methotrexate (MTX) or leflunomide in the treatment of RA at the time of diagnosis. This concept has not yet been fully accepted or integrated in the treatment of autoimmune ophthalmic diseases, though it has clearly been entertained [2, 3].

Antimetabolites

MTX and Mycophenolate (MMF) are frequently the first agents utilized when an acceptable steroid dose is deemed ineffective and/or toxic. Methotrexate is an antimetabolite that inhibits dihydrofolate reductase, an enzyme that participates in tetrahydrofolate synthesis. It is used in the treatment of cancer, autoimmune diseases, and for the induction of abortions. MTX acts by inhibiting the metabolism of folic acid which is needed for the de novo synthesis of thymidine, required for DNA synthesis. Folate is essential for purine and pyrimidine base biosynthesis. This impediment leads to the accumulation of adenosine with subsequent inhibition of T cell activation.

The first descriptions of MTX use in uveitis were in a 2 small cohorts of patients in 1969 [4, 5]. There is an established literature on the use of MTX both in adults with a variety of autoimmune ophthalmic diseases [2, 3, 6–14] and in Juvenile Idiopathic Arthritis (JIA) associated uveitis [15–21]. Interestingly, in one study, early use of MTX in children with JIA who did not have uveitis resulted in a lower probability of developing uveitis [22], perhaps exemplifying the operational concept of a "window of opportunity" to prevent the occurrence of uveitis in an at risk group. Therapy with MTX requires dosages between 15 and 25 mg weekly, administered either orally or parenterally [2, 14]. Twenty milligrams per week is both the mean and median dose of MTX used by ophthalmologists queried from the American Uveitis Society [14].

In a retrospective, non-comparative interventional case series that evaluated 160 patients with chronic noninfectious uveitis unresponsive to conventional anti-inflammatory therapy who were treated with MTX, control of inflammation was achieved in 76.2 % of patients, a steroid-sparing effect was achieved in 56 % and visual acuity was maintained or improved in 90 %. Side effects requiring discontinuation of MTX occurred in 18 % of patients and serious adverse events occurred in 8.1 % [10]. In a smaller study of 14 steroid resistant patients with active chronic uveitis two different MTX therapeutic paradigms were evaluated. In 8 patients, a dose of 40 mg was given intravenously once weekly for 4 weeks followed by 15 mg/week given orally whereas 6 subjects were treated with only 15 mg/week orally. During a follow-up period of 3–24 months, intraocular inflammation improved in all patients as did visual acuity in 11 patients [6, 13]. In a large cohort of 257 patients with inflammatory eye disease seen at a single center 90 patients with inflammatory eye disease were treated with MTX. Sixty-seven percent of these patients had uveitis and the median time to treatment success was 6.5 months for MTX treatment group [11]. Intraocular MTX is infrequently used to treat uveitis but has been studied in two case series. In patients with uveitis and uveitic cystoid macular edema (CME), intravitreal MTX improves visual acuity and reduces CME. Recurrence of inflammation is not uncommon in these cohorts; however, patients respond to reinjection [23, 24].

Adverse events from systemic MTX include alopecia, stomatitis, rashes, infections, nausea, abdominal pain, fatigue, fever, dizziness, acute pneumonitis, hepatic and pulmonary fibrosis, and kidney failure. Common adverse events include cytopenias and abnormal liver function tests. Malignancies including lymphoma have been described with use of this medication.

MMF has become an increasingly popular therapy to treat recalcitrant uveitis. MMF is a prodrug of mycophenolic acid that is used predominantly in transplant medicine. It is also used in the treatment of autoimmune diseases, such as systemic lupus erythematosus, Behçet's disease, and pemphigus vulgaris. It is a reversible inhibitor of inosine monophosphate dehydrogenase which is required in purine biosynthesis and is necessary for the development of T and B cells. Dosing generally requires 1–3 g/day in divided doses.

This medication has been used in JIA associated uveitis, systemic illnesses associated with uveitis and in ocular immune mediated syndromes generally in the setting of steroid failure or toxicity [25–38]. In a relatively robust long-term study of 60 patients followed for at least 5 years that assessed the efficacy and tolerability of MMF in patients with chronic noninfectious uveitis, outcome measures evaluated included control of inflammation, corticosteroid-sparing potential, ability to stop or taper MMF and safety. Control of intraocular inflammation was achieved in 43 of 60 patients (72 %) after 1 year and in 45 of 55 patients (82 %) after 2 years. An improvement or stabilization of visual acuity was observed in 49 patients (82 %), and a worsening in 11 patients (18 %, 95 % CI: 10–30 %). At 5 years of therapy the probability of discontinuing corticosteroids was 40 %. Treatment was stopped because of inefficacy in 12 patients (rate: 0.05/PY) and because of side effects in four patients [33].

No definitive prospective, superiority, masked, head-to-head studies have been successfully completed comparing the different potentially steroid-sparing medications. There have been a number of retrospective studies comparing MTX and mycophenolate. In a series of 257 patients with inflammatory eye disease treated at one center, 90 patients with inflammatory eye disease were treated with methotrexate, 38 with azathioprine, and 129 with mycophenolate. Uveitis accounted for the majority of the diagnoses between 66 and 68 % in each group. The median time to treatment success was 4.0, 4.8, and 6.5 months for the MMF, azathioprine, and MTX treatment groups respectively ($P = 0.02$, log-rank test). These data suggest that the time to control of ocular inflammation is faster with mycophenolate than with MTX [11]. In a separate study of 80 patients with noninfectious intermediate, posterior, or panuveitis requiring corticosteroid-sparing therapy, patients were randomized to receive 25 mg weekly oral MTX or 1000 mg BID of MMF. Oral prednisone and topical corticosteroids were tapered. The primary outcome of treatment success was defined by: (1) ≤0.5+ anterior chamber cells, ≤0.5+ vitreous cells, ≤0.5+ vitreous haze and no active retinal/choroidal lesions in both eyes, (2) ≤10 mg of prednisone and ≤2 drops of prednisolone acetate 1 % a day, and (3) no declaration of treatment failure because of intolerability or safety. Additional outcomes included time to sustained corticosteroid-sparing control of inflammation, change in best spectacle-corrected visual acuity, resolution of macular edema and adverse events. Thirty five MTX treated patients and 32 MMF treated patients completed the study. Sixty-nine percent of patients achieved treatment success with MTX and 47 % with MMF ($P = 0.09$). There were no differences between treatment groups in time to corticosteroid-sparing control of inflammation ($P = 0.44$), change in best spectacle-corrected visual acuity ($P = 0.68$), or resolution of macular edema ($P = 0.31$). Treatment failure from adverse events or tolerability was not different by treatment arm ($P = 0.99$) [29]. There is currently a comparative MTX versus MMF effectiveness study ongoing entitled: First-line Antimetabolites as Steroid-sparing Treatment (clinicaltrials.gov).

Potential toxicities of MMF include hyperlipidemia, abnormal liver function tests, hypomagnesemia, hypocalcemia, hyperkalemia, and an increase in BUN. Leukopenia, anemia and thrombocytopenia have been described. Patients are at risk for infections and cases of progressive multifocal leukoencephalopathy have been described. Pulmonary toxicity including pleural effusions and pulmonary fibrosis have been noted. Malignancies including skin cancers, melanoma and lymphoma have occurred. Common and potentially troublesome side effects include rashes, headaches, fever and diarrhea.

Although azathioprine has been used to treat different forms of uveitis [39–43], a prominent role for this therapy is not established given the lack of large published studies. In one small study of 27 patients with various forms of uveitis (3 with anterior uveitis, 1 pars planitis, 4 idiopathic panuveitis, 8 Vogt-Koyonagi-Harada syndrome, 3 Behcet's disease, and 8 choroidoretinopathies), complete response was observed in 92 %. Eleven patients had well-tolerated minor side effects [40]. Azathioprine is a prodrug that is converted into 6-mercaptopurine which blocks purine metabolism and DNA synthesis suppressing leukocyte cellular proliferation. Significant adverse reactions can include an increased risk of infection, bone marrow suppression, hepatotoxicity, pancreatitis, and increased risk of lymphoma. Common adverse reactions include nausea, vomiting, anorexia, and fever. The enzyme thiopurine S-methyltransferase (TPMT) deactivates 6-mercaptopurine. Patients who have low TMPT activity (<10 %) are at increased risk of drug induced bone marrow suppression.

T Cell Inhibitors

Cyclosporin [44–55] and tacrolimus [56–62] have been utilized in dosages of 2.5–5 mg/kg/day and 0.03–0.08 mg/kg/day respectively to treat recalcitrant uveitis. Cyclosporin is an immunosuppressant drug used in organ transplantation to prevent rejection. Its mode of action is thought to be due to the binding to the cytosolic protein cyclophilin of lymphocytes which inhibits calcineurin. This results in the inhibition of lymphokine production and interleukin release. Tacrolimus has similar indications and similar immunosuppressive properties to cyclosporine but is much more potent. It is a macrolide that binds to the immunophilin FK506 binding protein creating a complex that interacts with and inhibits calcineurin thus inhibiting both T lymphocyte signal transduction and IL-2 transcription.

In a prospective randomized study of 37 patients with posterior uveitis that required a second-line agent, the efficacy of tacrolimus and cyclosporine was assessed. The effect on peripheral blood CD4 (+) T-cell was also evaluated. The main outcomes were visual acuity, indirect ophthalmoscopy score, quality of life, and adverse events. Thirteen patients (68 %) taking tacrolimus and 12 patients (67 %) taking cyclosporine responded to treatment. No significant difference was detected with regard to effect on quality of life. Cyclosporine was associated with slightly greater toxicity with regards to blood pressure and serum cholesterol levels. No significant difference was detected with regard to effect on CD4 (+) T-cell phenotype [58]. In another retrospective study supporting the use of tacrolimus for the treatment of uveitis, 62 consecutive patients with noninfectious uveitis treated with tacrolimus at a single academic center successfully tapered prednisone to 10 mg daily at an average rate of 1.62 per patient-year (PY), with an 85 % probability of achieving ≤10 mg after 1 year 2 months of treatment. Tacrolimus was discontinued due to intolerance at a rate of 0.13/PY. This was predominantly due to noncardiovascular adverse events. Creatinine rises of ≥30 % were uncommon (0.05/PY). It was felt by the investigators that tacrolimus's efficacy for the treatment of uveitis is maintained long term and that the cardiovascular risk profile is acceptable [61].

Potential side effects of cyclosporine include fever, vomiting, diarrhea, gingival hyperplasia, peptic ulcers, pancreatitis, seizures, confusion, hypercholesterolemia, dyspnea, paresthesia, pruritus, hypertension, hyperkalemia, kidney and liver dysfunction and an increased vulnerability to opportunistic fungal and viral infections. Potential adverse events from tacrolimus include infection, hypertension, electrolyte abnormalities, renal, pulmonary, cardiac and hepatic toxicity and several neurologic and psychiatric illnesses. Skin cancers and lymphoma have been reported.

Alkylating Agents

Cyclophosphamide [63–66] and chlorambucil [67–73] have been used to treat recalcitrant uveitis but only in circumstances where all other therapy has failed. With the current availability of biologic therapies these two medications are only rarely used to treat uveitis. Cyclophosphamide and chlorambucil are alkylating agents which covalently bind and crosslink a variety of macromolecules including deoxyribonucleic acid (DNA), ribonucleic acid (RNA), and proteins. DNA crosslinking impairs DNA replication and transcription, ultimately leading either to cell death or to altered cellular function [74]. The degree of immune suppression is dose and duration of treatment dependent. Toxicities include risk of infection, bone marrow suppression, gonadal dysfunction/sterility, increased risk of secondary malignancies (including lymphoma and lymphoma). Cyclophosphamide also carries the additional risk of potentially inducing hemorrhagic cystitis and bladder cancer.

Biologic Agents

Biologic therapies have been introduced for the therapy of recalcitrant uveitis over the last two decades. These compounds are defined as bioengineered chimeric and monoclonal antibodies, cytokine receptors, Fab fragments and agents such as interferons that influence the expression of cells and pro- and anti-inflammatory constituents of the immune system.

Biologic therapies were initially introduced to treat more common autoimmune illnesses such as Crohn's disease, rheumatoid arthritis, organ transplant rejection and malignancies. As the use of these therapies has evolved, they have become increasingly employed in the management to treat both idiopathic ocular inflammatory disease and uveitis associated with known underlying systemic illnesses. Recognized difficulty in interpreting published data is due to the lack of prospective, double masked, randomized trials and a deficiency of more strict definitions of the autoimmune ophthalmic disease being studied. Therefore, the published literature is comprised of predominantly case series. Biological therapies used to date include a broad range of agents: anti-TNF, anti-IL1, anti-IL2 receptor, anti-IL6 receptor, anti-IL17, co-stimulatory blockade, interferon, and CD-20 B cell-directed therapy. It is of important note that every one of these therapies were developed for the treatment of conditions other than uveitis.

There are currently five anti-TNF agents approved for the treatment of autoimmune diseases and although most of these have been used in autoimmune ophthalmic diseases none of these therapies are yet approved for the treatment of uveitis. Adalimumab was recently granted "orphan drug status" by the FDA for the treatment of noninfectious intermediate, posterior, or panuveitis, or chronic noninfectious anterior uveitis. For the most part, anti-TNF therapies have been studied in a retrospective manner although some prospective studies have been successfully completed. There are a number of studies that target one underlying systemic disease or form of uveitis; however, most reports combine different underlying systemic diseases and include idiopathic uveitis.

Infliximab

Based on published literature, infliximab appears to be the most frequently used biological therapy to treat recalcitrant uveitis. It is a chimeric mouse/human monoclonal antibody with a murine variable region that binds to the soluble and transmembrane forms of TNF-α. In the United States it is approved for Crohn's disease (in both adults and children), rheumatoid arthritis, ankylosing spondylitis, psoriatic arthritis, plaque psoriasis and ulcerative colitis (in both children and adults). It is not approved in JIA. In Japan, infliximab is approved for the treatment of Behçet's associated uveitis.

Infliximab is unique in that it is approved for different systemic diseases with or without MTX and in a wide range of doses and thus, provides dosing flexibility that can range from 3 mg/kg every eight weeks to 10 mg/kg every four weeks. Given the potential impediment of the blood ocular barrier and the need for high-dose medications to treat ocular inflammatory disease, this appears to be a significant advantage over other biologics. It must be recognized however, that at a higher dose infliximab does incur a higher risk of serious infections [75].

There are a number of conditions for which infliximab is approved that have a significance incidence of uveitis. Foremost amongst these are Ankylosing Spondylitis [76, 77], Psoriatic Arthritis and Crohn's disease [78, 79]. It has additionally been used in uveitis associated with JIA [80–87], sarcoidosis [85, 88] and Behçet's Disease.

In one of the few prospective studies on the use of infliximab in recalcitrant uveitis, 31 patients with various underlying etiologies were enrolled and 78 % of patients met criteria for clinical success at week 10 as judged by a composite clinical end point of visual acuity, control of intraocular inflammation, ability to taper concomitant therapy, and improvement of fluorescein angiography and/or ocular coherence tomography. This study was unique however as there were an inordinate number of serious adverse events that were potentially related to infliximab. These included: lupus-like reaction in two patients, pulmonary embolus, congestive heart failure, and vitreous hemorrhage in two patients. Although infliximab was effective, the number of potential toxicities in this study was dramatically different than any other study published across all indications for this medication. In a 2-year follow-up a 60 % retention rate for maintenance of infliximab therapy was observed [89].

In a large retrospective analysis of 88 patients with resistant uveitis from a single center treated with infliximab, 81.8 % of the patients achieved clinical remission but 58.3 % required additional immunomodulatory medications. In this study 36.4 % of the patients experienced at least one side effect and 19.3 % discontinued treatment due to toxicity. Interestingly, even in this study in contrast to the Suhler study [90], potential serious adverse events were not common and included only one case of autoimmune hepatitis, two of chronic infections and one of drug-induced lupus [91].

Although not approved for JIA, infliximab has been frequently used to treat uveitis in children [80–87]. In an interesting retrospective study stressing the importance of aggressive therapy to control recalcitrant uveitis in children, seventeen children with chronic uveitis were administered high-dose infliximab (10–20 mg/kg/dose). All 17 patients demonstrated a dramatic, rapid response, with no observed inflammation in 13 patients after the second infusion. Four patients required three to seven infusions to achieve disease control [80]. This therapeutic dose is not approved as a starting therapy for any condition and is very uncommonly used to treat any autoimmune disease. In a more traditionally dosed retrospective review of infliximab use in JIA in six patients with both ocular and musculoskeletal involvement, five of whom had been treated with other anti-TNF agents, drug induced remission occurred in three patients, with improvement of ocular inflammation in two more patients. Resolution of joint involvement occurred in five of six patients [84].

Adalimumab

Adalimumab, a recombinant human Ig G 1 monoclonal antibody targeting TNF approved for the therapy of many autoimmune diseases, has also been used to treat recalcitrant uveitis [85, 87, 92–120]. It is currently approved for RA, Crohn's disease, ulcerative colitis, ankylosing spondylitis, psoriatic arthritis, psoriasis and JIA. The medication is used at a dosage of 40 mg every two weeks for RA with or without methotrexate. The dose can be increased to 40 mg per week. It has been demonstrated that in RA combination therapy of adalimumab and methotrexate is superior to monotherapy with adalimumab alone [121].

In a prospective, multicenter, open-label trial to assess the effectiveness and safety of adalimumab in treating refractory uveitis patients with multiple underlying systemic conditions, 68 % of patients were responders at ten weeks and 39 % exhibited durable response at 50 weeks. No patients experienced treatment-limiting toxicity [96]. In a large study comprising of 1250 patients with ankylosing spondylitis treated with adalimumab the rates of anterior uveitis flares per 100 patient years (PYs) reported during the year before adalimumab treatment were compared to rates during adalimumab treatment. Flare rates before adalimumab treatment were 15/100 PYs in all patients. During adalimumab treatment, the rate was reduced by 51 %. Additionally, flares during adalimumab treatment were predominantly mild. Two patients with periods of high ankylosing spondylitis disease activity had new-onset anterior uveitis during the treatment period.

In the largest retrospective series of JIA patients with uveitis treated with adalimumab studied to date, composed of 54 patients, 66 % achieved good clinical control. There was, however, worsening of disease activity in 13 % of patients [109]. A current prospective randomized controlled trial of the clinical effectiveness, safety, and cost-effectiveness of adalimumab in combination with methotrexate to treat JIA associated uveitis is ongoing [102].

In an interesting study, comparing infliximab to adalimumab, a greater benefit for adalimumab was demonstrated; however, caution needs to be exercised in interpretation of this study given the trial design and small numbers of patients [87]. There is currently an ongoing prospective sponsored trial entitled Efficacy and Safety of Adalimumab in Subjects with Active Uveitis (VISUAL 1) that is enrolling patients (ClinicalTrials.gov).

Golimumab

Golimumab, a fully human anti-TNF IgG1 monoclonal antibody, has been used to treat autoimmune uveitis in small studies [122–127]. It is available as a subcutaneous preparation dosed at 50 mg per month and as an intravenous preparation dosed at 2 mg/kg every 2 months. The medication is approved for a number of autoimmune diseases. As a subcutaneous medication it is approved both with and without methotrexate depending on the indication (RA, ankylosing spondylitis psoriatic arthritis, and ulcerative colitis). As an intravenous medication it is only approved for RA with MTX.

In a small series combining patients with JIA and HLA B-27 associated uveitis (13 patients with JIA, 4 with HLA-B27) who had failed other biologics, of 17 patients treated, response at last visit was noted in 12 patients [123]. There are ongoing studies on this agent [124].

Etanercept

Etanercept a fusion protein produced by recombinant DNA technique that expresses the p75 TNF receptors attached to an IgG1 Fc. It can be administered as a once a week 50 mg dose or 25 mg twice a week. It is approved for RA, psoriatic arthritis, psoriasis, ankylosing spondylitis, and JIA both with and without MTX. Although etanercept was first thought to have a potential role in treating resistant uveitis [76, 128–130], further studies have not substantiated a definitive benefit in uveitis [131, 132]. A controversial area that requires clarification and further study is the potential paradoxical role of anti-TNF agents as a cause of uveitis. Uveitis has not been the only potential paradoxical reaction to anti-TNF therapy; indeed, psoriasis, inflammatory bowel disease, scleritis, and sarcoidosis have been reported in case studies as potential consequence of anti-TNF therapy. A pivotal study on this subject clarifies the potential causative role of anti-TNF therapies on the development of uveitis by demonstrating that while the incidence of uveitis is higher in etanercept-treated patients than those treated with infliximab or adalimumab, the overall incidence of new-onset uveitis with the first three anti-TNF agents approved is very low, and if indeed there was an association between any one of these agents and uveitis, the incidence of uveitis should have been much higher [133].

A difficult question that remains however is whether to use etanercept in patients with underlying diseases that in and of themselves have a risk for the development of uveitis. It is well accepted that uveitis can occur in 20–40 % of patients with any of the HLA B-27 associated inflammatory conditions [134]. In the published literature it has been found that in the ankylosing spondylitis trials in which etanercept was used, there was no observation of a higher incidence of uveitis [135].

A recent expert panel has published recommendations for the use of anti-TNF agents in ocular inflammatory diseases with a focus on infliximab and adalimumab. Both of these agents can be considered as first line for the treatment of ocular manifestations of Behçet's disease. Additionally, these medications can be considered as second line for the treatment of uveitis associated with JIA and for severe ocular inflammatory conditions including posterior uveitis, panuveitis, severe uveitis associated with seronegative spondyloarthropathy, and scleritis in patients who have failed or who are not candidates for antimetabolite or calcineurin inhibitor immunomodulation [136].

There are overlapping but not completely identical potential side effects of anti-TNF therapies. These include increased susceptibility to routine and opportunistic infections (Tuberculosis, Listeria Mycosis, Histoplasmosis, Coccidiomycosis, reactivation of Hepatitis B), other autoimmune diseases such as paradoxical psoriasis, uveitis is listed as one of the potential risks in patients treated with etanercept, congestive heart failure, neurological complications (particularly multiple sclerosis), skin cancers, lymphoma, and malignancies in general. Adalimumab and infliximab have also had a number of cases reported of hepatosplenic T-cell lymphoma—an uncommon malignancy reported in patients with inflammatory bowel disease and concomitant therapy with purine inhibitors

Interleukin Blockers

Daclizumab, a humanized monoclonal antibody of IgG1 subtype that binds to the Tac epitope on the interleukin-2 receptor α-chain55k subunit has been used for the prevention of organ transplant rejection, multiple sclerosis and HTLV-1 associated lymphoma [137]. It is available as both an intravenous and as subcutaneous formulation and administered at 2 mg/kg every 2 weeks for two doses then 1 mg/kg every 2 weeks or intravenously at 1 mg/kg every 4 weeks [138, 139] Initial reports on the use of this agent in patients with uveitis were published in 1999 [140] with subsequent supporting efficacy data [141].

One of the largest published retrospective studies on the use of daclizumab included 39 patients with an average follow-up of 40 months. Different formulations and dosages were evaluated. Twenty-nine patients underwent intravenous administration with the standard regimen, five patients received a high-dose intravenous regimen and five patients received subcutaneous administration. Visual acuity improved by two lines or more in seven patients and worsened by two lines or more in six patients. The mean number of flares was 0.62 per patient-year. The mean number of other immunosuppressant therapies decreased from 1.89 per patient at baseline to 1.17 medications [142].

Daclizumab is generally very well tolerated with the most common adverse event being a cutaneous reaction. Other reported side effects include infections, elevated liver function tests, transient leukopenia, neuralgia, edema, palpitations, lymphadenopathy and cramping. In a retrospective review by Wroblewski, 4 cases of malignancy were reported in 39 patients studied and one patient with Behçet's disease treated with daclizumab who terminated the medication acutely, developed cerebellar herniation [142]. The drug was voluntarily removed from the United States market in 2009 (although still available in Europe) and currently undergoing clinical trials in the treatment of relapsing, remitting multiple sclerosis.

Il-17 has recently been demonstrated to be a critical cytokine in autoimmune dysregulation. A number of biologic therapies are currently in development that target IL-17 for a number of autoimmune diseases. Upregulation of IL-23 and IL-17A occurs in patients with various forms of uveitis [143]. Secukinumab a fully human monoclonal antibody that targets interleukin-17A has been studied in three independent studies to evaluate efficacy and safety. 118 patients with Behçet's uveitis (SHIELD study); 31 noninfectious, active non-Behçet's uveitis (INSURE study); and 125 patients with quiescent, noninfectious, non-Behçet's uveitis (ENDURE study) were studied. Reductions of uveitis recurrence or vitreous haze score during withdrawal of concomitant immunosuppressive medication were the main outcomes studied. The primary efficacy end points of the three studies were not met [144]. The safety profile for this agent has not yet been fully delineated, but there does appear to be a slightly greater risk of infections [145]. Other therapies targeting IL-17 remain as potential therapeutic agents for the treatment of recalcitrant uveitis.

IL-1 is a potent inflammatory cytokine that plays an important role in a number of autoimmune diseases and has been a successful target in conditions such as Still's disease [146]. In uveitis it has been found that this is one of the cytokines that is expressed in the vitreous fluid of patients with active uveitis [147]. Two therapies that target IL-1 have been published for the treatment of uveitis. Anakinra, a glycosylated version of human IL-1 receptor antagonist has been studied in only a small number of patients with uveitis and therefore definitive statements about efficacy are difficult to determine at this time [148, 149]. It is used at a dose of 100 mg daily by subcutaneous injection or 1–2 mg/kg daily in children. Potential significant risks of Anakinra include injection site reactions and infections.

Gevokizumab, a recombinant, humanized IgG2 monoclonal antibody that binds IL-1β, is a modulating antibody that reduces the affinity for IL-1RI, IL-1RAcP signaling, and thus downregulates IL-1β activity. In 2012 it was granted Orphan Drug Designation for the treatment of noninfectious intermediate, posterior and panuveitis, or chronic noninfectious anterior uveitis. Seven patients with acute posterior or panuveitis, and/or retinal vasculitis resistant to azathioprine and/or cyclosporine were enrolled. Immunosuppressive agents were discontinued at baseline and patients received a single infusion of gevokizumab. All patients responded and no serious adverse events were reported [150]. Larger multicenter studies are currently enrolling patients (ClinicalTrials.gov).

IL-6 has been identified as one of the cytokines overexpressed in patients with uveitis [151]. Tocilizumab, a recombinant humanized anti-human IgG1 IL-6 receptor monoclonal antibody with approved indications in RA, polyarticular JIA and systemic onset JIA has been reported as an effective therapy to treat uveitis in a small number of patients. It is available as both and IV preparation dosed at 4 mg or 8 mg/kg monthly or as a subcutaneous medication dosed at 162 mg every 2 weeks or weekly. It can be given with or without MTX. Patients with uveitis and various underlying illnesses previously treated with remittive medications, anti-TNF agents and abatacept have been successfully treated with tocilizumab. In a series of patients with JIA, Adan published five patients with uveitis refractory to conventional therapy including at least 1 biologic agent [152]. The patients received tocilizumab 8 mg/kg every 4 weeks. At mean follow-up of 8.4 months, 50 % of the affected eyes studied had improvement in visual acuity and 25 % of affected eyes remained stable. All patients sustained uveitis remission for the 6-month follow-up period. Most of the studies did not find toxicity with Tocilizumab administration, although neutropenia has been described. The most common adverse effects observed in clinical trials have been upper respiratory tract infections, headache, and high blood pressure. Abnormal liver function tests and elevations in cholesterol levels were common. Among the less common side effects dizziness, various infections, as well as reactions of the skin and mucosae like mild rashes, gastritis, and mouth ulcers. Rare but severe reactions of gastrointestinal perforations and anaphylaxis have been described.

Interferon Blockers

Interferons (IFN) have a number of immune regulatory functions including the capacity to increase regulatory T cells. There are numerous published series and reports that define a beneficial role for IFN-α in the treatment of Behçet's disease and other types of uveitis. In a small prospective study of 12 patients with sight-threatening uveitis that failed to respond to one or more immunosuppressive therapies, human IFN-alpha-2b was administered subcutaneously daily. After a mean observational period of 11 months a favorable clinical response was observed in 83 % of patients [153]. Potential side effects of interferon include infections, neuropsychiatric illnesses, cardiovascular events, and other autoimmune disorders. Injection site reactions and a flu-like syndrome are also frequently noted.

Other Targets

Other biologic agents have been utilized to treat uveitis, include abatacept [154], and rituximab [155, 156].

In selected cases, abatacept, an agent that blocks the costimulatory signaling that normally leads to T cell activation, has been used to treat autoimmune uveitis. It is a fusion protein composed of the Fc region of the immunoglobulin IgG1 fused to the extracellular domain of CTLA-4. It binds to CD80. This agent is currently approved for the treatment of rheumatoid arthritis as both an intravenous and subcutaneous medication.

In the largest published series of seven patients with JIA and uveitis, abatacept was found to be efficacious in maintaining clinical remission in six of the seven patients during a period 9.2 months [157]. The patients were found to have decreased uveitis flares after 6 months of therapy. One patient, however, relapsed after 12 months with both arthritis and uveitis, and two patients required continued methotrexate. There have been other smaller series of reports using abatacept to treat uveitis and interestingly this medication has been effective in a few patients who have failed or been intolerant of anti-TNF agents [154, 158, 159]. Side effects have been reported, with a case of oral mycosis [157] and interestingly arthritis flare [154]. Given the small sample size of the study, abatacept use needs to be investigated further. The most serious adverse reactions are serious infections and malignancies. The most commonly reported adverse events include headache, upper respiratory tract infection, nasopharyngitis, and nausea.

Although the role of B cells is unknown in uveitis, in a pathologic study of an enucleated eye of a patient with JIA associated uveitis, focal aggregates of CD20 positive cells with CD3 and CD8 positive cells were noted [160]. Therefore, there may be rationale for using anti-B cell therapy and rituximab has been reported as a successful treatment for noninfectious uveitis. In one study of eight patients with JIA associated uveitis, seven patients attained a response [155]. In another publication ten patients with JIA and severe uveitis with vision threatening complications resistant to traditional therapy, including anti-TNF agents, responded after one cycle of rituximab. Uveitis became inactive in seven patients for a mean period of 11 months. It then recurred in four patients, though retreatment with rituximab resulted in disease inactivity in three of the four patients [161]. Other case studies of rituximab use have been published [156, 162]. Listed side effects for rituximab include infusion reactions, mucocutaneous reactions, Hepatitis B reactivation, progressive multifocal leukoencephalopathy, tumor lysis syndrome, infections, and renal toxicity. The most common adverse reactions of Rituxan (incidence ≥25 %) observed in clinical trials of patients with NHL were infusion reactions, fever, lymphopenia, chills, infection, and asthenia.

Although approved for the therapy of severe acute and chronic allergic and inflammatory processes involving the eye and its adnexa such as keratitis, iritis, iridocyclitis, diffuse posterior uveitis and choroiditis, optic neuritis, chorioretinitis, and anterior segment inflammation, ACTHAR Gel, an adrenocorticotropic hormone (ACTH) analogue does not have any published data on use in uveitis.

Intravitreal infliximab and adalimumab have been studied in animal models and patients with uveitis [163–167]. In a study of seven patients with anterior and posterior uveitis that was unresponsive to conventional treatments, 1.5 mg of infliximab in 0.15 cc was injected intravitreally and patients were followed for six months. Interestingly this approach has not resulted in dramatic response and the authors concluded that infliximab probably improves vision and decreases macular edema but the observed effect is only temporary [166].

Conclusion

The therapeutic armamentarium to treat patients with autoimmune ophthalmic disease is diverse and includes medications in different classes with individually unique modes of action. These include corticosteroids, antiproliferative therapies, and targeted biological agents. New classes of therapies including small molecules and perhaps medications that will alter the microbiome may in the future continue to expand the therapeutics available to treat this group of diseases. Challenges remain in terms of better understanding the immunology of autoimmune ophthalmic disease, defining the phenotype of individual disease entities, constructing prospective trials of comparative efficacy, developing genetic and biomarkers to provide guidance in choosing a specific therapy for a unique patient.

References

1. Resman-Targoff BH, Cicero MP. Aggressive treatment of early rheumatoid arthritis: recognizing the window of opportunity and treating to target goals. Am J Manag Care. 2010;16(9 Suppl):S249–58.
2. Kaplan-Messas A, et al. Methotrexate as a first-line corticosteroid-sparing therapy in a cohort of uveitis and scleritis. Ocul Immunol Inflamm. 2003;11(2):131–9.
3. Jabs DA, et al. Guidelines for the use of immunosuppressive drugs in patients with ocular inflammatory disorders: recommendations of an expert panel. Am J Ophthalmol. 2000;130(4):492–513.
4. Giles CL. The use of methotrexate in the treatment of uveitis. Univ Mich Med Cent J. 1969;35(1):30–1.
5. Lazar M, Weiner MJ, Leopold IH. Treatment of uveitis with methotrexate. Am J Ophthalmol. 1969;67(3):383–7.
6. Holz FG, et al. Low-dose methotrexate treatment in noninfectious uveitis resistant to corticosteroids. Ger J Ophthalmol. 1992;1(3–4):142–4.
7. Shah SS, et al. Low-dose methotrexate therapy for ocular inflammatory disease. Ophthalmology. 1992;99(9):1419–23.
8. Dev S, McCallum RM, Jaffe GJ. Methotrexate treatment for sarcoid-associated panuveitis. Ophthalmology. 1999;106(1):111–8.
9. Bom S, Zamiri P, Lightman S. Use of methotrexate in the management of sight-threatening uveitis. Ocul Immunol Inflamm. 2001;9(1):35–40.
10. Samson CM, et al. Methotrexate therapy for chronic noninfectious uveitis: analysis of a case series of 160 patients. Ophthalmology. 2001;108(6):1134–9.
11. Galor A, et al. Comparison of antimetabolite drugs as corticosteroid-sparing therapy for noninfectious ocular inflammation. Ophthalmology. 2008;115(10):1826–32.
12. Gangaputra S, et al. Methotrexate for ocular inflammatory diseases. Ophthalmology. 2009;116(11):2188–98 e1.
13. Munoz-Fernandez S, et al. Methotrexate: an option for preventing the recurrence of acute anterior uveitis. Eye (Lond). 2009;23(5):1130–3.
14. Ali A, Rosenbaum JT. Use of methotrexate in patients with uveitis. Clin Exp Rheumatol. 2010;28(5 Suppl 61):S145–50.
15. Weiss AH, Wallace CA, Sherry DD. Methotrexate for resistant chronic uveitis in children with juvenile rheumatoid arthritis. J Pediatr. 1998;133(2):266–8.
16. Foeldvari I, Wierk A. Methotrexate is an effective treatment for chronic uveitis associated with juvenile idiopathic arthritis. J Rheumatol. 2005;32(2):362–5.
17. Malik AR, Pavesio C. The use of low dose methotrexate in children with chronic anterior and intermediate uveitis. Br J Ophthalmol. 2005;89(7):806–8.
18. Chan AY, Liu DT. Methotrexate and chronic uveitis associated with juvenile idiopathic arthritis. J Rheumatol. 2006;33(1):198; author reply 198.
19. Heiligenhaus A, et al. Methotrexate for uveitis associated with juvenile idiopathic arthritis: value and requirement for additional anti-inflammatory medication. Eur J Ophthalmol. 2007;17(5):743–8.
20. Kalinina Ayuso V et al. Relapse rate of uveitis post-methotrexate treatment in juvenile idiopathic arthritis. Am J Ophthalmol. 2011;151(2):217–22.
21. Simonini G, et al. Current evidence of methotrexate efficacy in childhood chronic uveitis: a systematic review and meta-analysis approach. Rheumatology (Oxford). 2013;52(5):825–31.
22. Papadopoulou C, et al. Methotrexate therapy may prevent the onset of uveitis in juvenile idiopathic arthritis. J Pediatr. 2013;163(3):879–84.
23. Taylor SR, et al. Intraocular methotrexate in the treatment of uveitis and uveitic cystoid macular edema. Ophthalmology. 2009;116(4):797–801.
24. Taylor SR, et al. Intraocular methotrexate can induce extended remission in some patients in noninfectious uveitis. Retina. 2013;33(10):2149–54.
25. Teoh SC, et al. Mycophenolate mofetil for the treatment of uveitis. Am J Ophthalmol. 2008;146(5):752–60, 760 e1–3.
26. Sobrin L, Christen W, Foster CS. Mycophenolate mofetil after methotrexate failure or intolerance in the treatment of scleritis and uveitis. Ophthalmology. 2008;115(8):1416–21, 1421 e1.
27. Siepmann K, et al. Mycophenolate mofetil is a highly effective and safe immunosuppressive agent for the treatment of uveitis: a retrospective analysis of 106 patients. Graefes Arch Clin Exp Ophthalmol. 2006;244(7):788–94.
28. Rathore VM, et al. Mycophenolate mofetil therapy in uveitis: analysis of eight cases in a tertiary ophthalmic care centre in India. Int Ophthalmol. 2009;29(2):117–22.

29. Rathinam SR, et al. A randomized clinical trial comparing methotrexate and mycophenolate mofetil for noninfectious uveitis. Ophthalmology. 2014.
30. Neri P, et al. Long-term control of cystoid macular oedema in noninfectious uveitis with mycophenolate mofetil. Int Ophthalmol. 2009;29(3):127–33.
31. Klisovic DD. Mycophenolate mofetil use in the treatment of noninfectious uveitis. Dev Ophthalmol. 2012;51:57–62.
32. Kilmartin DJ, Forrester JV, Dick AD. Rescue therapy with mycophenolate mofetil in refractory uveitis. Lancet. 1998;352(9121):35–6.
33. Doycheva D, et al. Long-term results of therapy with mycophenolate mofetil in chronic non-infectious uveitis. Graefes Arch Clin Exp Ophthalmol. 2011;249(8):1235–43.
34. Doycheva D, et al. Mycophenolate mofetil in the treatment of uveitis in children. Br J Ophthalmol. 2007;91(2):180–4.
35. Deuter CM, et al. Mycophenolate sodium for immunosuppressive treatment in uveitis. Ocul Immunol Inflamm. 2009;17(6):415–9.
36. Chang PY, et al. Mycophenolate mofetil monotherapy in the management of paediatric uveitis. Eye (Lond). 2011;25(4):427–35.
37. Bhat P, et al. Mycophenolate mofetil therapy for sarcoidosis-associated uveitis. Ocul Immunol Inflamm. 2009;17(3):185–90.
38. Abu El-Asrar AM, et al. The outcomes of mycophenolate mofetil therapy combined with systemic corticosteroids in acute uveitis associated with Vogt-Koyanagi-Harada disease. Acta Ophthalmol. 2012;90(8):e603–8.
39. Saadoun D, et al. Azathioprine in severe uveitis of Behcet's disease. Arthritis Care Res (Hoboken). 2010;62(12):1733–8.
40. Pacheco PA, et al. Azathioprine in the management of autoimmune uveitis. Ocul Immunol Inflamm. 2008;16(4):161–5.
41. Newell FW, Krill AE. Treatment of uveitis with azathioprine (Imuran). Trans Ophthalmol Soc UK. 1967;87:499–511.
42. Hamuryudan V, et al. Interferon alfa combined with azathioprine for the uveitis of Behcet's disease: an open study. Isr Med Assoc J. 2002;4(11 Suppl):928–30.
43. Goebel JC, et al. Azathioprine as a treatment option for uveitis in patients with juvenile idiopathic arthritis. Br J Ophthalmol. 2011;95(2):209–13.
44. Karjalainen K. Cyclosporin A treatment for chronic uveitis associated with retinitis. Acta Ophthalmol (Copenh). 1984;62(4):631–5.
45. Graham EM, et al. Cyclosporin A in the treatment of posterior uveitis. Trans Ophthalmol Soc UK. 1985;104(Pt 2):146–51.
46. Nissen C, et al. The treatment of presumed non-infective uveitis with Cyclosporin A. Acta Ophthalmol Suppl. 1985;173:72–3.
47. Binder AI, et al. Cyclosporin A in the treatment of severe Behcet's uveitis. Br J Rheumatol. 1987;26(4):285–91.
48. Towler HM, et al. Low dose Cyclosporin A therapy in chronic posterior uveitis. Eye (Lond). 1989;3(Pt 3):282–7.
49. de Vries J, et al. Cyclosporin in the treatment of severe chronic idiopathic uveitis. Br J Ophthalmol. 1990;74(6):344–9.
50. Cohen E, et al. Low-dose Cyclosporin A in uveitis a long-term follow-up. Ocul Immunol Inflamm. 1993;1(3):195–202.
51. Vitale AT, Rodriguez A, Foster CS. Low-dose Cyclosporin A therapy in treating chronic, noninfectious uveitis. Ophthalmology. 1996;**103**(3):365–73; discussion 373–4.
52. Dick AD, Azim M, Forrester JV. Immunosuppressive therapy for chronic uveitis: optimising therapy with steroids and Cyclosporin A. Br J Ophthalmol. 1997;81(12):1107–12.
53. Kilmartin DJ, Forrester JV, Dick AD. Cyclosporin A therapy in refractory non-infectious childhood uveitis. Br J Ophthalmol. 1998;82(7):737–42.
54. Sullu Y, et al. Cyclosporin-A therapy in severe uveitis of Behcet's disease. Acta Ophthalmol Scand. 1998;76(1):96–9.
55. Mathews D, Mathews J, Jones NP. Low-dose cyclosporine treatment for sight-threatening uveitis: efficacy, toxicity, and tolerance. Indian J Ophthalmol. 2010;58(1):55–8.
56. Taddio A, et al. Childhood chronic anterior uveitis associated with vernal keratoconjunctivitis (VKC): successful treatment with topical tacrolimus. Case series. Pediatr Rheumatol Online J. 2011;9(1):34.
57. Sloper CM, Powell RJ, Dua HS. Tacrolimus (FK506) in the treatment of posterior uveitis refractory to cyclosporine. Ophthalmology. 1999;106(4):723–8.
58. Murphy CC, et al. Cyclosporine vs tacrolimus therapy for posterior and intermediate uveitis. Arch Ophthalmol. 2005;123(5):634–41.
59. Lee RW, et al. A randomized trial of tacrolimus versus tacrolimus and prednisone for the maintenance of disease remission in noninfectious uveitis. Ophthalmology. 2012;119(6):1223–30.
60. Kilmartin DJ, Forrester JV, Dick AD. Tacrolimus (FK506) in failed Cyclosporin A therapy in endogenous posterior uveitis. Ocul Immunol Inflamm. 1998;6(2):101–9.
61. Hogan AC, et al. Long-term efficacy and tolerance of tacrolimus for the treatment of uveitis. Ophthalmology. 2007;114(5):1000–6.
62. Figueroa MS, Ciancas E, Orte L. Long-term follow-up of tacrolimus treatment in immune posterior uveitis. Eur J Ophthalmol. 2007;17(1):69–74.
63. Taheri S, Taheri D. Short course of cyclophosphamide therapy may reduce recurrence in patients

with tubulointerstitial nephritis and uveitis syndrome. Saudi J Kidney Dis Transpl. 2009;20(4):655–7.
64. Rosenbaum JT. Treatment of severe refractory uveitis with intravenous cyclophosphamide. J Rheumatol. 1994;21(1):123–5.
65. Buckley CE 3rd, Gills JP Jr. Oral cyclophosphamide in the treatment of uveitis. Trans Am Acad Ophthalmol Otolaryngol. 1970;74(3):505–8.
66. Buckley CE 3rd, Gills JP Jr. Cyclophosphamide therapy of peripheral uveitis. Arch Intern Med. 1969;124(1):29–35.
67. Zaghetto JM, et al. Chlorambucil and Cyclosporine A in Brazilian patients with Behcet's disease uveitis: a retrospective study. Arq Bras Oftalmol. 2010;73(1):40–6.
68. Palmer RG, Kanski JJ, Ansell BM. Chlorambucil in the treatment of intractable Uveitis associated with juvenile chronic arthritis. J Rheumatol. 1985;12(5):967–70.
69. O'Duffy JD, Robertson DM, Goldstein NP. Chlorambucil in the treatment of uveitis and meningoencephalitis of Behcet's disease. Am J Med. 1984;76(1):75–84.
70. Mudun BA, et al. Short-term chlorambucil for refractory uveitis in Behcet's disease. Ocul Immunol Inflamm. 2001;9(4):219–29.
71. Miserocchi E, et al. Efficacy and safety of chlorambucil in intractable noninfectious uveitis: the Massachusetts Eye and Ear Infirmary experience. Ophthalmology. 2002;109(1):137–42.
72. Godfrey WA, et al. The use of chlorambucil in intractable idiopathic uveitis. Am J Ophthalmol. 1974;78(3):415–28.
73. Dinning WJ, Perkins ES. Immunosuppressives in uveitis. A preliminary report of experience with chlorambucil. Br J Ophthalmol. 1975;59(8):397–403.
74. Hall AG, Tilby MJ. Mechanisms of action of, and modes of resistance to, alkylating agents used in the treatment of haematological malignancies. Blood Rev. 1992;6:163.
75. Westhovens R, et al. The safety of infliximab, combined with background treatments, among patients with rheumatoid arthritis and various comorbidities: a large, randomized, placebo-controlled trial. Arthritis Rheum. 2006;54(4):1075–86.
76. Braun J, et al. Decreased incidence of anterior uveitis in patients with ankylosing spondylitis treated with the anti-tumor necrosis factor agents infliximab and etanercept. Arthritis Rheum. 2005;52(8):2447–51.
77. Matsuda J, et al. Treatment of recurrent anterior uveitis with infliximab in patient with ankylosing spondylitis. Jpn J Ophthalmol. 2013;57(1):104–7.
78. Ally MR, Veerappan GR, Koff JM. Treatment of recurrent Crohn's uveitis with infliximab. Am J Gastroenterol. 2008;103(8):2150–1.
79. Fries W, et al. Treatment of acute uveitis associated with Crohn's disease and sacroileitis with infliximab. Am J Gastroenterol. 2002;97(2):499–500.
80. Kahn P, et al. Favorable response to high-dose infliximab for refractory childhood uveitis. Ophthalmology. 2006;113(5):860–4 e2.
81. Mangge H, et al. Therapeutic experience with infliximab in a patient with polyarticular juvenile idiopathic arthritis and uveitis. Rheumatol Int. 2003;23(5):258–61.
82. Rajaraman RT, et al. Retrospective case review of pediatric patients with uveitis treated with infliximab. Ophthalmology. 2006;113(2):308–14.
83. Richards JC, et al. Infliximab for juvenile idiopathic arthritis-associated uveitis. Clin Exp Ophthalmol. 2005;33(5):461–8.
84. Sharma SM, et al. Use of infliximab in juvenile onset rheumatological disease-associated refractory uveitis: efficacy in joint and ocular disease. Ann Rheum Dis. 2007;66(6):840–1.
85. Simonini G, et al. Prevention of flare recurrences in childhood-refractory chronic uveitis: an open-label comparative study of adalimumab versus infliximab. Arthritis Care Res (Hoboken). 2011;63(4):612–8.
86. Tynjala P, et al. Infliximab and etanercept in the treatment of chronic uveitis associated with refractory juvenile idiopathic arthritis. Ann Rheum Dis. 2007;66(4):548–50.
87. Zannin ME, et al. Safety and efficacy of infliximab and adalimumab for refractory uveitis in juvenile idiopathic arthritis: 1-year followup data from the Italian Registry. J Rheumatol. 2013;40(1):74–9.
88. Benitez-del-Castillo JM, et al. Long-term treatment of refractory posterior uveitis with anti-TNFalpha (infliximab). Eye (Lond). 2005;19(8):841–5.
89. Suhler EB, et al. Infliximab therapy for refractory uveitis: 2-year results of a prospective trial. Arch Ophthalmol. 2009;127(6):819–22.
90. Suhler EB, et al. A prospective trial of infliximab therapy for refractory uveitis: preliminary safety and efficacy outcomes. Arch Ophthalmol. 2005;123(7):903–12.
91. Kruh JN, et al. Infliximab for the treatment of refractory noninfectious Uveitis: a study of 88 patients with long-term follow-up. Ophthalmology. 2014;121(1):358–64.
92. Vazquez-Cobian LB, Flynn T, Lehman TJ. Adalimumab therapy for childhood uveitis. J Pediatr. 2006;149(4):572–5.
93. Tynjala P, et al. Adalimumab in juvenile idiopathic arthritis-associated chronic anterior uveitis. Rheumatology (Oxford). 2008;47(3):339–44.
94. Turel Ermertcan A, et al. Psoriatic uveitis responding to adalimumab therapy. Int J Dermatol. 2013.
95. Takase K, et al. Successful switching to adalimumab in an infliximab-allergic patient with severe Behcet disease-related uveitis. Rheumatol Int. 2011;31(2):243–5.

96. Suhler EB, et al. Adalimumab therapy for refractory uveitis: results of a multicentre, open-label, prospective trial. Br J Ophthalmol. 2013;97(4):481–6.
97. Soheilian M, et al. Bilateral uveitis after phakic intraocular lens implantation and management with adalimumab. J Cataract Refract Surg. 2012;38 (6):1094–6.
98. Simonini G, et al. Superior efficacy of Adalimumab in treating childhood refractory chronic uveitis when used as first biologic modifier drug: Adalimumab as starting anti-TNF-alpha therapy in childhood chronic uveitis. Pediatr Rheumatol Online J. 2013;11(1):16.
99. Seve P, et al. Sarcoid-related uveitis occurring during adalimumab therapy. Ocul Immunol Inflamm. 2012;20(1):59–60.
100. Sen ES, et al. Use of adalimumab in refractory non-infectious childhood chronic uveitis: efficacy in ocular disease–a case cohort interventional study. Rheumatology (Oxford). 2012;51(12):2199–203.
101. Rudwaleit M, et al. Adalimumab effectively reduces the rate of anterior uveitis flares in patients with active ankylosing spondylitis: results of a prospective open-label study. Ann Rheum Dis. 2009;68 (5):696–701.
102. Ramanan AV, et al. A randomised controlled trial of the clinical effectiveness, safety and cost-effectiveness of adalimumab in combination with methotrexate for the treatment of juvenile idiopathic arthritis associated uveitis (SYCAMORE Trial). Trials. 2014;15:14.
103. Mushtaq B, et al. Adalimumab for sight-threatening uveitis in Behcet's disease. Eye (Lond). 2007;21 (6):824–5.
104. Martel JN, et al. Infliximab and adalimumab for uveitis. Ocul Immunol Inflamm. 2012;20(1):18–26.
105. Mansour AM. Adalimumab in the therapy of uveitis in childhood. Br J Ophthalmol. 2007;91(3):274–6.
106. Magli A, et al. Adalimumab for juvenile idiopathic arthritis-associated uveitis. Graefes Arch Clin Exp Ophthalmol. 2013;251(6):1601–6.
107. Li SY, Birnbaum AD, Goldstein DA. Optic neuritis associated with adalimumab in the treatment of uveitis. Ocul Immunol Inflamm. 2010;18(6):475–81.
108. Leccese P, et al. Efficacy of switching to adalimumab in a patient with refractory uveitis of Behcet's disease to infliximab. Clin Exp Rheumatol. 2011;29(4 Suppl 67):S93.
109. Kotaniemi K, Saila H, Kautiainen H. Long-term efficacy of adalimumab in the treatment of uveitis associated with juvenile idiopathic arthritis. Clin Ophthalmol. 2011;5:1425–9.
110. Garcia-De-Vicuna C, et al. Usefulness of adalimumab in the treatment of refractory uveitis associated with juvenile idiopathic arthritis. Mediators Inflamm. 2013;2013:560632.
111. Erckens RJ, et al. Adalimumab successful in sarcoidosis patients with refractory chronic non-infectious uveitis. Graefes Arch Clin Exp Ophthalmol. 2012;250(5):713–20.
112. Dobner BC, et al. A three-centre experience with adalimumab for the treatment of non-infectious uveitis. Br J Ophthalmol. 2013;97(2):134–8.
113. Diaz-Llopis M, et al. Treatment of refractory uveitis with adalimumab: a prospective multicenter study of 131 patients. Ophthalmology. 2012;119 (8):1575–81.
114. Diaz-Llopis M, et al. Adalimumab therapy for refractory uveitis: a pilot study. J Ocul Pharmacol Ther. 2008;24(3):351–61.
115. Cordero-Coma M, et al. Serum cytokine profile in adalimumab-treated refractory uveitis patients: decreased IL-22 correlates with clinical responses. Ocul Immunol Inflamm. 2013;21(3):212–9.
116. Callejas-Rubio JL, et al. Adalimumab therapy for refractory uveitis: a pilot study. J Ocul Pharmacol Ther. 2008;24(6):613–4; author reply 614.
117. Calleja S, et al. Adalimumab specifically induces CD3(+) CD4(+) CD25(high) Foxp3(+) CD127(-) T-regulatory cells and decreases vascular endothelial growth factor plasma levels in refractory immuno-mediated uveitis: a non-randomized pilot intervention study. Eye (Lond). 2012;26(3):468–77.
118. Brávo-Ljubetic L, et al. Adalimumab therapy for refractory childhood uveitis. J AAPOS. 2013;17 (5):456–9.
119. Biester S, et al. Adalimumab in the therapy of uveitis in childhood. Br J Ophthalmol. 2007;91 (3):319–24.
120. Androudi S, et al. Intravitreal adalimumab for refractory uveitis-related macular edema. Ophthalmology. 2010;117(8):1612–6.
121. Breedveld FC, et al. The PREMIER study: a multicenter, randomized, double-blind clinical trial of combination therapy with adalimumab plus methotrexate versus methotrexate alone or adalimumab alone in patients with early, aggressive rheumatoid arthritis who had not had previous methotrexate treatment. Arthritis Rheum. 2006;54 (1):26–37.
122. William M, et al. Golimumab for the treatment of refractory juvenile idiopathic arthritis-associated uveitis. J Ophthalmic Inflamm Infect. 2012;2 (4):231–3.
123. Miserocchi E, et al. Long-term treatment with golimumab for severe uveitis. Ocul Immunol Inflamm. 2013.
124. Miserocchi E, et al. Golimumab treatment for complicated uveitis. Clin Exp Rheumatol. 2013;31 (2):320–1.
125. Mesquida M, et al. Behcet disease-associated uveitis successfully treated with golimumab. Ocul Immunol Inflamm. 2013;21(2):160–2.
126. Faez S, et al. Treatment of seronegative spondyloarthropathy-associated uveitis with golimumab: retrospective case series. Clin Exp Ophthalmol. 2013.

127. Cordero-Coma M, et al. Golimumab for uveitis. Ophthalmology. 2011;118(9):1892 e3–4.
128. Reiff A, et al. Etanercept therapy in children with treatment-resistant uveitis. Arthritis Rheum. 2001;44(6):1411–5.
129. Smith BJ, McMillan VM, Newton JS. Corticosteroid-sparing effect of etanercept in idiopathic panuveitis resistant to immunosuppressive therapy. J Clin Rheumatol. 2001;7(3):175–8.
130. Foster CS, et al. Efficacy of etanercept in preventing relapse of uveitis controlled by methotrexate. Arch Ophthalmol. 2003;121(4):437–40.
131. Schmeling H, Horneff G. Etanercept and uveitis in patients with juvenile idiopathic arthritis. Rheumatology (Oxford). 2005;44(8):1008–11.
132. Smith JA, et al. A randomized, placebo-controlled, double-masked clinical trial of etanercept for the treatment of uveitis associated with juvenile idiopathic arthritis. Arthritis Rheum. 2005;53(1):18–23.
133. Lim LL, Fraunfelder FW, Rosenbaum JT. Do tumor necrosis factor inhibitors cause uveitis? A registry-based study. Arthritis Rheum. 2007;56 (10):3248–52.
134. Zeboulon N, Dougados M, Gossec L. Prevalence and characteristics of uveitis in the spondyloarthropathies: a systematic literature review. Ann Rheum Dis. 2008;67(7):955–9.
135. Sieper J, et al. Analysis of uveitis rates across all etanercept ankylosing spondylitis clinical trials. Ann Rheum Dis. 2010;69(1):226–9.
136. Levy-Clarke G, et al. Expert panel recommendations for the use of anti-tumor necrosis factor biologic agents in patients with ocular inflammatory disorders. Ophthalmology. 2013.
137. Waldmann TA. Anti-Tac (daclizumab, Zenapax) in the treatment of leukemia, autoimmune diseases, and in the prevention of allograft rejection: a 25-year personal odyssey. J Clin Immunol. 2007;27(1):1–18.
138. Yeh S, et al. High-dose humanized anti-IL-2 receptor alpha antibody (daclizumab) for the treatment of active, non-infectious uveitis. J Autoimmun. 2008;31(2):91–7.
139. Nussenblatt RB, et al. Initial evaluation of subcutaneous daclizumab treatments for noninfectious uveitis: a multicenter noncomparative interventional case series. Ophthalmology. 2005;112(5):764–70.
140. Nussenblatt RB, et al. Treatment of noninfectious intermediate and posterior uveitis with the humanized anti-Tac mAb: a phase I/II clinical trial. Proc Natl Acad Sci USA. 1999;96(13):7462–6.
141. Nussenblatt RB, et al. Humanized anti-interleukin-2 (IL-2) receptor alpha therapy: long-term results in uveitis patients and preliminary safety and activity data for establishing parameters for subcutaneous administration. J Autoimmun. 2003;21(3):283–93.
142. Wroblewski K, et al. Long-term daclizumab therapy for the treatment of noninfectious ocular inflammatory disease. Can J Ophthalmol. 2011;46 (4):322–8.
143. Chi W, et al. IL-23 promotes CD4+ T cells to produce IL-17 in Vogt-Koyanagi-Harada disease. J Allergy Clin Immunol. 2007;119(5):1218–24.
144. Dick AD, et al. Secukinumab in the treatment of noninfectious uveitis: results of three randomized, controlled clinical trials. Ophthalmology. 2013;120 (4):777–87.
145. Genovese MC, et al. One-year efficacy and safety results of secukinumab in patients with rheumatoid arthritis: phase II, dose-finding, double-blind, randomized, placebo-controlled study. J Rheumatol. 2014;41(3):414–21.
146. Giampietro C, et al. Anakinra in adult-onset Still's disease: long-term treatment in patients resistant to conventional therapy. Arthritis Care Res (Hoboken). 2013;65(5):822–6.
147. Ooi KG, et al. Cytokines and chemokines in uveitis: is there a correlation with clinical phenotype? Clin Med Res. 2006;4(4):294–309.
148. Emmi G, et al. Anakinra for resistant Behcet uveitis: why not? Clin Exp Rheumatol. 2013;31(3 Suppl 77):152–3.
149. Teoh SC, et al. Tailoring biological treatment: anakinra treatment of posterior uveitis associated with the CINCA syndrome. Br J Ophthalmol. 2007;91(2):263–4.
150. Gul A, et al. Interleukin-1beta-regulating antibody XOMA 052 (gevokizumab) in the treatment of acute exacerbations of resistant uveitis of Behcet's disease: an open-label pilot study. Ann Rheum Dis. 2012;71(4):563–6.
151. Petrinovic-Doresic J, et al. Interleukin 6 and its soluble receptor are elevated in aqueous humor of patients with uveitis. Ocul Immunol Inflamm. 1999;7(2):75–84.
152. Adan A, et al. Tocilizumab treatment for refractory uveitis-related cystoid macular edema. Graefes Arch Clin Exp Ophthalmol. 2013;251(11):2627–32.
153. Plskova J, Greiner K, Forrester JV. Interferon-alpha as an effective treatment for noninfectious posterior uveitis and panuveitis. Am J Ophthalmol. 2007;144 (1):55–61.
154. Kenawy N, et al. Abatacept: a potential therapy in refractory cases of juvenile idiopathic arthritis-associated uveitis. Graefes Arch Clin Exp Ophthalmol. 2011;249(2):297–300.
155. Miserocchi E, Modorati G. Rituximab for noninfectious uveitis. Dev Ophthalmol. 2012;51:98–109.
156. Miserocchi E, et al. Rituximab for uveitis. Ophthalmology. 2011;118(1):223–4.
157. Zulian F, et al. Abatacept for severe anti-tumor necrosis factor alpha refractory juvenile idiopathic arthritis-related uveitis. Arthritis Care Res (Hoboken). 2010;62(6):821–5.
158. Angeles-Han S, Flynn T, Lehman T. Abatacept for refractory juvenile idiopathic arthritis-associated uveitis- a case report. J Rheumatol. 2008;35 (9):1897–8.
159. Elhai M, Deslandre CJ, Kahan A. Abatacept for refractory juvenile idiopathic arthritis-associated

uveitis: two new cases. Comment on the article by Zulian et al. Arthritis Care Res (Hoboken), 2011;63 (2):307–8; author reply 308.
160. Parikh JG, Tawansy KA, Rao NA. Immunohistochemical study of chronic nongranulomatous anterior uveitis in juvenile idiopathic arthritis. Ophthalmology. 2008;115(10):1833–6.
161. Heiligenhaus A, et al. Treatment of severe uveitis associated with juvenile idiopathic arthritis with anti-CD20 monoclonal antibody (rituximab). Rheumatology (Oxford). 2011;50(8):1390–4.
162. Tappeiner C, et al. Rituximab as a treatment option for refractory endogenous anterior uveitis. Ophthalmic Res. 2007;39(3):184–6.
163. Yuksel E, et al. Comparison of acute effect of systemic versus intravitreal infliximab treatment in an experimental model of endotoxin-induced uveitis. J Ocul Pharmacol Ther. 2014;30(1):74–80.
164. Markomichelakis N, et al. Intravitreal infliximab for sight-threatening relapsing uveitis in Behcet disease: a pilot study in 15 patients. Am J Ophthalmol. 2012;154(3):534–541 e1.
165. Hosseini H, et al. Intravitreal infliximab in experimental endotoxin-induced uveitis. Eur J Ophthalmol. 2009;19(5):818–23.
166. Farvardin M, Afarid M, Shahrzad S. Long-term effects of intravitreal infliximab for treatment of sight-threatening chronic noninfectious uveitis. J Ocul Pharmacol Ther. 2012;28(6):628–31.
167. Farvardin M, et al. Intravitreal infliximab for the treatment of sight-threatening chronic noninfectious uveitis. Retina. 2010;30(9):1530–5.

Surgical Therapy: Retisert Implant

45

Cynthia X. Qian and Dean Eliott

General Principles

The use of corticosteroids to treat ocular inflammation remains the first line of treatment in halting acute uveitic crises and the persistent ocular structural damage caused by chronic uveitis. The Retisert™ fluocinolone acetonide (FA) 0.59-mg implant is a sustained-release corticosteroid device developed by pSivida (pSivida Corp, Watertown, MA) and marketed under license by Bausch and Lomb (Bausch and Lomb, Rochester, NY) [1, 2]. Although the indications for the implant have widened since its inception [3–5], it was specifically developed for the treatment of non-infectious posterior uveitis (NIPU). It is the first drug delivery device approved by the Food and Drug Administration (FDA) for this indication [6]. Its unique design sought to provide better drug bioavailability to the target tissue and to sustain constant therapeutic levels of medication without repeated dosing, while limiting the widespread effects of systemic corticosteroid administration [7–12]. Systemic FA levels after intravitreal implantation were shown in various studies to be below the threshold of detection, implying minimal systemic absorption [7, 9, 11]. This contrasts with traditional systemic and local delivery methods, where even a periocular injection with a repository located outside Tenon's space can produce serum levels comparable to a 50-mg oral dose of prednisolone [9], leading to systemic adverse effects such as hyperlipidemia, diabetes mellitus, hypertension, osteoporosis, fractures, and blood count/chemistry abnormalities.

Pharmacokinetics

The implant contains a silicone-based elastomer cup encasing a 1.5 mm drug core with a releasing orifice at one end. FA is a synthetic corticosteroid that has 1/24 the solubility of dexamethasone, theoretically allowing for extended drug release. A 98 % hydrolyzed polyvinyl alcohol (PVA) membrane across the opening of the pellet orifice allows for steady drug diffusion. Since silicone is impermeable to FA, the drug is only able to slowly diffuse across the polyvinyl alcohol diffusion port [2, 13].

Early in vitro studies of the drug delivery device containing 2- and 15-mg of FA were

C.X. Qian
Department of Ophthalmology, Retina Service, Massachusetts Eye and Ear Infirmary, 12th Floor, 243 Charles Street, Boston, MA 02114, USA
e-mail: cynthia_qian@meei.harvard.edu

D. Eliott (✉)
Department of Ophthalmology, Massachusetts Eye and Ear Infirmary, 243 Charles Street, Boston MA 02114, USA
e-mail: dean_eliott@meei.harvard.edu

G.N. Papaliodis (ed.), *Uveitis*,
DOI 10.1007/978-3-319-09126-6_45

tested in both protein-free buffer or buffer containing 50 % plasma protein [7]. The release rate was 1.9 ± 0.25-μg/day for the 2-mg device and 2.2 ± 0.6-μg/day for the 15-mg device. This rate remained linear over the testing period and was 20 % higher when the devices were transferred from protein-free buffer-to-buffer containing protein. This release kinetic related to protein concentration was hypothesized to be advantageous in the management of active uveitis, where blood ocular barrier breakdown and more protein in the eye may trigger a larger dose-appropriate amount of drug to be released.

Early in vivo rabbit experiments were also performed to assess the pharmacokinetics of FA. Fourteen rabbit right eyes were implanted with the 15-mg FA implant and were analyzed post-enucleation at 4, 20 and 54 weeks for release rate and toxicity studies [7]. Relatively constant vitreous levels were measured at each of these time points. No drug was detected in the aqueous humor during these time periods and there was no evidence of drug toxicity by clinical examination, electroretinography or histologic examination when compared to the control fellow non-implanted eye.

Surgical Procedure

The implant is inserted through a pars plana incision and the silicone strut is fixated to the sclera such that the drug pellet with the polyvinyl alcohol diffusion port is in contact with the vitreous. The following is a brief description of the implantation procedure: After appropriate anesthesia is obtained, the operative eye is prepared and draped in a sterile manner prior to insertion of a lid speculum. A pars plana infusion is not usually necessary. The implant is usually positioned in the inferonasal or inferotemporal quadrant after confirming the absence of severe vitreoretinal pathology in the quadrant via indirect ophthalmoscopy. A conjunctival peritomy is made in the quadrant of interest followed by a full thickness scleral incision with a 20-Ga MVR knife 3.5- to 4.0-mm posterior to the limbus, measuring 3- to 3.5-mm in length parallel to the limbus. Cautery may be used on the edge of the wound to prevent bleeding. A limited vitrectomy may also be performed. The implant is grasped using a locking needle holder and a double-armed 8-0 polypropylene suture is passed through the suture strut. A first knot is made around the strut. The sclera wound is carefully opened with forceps and the implant is inserted with the drug pellet facing the front of the eye. The double arms of the suture are then passed through 90 % thickness of the sclera on either side of the incision [14]. The remaining portion of the scleral wound is closed with interrupted sutures of 9-0 polypropylene before conjunctiva is re-apposed.

When placing a second implant, a pars plana infusion may be placed to control intraocular pressure and prevent intraoperative hypotony and bleeding. If the second implant is placed after depletion of the first implant, the original implant may or may not be removed. If it is placed for other indications such as spontaneous implant dissociation or scleral thinning and implant extrusion, the original implant is first removed. This is done by severing all scleral wound sutures except for the anchoring suture at the strut. The wound is then partially opened by an MVR blade, and the implant is first grasped with a toothed forceps or a needle holder by the suture strut before the anchoring suture is cut. This prevents the slippage and displacement of the implant into the vitreous cavity. When the wound is completely open, the original implant is removed and replaced by a secondary implant, which may be placed in the same location as the original implant [15]. Due to the possible need for re-implantation and the effect of FA on scleral wound healing, it is advised to use non-biodegradable sutures to close the scleral wound to avoid wound dehiscence and implant extrusion.

Clinical Trials

After a proof of concept pilot study on 7 eyes of 5 patients demonstrating the safety and promise of the FA implant for severe posterior uveitis [8],

Jaffe and colleagues completed the first randomized, dose-masked, prospective interventional series comparing 0.59- to 2.1-mg FA implants in 36 eyes in 2005 [9]. Outcomes studied included post-implant control of inflammation, recurrence rate and delay to recurrence, need for adjunctive therapy, visual acuity (VA) changes and adverse events. Over a 30 month period, best corrected visual acuity (BCVA) in implanted eyes improved from 1.1 logarithm of the minimum angle of resolution (LogMAR) to 0.81 LogMAR with effective control of inflammation during this period. Visual acuity stabilized or improved in most patients, with >60 % of eyes gaining ≥3 lines at 24 months, which is significantly longer than the transient gains reported with other short lived treatments such as periocular or intraocular injections. Favorable outcomes were also observed for other variables including reduction in use of topical, periocular and systemic adjunctive medication.

Callanan et al. [10] also initiated the Fluocinolone Acetonide Uveitis Study Group and published their 3-year multicenter data to evaluate the safety and efficacy of the 0.59- and 2.1-mg implants. A total of 278 subjects were randomized in a ratio of 2:3 to receive the 0.59-mg or 2.1-mg FA implants. Eligibility criteria included currently quiescent eyes with ≥1 year-history of recurrent NIPU previously treated with systemic medication for at least 3 months or had ≥2 recurrences in a 6-month period. Results were pooled from 27 clinical centers. Interim results on safety and efficacy were reported at 34 weeks [9]. Topical uveitis medications were slowly tapered in the implanted eye. Systemic corticosteroid doses were decreased by 30 % per week and were then discontinued. Immunosuppressive agents were also discontinued or tapered within 6 weeks of FA implantation. In patients with bilateral uveitic diseases, patients were only enrolled if the investigator felt it would be possible to control the fellow non-implanted eye with local therapy alone. At 34 weeks, FA implant reduced recurrence rate from 51.4 % at baseline to 6.1 %. Recurrence was defined by one of the following criteria: (1) 2-step or more increase in anterior chamber cell from baseline, (2) 2-step or more increase in vitreous haze compared to baseline, (3) loss of ≥0.30 LogMAR in VA from baseline without any other etiology, and (4) intraocular inflammation that necessitated modification of therapy. Visual acuity was either stable or improved in 87 % of implanted eyes. The need for adjunctive treatment with topical, periocular, and systemic corticosteroids decreased dramatically from 52.9, 63.0, and 35.7 % to 12.1, 2.2, and 16.5 %, respectively. Final 3-year results showed that implants at both concentrations significantly reduced uveitis recurrence. For the 0.59-mg group, the 1-, 2-, and 3-year post-implantation recurrence rates were 4, 10, and 20 %, respectively, compared with the pre-implantation rate of 62 %. For the 2.1-mg group, the 1-, 2-, and 3-year postimplantation recurrence rates were 7, 17, and 41 %, respectively, compared with the pre-implantation rate of 58 %. The need for adjunctive treatment while on FA implant also decreased considerably, with an 80 % reduction in the number of patients requiring systemic medications during the study period. In comparison to the fellow non-implanted eye in patients with bilateral uveitis and unilateral FA implant, the rate of recurrence, need for periocular injection or topical corticosteroids were all significantly lower for the implanted eye. The mean LogMAR BCVA was maintained at baseline levels in both dose groups while the non-implanted eye was noted to deteriorate over the course of the study. In addition, there was a significant reduction in the area of cystoid macular edema (CME) in the FA implant groups and this reduction was directly correlated with final visual acuity (86 % reduction of CME at 1 year and 73 % at 3 years with the 0.59-mg group compared with 28 and 28 % reduction in the control fellow eye group; and 70 and 45 % reduction in CME with the 2.1-mg group versus 27 and 22 % in the control fellow eye group). In all instances, there was no significant difference in recurrence rates between eyes receiving the 0.59-mg and the 2.1-mg implants. These studies were crucial for the 2005 approval of the 0.59-mg implant by the

FDA for the treatment of intermediate, posterior and panuveitis with a single implant lasting up to 3 years. The implant releases FA at an initial rate of 0.6-μg/day in the first month, then decreasing to a steady state of 0.3–0.4-μg/day thereafter [6, 16, 17].

Fluocinolone Acetonide Versus Standard Systemic Therapy

Pavesio et al. [18] evaluated the safety and efficacy of the FA implant compared with standard systemic therapy (defined as standard of care, SOC) consisting of either systemic prednisolone, equivalent corticosteroid as monotherapy, or with immunosuppressive agents. In this European phase IIB/III study, 140 patients were enrolled to receive either 0.59-mg FA or standard of care at a 1:1 ratio. Patients with bilateral disease randomized to the FA implant group were implanted in their more severely affected eye, with the contralateral eye expected to be controlled with periocular corticosteroid injections alone. Results demonstrated that the FA implant provided better control of inflammation with longer delay to recurrence and lower rate of uveitis recurrence (18.2 % vs. 63.5 %) without any nonocular adverse events (0 % vs. 25.7 % in the systemic treatment group which included arthralgia and hypertension). None of these adverse events were considered severe and none required additional treatment. VA was maintained and improved by similar percentages in both groups. At 2 years, reduction in the area of CME (>1 mm^2 by fluorescein angiography) in the implant group was greater than in the SOC group (86.5 % vs. 74.4 %). Shen et al. [19] specifically analyzed the early changes in macular edema on optical coherence tomography (OCT) after fluocinolone implantation (within 90 days of implantation). Twelve eyes of 7 patients were included in this retrospective study. Consistent with the proposed mechanism of the drug, spectral domain OCT measurements of central subfield thickness (−234 μm), cube volume (−1 mm^3), cube average thickness (−39 μm), and CME grade (−3) were all reduced significantly.

Similarly, the Multicenter Uveitis Steroid Treatment (MUST) Trial was a NIH-funded trial designed to study 255 patients with a total of 479 uveitic eyes randomized to the fluocinolone implant vs systemic therapy over 24 months of treatment for intermediate, posterior or panuveitis [20]. Patients were randomized to a 1:1 ratio to receive systemic or implant therapy at 23 centers. Outcomes studied were BCVA and reported quality of life, uveitic activity, and complications from therapy. Over 24 months, the results revealed the non-inferiority of implants compared to systemic therapy and steroid-sparing immunosuppressive agents with no detectable superiority of either approach. VA improvement in both groups was +6.0 letters versus +3.2 letters, and quality of life improvement was +11.4 and +6.8 units, respectively, for the implant and the systemic groups. Macular edema also decreased in both groups, from 41 and 39 % at baseline to 20 and 34 % at 6 months and 22 % versus 30 % at 24 months for the implant and the systemic groups, respectively. None of these values reached a statistical significant difference between the 2 groups.

Fluocinolone Acetonide Implant for Specific Diagnoses

Table 45.1 summarizes the findings from various studies detailing the treatment and response of patients with specific uveitic conditions to the FA implant. These include serpiginous choroiditis, Vogt–Koyanagi–Harada disease (VKH), sympathetic ophthalmia, birdshot chorioretinopathy, and Behçet's disease [21–27]. Since severe loss of vision often occurs in these conditions due to the waxing and waning nature of inflammation and CME; episodic treatment is not always ideal. The FA implant's ability to deliver a continuous low therapeutic dose over a long period of time may offer excellent long-term control of these disorders.

The results from the case reports seem to indicate that most uveitic conditions respond well to treatment with the FA implant alone (without systemic medications). However, the

Table 45.1 Table of studies on response of different uveitic conditions to the fluocinolone acetonide implant

Uveitic condition	Author	Yr	N[a]	Results	Adverse effects
Serpiginous choroiditis [21]	Seth	2008	1/1	• At 14 mon, VA increased from 20/70 to 20/50, quiescent eye	• Intractable OHT, trab
VKH [22]	Khalifa	2009	2/4	• Bilateral FA implants • With systemic corticosteroid tapering, serous RD recurred in one at 2 and 6 mon, and panuveitis returned in the other at 3 mon during steroid taper	• N/A
Sympathetic ophthalmia [23, 24]	Mahajan	2009	8/8	• Reduction in systemic medication in all patients • 3/8 had recurrent inflammation necessitating concurrent IMT • VA stable in 5 and improved in 3	• 2 IOP elevations needing trab • 1 had RD 47 weeks post-implant, needed PPV and SO
	Jonas	2008	1/1	• 2.1-mg FA implant • 11 mon follow-up, IOP stable 12–18 mmHg and VA at 0.4–0.5 LogMAR • IMT stopped	• N/A
Birdshot chorioretinopathy [25, 26]	Rush	2011	22/36	• At 12 mon, 32 eyes followed up • Mean VA improved from 20/50 to 20/30 • IMT use from 82 to 5 % • 0 vitreous haze from 26 to 100 % • CME decreased from 36 to 6 %	• 100 % OHT • 19 eyes underwent CE
	Burkholder	2013	28/48	• 20 birdshot and 28 panuveitis eyes • 37 mon follow-up, loss of ≥3 lines 0.16/eye-yr in birdshot vs 0.39/eye-yr in other panuveitis	• Birdshot had more increase in IOP in first 4 mon post-FA implant ($p = 0.04$) versus other panuveitis • More birdshot eyes required glaucoma surg (0.42/eye-yr vs 0.11/eye-yr, mean time 15.5 mon vs 31.5 mon) • Cataract surgery 0.75/EY and 0.88/EY for birdshot and others • 7 had VH
Behçet [27]	Oh	2014	7/8	• Over 47.8 mon follow-up, VA improved ≥3 lines in 75 %	• 75 % had IOP ≥30 mmHg • 5 patients needed glaucoma filtering surgery

(continued)

Table 45.1 (continued)

Uveitic condition	Author	Yr	N^a	Results	Adverse effects
				• 5 patients discontinued all systemic meds after mean of 13.4 mon • Decrease in IMT need in both groups and decrease in CME at mon 24 in birdshot eyes	• Phakic eye developed cataract • 1 case of postop CMV endotheliitis

[a]First digit indicates number of patients, second digit indicates number of eyes; *CE* Cataract extraction; *CME* Cystoid macular edema; *CMV* Cytomegalovirus; *FA* Fluocinolone acetonide; *IMT* Immunosuppressive therapy; *IOP* Intraocular pressure; *Mon* Months; *N* Number of patients/eyes; *N/A* Not applicable; *OHT* Ocular hypertension; *Postop* Post-operative; *PPV* Pars plana vitrectomy; *RD* Retinal detachment; *Trab* Trabeculectomy; *SO* Silicone oil; *VA* Visual acuity; *VH* Vitreous hemorrhage; *VKH* Vogt-Koyanagi-Harada disease; *Yr* Year of publication

results in eyes with VKH offer mixed response and only temporary quiescence when weaned off systemic corticosteroids.

Reimplantation

The FDA lists the duration of the FA implant in the eye at 30–36 months. This is significant as uveitis may recur after the depletion of the medication. Several case series have analyzed the outcome of FA re-implantation. In the continuing study of the same 3-year multicenter patient cohort by Callanan and Jaffe, 26 eyes of 22 patients in the entire cohort of 118 FA implanted eyes manifested recurrence inflammation on follow-up [28]. Jaffe et al. studied 17 eyes in 14 patients for whom FA implant reinsertion was performed. The majority of patients had idiopathic panuveitis (6 of 14 patients) or sarcoid panuveitis (4 of 14 patients). The mean time from initial FA implant to recurrence was 38 months. In the follow-up after the second implantation, only one eye experienced recurrence 3 years later. In nearly all cases, FA implantation and re-implantation drastically decreased or eliminated other ocular and systemic anti-inflammatory therapy. Re-implantation also did not seem to affect the rate of IOP control or cataract formation from baseline established by the first implant. Complications related to re-implantation were rare and suture strut protrusion and wound dehiscence were not reported in this small series. One case of staphylococcus endophthalmitis, which responded favorably to treatment, and one case of tractional retinal detachment, occurred in this series. Another study of 10 eyes from 10 patients noted uveitis recurrence at a median of 32.5 months post initial FA implantation [15]. Once again, the majority of patients had a diagnosis of idiopathic panuveitis (30 %) or sarcoid panuveitis (20 %). After placement of the second implant, patients were followed for an additional 16.8 months. During this time, visual acuity was noted to stabilize or improve in all patients, with recurrences occurring in 4 of 10 patients at around month 18. Kaplan–Meier analysis of time to recurrence for all patients combined reveals a mean recurrence time between 25 and 30 months, within the range of effectiveness paralleling in vitro pharmacokinetics studies. In a third study of 8 patients, the average time to second implant was 42.7 months [29]. Two patients received a third implant, with average time from second to third implant being 30.1 months. Final VA showed that 4 of 8 patients improved visually and one was stable.

Complications

Complications after FA implantation are not infrequent and directly related to the chronic exposure to intraocular steroids. The most common side effects are cataract formation and increased intraocular pressure. Adverse events within the immediate perioperative period include eye pain, ptosis, eyelid edema, corneal edema, vitreous opacities, vitreous hemorrhage, macular edema, retinal hemorrhage, hypotony, and choroidal detachment. Approximately 35–40 % of patients report conjunctival injection, reduced visual acuity and conjunctival hemorrhage [30]. According to the Bausch and Lomb product insert, the most common nonocular event reported is headache (>33 %) [31]. Other complications reported in literature which manifest over time include spontaneous dissociation of the implant, nonfunctional implant [15, 32], endophthalmitis (0.4–4.5 %) [9, 18, 20], retinal detachment (1.5–5.0 %) [9, 18, 20], vitreous bands [30], necrotizing scleritis and thinning in the area of the implant [33], viral retinitis, viral endotheliitis [34, 35], and chronic hypotony (11–15 %) [18]. The most common adverse events will be detailed below.

Intraocular Pressure

The FA implant had a high incidence of increased IOP requiring topical therapy or glaucoma surgery. In the 30-month long pilot study by Jaffe and colleagues, the most common side effect was elevated IOP, for which 11–56 % of eyes needed an average of 3.3 IOP-lowering medications on follow-up. Filtering procedures were performed in 19.4 % of patients over time, most often between 1.5 and 2.5 years postimplantation. The investigators hypothesized that this increase in IOP may be multifactorial in origin from a combination of steroid response, increased aqueous production from improvement of ciliary body function after control of inflammation, and permanent long-standing trabecular meshwork damage due to chronic inflammation.

The extended full 3-year study by Callanan, Jaffe and colleagues confirmed trends observed at 34 weeks. At 34 weeks, 51.1 % of treated eyes needed IOP-lowering therapy, with 59 % of all implanted eyes demonstrating ≥10 mmHg IOP increase, and 5.8 % underwent glaucoma filtering surgery [9]. At 3 years, 67 % of eyes receiving the 0.59-mg implant and 79 % of eyes with the 2.1-mg implant had an IOP elevation recorded as ≥10 mmHg from baseline, and 78 % of all implanted eyes required IOP-lowering drops as compared to 36 % in the fellow non-implanted eyes. In addition, 40 % of all implanted eyes required further IOP-lowering surgery compared with 2 % of fellow eyes. Six of these eyes needed FA explantation due to intractable IOP elevation.

The largest pooled analysis of 584 eyes from 3 studies (ClinicalTrials.gov Identifier: NCT00407082, NCT00468871, and NCT00456482) showed that 75 % of eyes required IOP-lowering treatment during the course of the 3-year study [16, 36]. These results noted a ≥10 mmHg IOP rise from baseline in 71.0 % of eyes 3 years after implantation, and 55.1 % of eyes also reached an IOP ≥30 mmHg [16]. Topical IOP-lowering medication was used in 74.8 % of implanted eyes while IOP-lowering surgery was performed in 36.6 % of eyes. Most of these surgeries were trabeculectomies (76.2 %) and glaucoma drainage device implantation (20.6 %). The mean time from FA implantation to initiation of new IOP-lowering therapy was 409.3 ± 18.7 days while the mean time from implantation to IOP-lowering surgery was 870.5 ± 13.9 days. Complete surgical success, defined as post-operative IOP of 6-21 mmHg without any additional medication, was 50.0 % at 12 months and qualified success was 35.1 % at 12 months.

In the study by Pavesio et al. [18], 55.4 % of eyes had an IOP increase of ≥10 mmHg from baseline versus 10.8 % in the SOC group. IOP-lowering medication was needed in 62.1 % of implanted eyes versus 20.3 % of SOC eyes. IOP-lowering surgery was performed in 21.2 % of implanted eyes versus 2.7 % of SOC eyes. Hypotony was also higher in the implanted eyes, at 19.7 %, versus 1.4 % in SOC eyes.

Friedman et al. [37] examined the risk of IOP elevation and glaucoma in the MUST trial 2 years after enrollment. The MUST study showed that the implant group had an overall 4-fold increase in IOP elevation ≥10 mmHg (65 % post-FA implant vs. 24 % post systemic treatment), absolute IOP above 30 mmHg (49 % vs. 11 %) and need for treatment of elevated IOP compared with the systemic treatment group (69 % vs. 26 %) [20]. The incidence of glaucoma was 17 and 4.0 % after 24 weeks in the 2 groups respectively. At 3 years follow-up of the MUST cohort, glaucoma surgery was needed in 40 % of implanted eyes versus 2 % of non-implanted eyes.

Although early IOP elevations can be expected within the first year, more recent studies indicate that extreme elevations may be expected as late as the third year after implantation. The longest follow-up post-FA implantation reported is a case series of 42 eyes over an 8-year period [38]. In this study, 45 % of eyes (19 of 42) required glaucoma surgery, with success achieved in 92 % at 24 months. Seven of these 19 eyes received multiple FA implants and most underwent IOP-lowering surgery (58 % glaucoma drainage device and 42 % trabeculectomy) after placement of the first implant.

To mitigate the high likelihood of future glaucomatous damage, regular IOP monitoring as often as every 2 months is advocated, as is combined FA implant and filtering surgery in those at high risk of glaucomatous optic neuropathy [15, 29, 39, 40]. Malone and colleagues studied a group of 5 patients (7 eyes) with preexisting chronic non-infectious posterior uveitis and elevated IOP on maximum tolerated medical therapy who then underwent combined FA implantation and glaucoma tube shunt placement in one surgical session [41]. Three eyes also underwent concurrent phacoemulsification and lens implantation. Mean Snellen visual acuity improved from 20/400 pre-implant to 20/114 at 12 months. Average IOP decreased from 27.3 mmHg at baseline to 14.6 mmHg at 12 months. Adjunctive anti-inflammatory therapy use decreased, with all patients off topical prednisolone and 3 patients with reduced doses of systemic anti-inflammatory therapy. None of the eyes with follow-up for more than 30 months had any inflammatory recurrence.

Cataract

Cataract formation is a near universal complication of FA implantation for phakic eyes. Callanan, Jaffe, et al. found that after 3 years, 67 % of phakic implanted eyes as compared with 18 % of fellow phakic non-implanted eyes developed posterior subcapsular cataract progression. Pavesio et al. reported a change >2 grades in lens opacity in 89.6 % of their phakic patients at 2 years versus 23.3 % of patients on systemic SOC treatment. A total of 87.8 % of implanted eyes underwent cataract extraction versus 19.3 % in the SOC study eyes [18]. The MUST study group incurred a higher cumulative risk of cataract progression and cataract surgery after implant (91 and 80 %) in contrast to systemic treatment (45 and 1 %). Due to the high likelihood of cataract after FA implantation some researchers have advocated for combined lens extraction at the time of implant placement [39, 42].

Sheppard et al. [43] initiated a post hoc analysis on a subset of eyes from the main Fluocinolone Acetonide Study Group consisting of 278 patients who underwent cataract surgery after FA implantation. They found that 132 of 142 phakic implanted eyes and 39 of 186 phakic non-implanted eyes underwent cataract surgery. The groups were compared for VA, inflammation, rate of uveitis recurrence and postoperative complications. Mean VA improvement post cataract extraction was greater in the implanted groups at 1 and 3 months postoperatively. Statistically significant less anterior chamber and vitreous inflammation were also noted in the implanted eyes compared with non-implanted eyes at the same time points. Post-surgical uveitis recurrence was 26.5 % versus 44.4 % and glaucoma rates were 19.7 % versus 0 % in the 2 groups. These results indicate that cataractogenesis post-FA implant is a common but manageable complication and good visual outcomes may be achieved post surgery without triggering a recurrence of inflammation, although glaucoma did occur more frequently in these eyes.

Implant Dissociation

Dissociation of the medication reservoir from the anchoring strut has been reported in several instances, either spontaneously [44, 45] or most often at the time of explantation [10, 45, 46]. The process has been attributed to the defective adhesive agent compounding both parts together. This older implant model has since been modified. The multicenter study of 278 patients by Callanan and Jaffe reported three cases of spontaneous FA implant dissociation [10]. Taban et al. described two incidences wherein the reservoir separated from the anchoring strut. However, both were easily removed with limited vitrectomy and without the need for intraocular foreign body removal techniques [15]. In another case series with three implant dissociations from the newer model batch, one necessitated a pars plana vitrectomy with perfluorocarbon instillation in order to float the posteriorly displaced strut up toward the wound [47]. Nicholson and colleagues discovered that length of time the implant has resided in the eye correlated significantly with the rate of implant cup dissociation [46]. In their study of 27 procedures, dissociated implants resided a mean of 47.4 months versus intact implants with a mean of 32.5 months. Late onset spontaneous dissociation years (>6–7 years) after implantation with dislocation of the reservoir either posteriorly into the vitreous or anteriorly into the anterior chamber is also possible, and surgeons should be aware of this possibility since not all reservoirs are retrieved from the eye once the drug has been depleted [48]. In these cases, the surgeon should also be prepared to employ vitrectomy and intraocular foreign body removal techniques for its retrieval. Another strategy described is to use a high infusion rate with a bottle height of up to 80 mmHg to exert pressure by flowing out of the incision and to "buoy" the dissociated component and its tendency to fall backward [49].

Viral Retinitis and Endotheliitis

While uncommon, viral retinitis development or reactivation has been a reported complication following intraocular or periocular corticosteroid administration. Cytomegalovirus (CMV) is the most frequent causative agent, followed by the herpes simplex virus. Three cases in the literature have been attributed to FA implants with a mean presentation time of 10.3 months after implantation [35, 50, 51]. Although systemic and intravitreal antiviral agents may control the spread of retinitis, vision is usually poor at follow-up due to retinal atrophy and the development of rhegmatogenous retinal detachment.

Polymerase chain reaction-proven CMV endotheliitis without any signs of concurrent retinitis has been described in two separate immunocompetent patients. Both patients had a diagnosis of Behçet's disease; one manifested symptoms 4 months and the other 2 years after FA implantation [52, 53]. Despite prompt treatment by FA explantation followed by systemic valganciclovir therapy, the visual outcome was poor due to endothelial decompensation.

Conclusion

Chronic non-infectious posterior uveitis is a severe illness with an economic cost of blindness akin to that of diabetes. The fluocinolone acetonide sustained-release implant has been shown to be effective in controlling intraocular inflammation, decreasing adjunctive therapy, and stabilizing and improving vision for long periods of time with one single drug administration. However, adverse effects do occur. Notably, the use of the implant is associated with extremely high rates of cataract development/progression and intraocular pressure increase. Therefore, the positive attributes of this treatment modality need to be balanced against its disadvantages and carefully adapted to each patient's individual clinical circumstances.

References

1. Fluocinolone acetonide ophthalmic–Bausch & Lomb: fluocinolone acetonide Envision TD implant. Drugs R D. 2005;6:116–9.
2. Lim L, Smith J, Rosenbaum J. Retisert (Bausch & Lomb/Control Delivery Systems). Curr Opin Investig Drugs. 2005;6:1159–67.
3. Jain N, Stinnett SS, Jaffe GJ. Prospective study of a fluocinolone acetonide implant for chronic macular

edema from central retinal vein occlusion: thirty-six-month results. Ophthalmology. 2012;119: 132–7.
4. Pearson PA, Comstock TL, Ip M, et al. Fluocinolone acetonide intravitreal implant for diabetic macular edema: a 3-year multicenter, randomized, controlled clinical trial. Ophthalmology. 2011;118:1580–7.
5. Campochiaro PA, Brown DM, Pearson A, et al. Sustained delivery fluocinolone acetonide vitreous inserts provide benefit for at least 3 years in patients with diabetic macular edema. Ophthalmology. 2012;119:2125–32.
6. Callanan DG. Novel intravitreal fluocinolone acetonide implant in the treatment of chronic noninfectious posterior uveitis. Expert Rev Ophthalmol. 2007;2:33–44.
7. Jaffe GJ, Yang CH, Guo H, Denny JP, Lima C, Ashton P. Safety and pharmacokinetics of an intraocular fluocinolone acetonide sustained delivery device. Invest Ophthalmol Vis Sci. 2000;41: 3569–75.
8. Jaffe GJ, Ben-nun J, Guo H, Dunn JP, Ashton P. Fluocinolone acetonide sustained drug delivery device to treat severe uveitis. Ophthalmology. 2000;107: 2024–33.
9. Jaffe GJ, Martin D, Callanan D, Pearson PA, Levy B, Comstock T. Fluocinolone acetonide implant (Retisert) for noninfectious posterior uveitis: thirty-four–week results of a multicenter randomized clinical study. Ophthalmology. 2006;113:1020–7.
10. Callanan DG, Jaffe GJ, Martin DF, Pearson PA, Comstock TL. Treatment of posterior uveitis with a fluocinolone acetonide implant: three-year clinical trial results. Arch Ophthalmol. 2008;126:1191–201.
11. Brumm M, Nguyen Q. Fluocinolone acetonide intravitreal sustained release device–a new addition to the armamentarium of uveitic management. Int J Nanomedicine. 2007;2:55–64.
12. Yeh S, Nussenblatt RB. Fluocinolone acetonide for the treatment of uveitis: weighing the balance between local and systemic immunosuppression. Arch Ophthalmol. 2008;126:1287–9.
13. Kuno N, Fujii S. Biodegradable intraocular therapies for retinal disorders. Drugs Aging. 2010;27:117–34.
14. Berger BB, Mendoza W. Sclerotomy closure for Retisert implant. Retina. 2013;33:436–8. doi:10. 1097/IAE.0b013e3182759fdb.
15. Taban M, Lowder CY, Kaiser PK. Outcome of fluocinolone acetonide implant (Retisert™) reimplantation for chronic noninfectious posterior uveitis. Retina. 2008;28:1280–8.
16. Goldstein D, Godfrey D, Hall A, et al. Intraocular pressure in patients with uveitis treated with fluocinolone acetonide implants. Arch Ophthalmol. 2007;125:1478–85.
17. Campochiaro PA, Nguyen QD, Hafiz G, et al. Aqueous levels of fluocinolone acetonide after administration of fluocinolone acetonide inserts or fluocinolone acetonide implants. Ophthalmology. 2013;120:583–7.
18. Pavesio C, Zierhut M, Bairi K, Comstock TL, Usner DW. Evaluation of an intravitreal fluocinolone acetonide implant versus standard systemic therapy in noninfectious posterior uveitis. Ophthalmology. 2010;117(567–75):e1.
19. Shen BY, Punjabi OS, Lowder CY, Sears JE, Singh RP. Early treatment response of fluocinolone (Retisert) implantation in patients with uveitic macular edema: an optical coherence tomography study. Retina. 2013;33:873–7.
20. Kempen JH, Altaweel MM, Holbrook JT, et al. Randomized comparison of systemic anti-inflammatory therapy versus fluocinolone acetonide implant for intermediate, posterior, and panuveitis: the multicenter uveitis steroid treatment trial. Ophthalmology. 2011;118:1916–26.
21. Seth RK, Gaudio PA. Treatment of serpiginous choroiditis with intravitreous fluocinolone acetonide implant. Ocul Immunol Inflamm. 2008;16:103–5.
22. Khalifa Y, Loh AR, Acharya NR. Fluocinolone acetonide intravitreal implants in Vogt-Koyanagi-Harada disease. Ocul Immunol Inflamm. 2009;17:431–3.
23. Mahajan VB, Gehrs KM, Goldstein DA, Fischer DH, Lopez JS, Folk JC. Management of sympathetic ophthalmia with the fluocinolone acetonide implant. Ophthalmology. 2009;116(552–7):e1.
24. Jonas J, Rensch F. Intravitreal steroid slow-release device replacing repeated intravitreal triamcinolone injections for sympathetic ophthalmia. Eur J Ophthalmol. 2008;18:834–6.
25. Burkholder BM, Wang J, Dunn JP, Nguyen QD, Thorne JE. Postoperative outcomes after fluocinolone acetonide implant surgery in patients with birdshot chorioretinitis and other types of posterior and panuveitis. Retina. 2013;33:1684–93.
26. Rush RB, Goldstein DA, Callanan DG, Meghpara B, Feuer WJ, Davis JL. Outcomes of birdshot chorioretinopathy treated with an intravitreal sustained-release fluocinolone acetonide-containing device. Am J Ophthalmol. 2011;151:630–6.
27. Oh EK, Lee EK, Yu HG. Long-term results of fluocinolone acetonide intravitreal implant in Behçet intractable posterior uveitis. Can J Ophthalmol (J Can Ophtalmol). 2014;49:273–8.
28. Jaffe GJ. Reimplantation of a fluocinolone acetonide sustained drug delivery implant for chronic uveitis. Am J Ophthalmol 2008;145:667–75.e1.
29. Allen R, Suhler E, Flaxel C, Chen Z, Choi D. Long-term follow-up of patients treated with multiple fluocinolone acetonide implants for noninfectious uveitis. J Ophthalmic Inflamm Infect. 2012;2: 177–82.
30. Galor A, Margolis R, Kaiser PK, Lowder CY. VItreous band formation and the sustained-release, intravitreal fluocinolone (Retisert) implant. Arch Ophthalmol. 2007;125:836–8.
31. Bausch and Lomb. Retisert. Retisert website. http://www.retisert.com/retisert_implant.html. Accessed 10 Sep 2014.

32. Hebson CB, Srivastava SK. A functional, nonfunctioning Retisert implant. Ocul Immunol Inflamm. 2011;19:210–1.
33. Taban M, Lowder CY, Ventura AACM, et al. Scleral thickness following fluocinolone acetonide implant (Retisert). Ocul Immunol Inflamm. 2010;18:305–13.
34. Sallam A, Taylor SR, Lightman S. Review and update of intraocular therapy in noninfectious uveitis. Curr Opin Ophthalmol. 2011;22:517–22.
35. Ufret-Vincenty RL, Singh RP, Lowder CY, Kaiser PK. Cytomegalovirus retinitis after fluocinolone acetonide (Retisert™) implant. Am J Ophthalmol. 2007;143:334–5.
36. Bollinger KE, Smith SD. Prevalence and management of elevated intraocular pressure after placement of an intravitreal sustained-release steroid implant. Curr Opin Ophthalmol. 2009;20:99–103. doi:10.1097/ICU.0b013e32831d7f3a.
37. Friedman DS, Holbrook JT, Ansari H, et al. Risk of elevated intraocular pressure and glaucoma in patients with uveitis: results of the multicenter uveitis steroid treatment trial. Ophthalmology. 2013;120:1571–9.
38. Bollinger K, Kim J, Lowder CY, Kaiser PK, Smith SD. Intraocular pressure outcome of patients with fluocinolone acetonide intravitreal implant for noninfectious uveitis. Ophthalmology. 2011;118:1927–31.
39. Ahmad ZM, Hughes BA, Abrams GW, Mahmoud TH. Combined posterior chamber intraocular lens, vitrectomy, Retisert, and pars plana tube in noninfectious uveitis. Arch Ophthalmol. 2012;130:908–13.
40. Ansari H, Kempen JH. Proof of concept for combined insertion of fluocinolone acetonide and glaucoma drainage implants for eyes with uveitis and glaucoma. Am J Ophthalmol. 2010;149:699–700.
41. Malone PE, Herndon LW, Muir KW, Jaffe GJ. Combined fluocinolone acetonide intravitreal insertion and glaucoma drainage device placement for chronic uveitis and glaucoma. Am J Ophthalmol. 2010;149 (800.e1):806.e1.
42. Chieh JJ, Carlson AN, Jaffe GJ. Combined fluocinolone acetonide intraocular delivery system insertion, phacoemulsification, and intraocular lens implantation for severe uveitis. Am J Ophthalmol. 2008;146(589–94):e1.
43. Sheppard J Jr, Nguyen Q, Usner D, Comstock T. Post-cataract outcomes in patients with noninfectious posterior uveitis treated with the fluocinolone acetonide intravitreal implant. Clin Ophthalmol. 2012;6:79–85.
44. Rofagha S, Prechanond T, Stewart JM. Late spontaneous dissociation of a fluocinolone acetonide implant (Retisert). Ocul Immunol Inflamm. 2013;21:77–8.
45. Akduman L, Cetin EN, Levy J, Becker MD, Mackensen F, Lim LL. Spontaneous dissociation and dislocation of Retisert pellet. Ocul Immunol Inflamm. 2013;21:87–9.
46. Nicholson BP, Singh RP, Sears JE, Lowder CY, Kaiser PK. Evaluation of fluocinolone acetonide sustained release implant (Retisert) dissociation during implant removal and exchange surgery. Am J Ophthalmol 2012;154:969–73.e1.
47. Yeh S, Cebulla C, Witherspoon S, et al. Management of fluocinolone implant dissociation during implant exchange. Arch Ophthalmol. 2009;127:1218–21.
48. Chang PY, Kresch Z, Samson CM, Gentile RC. Spontaneous dissociation of fluocinolone acetonide sustained release implant (Retisert) with dislocation into the anterior chamber. Ocul Immunol Inflamm. 2014;23:454–57.
49. Wan W, Stewart JM. Use of a high infusion rate to prevent posterior dislocation of fluocinolone acetonide implant during surgical removal. Ocul Immunol Inflamm. 2011;19:214–5.
50. Takakura A, Tessler HH, Goldstein DA, et al. Viral retinitis following intraocular or periocular corticosteroid administration: a case series and comprehensive review of the literature. Ocul Immunol Inflamm. 2014;22:175–82.
51. Ramaiya KJ, Rao PK. Herpetic necrotizing retinitis following fluocinolone acetonide intravitreal implant. Ocul Immunol Inflamm. 2011;19:72–4.
52. Sims JL, Chee SP. Cytomegalovirus endotheliitis following fluocinolone acetonide (Retisert) implant. Eye. 2009;24:197–8.
53. Park UC, Kim SJ, Yu HG. Cytomegalovirus endotheliitis after fluocinolone acetonide (Retisert) implant in a patient with behçet uveitis. Ocular Immunology and Inflammation. 2011;19:282–3.

Surgical Therapy: Dexamethasone Biodegradable Intravitreal Implant (Ozurdex®)

46

Robert Wang

Introduction

The treatment of uveitis has always been a delicate balancing act of managing complications of the disease and the toxicity of the ensuing therapy. Systemic medications have potential side effects to various organ systems in the body and the inherent risk of infectious complications. Therapies such as topical or injection of local steroids can potentially induce glaucoma and cataract formation but have the advantage of limited systemic complications. While long sustained local therapy has been technologically established such as Vitrasert® (intravitreal ganciclovir) for the treatment of CMV retintitis [1–3], and Retisert® (intravitreal fluocinolone acetonide) for uveitis, these therapies have the disadvantage of requiring insertion in the operating room. Additionally, Retisert has a high incidence of cataract development and glaucoma [4–6]. The advent of an office placed low risk dexamethasone implant has provided a new treatment in our armamentarium against uveitis.

R. Wang (✉)
Department of Ophthalmology, Texas Retina Associates, UT Southwestern, Dallas, TX, USA
e-mail: rwang@texasretina.com

G.N. Papaliodis (ed.), *Uveitis*,
DOI 10.1007/978-3-319-09126-6_46

Design Concepts of the Ozurdex® Implant

The Ozurdex® implant develop by Allergan, Inc. is a novel drug delivery system that can be placed in an office setting via a 22 gauge needle thru the pars plana into the vitreous cavity. The injection device delivers an implant that is completely biodegradable, slowly releasing dexamethasone over 90 days. Originally developed by Oculex Pharmaceuticals, the Novadur® drug delivery system uses a D,L-lactide-co-glycolide (PLG) biodegradable polymer matrix that slowly devolves to lactic acid and glycolic acid releasing dexamethasone (Fig. 46.1). The lactic acid and glycolic acid further degrade into carbon dioxide and water (Figs. 46.2 and 46.3). The platform is loaded with 0.7 mg of dexamethasone in a 400 μg diameter cylinder. The implant is FDA approved for the treatment of uveitis, macular edema following branch or central retinal vein occlusion, and more recently diabetic macular edema. The injection device itself is a novel design delivery device unlike a traditional injection needle. The injection device has a "safety pin" that is first removed, then the protective cap from the needle. Instead of pushing a "plunger" to deliver the drug, a push button activates a pin that pushes the drug out thru the bore of the needle and into the eye. The push button has a hard fixed stop with a mild "click"

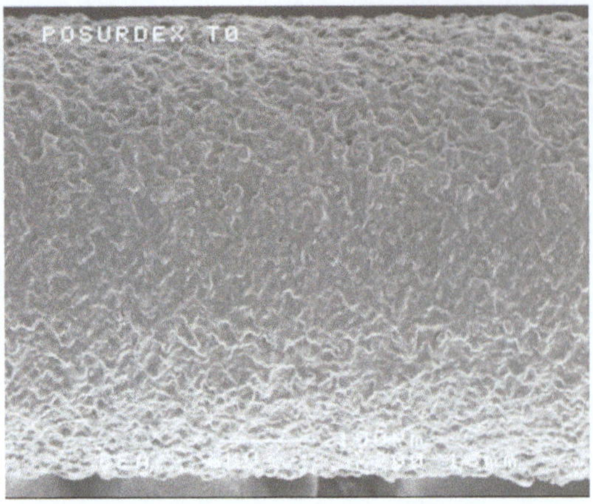

Fig. 46.1 Microscopic appearance of complete Ozurdex implant *courtesy Allergan

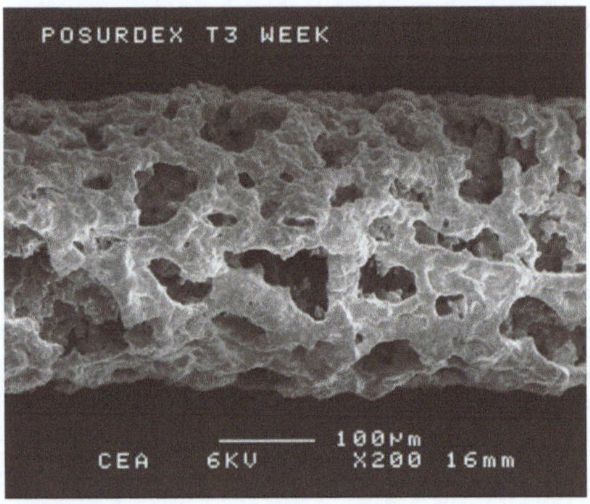

Fig. 46.2 Microscopic appearance of Ozurdex after dissolving for 3 weeks *courtesy Allergan

when the button has been fully depressed and drug delivered (Fig. 46.4).

Clinical Studies

The first large study published reported the efficacy and safety of Ozurdez in the treatment of macular edema (causes of macular included diabetic retinopathy, retinal vein occlusions, uveitis, or Irvine-Gass syndrome with persistent macular edema). This was a 6 month, multi-center trial with 315 patients enrolled. Of the patients randomized to the 0.7 mg dexamethasone implant, 35 % demonstrated a 10 or more letter improvement (via ETDRS testing) at 90 days from injection compared to 13 % of the control group (sham injection). Improvement in BCVA (best corrected visual acuity) of 15 letters or more was achieved in 18 % of patients versus 6 % in controls. Additionally, the concern regarding intraocular pressure (IOP) elevation was lower than expected with 11 % of patients developing a 10 mm hg or higher rise in IOP compared to 2 % of controls.

During the study, OCTs were used to monitor response with a dramatic improvement/resolution of macular edema in those treated with Ozurdex [8]. However, in the entire study, there were only 5 patients with uveitis enrolled.

To further expand the possible benefit of the implant specifically in patients with uveitis, a large scale randomized clinical trial was completed to evaluate the efficacy of the

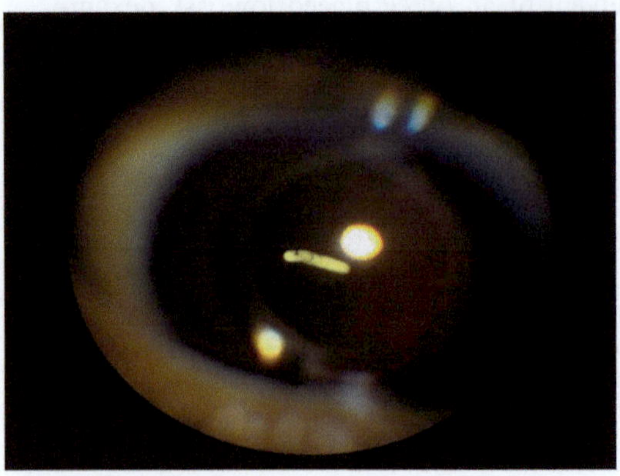

Fig. 46.3 Dissolving Ozurdex 72 days after implantation in human eye

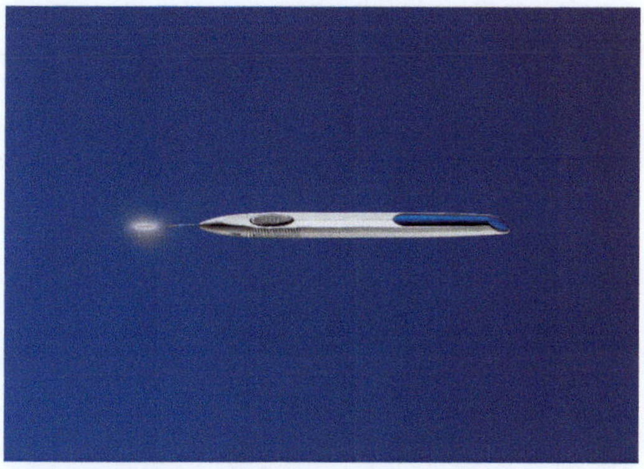

Fig. 46.4 Ozurdex® injector device with dexamethasone pellet highlighted

dexamethasone implant in patients with non-infectious posterior uveitis (Huron Study). Patients were randomized to sham injection or one of two dexamethasone dosages (0.35, 0.7 mg).

In this study, 229 patients from 18 countries were enrolled. 81 % had the diagnosis of intermediate uveitis with the remainder having various forms of posterior uveitis. Those patients receiving the 0.7 mg injection had a dramatic improvement in vitreous haze (Fig. 46.5) with nearly half of the patients achieving a haze score of "0". 90 % had a one step improvement in haze and a significant portion had a two step improvement (Figs. 46.6 and 46.7) with the effect continuing for 6 months.

Fortunately, the complications of the sustained release dexamethasone implant were lower than those reported for Retisert. The rate of cataract formation in the implant group was 11.8 % compared to 5.3 % in those receiving sham injection. Additionally, IOP elevation of 10 mm hg over baseline was only seen in 15–20 % of patients, with the majority of patient not requiring IOP lowering medications. With those that required therapy, most only needed one topical drop (Fig. 46.8) compared to 40 % or greater in patients receiving the Retisert® implant.

Since these initial studies and the subsequent FDA approval, the familiarity and clinical use has become more common in clinical practice.

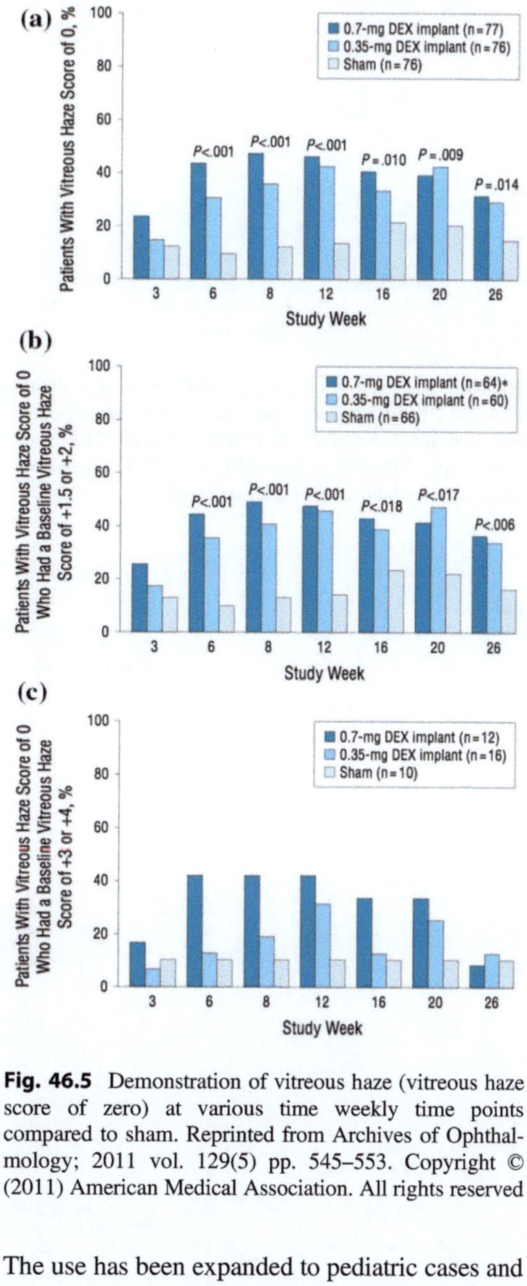

Fig. 46.5 Demonstration of vitreous haze (vitreous haze score of zero) at various time weekly time points compared to sham. Reprinted from Archives of Ophthalmology; 2011 vol. 129(5) pp. 545–553. Copyright © (2011) American Medical Association. All rights reserved

The use has been expanded to pediatric cases and also as a pre-treatment prior to cataract removal [9, 10]. However, there have been reported cases of a higher than expected IOP rise occasionally necessitating removal [11]. Caution should always be taken in the usage in the pediatric population.

In adults, the implant has shown similar success as was demonstrated in the preliminary studies, with newer small clinical studies

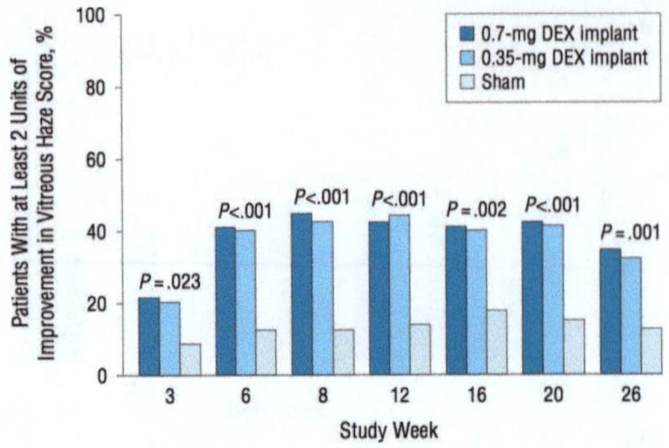

Fig. 46.6 Percentage of patients with at least a 2 unit improvement in vitreous haze at weekly time points. Reprinted from Archives of Ophthalmology; 2011 vol. 129(5) pp. 545–553. Copyright © (2011) American Medical Association. All rights reserved

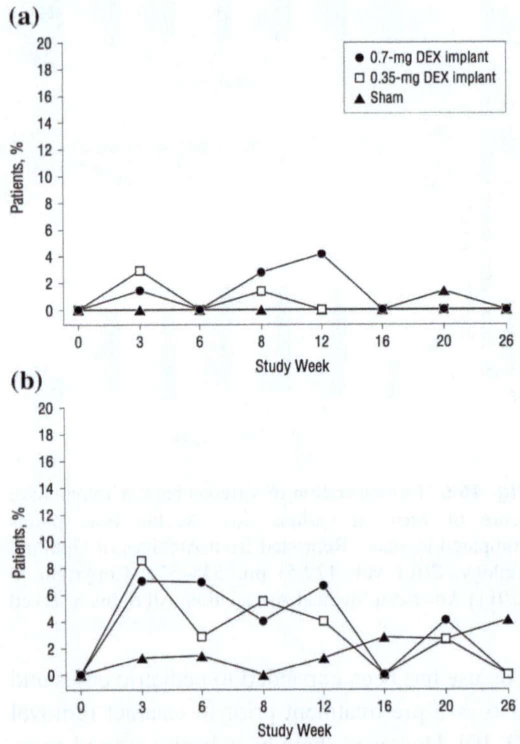

Fig. 46.7 Percentage of patients with a >25 mmHg increase in IOP at weekly time points. Reprinted from Archives of Ophthalmology; 2011 vol. 129(5) pp. 545–553. Copyright © (2011) American Medical Association. All rights reserved

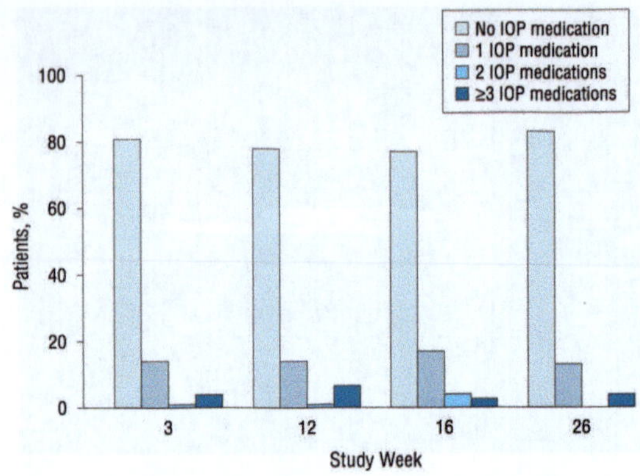

Fig. 46.8 Number of IOP lowering medications required by patients reveiving the Ozurdex implant at various time points. Reprinted from Archives of Ophthalmology; 2011 vol. 129(5) pp. 545–553. Copyright © (2011) American Medical Association. All rights reserved

showing benefit in cases with persistent macular edema [12] and long term uveitic disease [13]. The only new complication that has been described has been the anterior migration of the implant into the anterior chamber in a pseudophakic eyes [14], but this appears extremely uncommon.

Injection Technique and Clinical Use

The eye is prepped in steroid fashion. Topical betadine preparation of the eye with an eyelid speculum is used. Due to the size of the injection needle (22 gauge) subconjunctival lidocaine usually is more comfortable, though topical anesthesia can also be utilized.

Due to the occasional resistance of the needle going thru the scleral and possible reflux of intraocular fluid thru the wound, a toothed forcep helps with counter traction and to pinch the wound closed after the needle is removed.

The needle of the Ozurdex® injection device has a collar to indicate the depth needed before injection of the drug. Typically, the needle is inserted at an angle in a beveled manner after the "safety pin" and cap are removed. Once the needle has been inserted to the collar, the push button is fully depressed injecting the drug.

While the injection technique is extremely easy, the clinical use still requires the "art of medicine" in clinical use. Though it is tempting to use the injection for anterior uveitis, one must remember that the implant has only been FDA approved for the use in posterior segment disease. With most cases of anterior uveitis, inflammation is generally easily controlled with topical drops or local therapy.

With posterior disease the treatment varies. While the initial studies did guide the use, uveitis tends to be a widely varying disease that requires a more balanced management. Typically, in patients with pars planitis, that might wax and wane with occasional cystoid macular edema. Ozurdex tends to be a great treatment protocol as the injection tend to be infrequent with very low chance of cataract or glaucoma development. However, in more serious posterior disease, Ozurdex might not be indicated such as in cases of Behcet's where long term sustain therapy is more ideal due to possible loss of vision from gaps in treatment such as when the concentration of dexamethasone is at its lowest around 90 days. However, sometimes Ozurdex can be used as a "bridge" in these more serious conditions to rapidly gain control of inflammation or resolve macular edema while systemic therapies are initiated, that typically take 3–4 weeks to become effective.

The most difficult clinical decision is deciding on treatment for chronic, aggressive posterior disease. The typical decision is a tough choice between longterm oral therapy, Retisert® implantation, or repeated Ozurdex. Sometimes the choice can be pretty straightforward, such as a young phakic patient where oral therapy would be more favorable, or a young female trying to have children, where Ozurdex® or Retisert® would be more logical. While longterm repeated Ozurdex has been used successfully with a lower incidence of IOP rise compared to Retisert®, one still worries about aggressive disease and the nadir that occurs every 3 months as the drug runs out subjecting a patient to a possible uveitis flare and irrecoverable loss of vision.

Understanding the clinical disease, the benefits and risk of treatment help guide the clinician in the choice of treatment. The Ozurdex® implant has greatly expanded that choice.

Conclusion

Uveitis tends to be a chronic, smoldering disease. The development of the Ozurdex® implant has allowed a very effective therapy for the treatment of uveitis with a better side effect profile compared to the operating room placed Retisert® implant. The novel development of the polymer used in the implant has the benefit of not leaving any residual implanted material in the eye, dissolving to just water and carbon dioxide. As sustained intraocular delivery of drugs continue to evolve, Ozurdex® represents a significant step in this evolution and treatment of uveitis.

References

1. Martin DF, Parks DJ, Mellow SD, et al. Treatment of cytomegalovirus retinitis with an intraocular sustained-release ganciclovir implant. A randomized controlled clinical trial. Arch Ophthalmol. 1994;112 (12):1531–9.
2. Musch DC, Martin DF, Gordon JF, Davis MD, Kuppermann BD. Treatment of cytomegalovirus retinitis with a sustained-release ganciclovir implant. The Ganciclovir Implant Study Group. N Engl J Med. 1997;337(2):83–90.
3. Sanborn GE, Anand R, Torti RE, et al. Sustained-release ganciclovir therapy for treatment of cytomegalovirus retinitis. Use of an intravitreal device. Arch Ophthalmol. 1992;110(2):188–95.
4. Callanan DG, Jaffe GJ, Martin DF, Pearson PA, Comstock TL. Treatment of posterior uveitis with a fluocinolone acetonide implant: three-year clinical trial results. Arch Ophthalmol. 2008;126(9):1191–201.
5. Goldstein DA, Godfrey DG, Hall A, et al. Intraocular pressure in patients with uveitis treated with fluocinolone acetonide implants. Arch Ophthalmol. 2007;125(11):1478–85.
6. Jaffe GJ, Martin D, Callanan D, Pearson PA, Levy B, Comstock T. Fluocinolone acetonide implant (Retisert) for noninfectious posterior uveitis: thirty-four-week results of a multicenter randomized clinical study. Ophthalmology. 2006;113(6):1020–7.
7. Williams GA, Haller JA, Kuppermann BD, et al. Dexamethasone posterior-segment drug delivery

system in the treatment of macular edema resulting from uveitis or Irvine-Gass syndrome. Am J Ophthalmol. 2009;147(6):1048–54, 1054.e1.
8. Bratton ML, He YG, Weakley DR. Dexamethasone intravitreal implant (Ozurdex) for the treatment of pediatric uveitis. J AAPOS. 2014;18 (2):110–3.
9. Cordero-Coma M, Garzo I, Calleja S, Galan E, Franco M, Ruiz de Morales JG. Preoperative cataract surgery use of an intravitreal dexamethasone implant (Ozurdex) in a patient with juvenile idiopathic arthritis and chronic anterior uveitis. J AAPOS. 2013;17(6):632–4.
10. Kumari N, Parchand S, Kaushik S, Singh R. Intractable glaucoma necessitating dexamethasone implant (Ozurdex) removal and glaucoma surgery in a child with uveitis. BMJ Case Rep. 2013;2013.
11. Cao JH, Mulvalhill M, Zhang L, Joondeph BC, Dacey MS. Dexamethasone Intravitreal Implant in the treatment of persistent uveitic macular edema in the absence of active inflammation. Ophthalmology 2014.
12. Tomkins-Netzer O, Taylor SR, Bar A, et al. Treatment with repeat dexamethasone implants results in long-term disease control in eyes with noninfectious uveitis. Ophthalmology 2014.
13. Malcles A, Janin-Manificat H, Yhuel Y, et al. Anterior chamber migration of intravitreal dexamethasone implant (Ozurdex(R)) in pseudophakic eyes: report of three cases. J Fr Ophtalmol. 2013;36 (4):362–7.

Part V
Complications

Cataracts

47

George N. Papaliodis

Introduction

Cataracts are a leading cause of blindness worldwide and remain an important cause of visual impairment and blindness in the United States accounting for approximately 50 % of visual impairment in adults over the age of 40 [1]. By age 80, over 50 % of all Americans will have cataracts [2]. Cataracts are a common complication associated with uveitis as the intraocular inflammation and the most commonly used therapy for the management of the disorder, corticosteroids, can both induce lenticular opacification. In a large retrospective study from the UK evaluating complications associated with uveitis management and following these patients for 22 years, the most common reported complication was the development of cataract (35 % of patients) [3]. Other case series have documented the incidence of cataracts in patients with uveitis ranges from 30 to 78 % (more common in patients with Fuchs heterochromic iridocyclitis and juvenile idiopathic arthritis and uveitis syndrome). The development of lenticular changes is influenced by the chronicity and severity of intraocular inflammation, the frequency and duration of steroid use, and the underlying diagnosis.

G.N. Papaliodis (✉)
Department of Ophthalmology, Harvard Medical School, Massachusetts Eye and Ear Infirmary, Boston, MA, USA
e-mail: George_Papaliodis@meei.harvard.edu

G.N. Papaliodis (ed.), *Uveitis*,
DOI 10.1007/978-3-319-09126-6_47

Risk Factors

The risk factors for the development of cataracts have been well described and include: advanced age, diabetes, steroid use (inhaled, systemic, periocular, intraocular, topical ophthalmic), family history of cataracts, UV light exposure, ionizing radiation, ocular trauma, prior intraocular surgery, intraocular inflammation, and tobacco use [4–6]. Patients who develop uveitic cataracts often have multiple mechanisms that may contribute to cataractogenesis and progression. The two most commonly implicated predisposing factors for uveitic cataracts include the presence of intraocular inflammation and the use of corticosteroids.

Decision to Operate

The decision to operate on a patient with a uveitic cataract is not a simple determination. There are multiple considerations that must be assessed and discussed with the patient. Objective measures such as visual acuity, the status of the inflammatory disease, and the presence of lenticular opacification can be evaluated via clinical exam. Equally important are the patient's subjective symptoms including blurry vision at distance/intermediate/near, glare with bright lights and oncoming headlights while driving and specific limitations that impair quality of life (e.g. avoiding night driving, difficulty reading, inability to play sports, etc.). Foster and Rashid have described 4 clinical indications for cataract surgery in patients with uveitis including: phacoantigenic uveitis, visually significant cataract in a quiet eye with good visual prognosis, cataract impairing posterior segment examination, and cataract impairing the ability to perform posterior segment surgery [7]. The benefits of cataract surgery have been extensively studied including improvement in visual acuity, improvement in the performance of activities of daily living, reduction of risk of injury from falls, improved mental health, and general sense of well-being. In observational studies after cataract surgery, up to 90 % of patients undergoing first eye cataract surgery noted improvement in functional status and satisfaction with vision [8].

Perioperative Management

The recommendations for perioperative management are based on cohort studies demonstrating successful surgical outcomes with uveitic cataracts [9]. The following are general principles extrapolated from these sources:

- for elective procedures like cataract surgery, the patient should have no evidence of active uveitis by standard criteria for 3 months preceding the surgery
- if immunosuppressive medications were required for disease control, these should be continued through the perioperative period
- prophylactic topical steroids initiated one week prior to surgery are associated with decreased post-operative inflammation (the frequency of administration ranges from QID to q 1 h while awake as dictated by severity of ocular inflammatory disease); some surgeons have advocated for prophylactic topical NSAIDs for one week prior to surgery to reduce incidence of cystoid macular edema (but the data is less compelling)
- for patients with severe, difficult to control ocular inflammatory disease (Behcet's, juvenile idiopathic arthritis and uveitis syndrome), prophylactic systemic corticosteroids (Prednisone one mg/kg/day) can be prescribed for one week prior to surgery and tapered after the procedure as guided by the degree of ocular inflammation
- intravenous methylprednisolone in doses of 500–1000 mg administered at the time of surgery has also demonstrated efficacy in reduction of post-operative inflammation
- intraocular triamcinolone (0.05–0.1 cc of 40 mg/ml concentration) injected in the vitreous or anterior chamber has been correlated with reduction of post-operative cystoid macular edema and intraocular inflammation
- post-operative regimens vary considerably but generally include a topical steroid, topical non-steroidal anti-inflammatory agent, and topical antibiotic.

Surgery

Surgical procedures for cataract removal have tremendously improved over the last 60 years and continue to evolve. With the advent of phacoemulsification, injectable intraocular lens implants and small incision cataract surgery, patients can appreciate rapid visual rehabilitation, restoration of excellent visual acuity, and few post-operative restrictions. Multiple studies have demonstrated that cataract extraction via phacoemulsification causes less overall inflammation and fewer complications compared to traditional extracapsular cataract extraction in uveitic cataracts [10]. The goals of the surgical procedure include:

- construction of a small incision wound that allows for adequate fluidically stable anterior chamber during surgery [11]
- minimal manipulation of the iris if avoidable (in patients with posterior synechiae this may not be possible as synechialysis and placement of iris retraction instruments may be required for adequate visualization of the lens)
- complete removal of all lens material (any residual lens particles may induce post-operative inflammation)
- implantation of a posterior chamber intraocular lens within the capsular bag (lens implants in the sulcus and anterior chamber are associated with greater degree of intraocular inflammation)
- a secure, watertight incision that does not induce surgical astigmatism and may reduce pre-existing corneal astigmatism.

A new advance to cataract surgery, the femtosecond laser, can be used to construct corneal incisions, perform anterior capsulotomy, and fragment the nucleus. At the time of this publication, there is inadequate data in patients with uveitic cataracts who have used this modality of augmented cataract surgery to determine superiority versus traditional phacoemulsification.

Complications of Cataract Surgery

In general, complications of cataract surgery are relatively uncommon and patients have a high expectation of visual improvement after surgery. Stein et al. reviewed cataract surgery in Medicare recipients in 2005–2006 and found that the overall rate of severe complications (defined as endophthalmitis, suprachoroidal hemorrhage and retinal detachment) was 0.4 % [12]. The uveitic cataract poses greater challenge and has been associated with higher complication rates.

Yamane et al. published one of the largest retrospective case series of 242 uveitic eyes who underwent cataract surgery by phacoemulsification. Recurrence of uveitis was the most common postoperative complication seen in 73 eyes (30.16 %). Other postoperative complications included iris atrophy (28.51 %), ocular hypertension (28.09 %), epiretinal membrane (26.44 %), posterior capsule opacification (19 %), cystoid macular edema (13.63 %), ocular hypotony (12.80 %), optic disc atrophy (8.67 %) and posterior synechiae (6.61 %) [13]. Of note, 10.7 % of patients in this study lost vision compared to pre-operative visual acuity with the presence of the cataract [13].

Despite these issues, cataract surgery remains highly successful in this patient population. Mehta et al. published a meta-analysis of uveitic cataract surgical series and reported that 68 % of uveitis patients who underwent phacoemulsification and had quiet or nearly quiet disease prior to surgery had 20/40 visual acuity or better following the procedure [14].

Lens Implant Selection

The decision regarding selection of lens implant material and style to achieve superior surgical results in uveitis patients is complicated and remains largely unresolved. Proponents of hydrophilic lens implant materials argue that these lenses can be inserted through a smaller incision reducing tissue trauma but have a higher propensity to induce posterior capsular opacification compared to hydrophobic lens implants. Hydrophobic lens implants have good uveal and excellent capsular biocompatibility but may require a larger incision for insertion.

Heparin surface modification (HSM) of lens implant materials has been demonstrated in multiple studies to be associated with reduced intraocular inflammation [15, 16]. The binding of heparin to the lens implant is thought to prevent attachment of bacteria, corneal endothelial cells, and lens epithelial cells. Lin et al. performed cataract surgery in high risk patients (defined as having a diagnosis of either diabetes, glaucoma or uveitis) and randomized the study participants into 1 of 2 groups: heparin surface modified intraocular lens versus traditional PMMA lens implant. Short term clinical follow up demonstrated significantly less anterior chamber cell in the HSM IOL group compared to the traditional PMMA group. When these patients were followed long term, there was no statistically significant difference between the 2 groups in visual acuity, corneal edema, anterior chamber reaction, and amount of posterior synechia formation and IOL deposits [16].

Silicone was the first material available for foldable intraocular lens implants. While silicone has a very low rate of posterior capsular opacification compared to others [17], the use of this implant material has steadily declined over the last 10 years. There are multiple reasons this implant material has become less popular despite the excellent biocompatibility profile. In the era of small incision cataract surgery (wound size less than 2.8 mm) and preloaded lens injectors, there is a risk of tearing of the optic at the optic—haptic junction or kinking of the haptics. Additionally, if the patient develops a retinal detachment in the future requiring silicone oil, there have been case reports of silicone oil droplets adherent to the posterior surface of the silicone lens implant [18].

Leung et al. pooled data from 4 randomized control trials comparing hydrophilic or hydrophobic acrylic lenses, silicone lenses, polymethyl methacrylate (PMMA) lens implants with or without HSM. The review included 216 patients with substantial heterogeneity with respect to ages of participants and etiology of uveitis. Patient outcome measures included visual acuity, posterior capsular opacification, cystoid macular edema, corneal edema, and lens decentration. Based on this review, the authors concluded that it is still uncertain which implant material provided the best visual and clinical outcomes in patients with uveitis undergoing cataract surgery [19].

Conclusion

The development of cataract is the most common complication in patients with uveitis as both intraocular inflammation and corticosteroids (the most frequently employed treatment) can induce progressive opacification of the lens. The surgical procedure can be technically difficult given multiple potentially challenging issues including corneal opacities, poor dilation, posterior synechiae, unstable zonules, capsular abnormalities, etc. Aside from navigating these demanding surgical problems, the resultant post-operative inflammation can negate any potential visual improvement that may be derived by the removal of the lens. Despite these limitations, cataract surgery remains highly successful even in patients with uveitis.

There are many unresolved controversies including:

1. What is the best intraocular lens material with lowest rates of posterior capsular opacification, biocompatibility, and macular edema?
2. Should intraocular lens implants be used in all uveitis patients including those with Behcet's disease and juvenile idiopathic arthritis and uveitis syndrome?
3. Are multifocal intraocular lens implants appropriate for uveitis patients?
4. Is the femtosecond laser a less traumatic and thus safer manner to assist with lens removal in uveitis patients?
5. What is the most effective perioperative and postoperative management strategy to avoid significant post operative inflammation?

In an effort to practice evidence based medicine, there is continued need for large cohort studies and/or randomized clinical trials to scientifically address these issues.

References

1. Congdon N, Vingerling JR, Klein BE, et al. Prevalence of cataract and pseudophakia/aphakia among adults in the United States. Arch Ophthalmol. 2004;122:487–94.
2. Prevent Blindness America. Vision problems in the US: prevalence of adult vision impairment and age-related eye disease in America. In: 2008 update to the fourth edition. Chicago, IL: Prevent Blindness America; 2008. p. 23.

3. Jones NP1. The Manchester Uveitis Clinic: the first 3000 patients, 2: uveitis manifestations, complications, medical and surgical management. Ocul Immunol Inflamm. 2014:1–8.
4. West SK, Valmadrid CT. Epidemiology of risk factors for age-related cataract. Surv Ophthalmol. 1995;39:323–34.
5. Cumming RG, Mitchell P, Leeder SR. Use of inhaled corticosteroids and the risk of cataracts. N Engl J Med. 1997;337:8–14.
6. Urban RC Jr, Cotlier E. Corticosteroid-induced cataracts. Surv Ophthalmol. 1986;31:102–10.
7. Foster CS, Rashid S. Management of coincident cataract and uveitis. Curr Opin Ophthalmol. 2003;14:1–6.
8. Mangione CM, Phillips SR, Lawrence MG, et al. Improved visual function and attenuation of declines in health-related quality of life after cataract extraction. Arch Ophthalmol. 1994;112:1419–52.
9. Foster CS, Fong LP, Singh G. Cataract surgery and intraocular lens implantation in patients with uveitis. Ophthalmology 1989;(96)3:281–88.
10. Estafanous MF, Lowder CY, Meisler DM, et al. Phacoemulsification cataract extraction and posterior chamber lens implantation in patients with uveitis. Am J Ophthalmol. 2001;131:620–5.
11. Liyanage SE, Agunawela RI, et al. Anterior chamber instability caused by incisional leakage in coaxial phacoemulsification. J Cataract Refract Surgery. 2009;35:1003–5.
12. Stein JD, Grossman DS, et al. Severe adverse events after cataract surgery among medicare beneficiaries. Ophthalmology. 2011;118:1716–23.
13. Yamane Cde L1, Vianna RN, Cardoso GP, Deschênes J, Burnier MN Jr. Cataract extraction using the phacoemulsification technique in patients with uveitis. Arq Bras Oftalmol. 2007;70(4):683–8.
14. Mehta S1, Linton MM2, Kempen JH3. Outcomes of cataract surgery in patients with uveitis: a systematic review and meta-analysis. Am J Ophthalmol. 2014;158(4):676–692.e7. doi:10.1016/j.ajo.2014.06.018. Epub 2014 Jun 28.
15. Percival SPC, Pai V. Heparin-modified lenses for eyes at risk for breakdown of the blood-aqueous barrier during cataract surgery. J Cataract Refract Surg. 1993;19:760–5.
16. Lin CL, Wang AG, Chou JC, Shieh G, Liu JH. Heparin-sur-face-modified intraocular lens implantation in patients with glaucoma, diabetes, or uveitis. J Cataract Refract Surg. 1994;20:550–3.
17. Findl O, Menapace R, Sacu S, et al. Effect of optic material on posterior capsule opacification in intraocular lenses with sharp-edge optics: randomized clinical trial. Ophthalmology. 2005;112(1):67–72.
18. Bartz-Schmidt KU1, Konen W, Esser P, Walter P, Heimann K. Intraocular silicone lenses and silicone oil. Klin Monbl Augenheilkd. 1995;207(3):162–6.
19. Leung TG1, Lindsley K, Kuo IC. Types of intraocular lenses for cataract surgery in eyes with uveitis. Cochrane Database Syst Rev. 2014;3:CD007284. doi:10.1002/14651858.CD007284.pub2

Macular Edema

48

Cynthia X. Qian and Lucia Sobrin

Introduction

Macular edema (ME) is a common complication and cause of visual impairment in patients with noninfectious uveitis, occurring in 33–46 % of all patients [1]. It is a challenging condition to treat. As compared to ME secondary to intraocular surgery, uveitic ME is much less likely to resolve spontaneously and can persist after control of inflammation is established, causing long-standing irreversible changes and photoreceptor damage. In recent years, use of optical coherence tomography (OCT) imaging has revolutionized our understanding and diagnosis of this condition. The concurrent investigation of novel pharmacological agents has expanded treatment options for this condition.

C.X. Qian
Department of Ophthalmology, Retina Service, Massachusetts Eye and Ear Infirmary, 12th Floor, 243 Charles Street, Boston, MA 02114, USA
e-mail: cynthia_qian@meei.harvard.edu

L. Sobrin (✉)
Department of Ophthalmology, Harvard Medical School, Massachusetts Eye and Ear Infirmary, 243 Charles Street, 12th Floor, Boston, MA 02114, USA
e-mail: lucia_sobrin@meei.harvard.edu

G.N. Papaliodis (ed.), *Uveitis*,
DOI 10.1007/978-3-319-09126-6_48

Diagnosis

ME may arise with uveitis from any location or etiology, although it is more common with intermediate and posterior uveitis [2–4]. Fundus examination at the slit lamp with a contact lens has now also been aided by ancillary tests for ME detection. While fluorescein angiography (FA) still holds a role in ME, this imaging modality has been largely supplanted by optical coherence tomography (OCT). This technology is fast, noninvasive, and highly reproducible from visit to visit and from examiner to examiner [5]. OCT allows identification of various patterns of ME: diffuse edema, cystoid edema, and presence of serous retinal detachment (SRD) (Fig. 48.1) [6]. OCT also can reveal vitreomacular traction (VMT) and epiretinal membranes (ERM), two entities that can cause ME and may need to be addressed in addition to uveitic inflammation control to eliminate ME. Central subfield macular thickness (CSMT) measurements from OCT can be followed to quantitatively assess response to treatment. FA's role is most useful in detecting cases of isolated "angiographic" edema—cases where there is leakage on FA but no thickening on OCT. This scenario can appear at any point in the course of disease but may be more common when the retina becomes atrophic and macular edema can no longer manifest as cystic changes. FA is also valuable in determining the presence of angiographic retinal vasculitis when evidence of vasculitis is not seen on examination (Fig. 48.2). Detection of such vasculitis suggests the need for

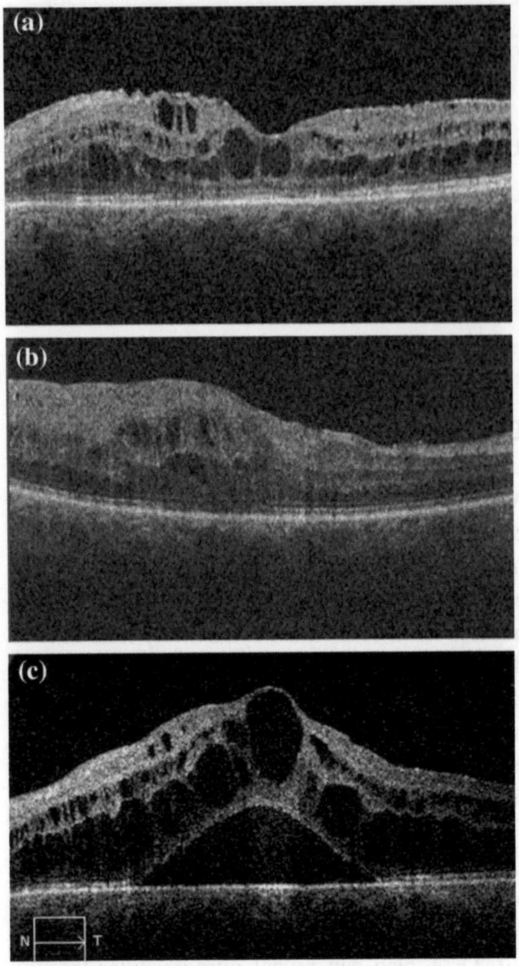

Fig. 48.1 Different patterns of uveitic macular edema. **a** Cystoid macular edema (CME). Optical coherence tomography (OCT) shows well-defined intraretinal cystoid spaces in the central macula. **b** Diffuse macular edema (DME). OCT shows sponge-like thickening of the macula. **c** CME with serous retinal detachment. OCT shows well-defined cystoid spaces and fluid under the neurosensory retina

more aggressive anti-inflammatory therapy to control the intraocular inflammation and associated ME [6, 7].

Treatments

The pathophysiology underlying uveitic ME is complex and poorly understood. It is thought that vascular permeability in the inner blood–retinal barrier (BRB) of the macular area and retinal pigment epithelial dysfunction within the outer blood–retinal barrier may play a role. In addition, intraocular inflammation from systemic diseases may also induce the release of diverse inflammatory mediators and cytokines such as interleukins, tumor necrosis factor-alpha (TNF-alpha), and vascular endothelial growth factor (VEGF), influencing both BRBs. All these sites and molecules are possible targets for treatment [2, 8].

It is generally advisable to follow and treat any uveitic ME promptly. Better visual acuity at baseline, younger age, and short duration of ME are all prognostic factors of favorable functional and anatomical outcome [4, 9–11]. The most important principle in treating uveitic macular edema is to ensure that the uveitis is completely controlled. Subclinical uveitic inflammation is often the reason for recalcitrant or recurrent macular edema. Searching for subclinical vasculitis with FA as described above is one way to uncover occult inflammation that needs to be more aggressively treated. However, ME can also be found in quiescent uveitic eyes. ME in quiescent eyes can be quite difficult to treat, as the ME is often chronic and associated with irreparable damage to the BRB [9, 12].

There are many different ways to classify the different treatment modalities of noninfectious uveitic ME. The most common way of separating treatments is by delivery mode: topical, local, and systemic. The general approach is to use topical or local treatment as the first-line but not to delay using systemic therapy when the disease is severe at the onset or persistent with regional therapy. Each category will be covered below. These treatment options are summarized in Table 48.1.

Topical Therapy

Topical NSAIDs

While topical non-steroidal anti-inflammatory drugs (NSAIDs) have proven very useful in pseudophakic ME, studies have shown that there

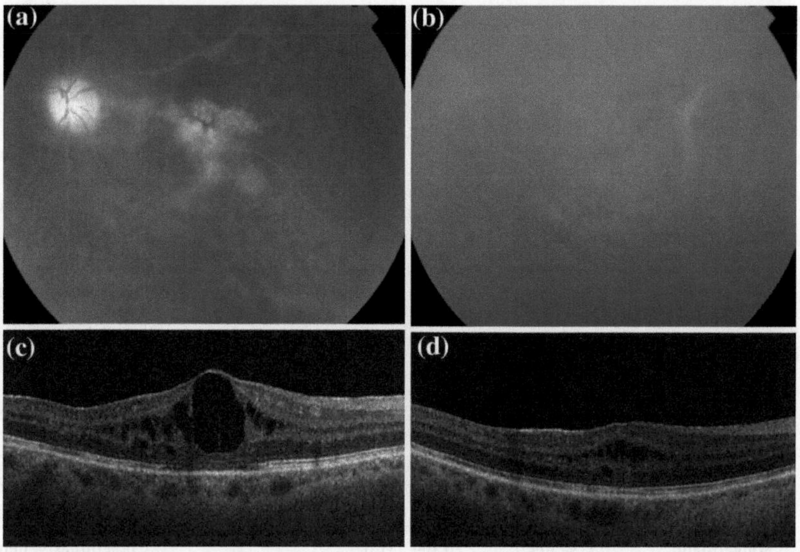

Fig. 48.2 A 58 year-old woman with idiopathic panuveitis and persistent macular edema in her left eye. Vision in the left eye was 20/50. Edema had failed to respond or recurred with intravitreal triamcinolone, intravitreal bevacizumab, and pars plana vitrectomy. Uveitis was being treated with methotrexate. **a** Late-phase fluorescein angiogram shows petalloid leakage in the macula consistent with macular edema. In addition, there is disc staining suggesting ongoing uveitis activity. **b** Peripheral fluorescein angiogram frame shows perivascular leakage suggesting subclinical, ongoing retinal vasculitis as a cause for the patient's persistent macular edema. **c** OCT shows significant cystic changes. **d** The patient was switched from methotrexate to infliximab. After 6 months of infliximab therapy, and without any additional treatment for the macular edema, her macular edema improved significantly and vision increased to 20/32

Table 48.1 Adjunctive treatments for uveitic macular edema

Name	Trade name	Route	Dosage	Note	Side effects
Corticosteroids					
Prednisone	Prednisone, Deltasone	Oral	0.5–1 mg/kg		Weight gain, hypertension, diabetes, cardiovascular events, ischemic necrosis hip, osteoporosis, cataract, glaucoma
Triamcinolone acetate	Kenalog, Triescence (Preservative-Free)	Intravitreal	1–4 mg		Cataract, glaucoma, endophthalmitis, retinal detachment
		Sub-Tenon's or inferior trans-septal	40 mg/1 ml		Ptosis with sub-Tenon's injection, fat prolapse through septum with inferior trans-septal injection
Fluocinolone acetonide sustained release	Retisert	Intravitreal implant	0.59 mg/implant	Duration approx. 30 month	High rate of cataract, glaucoma
Dexamethasone sustained release	Ozurdex	Intravitreal implant	0.7 mg/implant	Longer duration than IVTA in vitrectomized eyes	Cataract, glaucoma

(continued)

Table 48.1 (continued)

Name	Trade name	Route	Dosage	Note	Side effects
Non-corticosteroid intravitreal drugs					
Ranibizumab	Lucentis	Intravitreal	0.5 mg	Duration 6–8 week	Transient IOP rise, endophthalmitis, cataract, possible small increased risk of CVA, MI and other thromboembolic events
Bevacizumab	Avastin	Intravitreal	1.25 mg or 2.5 mg	Duration 6–8 week	
Methotrexate		Intravitreal	400 μg	Repeat q 4 month	Corneal epitheliopathy, band keratopathy, cataract progression, IOP rise, endophthalmitis
Non-steroidal anti-inflammatory drugs					
Naproxen	Naprosyn	Systemic	250 mg po BID	Limited efficacy in uveitic ME	GI upset, nausea
Somatostatin and somatostatin analogue					
Somatostatin	Somatostatin	Systemic	100 μg SC TID		Cutaneous flush, nausea, diarrhea, elevated LFTs hypothyroidism,
Octreotide Long Acting Repeatable (LAR)	Somatostatin analogue	Systemic	20 mg IM q mon		Cholelithiasis, ileus, dysglycemia
Carbonic anhydrase inhibitor					
Acetazolamide	Diamox	Systemic	500 mg po BID or QD	May need long-term maintenance dosage at 125–250 mg QD	Paresthesia, nausea, GI, fatigue, weight loss, polyuria, rash
Interferons					
IFN alpha 2a IFN alpha 2b	Roferon A Intron A	Systemic	3–6 million IU SC QD initially	Maintenance dosing is 2–3 times/week	Flu-like sx, depression
IFN beta	Avonex	Systemic	44 mg SC 3 times/week	Intermediate uveitis, MS-associated ME	Flu-like sx, elevated LFTs, alopecia

CVA Cerebrovascular accident; *GI* gastrointestinal; *IM* intramuscular; *Ini* initial dosage; *IU* International Units; *LFTs* liver function tests; *Max* maximum dosage; *MI* myocardial infarction; *MS* multiple sclerosis; *N/V* nausea/vomiting; *SC* subcutaneous; *Sx* symptoms

is limited to no role for topical NSAID monotherapy in the treatment of inflammatory ME. This class of medications may have a weak synergistic effect when used in conjunction with other local therapies such as intravitreal triamcinolone acetate (IVTA) or intravitreal anti-VEGF, prolonging the effect of CSMT reduction [13]. There is a higher concentration NSAID, indomethacin 0.5 %, which when administered 4 times daily, has shown some early promise in uveitic ME [14].

Topical Corticosteroids

Topical prednisolone 1 % has shown more success than topical NSAIDs in decreasing vascular permeability and inflammatory-mediated reactions. However, its poor penetration to the posterior segment still limits its utility and the general principle is that topical corticosteroids may be used primarily for mild ME. There is a higher chance of achieving sufficient drug levels around the macula in pseudophakic or aphakic patients

More recently, difluprednate, a more potent topical corticosteroid, has become available. In the pediatric population, its use has been associated with an improvement in uveitic ME in 78 % (7/9) of studied eyes and a mean decrease in CSMT of 192 μm [15]. Because difluprednate is more potent, cataract and intraocular pressure (IOP) rise can occur earlier and be more severe than with topical prednisolone. Close monitoring for these side effects is important.

Local Corticosteroid Therapy

Periocular Corticosteroids

Periocular corticosteroid is often effective for treating uveitic ME and is a common first-line therapy. Triamcinolone acetate 40 mg injected into the posterior sub-Tenon's space or transeptally into the inferior orbital floor is one commonly used injectable steroid. The goal of periocular steroid injection is to bring the medication as immediately adjacent to the site of inflammation as possible. Hence, some have suggested that delivering the medication in the sub-Tenon's location may be more effective than orbital floor injection, but this has not been definitively proven. The sub-Tenon's injection is usually delivered using the Smith and Nozik method with lid retraction and drug delivery with a 16 mm 25-gauge needle into the posterior superotemporal space with the bevel facing the globe. A trans-septal injection is delivered at the lateral third of the inferior orbital rim with a 25- or 27-gauge needle [16]. A study looked at the location of the deposited steroid injection using ultrasound scanning immediately before and after sub-Tenon's corticosteroid injection [17]. It found that a superotemporal depot is more successful than an inferotemporal depot in delivering the medication to the macular area.

Leder et al. [18] reviewed the results of their experience over a decade for 156 eyes and found that 53 % of eyes treated with a single periocular corticosteroid injection had complete clinical resolution of ME within one month of injection. An additional 22 % of eyes needed repeated periocular injections in one month intervals to achieve resolution. In most depot cases, removal after instillation is very difficult. Hence, close follow-up for IOP control and cataract development is essential. Single injections have limited rates of complications, but with repeated applications these side effects will increase. There are also side effects specific to periocular delivery methods. Trans-septal injections may cause adipose tissue prolapse through the septum, particularly if multiple injections are given, while superior sub-Tenon's injections may lead to ptosis.

Intravitreal Corticosteroids

IVTA has been reported to be non-inferior if not superior to periocular corticosteroid use [19]. It is commonly used in cases of ME that are incompletely responsive to periocular corticosteroids. As with periocular corticosteroid injections, it can used as a fast-acting treatment for ME while waiting for longer acting systemic medication to take effect. A single injection of 4 mg/0.1 ml IVTA has clinical efficacy for approximately 2–6 months in non-vitrectomized eyes [20]. In some cases, just one IVTA can result in ME resolution without recurrence, but control of the underlying uveitis inflammation is imperative for this result. One large series in the literature followed 65 eyes over 8 months and detected a 83 % response rate to 4 mg of IVTA with significant visual improvement with 51 % of patients gaining >2 Snellen lines [11]. Half-dose IVTA (2 mg/0.05 ml) produced an 80 % resolution of ME in a 29-patient cohort, with 39 % of eyes gaining >2 Snellen lines [21]. Studies in diabetic patients have shown 4 mg IVTA to cause no additional retinotoxic effect [22]. However, benzyl alcohol at concentrations slightly higher than that which is present in some commercially available triamcinolone preparations caused histological damage to outer retinal structures in rabbits [23]. Therefore, removal of preservatives from a preservative-containing corticosteroid solution is recommendable. Currently, the preservative-free formulation of triamcinolone acetate (Triescence) is the agent of choice due to its design specifically for intraocular use [2]. Intravitreal injections have the associated risks of endophthalmitis (0.5–0.87 %), cataracts leading to cataract surgery (15–20 % of elderly patients within 1 year of injection), IOP spikes in about 30–40 % of eyes leading to surgical glaucoma intervention in about 1–2 % of cases and other retinal complications including retinal detachment [24, 25].

Corticosteroid Implants

Fluocinolone acetonide (Retisert) and dexamethasone (Ozurdex) intravitreal implants are both sustained-release corticosteroid devices. Both were designed in an attempt to create longer lasting local treatments for uveitis with a possibility of reducing dependency on systemic corticosteroids and immunosuppressive agents. They both also show efficacy in the treatment of uveitic ME. The 0.59 mg fluocinolone implant has been approved since 2005 by the FDA for the treatment of noninfectious intermediate, posterior and panuveitis. It releases fluocinolone acetonide at an initial rate of 0.6 μg/day in the first month, then decreasing to a steady state of 0.3–0.4 μg/day for approximately 3 years thereafter. This implant requires surgical placement in the operating room. While the main indication for fluocinolone implantation is to control uveitic inflammation, the implant is also efficacious in controlling the associated ME.

The implant was investigated for the treatment of uveitis and ME in a prospective randomized study of 278 patients. In the study, not only did the implants significantly reduce uveitis recurrence and decrease need for adjunctive treatment, of the 100 patients with uveitic ME, a quarter of eyes had a >3 line of sustained visual acuity improvement at 34 weeks [26]. The great efficacy of the fluocinolone implant is accompanied by significant rates of corticosteroid-related side effects. At three years after implantation, greater than 90 % of implanted phakic eyes will require cataract surgery [27] and a >10 mmHg IOP rise from baseline occurs in more than 70 % of eyes [28]. IOP-lowering surgery will be necessary in at least of third of eyes. In addition, there is also a small risk of retinal complications including detachment with the placement of the fluocinolone implant [29, 30]. In summary, in cases of uveitic ME where there is ongoing underlying uveitic inflammation, the fluocinolone implant is very likely to result in concurrent improvement or complete resolution of the ME but with a high likelihood of IOP rise and cataract formation.

The dexamethasone 0.7 mg implant is also approved for the treatment of noninfectious intermediate, posterior and panuveitis. Its duration of effect is 4–6 months. It can be injected intravitreally in the clinic, obviating the need to go to the operating room. With regards to ME, the dexamethasone intravitreal implant has been shown to significantly decrease CSMT in patients with uveitic ME, including pediatric patients and those previously refractory to treatment with IVTA, periocular corticosteroids or anti-VEGF [31, 32]. The improvement in visual acuity, which is due in large part to resolution of ME in these patients, has been shown to take effect with one single injection and to manifest in a best-corrected visual acuity (BCVA) gain of >2 lines in more than half of patients at 3 months and in more than a quarter of eyes at 2 years [32, 33]. With repeated dexamethasone intravitreal implant injections, the rates of cataract development and ocular hypertension were approximately 10 and 20 %, respectively, in one series [34]. The dexamethasone implant is particularly useful in treating ME in vitrectomized eyes where the duration of directly injected corticosteroid can be very short.

Local Non-corticosteroid Therapy

Intravitreal Anti-VEGF Compounds

Bevacizumab (Avastin) and ranibizumab (Lucentis), recombinant humanized monoclonal antibodies directed against VEGF, have both been used in the treatment of uveitic ME. It is believed that anti-VEGF drugs may inhibit the breakdown of the blood–retinal barrier and hence decrease vascular leakage and fluid accumulation leading to ME [2]. Ranibizumab 0.5 mg intravitreal injections can improve vision and reduce ME. In a small group of seven patients with refractory ME who failed corticosteroid treatment, all patients receiving intravitreal ranibizumab demonstrated improvement in vision by one month [35]. The mean gain of vision was 13 letters at the 6-month time point with monthly injections administered on an as needed basis. Similarly, many centers have studied the use of bevacizumab (1.25 mg or 2.5 mg) for the same purposes due to its wide availability and better cost competitiveness [36]. Single or repeated injections of intravitreal bevacizumab lead to a reduction in CSMT and improvement in vision of >2 Snellen lines in approximately 40–50 % of patients [36, 37]. Intravitreal anti-VEGF agents have the advantage over corticosteroids of causing less cataract and IOP rise. However, they are also more transient in effect and do not have any significant anti-inflammatory effect to treat concomitant uveitis [38–41]. In a randomized clinical trial of 31 eyes comparing use of 1–3 intravitreal bevacizumab injections to 1–3 injections of IVTA for refractory uveitic ME, the IVTA group did manifest better control of leakage and CSMT reduction [42].

Intravitreal NSAIDs

Diclofenac 500 μg/0.1 ml has been previously administered safely intravitreally in the eyes of some patients with uveitic ME with no signs of ocular toxicity at 8-week follow-up. However, when comparing IVTA and intravitreal diclofenac (IVD) head-to-head, it was found that while IVTA significantly reduced CSMT and increased mean BCVA at 6 and 24 months of study, the IVD group did not reach any statistically significant changes in these parameters [43]. Further study on intravitreal NSAIDs are needed to establish efficacy for uveitic ME.

Intravitreal Methotrexate

Locally, intravitreal methotrexate at a dose of 400 μg has been used in pilot studies with success as an alternative to intraocular steroid therapy in known steroid responders with uveitis and ME [44]. In one trial, 13 of 15 patients enrolled responded to a single intravitreal methotrexate injection with increase in acuity and decrease in macular thickness [45]. Mean macular thickness decreased from 425 to 275 μm and mean visual improvement was 4.5 lines at six months follow-up. The effect of the intravitreal drug lasted for an average of four months and may be repeated as needed. In the 2-year follow-up study, four patients achieved extended remission for longer than 12 months while four others experienced continued partial ME resolution [46]. The other five patients who had initially responded relapsed into bilateral reactivation and were switched to systemic corticosteroid rescue therapy. Intravitreal methotrexate holds promise as a treatment for uveitic ME, particularly in patients with a history of IOP rise with corticosteroids.

Systemic Therapy

Systemic NSAIDs

It has been suggested that systemic NSAID therapy may have a role in treating uveitic ME or preventing recurrence of ME after inflammation is controlled. However, there is no strong evidence that these agents are effective for this clinical problem. One study demonstrated a 52 % drop-out rate amongst 66 patients after 4 months of treatment with oral NSAIDs for ME due to adverse effects, inefficacy or both [47]. If oral NSAIDs are given for this indication, patients must be actively monitored for the risks of gastrointestinal ulceration and kidney and liver toxicity.

Corticosteroids

Systemic corticosteroids have been a mainstay in the treatment of both uveitic inflammation and ME, especially in cases not responsive to local treatment alone. Most commonly patients are treated with prednisone 0.5 mg–1 mg/kg with a taper over 2–3 months. A recent OCT study demonstrated that ME resolution was more rapid with systemic oral corticosteroids when compared with periocular steroid injections with significant visual acuity correlation [48]. The short-term side effects of corticosteroids that should be explained to patients are increased appetite and associated weight gain, difficulty sleeping and mood changes. If the patient's ME recurs with systemic corticosteroid tapering, it is important to consider advancing to a long-term local corticosteroid therapy or a systemic steroid-sparing agent as long-term side effects of systemic corticosteroids are multiple and significant, including diabetes and osteoporosis.

Traditional Steroid-Sparing Agents–Antimetabolites, T-Cell Inhibitors, and Alkylating Agents

When severe and refractory ME requires long-term treatment, the use of steroid-sparing immunosuppressive drugs is often the best solution. When these agents are invoked, they are usually being used primarily for uveitis control and not solely for ME. Because the resolution of ME is contingent on uveitis control, ME will often improve with the use of steroid-sparing agents, many times without the need for additional adjunctive therapy like local corticosteroids. In general, corticosteroid-sparing immunomodulatory drugs have an onset of action within a few weeks to months, and thus ME may take up to several months to resolve completely with these agents.

Steroid-sparing agents include antimetabolites, T-cell inhibitors, and alkylating agents. Biologic agents will be discussed separately. The antimetabolites most commonly used for ocular inflammation are azathioprine, methotrexate (MTX), and mycophenolate mofetil (MMF). T-cell inhibitors include cyclosporine and tacrolimus, and the two alkylating agents used for uveitis are cyclophosphamide and chlorambucil. Once a patient is initiated on an immunomodulatory drug with good response, this therapy is generally continued for 6–24 months, depending on the agent, at which time a careful taper or discontinuation may be attempted over a period of several months [49]. Most studies on immunosuppressive agents are focused on control of active ocular inflammatory disease rather than ME. One recent study looked at the role of MMF specifically in uveitic ME [50]. Patients were separated into those with preexisting ME and those with new onset ME during standard MMF treatment. It demonstrated that ME could develop in up to 39 % of patients on active MMF treatment and that MMF alone is not always sufficient in treating or preventing uveitic ME. When one agent is not successful in eliminating ME, combination therapy or switching to another therapy all together are strategies that should be employed.

Biological Agents

In recent years, interferons (IFN) and anti-TNF-alpha agents have been increasingly employed for the treatment of noninfectious uveitis and ME. IFN influences both innate and adaptive immune responses and is typically delivered as a subcutaneous injection three times per week. Deuter et al. [51, 52] hypothesized that IFN alpha-2a may have powerful antiexudative effects and set out to demonstrate its promise in patients with inactive uveitis and persistent ME. They treated 24 patients with IFN alpha-2a and noted complete resolution in 62.5 % and partial resolution in 25 % within 4 weeks. Effects waned when IFN therapy was terminated after 6 months, indicating that longer treatments may be needed to attain long-term remission. IFN beta has also been effective in uveitic ME, especially in patients with multiple sclerosis-associated or idiopathic intermediate uveitis [3, 53, 54]. A prospective randomized study of 19 patients has demonstrated the superiority of systemic IFN beta over methotrexate use over 12 months in the treatment of ME in the setting of intermediate uveitis [55]. The most common side effect of IFNs is flu-like symptoms but severe depression can occur. INF therapy is generally reserved for patients whose uveitis is well-controlled and whose ME has not responded to more traditional local therapy.

Anti-TNF-alpha agents, primarily infliximab (Remicade) and adalimumab (Humira), are increasingly used for cases of refractory uveitis [56], however, there is also specific evidence for their utility in the treatment of ME [56]. Markomichelakis et al. [57] showed sustained CSMT reduction at 6 months with a single dose of intravenous infliximab 5 mg/kg. Schaap-Fogler et al. [58] showed a favorable outcome at 1 year with anti-TNF-alpha treatment comparable to conventional immunosuppression regiment, with maximal macular thickness improvement at 6 months and maximal visual acuity at 3 months. Diaz-Llopis et al. showed complete resolution of edema in 70 and 54 % of patients at the 6-month and 12-month follow-up visits, respectively, with subcutaneous injections of adalimumab 40 mg every other week over 1 year [59, 60]. Anti-TNF-alpha agents show a promising role in the treatment of refractory uveitic ME specifically.

Carbonic Anhydrase Inhibitors

Oral carbonic anhydrase inhibitors (CAI) may be useful in some cases of refractory macular edema [61]. In a study of 52 eyes, patients were separated into two groups: (1) those without any signs of active inflammation and (2) those with active chronic inflammation necessitating systemic immunosuppressive therapy [62]. Acetazolamide 500 mg PO daily was administered to patients in both groups and response was monitored by improvement of >2 Snellen lines and by angiographic evidence of decreased leakage. About half the patients achieved anatomical and visual improvement by these criteria. As expected, patients without any signs of active inflammation responded better and could even be tapered partially or completely off acetazolamide while maintaining a ME-free state. Generally, CAIs are reserved treating edema in patients whose uveitis is well-controlled and whose ME has failed to respond to regional therapy.

Somatostatins

Somatostatin (SS) is a small neuropeptide intrinsically present in the central nervous system which acts as a potent hormone release inhibitor, blocking the production of growth hormone, insulin-like growth factor and VEGF. It is expressed within the neuroretina and retinal vascular endothelium, where it may have a positive effect on direction-oriented fluid transport, leading to interest and research on its use for treatment of edema in uveitis. It also aids in the restoration of the inner blood–retina barrier [63]. Individual case reports have documented some initial success in cases of chronic uveitic ME with octreotide (a SS analogue) 100 μg given subcutaneously three times daily. This has been typically given in conjunction with other systemic immunosuppressive therapy. Its effect on improved visual acuity and decreased angiographic leakage can persist up to 6 months after discontinuation of treatment [64]. In a study of 20 subjects with quiescent uveitis and active ME for greater than 7 months, longer acting octreotide was used after previous therapy (including systemic immunomodulators, regional corticosteroids, or acetazolamide) failed [63]. The investigators found a reduction in macular edema as calculated on serial OCT in 70 % of subject eyes within 3 months of intramuscular monthly treatment. Side effects are few and generally mild. They include nausea, gastrointestinal upset, steatorrhea and possible cholelithiasis. However, due to limited information available about this treatment modality, it is not currently commonly employed.

Surgery

Pars plana vitrectomy (PPV) with membrane peeling clearly has a role in the treatment of ME in patients with uveitis where ERM and VMT are playing a role in persistence of ME [65]. For this reason, it is imperative to examine the OCT carefully for ERM and VMT in patients with uveitic ME. In some cases, the ERM might be mild and it is not clear what component of the macular thickening is secondary to uveitic inflammation and how much is due to ERM traction. In these cases, aggressive control of uveitis inflammation and adjunctive treatment for inflammatory ME, if needed, should be executed first. If thickening persists despite these measures, the ERM is likely playing a significant role and removal should be considered.

However, PPV also has a role in cases of nonresponsive ME in the absence of vitreoretinal interface fibrosis or traction. The mechanism leading to ME regression after PPV in these cases is unclear. Some have proposed that removal of the inflammatory mediators and cytokines found within the vitreous gel may have a beneficial effect by the ME-inducing agents. However, findings are confounded by the small size of studies and the possible improvement of vision from improved media clarity. Earlier studies did not always specify the presence of ERM or VMT due to the lack of imaging modalities which could discern these findings. A recent study compared the effect of PPV versus systemic immunomodulatory therapy on the clinical course of uveitic patients without ERM or VMT [66]. After PPV, 3/11 patients who had pre-operative ME had persistent total resolution of ME at last follow-up (mean = 5.9 years).

Conclusion

Uveitic ME is often the factor dictating long-term visual outcome in chronic uveitis. The critical treatment principle for uveitic ME is to ensure that the underlying uveitic process is completely controlled. Sustained control of uveitis, sometimes requiring use of systemic immunomodulatory therapy, will often be sufficient to also eliminate ME. Conversely, if uveitis is not well-controlled ME is unlikely to resolve. If uveitis is well-controlled and ME persists, there are a variety of possible therapies available. In general topical or local therapies are employed for ME before systemic therapy. Some cases of uveitic ME may be recalcitrant and difficult to treat. In these instances, concerted efforts to titrate care on a case-by-case basis often involving several treatment modalities in series or simultaneously can achieve ME resolution and preserve vision.

References

1. Hunter RS, Skondra D, Papaliodis G, Sobrin L. Role of OCT in the diagnosis and management of macular edema from uveitis. Semin Ophthalmol. 2012;27:236–41.
2. Rothova A. Inflammatory cystoid macular edema. Curr Opin Ophthalmol. 2007;18:487–92.
3. Cho H, Madu A. Etiology and treatment of the inflammatory causes of cystoid macular edema. J Inflamm Res. 2009;2:37–43.
4. Tranos PG, Tsaousis KT, Vakalis AN, Asteriades S, Pavesio CE. Long-term follow-up of inflammatory cystoid macular edema. Retina. 2012;32:1624–8.
5. Sugar EA, Jabs DA, Altaweel MM, et al. Identifying a clinically meaningful threshold for change in uveitic macular edema evaluated by optical coherence tomography. Am J Ophthalmol. 2011;152:1044–52.
6. Sobrin L. Evolving therapies for macular edema. Ophthalmol Rounds. 2007;1:1–6.
7. Ossewaarde-van Norel J, Camfferman LP, Rothova A. Discrepancies between fluorescein angiography and optical coherence tomography in macular edema in uveitis. Am J Ophthalmol. 2012;154:233–9.
8. Okhravi N, Lightman S. Cystoid macular edema in uveitis. Ocular Immunol Inflamm. 2003;11:29–38.
9. Levin MH, Pistilli M, Daniel E, et al. Incidence of visual improvement in uveitis cases with visual impairment caused by macular edema. Ophthalmology. 2014;121:588–95.
10. van Kooij B, Probst K, Fijnheer R, Roest M, de Loos W, Rothova A. Risk factors for cystoid macular oedema in patients with uveitis. Eye. 2008;22:256–60.
11. Kok H, Lau C, Maycock N, McCluskey P, Lightman S. Outcome of intravitreal triamcinolone in uveitis. Ophthalmology 2005;112:1916.e1–7.
12. Maca SM, Abela-Formanek C, Kiss CG, Sacu SG, Benesch T, Barisani-Asenbauer T. Intravitreal triamcinolone for persistent cystoid macular oedema in eyes with quiescent uveitis. Clin Exp Ophthalmol. 2009;37:389–96.
13. Radwan A, Arcinue C, Yang P, Artornsombudh P, Al-Fadl EA, Foster CS. Bromfenac alone or with

single intravitreal injection of bevacizumab or triamcinolone acetonide for treatment of uveitic macular edema. Graefe's Arch Clin Exp Ophthalmol. 2013;251:1801–6.
14. Allegri P, Murialdo U, Peri S, et al. Randomized, double-blind, placebo-controlled clinical trial on the efficacy of 0.5 % indomethacin eye drops in uveitic macular edema. Invest Ophthalmol Vis Sci. 2014;55:1463–70.
15. Slabaugh MA, Herlihy E, Ongchin S, van Gelder RN. Efficacy and potential complications of difluprednate use for pediatric uveitis. Am J Ophthalmol. 2012;153:932–8.
16. Roesel M, Gutfleisch M, Heinz C, Heimes B, Zurek-Imhoff B, Heiligenhaus A. Orbital floor triamcinolone acetonide injections for the management of active non-infectious uveitis. Eye. 2009;23:910–4.
17. Freeman G. Cystoid macular oedema in uveitis: an unsolved problem. Eye. 2001;15:12–7.
18. Leder HA, Jabs DA, Galor A, Dunn JP, Thorne JE. Periocular triamcinolone acetonide injections for cystoid macular edema complicating noninfectious uveitis. Am J Ophthalmol. 2011;152:441–8.
19. Choudhry S, Ghosh S. Intravitreal and posterior subtenon triamcinolone acetonide in idiopathic bilateral uveitic macular oedema. Clini Exp Ophthalmol. 2007;35:713–8.
20. van Kooij B, Rothova A, de Vries P. The pros and cons of intravitreal triamcinolone injections for uveitis and inflammatory cystoid macular edema. Ocular Immunol Inflamm. 2006;14:73–85.
21. Das-Bhaumik R, Jones N. Low-dose intraocular triamcinolone injection for intractable macular oedema and inflammation in patients with uveitis. Eye. 2006;20:934–7.
22. Lang Y, Leibu R, Shoham N, Miller B, Perlman I. Evaluation of intravitreal kenalog toxicity in humans. Ophthalmology. 2007;114:724–31.
23. Morrison VL, Koh HJ, Cheng L, Bessho K, Davidson MC, Freeman WR. Intravitreal toxicity of the kenalog vehicle (benzyl alcohol) in rabbits. Retina. 2006;26:339–44.
24. Cunningham MA, Edelman JL, Kaushal S. Intravitreal steroids for macular edema: the past, the present, and the future. Surv Ophthalmol. 2008;53:139–49.
25. Hogewind B, Zijlstra C, Klevering B, Hoyng C. Intravitreal triamcinolone for the treatment of refractory macular edema in idiopathic intermediate or posterior uveitis. Eur J Ophthalmol. 2008;18:429–34.
26. Jaffe GJ, Martin D, Callanan D, Pearson PA, Levy B, Comstock T. Fluocinolone acetonide implant (Retisert) for noninfectious posterior uveitis: thirty-four-week results of a multicenter randomized clinical study. Ophthalmology. 2006;113:1020–7.
27. Callanan DG, Jaffe GJ, Martin DF, Pearson PA, Comstock TL. Treatment of posterior uveitis with a fluocinolone acetonide implant: three-year clinical trial results. Arch Ophthalmol. 2008;126:1191.
28. Goldstein DA, Godfrey DG, Hall A, et al. Intraocular pressure in patients with uveitis treated with fluocinolone acetonide implants. Arch Ophthalmol. 2007;125:1478–85.
29. Callanan DG. Novel intravitreal fluocinolone acetonide implant in the treatment of chronic noninfectious posterior uveitis. Expert Rev Ophthalmol. 2007;2:33–44.
30. Kempen JH, Altaweel MM, Holbrook JT, et al. Randomized comparison of systemic anti-inflammatory therapy versus fluocinolone acetonide implant for intermediate, posterior, and panuveitis: the multicenter uveitis steroid treatment trial. Ophthalmology. 2011;118:1916–26.
31. Bourgault S, Aroichane M, Wittenberg LA, Lavallée A, Ma PE. Treatment of refractory uveitic macular edema with dexamethasone intravitreal implants in a pediatric patient with bilateral granulomatous idiopathic panuveitis: a case report. J Ophthalmic Inflamm Infect. 2013;3:1–5.
32. Adán A, Pelegrín L, Rey A, et al. Dexamethasone intravitreal implant for treatment of uveitic persistent cystoid macular edema in vitrectomized patients. Retina. 2013;33:1435–40.
33. Lowder C, Belfort R, Lightman S, et al. Dexamethasone intravitreal implant for noninfectious intermediate or posterior uveitis. Arch Ophthalmol. 2011;129:545–53.
34. Tomkins-Netzer O, Taylor SRJ, Bar A, et al. Treatment with repeat dexamethasone implants results in long-term disease control in eyes with noninfectious uveitis. Ophthalmology. 2014 (epub ahead of print).
35. Acharya NR, Hong KC, Lee SM. Ranibizumab for refractory uveitis-related macular edema. Am J Ophthalmol. 2009;148:303–9.
36. Mirshahi A, Namavari A, Djalilian A, Moharamzad Y, Chams H. Intravitreal bevacizumab (Avastin) for the treatment of cystoid macular edema in Behçet disease. Ocular Immunol Inflamm. 2009;17:59–64.
37. Cordero Coma M, Sobrin L, Onal S, Christen W, Foster CS. Intravitreal bevacizumab for treatment of uveitic macular edema. Ophthalmology. 2007;114:1574–9.
38. Sallam A, Taylor SR, Lightman S. Review and update of intraocular therapy in noninfectious uveitis. Curr Opin Ophthalmol. 2011;22:517–22.
39. Bae JH, Lee CS, Lee SC. Efficacy and safety of intravitreal bevacizumab compared with intravitreal and posterior sub-tenon triamcinolone acetonide for treatment of uveitic cystoid macular edema. Retina. 2011;31:111–8.
40. Lasave AF, Zeballos DG, El-Haig WM, Díaz-Llopis M, Salom D, Arevalo JF. Short-term results of a single intravitreal bevacizumab (avastin) injection versus a single intravitreal triamcinolone acetonide (kenacort) injection for the management of refractory noninfectious uveitic cystoid macular edema. Ocular Immunol Inflamm. 2009;17:423–30.

41. Cervantes-Castañeda RA, Giuliari GP, Gallagher MJ, et al. Intravitreal bevacizumab in refractory uveitic macular edema: one-year follow-up. Eur J Ophthalmol. 2008;19:622–9.
42. Soheilian M, Rabbanikhah Z, Ramezani A, Kiavash V, Yaseri M, Peyman GA. Intravitreal bevacizumab versus triamcinolone acetonide for refractory uveitic cystoid macular edema: a randomized pilot study. J Ocul Pharmacol Ther. 2010;26:199–206.
43. Soheilian M, Eskandari A, Ramezani A, Rabbanikhah Z, Soheilian R. A pilot study of intravitreal diclofenac versus intravitreal triamcinolone for uveitic cystoid macular edema. Ocular Immunol Inflamm. 2013;21:124–9.
44. Hardwig PW, Pulido JS, Erie JC, Baratz KH, Buettner H. Intraocular methotrexate in ocular diseases other than primary central nervous system lymphoma. Am J Ophthalmol. 2006;142:883–5.
45. Taylor SRJ, Habot-Wilner Z, Pacheco P, Lightman SL. Intraocular methotrexate in the treatment of uveitis and uveitic cystoid macular edema. Ophthalmology. 2009;116:797–801.
46. Taylor SRJ, Habot-Wilner Z, Pacheco P, Lightman S. Intravitreal methotrexate in uveitis. Ophthalmology. 2012;119:878–9.
47. van Kooij B, De Boer J, Ten Dam N, Fijnheer R, Rothova A. The effect of non-steroidal anti-inflammatory drugs on inflammatory cystoid macular edema. Am J Ophthalmol. 2005;140:563–4.
48. Venkatesh P, Abhas Z, Garg S, Vohra R. Prospective optical coherence tomographic evaluation of the efficacy of oral and posterior subtenon corticosteroids in patients with intermediate uveitis. Graefe's Arch Clin Exp Ophthalmol. 2007;245:59–67.
49. Jabs DA, Rosenbaum JT, Foster CS, et al. Guidelines for the use of immunosuppressive drugs in patients with ocular inflammatory disorders: recommendations of an expert panel. Am J Ophthalmol. 2000;130:492–513.
50. Doycheva D, Zierhut M, Blumenstock G, Stuebiger N, Deuter C. Mycophenolate mofetil in the therapy of uveitic macular edema-long-term results. Ocular Immunol Inflamm. 2012;20:203–11.
51. Deuter CME, Koetter I, Guenaydin I, Stuebiger N, Zierhut M. Interferon alfa-2a: a new treatment option for long lasting refractory cystoid macular edema in uveitis?: A pilot study. Retina. 2006;26:786–91.
52. Deuter CME, Kötter I, Günaydin I, Stübiger N, Doycheva DG, Zierhut M. Efficacy and tolerability of interferon alpha treatment in patients with chronic cystoid macular oedema due to non-infectious uveitis. Br J Ophthalmol. 2009;93:906–13.
53. Mackensen F, Max R, Becker MD. Interferons and their potential in the treatment of ocular inflammation. Clin Ophthalmol (Auckland, NZ). 2009;3:559.
54. Butler NJ, Suhler EB, Rosenbaum JT. Interferon alpha 2b in the treatment of uveitic cystoid macular edema. Ocular Immunol Inflamm. 2012;20:86–90.
55. Mackensen F, Jakob E, Springer C, et al. Interferon versus methotrexate in intermediate uveitis with macular edema: results of a randomized controlled clinical trial. Am J Ophthalmol. 2013;156:478–86.
56. Durrani K, Zakka FR, Ahmed M, Memon M, Siddique SS, Foster CS. Systemic therapy with conventional and novel immunomodulatory agents for ocular inflammatory disease. Surv Ophthalmol. 2011;56:474–510.
57. Markomichelakis NN, Theodossiadis PG, Pantelia E, Papaefthimiou S, Theodossiadis GP, Sfikakis PP. Infliximab for chronic cystoid macular edema associated with uveitis. Am J Ophthalmol. 2004;138:648–50.
58. Schaap-Fogler M, Amer R, Friling R, Priel E, Kramer M. Anti-TNF-α agents for refractory cystoid macular edema associated with noninfectious uveitis. Graefe's Arch Clin Exp Ophthalmol. 2014;252:633–40.
59. Diaz-Llopis M, García-Delpech S, Salom D, et al. Adalimumab therapy for refractory uveitis: a pilot study. J Ocul Pharmacol Ther. 2008;24:351–61.
60. Neri P, Zucchi M, Allegri P, Lettieri M, Mariotti C, Giovannini A. Adalimumab (Humira™): a promising monoclonal anti-tumor necrosis factor alpha in ophthalmology. Int Ophthalmol. 2011;31:165–73.
61. Whitcup SM, Csaky KG, Podgor MJ, Chew EY, Perry CH, Nussenblatt RB. A randomized, masked, cross-over trial of acetazolamide for cystoid macular edema in patients with uveitis. Ophthalmology. 1996;103:1054–62.
62. Schilling H, Heiligenhaus A, Laube T, Bornfeld N, Jurklies B. Long-term effect of acetazolamide treatment of patients with uveitic chronic cystoid macular edema is limited by persisting inflammation. Retina. 2005;25:182–8.
63. Missotten T, van Laar JAM, van der Loos TL, et al. Octreotide long-acting repeatable for the treatment of chronic macular edema in uveitis. Am J Ophthalmol. 2007;144:838–43.
64. Papadaki T, Zacharopoulos I, Iaccheri B, Fiore T, Foster CS. Somatostatin for uveitic cystoid macular edema (CME). Ocular Immunol Inflamm. 2005;13:469–70.
65. Tranos P, Scott R, Zambarajki H, Ayliffe W, Pavesio C, Charteris DG. The effect of pars plana vitrectomy on cystoid macular oedema associated with chronic uveitis: a randomised, controlled pilot study. Br J Ophthalmol. 2006;90:1107–10.
66. Quinones K, Choi JY, Yilmaz T, Kafkala C, Letko E, Foster CS. Pars plana vitrectomy versus immunomodulatory therapy for intermediate uveitis: a prospective, randomized pilot study. Ocular Immunol Inflamm. 2010;18:411–7.

Management of Glaucoma

49

Louis R. Pasquale

Introduction

Patients with uveitis can present with a spectrum of intraocular pressures (IOPs) ranging from low to high. Using a nationwide database in Taiwan, it was estimated that 8.5 % of patients had glaucoma when uveitis was diagnosed and another 6.7 % developed glaucoma in follow-up [1]. This vision threatening complication of uveitis can occur from a variety of mechanisms. The trabecular meshwork can be the primary site of inflammation as is often seen in herpetic eye disease [2]. Secondary obstruction of the trabecular meshwork with inflammatory cells and fibrin represents another open-angle mechanism of elevated IOP exhibited by uveitis patients. There can be pupillary block mechanisms due to 360° of posterior synechiae. With time permanent peripheral anterior synechiae can produce angle closure glaucoma. There can also be uveal effusion syndrome (such as in scleritis) with forward rotation of the iris lens diaphragm. Finally, treatment of uveitis with steroids can induce a secondary open-angle glaucoma. It is important to keep in mind that the proper treatment of uveitis can reverse the outflow pathology if treated early with approaches directed at the root cause of inflammation. Also, in some instances, there may be predisposition to either open-angle glaucoma or angle closure glaucoma independent of the uveitis.

Overall glaucoma is more common in anterior uveitis (iridocyclitis) than in intermediate (pars planitis) or posterior uveitis [3]. Glaucoma is more common in chronic anterior uveitis than in acute anterior uveitis. Chronic anterior uveitis entities prone to glaucoma include Fuchs' heterochromic iridocyclitis (FHIC), Posner-Schlossman syndrome (PSS), herpetic keratouveitis (HKU), and juvenile idiopathic arthritis (JIA). Of these entities JIA probably has the worse prognosis due to its indolent, intractable course with relentless inflammation. One cohort study noted that 49 % of JIA patients still had active intraocular inflammation after 24 years of follow-up [4].

Approach to the Uveitic Glaucoma Patient

In obtaining a history on a patient with uveitic glaucoma, get a sense of the etiology of the uveitis, whether the uveitis is controlled and the duration of ocular inflammation. Glaucoma in

L.R. Pasquale (✉)
Massachusetts Eye and Ear Infirmary,
Harvard Medical School, 243 Charles Street,
Boston, MA 02114, USA
e-mail: Louis_Pasquale@meei.harvard.edu

G.N. Papaliodis (ed.), *Uveitis*,
DOI 10.1007/978-3-319-09126-6_49

the setting of uncontrolled inflammation without an obvious cause represents a major challenge and suggests that it will be difficult to successfully lower IOP.

Check for orbital signs to rule out orbital pseudotumor on external exam. Rarely this condition can produce intraocular inflammation and secondary angle closure glaucoma [5] but if you are not thinking about this possible association you might miss it. Lid edema and erythema can also occur in uveitic glaucoma but it represents a nonspecific finding.

On slit lamp exam, ciliary flush is not a useful discriminating feature in the setting of uveitic glaucoma but the corneal and iris exam is of central importance particularly if the etiology of the uveitis is unknown. Corneal anesthesia, dendrites, or stromal scars may hint of herpetic eye disease. Stellate keratitic precipitate (KP) on the corneal endothelium may point to FHIC. Mutton fat KP may signify granulomatous disease like sarcoid, syphilis, or tuberculosis. A sentinel nonpigmented KP, a rare anterior cellular reaction, an open angle and IOP >40 mm Hg suggests PSS. The anterior chamber needs to be assessed for cell, flare, hyphema, and hypopyon. The iris should be examined for atrophy (as may occur in HKU). It should be noted that anterior uveitis and sectoral iris atrophy can occur without keratitis among patients with herpetic eye disease [6]. Nodules such as can occur in granulomatous disease, posterior synechiae, peripheral anterior synechiae, neovascularization, and heterochromia, such as can occur in FHIC represent other notable iris findings in uveitis patient with elevated IOP. Gonioscopy is essential to determine whether the angle is open or closed. Fine vessels in the angle may suggest FHIC. On occasion, the vessels in FHIC can spontaneously bleed, producing a hyphema [7]. Inflammatory nodules in the angle are suggestive of sarcoidosis. If there is diffuse shallowing of the anterior chamber without obvious iris bombe, ancillary testing with ultrasound biomicroscopy and B scan ultrasound can be useful to rule out an associated uveal effusion syndrome (see Table 49.1 for the differential diagnosis of the uveal effusion syndrome). Check the optic nerve for the degree of glaucomatous optic neuropathy. Also check for retinitis, choroidal infiltrates, folds, or retinal detachment.

Table 49.1 The differential diagnosis of the uveal effusion syndrome

Human immunodeficiency virus sydnrome
Systemic lupus erythematosis
Vogt koyanagi harada syndrome
Scleritis
Orbital pseudotumor
Sarcoid
Myelodysplastic syndrome and other blood dyscrasias

Principles of Medical Therapy in Uveitic Glaucoma

Targeted therapy that addresses the root cause of intraocular inflammation and prevents the development of posterior and peripheral anterior synechiae is critical to successful management of uveitic glaucoma. Unlike some primary ope-angle glaucoma cases, where there can be an inherent vulnerability to IOP in the normal range, the target IOP in uveitic glaucoma does not necessarily have to be particularly low especially if there is no preexisting optic nerve disease. Use of aqueous humor suppressants first line is recommended, particularly when the uveitis is active. Latanoprost, travoprost, and bimatoprost can all rarely induce uveitis in eyes that are not necessarily predisposed to inflammation [8–10]. Nonetheless, there is data to suggest that latanoprost and bimatoprost can be effective in lowering IOP in quiescent uveitis [11, 12]. Overall, prostaglandin analogs should be avoided when uveitis is active because they are ineffective in that setting [13]. When the IOP is very high, use oral carbonic anhydrase inhibitors to improve bioavailability of medicines to the target tissue (the ciliary body). Since it is well known that pilocarpine can exacerbate synechiae formation in the anterior segment [14], it is wise to avoid cholinergic agents in uveitic glaucoma.

Medical Strategies for Specific Uveitis Entities

Strategies to protect the optic nerve and avoid surgical interventions can vary by glaucoma-prone uveitic entity. Unless glaucoma develops in FHIC, this condition has a relatively benign course and steroids should be used sparingly for fear of inducing steroid-induced glaucoma. Overall, the success rate of medical therapy in the setting of FHIC is fairly high (77 % in one series [15]) and many of these patients can avoid surgery. PSS shares some features with FHIC in that both entities can produce heterochromia and cytomegalovirus has been implicated in both conditions [16, 17]. While the IOP episodes in PSS tend to be episodic and possibly self-limiting, the IOP levels achieved can reach alarmingly high levels (60–70 mm Hg). Frequently, these episodes happen sporadically and IOP between events is entirely normal. In these instances, I give the well-informed patient a small supply of topical dorzolamide-timolol and oral acetazolamide to be used as needed for symptoms consistent with elevated IOP (halos around light and brow ache) with the understanding they will return to the office if they feel they need to use these medicines at the earliest available opportunity. On the other hand, frequent recurrent attacks are worrisome and consideration to anterior chamber tap with assessment for viral infection (PCR for HSV, HZV, and CMV) should be considered. There is one retrospective report that chronic use of valganciclovir in PSS patients with CMV positive aqueous humor aspirates had fewer glaucomacyclitic crises [18].

HKU with secondary glaucoma is one entity where early and aggressive antiviral therapy can be effective in directly addressing trabecular meshwork dysfunction. As mentioned above, one needs to be vigilant regarding this diagnostic possibility as keratitis can be conspicuously absent when glaucoma occurs [6]. All herpetic viruses are highly successful obligate intracellular parasites and depending on the competency of the immune system, recurrent HKU attacks can irreversibly damage the outflow pathway. In these instances antiviral and glaucoma therapy can fail, leading to the need for filtration surgery. In my personal experience, herpetic trabeculitis can even become contiguous with endothelial cell involvement leading to corneal decompensation requiring Descemet's stripping endothelial keratoplasty. In the setting of HKU, one needs to use prostaglandin analogs cautiously under the cover of antiviral therapy, as these agents are known to be associated with ocular herpes viral reactivation [19–21].

Since low-grade inflammation in JIA can continue unabated for many years, it pays to aggressively lower IOP in order to protect vision long-term. This philosophy runs contrary to the view that most uveitic glaucoma patients do not necessarily need a low-target IOP. Foster and associates found topical therapy alone controls IOP only in a minority of cases and that oral carbonic anhydrase inhibitors are frequently needed to control IOP [22].

Steroid-Induced Glaucoma in the Setting of Uveitic Glaucoma

One needs to be vigilant for the development of steroid-induced glaucoma in the uveitis patient. One should resist making this diagnosis in the setting of active uveitis because mechanisms other than steroid-induced trabecular meshwork change could be operative in producing elevated IOP. In the setting of quiescent uveitis when steroids have been used and the angle is open, it is reasonable to entertain the diagnosis of steroid-induced glaucoma, especially since elevated IOP in one large series of eyes with uveitis was more likely to be related steroid-induced ocular hypertension than from other causes [23]. Withdrawing steroids should be considered but this maneuver alone may not necessarily lead to lowering of IOP. A typical pitfall to avoid is the situation where the patient cycles between a quiet eye with elevated IOP on steroids and an inflamed eye but acceptable IOP when steroids are withdrawn. If the uveitis is steroid dependent, then anti-inflammatory therapy should be maintained and alternative approaches to lower IOP need to be entertained. Of course steroid sparing anti-inflammatory therapy should be considered as deemed appropriate.

Laser Surgery in the Uveitic Glaucoma Patient

Because the trabeculum can be primarily or secondarily inflamed, there is probably little place for laser trabeculoplasty (LTP) in uveitic glaucoma. LTP can be effective in steroid-induced ocular hypertension outside the setting of uveitis despite very high preoperative IOPs [24, 25], but it is unknown whether LTP lowers IOP for steroid-induced glaucoma that occurs in uveitic glaucoma.

When it is critical to address pathological relative pupillary block it is best to adopt an efficient technique for creating a patent iridotomy. I advocate a dual laser technique where argon laser is used to seal any dilated iris vessels, thin the iris stroma and put the uveal tissue on stretch. An argon laser bed of peripheral iris tissue is treated with a series of low energy (200 mW), long duration (200 ms) burns with a relatively large spot size (200 μm). This base is thinned further using the argon laser employing short duration (100 ms) and small spot size (50 μm) burns with escalating power from 200 to 1000 mW. If power is escalated too rapidly, gas bubbles that obscure the base of the iridotomy will appear. The argon laser treatment is followed by YAG laser treatment, typically using a double pulse of 6 mJ (treatment parameters can vary depending on the response to the initial argon laser applications). In this setting, the YAG laser acts as a "hole-puncher" to create an iridotomy while minimizing bleeding and further dispersal of pigment and inflammatory debris.

In any situation where the uveal tract is actively inflamed, the disruption of the blood aqueous barrier laser treatment can contribute to rapid sealing of a patent iridotomy. When a laser peripheral iridotomy promptly closes in uveitic glaucoma associated with pupillary block consider performing a surgical iridectomy. The typical setting where one may encounter a laser iridotomy that promptly closes is in Behçet's disease. A clear corneal approach is recommended when performing a surgical iridectomy so that the conjunctiva is preserved should filtration surgery be required a later date.

It is important to recognize scenarios where LPI is not appropriate even though the angle is closed such as occurs in secondary angle closure glaucoma due to diffuse uveal tract inflammation that leads to forward rotation of the iris lens diaphragm. In this scenario, cycloplegia and appropriate anti-inflammatory therapy, and not laser iridotomy, may be appropriate treatment to facilitate deepening of the anterior chamber.

Principles of Filtration Surgery in Uveitic Glaucoma

There is probably no place for minimally invasive glaucoma surgery in uveitic glaucoma patients. There is a role for either trabeculectomy (TRX) with antimetabolite or glaucoma drainage device (GDD) implantation in medically uncontrolled uveitic glaucoma. A suggested approach is to consult with a uveitis expert regarding peri-operative management of inflammation when glaucoma filtration surgery is needed. If possible, defer surgery until the uveitis is quiescent. At times, both the uveitis and IOP are uncontrolled, and there may be no choice but to perform emergency glaucoma filtration surgery in order to protect the optic nerve. In this setting I favor emergency TRX with mitomcyin C, supplementing with postoperative subconjunctival 5-fluorouracil subconjunctival injections if the patient is phakic. In pseudophakic patients a GDD might be best. Overall, there is no evidence that GDD implantation is superior to TRX in uveitic glaucoma. Also, there is no evidence one type of GDD is better than another in uveitic glaucoma. Trans-scleral cyclophotocoagulation (TSCPC) can be tried if TRX or GDD fails and can achieve modest results in this setting [26].

Surgical Outcomes in Uveitic Glaucoma

There are no prospective randomized trials with uniform follow-up to judge the long-term surgical outcomes in uveitic glaucoma. Several non-comparative case series with heterogeneous patient groups and variable follow-up are available but only studies with longer follow-up and with a comparison group are mentioned here. Noble et al. found that after 52 months of follow-up, uveitic glaucoma patients were likely to need additional glaucoma medicines in comparison to glaucoma patients without uveitis [27]. In a long-term comparison study, uveitic glaucoma patients achieved comparable 30-month success rates to non-inflammatory high-risk open-angle glaucoma patients after implantation of an Ahmed valve (~60 %) [28]. In another long-term comparison study, inactive uveitic glaucoma patients achieved comparable 5-year-success rates to high-risk open-angle glaucoma patients after TRX with MMC (~55 %) [29].

Some surgeons have explored whether deep sclerectomy (DS), where a full thickness incision is not performed and aqueous humor is allowed to percolate through a Descemet window into a scleral lake, has any place in uveitic glaucoma. Again series describing results in comparison to TRX have variable follow-up but do suggest thatIOP lowering can be achieved with DS but the need for laser goniopuncture is common [30].

Surgical Management of Pediatric Uveitic Glaucoma

The majority of pediatric uveitic glaucoma is secondary to JIA. This form of glaucoma can be managed with goniotomy [31] suggesting that a fine inflammatory membrane grows over the trabecular meshwork. Not surprisingly goniotomy needs to be repeated in these cases but the 10 year-success rate after repeat goniotomy was 69 % [32]. This success rate is superior to TRX (38 % at 5 years in one series [33]) and given concerns about corneal endothelial cell loss after GDD implantation during childhood [34], careful consideration should be given to goniosurgery for childhood glaucoma in the setting of JIA.

Conclusions and Summary

The best chance of controlling glaucoma in the setting of uveitis starts with identifying the cause of inflammation when possible. It is also important to use appropriate types and amounts of anti-inflammatory therapy to quell intraocular inflammation. Next it is important to identify the mechanism of glaucoma and start therapy with aqueous humor suppressants. Liberal use of cycloplegia is important to prevent iridolenticular adhesions and peripheral anterior synechiae. Outflow procedures have modest success rates and should be considered when the IOP remains uncontrolled despite maximum tolerated medical therapy.

References

1. Hwang DK, Chou YJ, Pu CY, Chou P. Risk factors for developing glaucoma among patients with uveitis: a nationwide study in Taiwan. J Glaucoma. 2013; Nov 14 [Epub ahead of print].
2. Amano S, Oshika T, Kaji Y, Numaga J, Matsubara M, Araie M. Herpes simplex virus in the trabeculum of an eye with corneal endotheliitis. Am J Ophthalmol. 1999;127(6):721–2.
3. Bodaghi B, Cassoux N, Wechsler B, et al. Chronic severe uveitis: etiology and visual outcome in 927 patients from a single center. Medicine. 2001;80 (4):263–70.
4. Skarin A, Elborgh R, Edlund E, Bengtsson-Stigmar E. Long-term follow-up of patients with uveitis associated with juvenile idiopathic arthritis: a cohort study. Ocular immunol inflamm. 2009;17(2): 104–8.
5. Bernardino CR, Davidson RS, Maus M, Spaeth GL. Angle-closure glaucoma in association with orbital pseudotumor. Ophthalmology. 2001;108(9):1603–6.
6. Van der Lelij A, Ooijman FM, Kijlstra A, Rothova A. Anterior uveitis with sectoral iris atrophy in the absence of keratitis: a distinct clinical entity among herpetic eye diseases. Ophthalmology. 2000;107(6):1164–70.
7. Liesegang TJ. Clinical features and prognosis in Fuchs' uveitis syndrome. Arch Ophthalmol. 1982;100(10):1622–6.

8. Fechtner RD, Khouri AS, Zimmerman TJ, et al. Anterior uveitis associated with latanoprost. Am J Ophthalmol. 1998;126(1):37–41.
9. Chiam P. Travoprost induced granulomatous anterior uveitis. Case Rep Ophthalmol Med. 2011;2011: 507073.
10. Packer M, Fine IH, Hoffman RS. Bilateral nongranulomatous anterior uveitis associated with bimatoprost. J Cataract Refract Surg. 2003;29(11):2242–3.
11. Markomichelakis NN, Kostakou A, Halkiadakis I, Chalkidou S, Papakonstantinou D, Georgopoulos G. Efficacy and safety of latanoprost in eyes with uveitic glaucoma. Graefes Arch Clin Exp Ophthalmol. 2009;247(6):775–80.
12. Fortuna E, Cervantes-Castaneda RA, Bhat P, Doctor P, Foster CS. Flare-up rates with bimatoprost therapy in uveitic glaucoma. Am J Ophthalmol. 2008;146(6):876–82.
13. Smith SL, Pruitt CA, Sine CS, Hudgins AC, Stewart WC. Latanoprost 0.005 % and anterior segment uveitis. Acta Ophthalmol Scand. 1999;77(6):668–72.
14. Phillips CI, Clark CV, Levy AM. Posterior synechiae after glaucoma operations: aggravation by shallow anterior chamber and pilocarpine. Br J Ophthalmol. 1987;71(6):428–32.
15. You YA, Wu Y, Hu S. Surgical management of secondary glaucoma in Fuchs' heterochromic iridocyclitis. Graefes Arch Clin Exp Ophthalmol. 2013;251(7):1785–90.
16. Hedayatfar A, Chee SP. Posner-schlossman syndrome associated with cytomegalovirus infection: a case series from a non-endemic area. Int Ophthalmol. 2014; Mar 13 [epub ahead of print].
17. Chee SP, Jap A. Presumed fuchs heterochromic iridocyclitis and Posner-schlossman syndrome: comparison of cytomegalovirus-positive and negative eyes. Am J Ophthalmol. 2008;146(6):883–889 (e881).
18. Sobolewska B, Deuter C, Doycheva D, Zierhut M. Long-term oral therapy with valganciclovir in patients with Posner-Schlossman syndrome. Graefes Arch Clin Exp Ophthalmol. 2014;252(1):117–24.
19. Kroll DM, Schuman JS. Reactivation of herpes simplex virus keratitis after initiating bimatoprost treatment for glaucoma. Am J Ophthalmol. 2002;133 (3):401–3.
20. Wand M, Gilbert CM, Liesegang TJ. Latanoprost and herpes simplex keratitis. Am J Ophthalmol. 1999;127 (5):602–4.
21. Ekatomatis P. Herpes simplex dendritic keratitis after treatment with latanoprost for primary open angle glaucoma. Br J Ophthalmol. 2001;85(8):1008–9.
22. Foster CS, Havrlikova K, Baltatzis S, Christen WG, Merayo-Lloves J. Secondary glaucoma in patients with juvenile rheumatoid arthritis-associated iridocyclitis. Acta Ophthalmol Scand. 2000;78(5):576–579.
23. Sallam A, Sheth HG, Habot-Wilner Z, et al. Outcome of raised intraocular pressure in uveitic eyes with and without a corticosteroid-induced hypertensive response. Am J Ophthalmol. 2009;48:207–13.
24. Ricci F, Missiroli F, Parravano M. Argon laser trabeculoplasty in triamcinolone acetonide induced ocular hypertension refractory to maximal medical treatment. Eur J Ophthalmol. 2006;16:756–7.
25. Rubin B, Taglienti A, Rothman RF, et al. The effect of selective laser trabeculoplasty on intraocular pressure in patients with intravitreal steroid-induced elevated intraocular pressure. J Glaucoma. 2008;17:287–92.
26. Schlote T, Derse M, Zierhut M. Transscleral diode laser cyclophotocoagutaion for the threatment of refractory glaucoma secondary to inflammatory eye diseases. Br J Ophthalmol. 2000;84:999–1003.
27. Noble J, Derzko-Dzulynsky L, Rabinovitch T, Birt C. Outcome of trabeculectomy with intraoperative mitomycin C for uveitic glaucoma. Can J Ophthalmol. 2007;42:89–94.
28. Rachmiel R, Trope GE, Buys YM, et al. Ahmed valve implantation in uveitic glaucoma versus open-angle glaucoma patients. Can J Ophthalmol. 2008;43:462–7.
29. Kaburaki T, Koshino T, Kawashima H, et al. Initial trabeculectomy with mitomycin C in eyes with uveitic glaucoma with inactive uveitis. Eye (Lond). 2009;23:1509–17.
30. Dupas B, Fardeau C, Cassoux N et al. Deep sclerectomy and trabeculectomy in uveitic glaucoma. Eye(Lond). 2010;24:310–4.
31. Ho CL, Wong EY, Walton DS. Goniosurgery for glaucoma complicating chronic childhood uveitis. Arch Ophthalmol. 2004;122:838–44.
32. Bohnsack BL, Freedman SF. Surgical outcomes in childhood uveitic glaucoma. Am J Ophthalmol. 2013;155:134–42.
33. Wiese K, Heiligenhaus A, Heine C. Trabeculectomy in uveitis associated with juvenile idiopathic arthritis: long-term results in pediatric secondary glaucoma. Ophthalmologe. 2014;111:330–8.
34. Kalinina Ayuso V, Scheerlinck LM, de Boer JH. The effect of an Ahmed glaucoma valve implant on corneal endothelial cell density in children with glaucoma secondary to uveitis. Am J Ophthalmol. 2013;155:530–5.

Index

Note: Page numbers followed by *f* and *t* indicate figures and tables respectively

G.N. Papaliodis (ed.), *Uveitis*,
DOI 10.1007/978-3-319-09126-6

D

Q

R

MIX
Papier aus verantwortungsvollen Quellen
Paper from responsible sources
FSC® C105338
FSC
www.fsc.org

If you have any concerns about our products,
you can contact us on
ProductSafety@springernature.com

In case Publisher is established outside the EU,
the EU authorized representative is:
Springer Nature Customer Service Center GmbH
Europaplatz 3, 69115 Heidelberg, Germany

Printed by Libri Plureos GmbH
in Hamburg, Germany